MEDICAL TERMINOLOGY

A Programmed Systems Approach

Tenth Edition

Jean Tannis Dennerll

Phyllis E. Davis

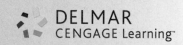

DELMAR
CENGAGE Learning™

Australia • Brazil • Japan • Korea • Mexico • Singapore • Spain • United Kingdom • United States

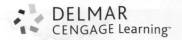
DELMAR
CENGAGE Learning™

Medical Terminology: A Programmed Systems Approach, Tenth Edition
Jean Tannis Dennerll, Phyllis E. Davis

Vice President, Career and Professional Editorial: Dave Garza

Director of Learning Solutions: Matthew Kane

Acquisitions Editor: Matthew Seeley

Managing Editor: Marah Bellegarde

Senior Product Manager: Debra Myette-Flis

Editorial Assistant: Samantha Zullo

Vice President, Career and Professional Marketing: Jennifer McAvey

Executive Marketing Manager: Wendy Mapstone

Senior Marketing Manager: Michele McTighe

Marketing Coordinator: Scott Chrysler

Production Director: Carolyn S. Miller

Content Project Manager: Thomas Heffernan

Senior Art Director: Jack Pendleton

Technology Project Manager: Patricia Allen

For product information and technology assistance, contact us at
Cengage Learning Customer & Sales Support, 1-800-354-9706

For permission to use material from this text or product,
submit all requests online at **www.cengage.com/permissions**
Further permissions questions can be emailed to
permissionrequest@cengage.com

Library of Congress Control Number: 2009931727

ISBN-13: 978-1-4354-3889-7

ISBN-10: 1-4354-3889-2

Delmar
Executive Woods
5 Maxwell Drive
Clifton Park, NY 12065
USA

Cengage Learning is a leading provider of customized learning solutions with office locations around the globe, including Singapore, the United Kingdom, Australia, Mexico, Brazil, and Japan. Locate your local office at **www.cengage.com/global**

Cengage Learning products are represented in Canada by Nelson Education, Ltd.

To learn more about Delmar, visit **www.cengage.com/delmar**

Purchase any of our products at your local bookstore or at our preferred online store **www.cengagebrain.com**

Notice to the Reader

Publisher does not warrant or guarantee any of the products described herein or perform any independent analysis in connection with any of the product information contained herein. Publisher does not assume, and expressly disclaims, any obligation to obtain and include information other than that provided to it by the manufacturer. The reader is expressly warned to consider and adopt all safety precautions that might be indicated by the activities described herein and to avoid all potential hazards. By following the instructions contained herein, the reader willingly assumes all risks in connection with such instructions. The publisher makes no representations or warranties of any kind, including but not limited to, the warranties of fitness for particular purpose or merchantability, nor are any such representations implied with respect to the material set forth herein, and the publisher takes no responsibility with respect to such material. The publisher shall not be liable for any special, consequential, or exemplary damages resulting, in whole or part, from the readers' use of, or reliance upon, this material.

Printed in the United States of America
6 7 8 19 18 17 16

CONTENTS

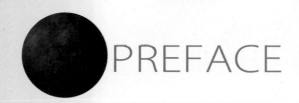# PREFACE

Medical Terminology: A Programmed Systems Approach, Tenth Edition, is a medical terminology textbook that teaches a word-building system using a programmed learning format. Thousands of medical words may be built by learning the Latin and Greek prefixes, suffixes, and word roots from which our English medical terms originate. Genevieve Smith and Phyllis Davis were the first to apply programmed learning to the teaching of medical terminology when they designed this textbook over 38 years ago. This system continues with the tenth edition to refine the process as well as to enhance this system using current educational technology.

Medical Terminology: A Programmed Systems Approach, Tenth Edition, is designed to provide a comprehensive entry-level study of medical language for health career learners with little or no previous experience. During 30 years of teaching medical terminology, I have been amazed by course assessment statistics showing positive results using this textbook. Instructor and student reviews also express their satisfaction and enthusiasm for using the materials in this textbook and its supplemental package.

ABBREVIATION USE WARNING

Use of correct medical abbreviations allows the healthcare provider to communicate concisely and quickly. However, use of incorrect, poorly written, confusing, and made-up abbreviations are dangerous. Poor quality care may result from errors made misusing medical abbreviations. The Joint Commission has issued an official *"do not use"* list of abbreviations and symbols. Visit the http://www.jointcommission.org Web site and search for "do not use list" to view the list. In addition to the Joint Commission list, the Institute for Safe Medication Practices (ISMP) has published *"ISMP's List of Error-Prone Abbreviations, Symbols, and Dosage Designations";* refer to Appendix A.

Medical Terminology: A Programmed Systems Approach, Tenth Edition will continue to include medical abbreviations as part of each unit. The rationale for this decision is that even though abbreviation use is being discouraged, its use continues in printed and electronic records and past medical records. It would be irresponsible for this text to exclude abbreviations from study. By continuing their presentation, this text hopes to increase the learner's awareness of correct use of abbreviations, the need for caution, and safe practices.

ORGANIZATION

This book contains fifteen units progressively organized by word-building subject matter and body systems that may be easily organized for semester assignments.

The programmed learning, word-building system format presents and reinforces word parts and word building with over 2,000 frames—more than any other programmed medical terminology textbook. This format requires active participation through reading, writing, answering questions, labeling, repetition, and providing immediate feedback.

Various types of tables offer word part summaries, medical report data, and additional information about subjects that may not be included in the frames. Abbreviation tables that appear at the end of each unit include correct medical abbreviations. Abbreviation lists are included in Appendix B and organized by subjects including weights and measures, chemical symbols, diagnoses, procedures, health professions and organizations, and charting.

Several special features in each unit enhance the learning of medical terminology. See "About This Programmed System" on pages xvii–xix for a detailed description of each feature.

LEARNING SUPPLEMENTS

The following supplements are included with your textbook to provide even more help as you study.

- **Flashcards.** Improve your knowledge and test your mastery by using the flashcards created from the cards provided in the last section of the book. Remove these perforated pages carefully and then separate the cards. Flashcards are an effective study aid for use even when you only have a small amount of time.
- **StudyWARE™ CD-ROM.** This interactive software packaged with the book offers an exciting way to gain additional practice (while having fun) through exercises, game activities, and audio for each chapter. See "How to Use StudyWARE™" on page xxi for details.

CHANGES TO THE TENTH EDITION

- **Extensive technical accuracy reviews** were performed on every aspect of the textbook and directly-linked ancillaries to ensure correctness of all terminology content and answers.
- **Over 50 NEW** images and line art illustrations were added to enhance your understanding of the content.
- **NEW** diagnostic imaging modalities; surgical techniques; and anatomy, physiology, and disease terminology updates can be found throughout the text.
- **NEW StudyWARE™ Connection** feature directs you to additional learning opportunities such as practice quizzes, animations, image labeling, and other interactive games included on the accompanying CD-ROM.
- **NEW Case Study Investigation (CSI)** in each unit features excerpts from actual medical records, and a vocabulary challenge provides "real-world" experience with analyzing medical terms, breaking down terms into their respective word parts, defining word parts, and defining abbreviations.
- **NEW Flashcards** in the back of the book are a convenient and portable study aide to help you master the important terms from each unit.
- **NEW Images for Professional Profiles** provide a visual with the description of the function and credentials of various allied health professions. These vignettes and photos provide information about possible career paths.
- **NEW Icons for feature frames** help you easily identify these special frames that point out interesting facts to help with retention, spelling tips and tricks, and dictionary exercises.
- **EXPANDED Glossaries** in each unit ensure you have all the latest terminology you'll need for the workplace.
- **Revised Review Activities** provide you with a variety of exercises to reinforce terms learned within the frames.
- **NEW** appendix lists error-prone abbreviations, symbols, and dose designations.
- **NEW Mobile Downloads** including audio for iPods, MP3 players, and cell phones allow you to study anywhere and at any time.
- **NEW instructor slides** created in PowerPoint® include images and animations and are designed to aid instructors in planning class lectures.

- **REVISED Audio CDs** provide practice for learning the definitions and proper pronunciation of 3500 word parts and terms and is presented with corresponding textbook frame references.
- **REVISED Instructor's Manual** in electronic format has numerous resources to help instructors prepare for class, including sample syllabi; course schedules; lesson plans; quizzes; exams; and word part activity sheets for each unit.

SPECIAL RESOURCES TO ACCOMPANY THE BOOK

Audio CDs ISBN: 1-4354-3893-0

Audio CDs to accompany *Medical Terminology: A Programmed Systems Approach,* Tenth Edition, includes specific frame references and pronunciation of most terms, presented in unit order. The Audio CDs are designed to allow learners to listen to the term, pronounce it aloud, and in many cases hear the term used in context or defined. The Audio CDs may also be used as dictation by listening to the term, writing the word, and then checking the spelling of the terms in the textbook.

Also Available: Text/Audio CDs Value Package ISBN: 1-1110-8036-4

Instructor Resources ISBN 1-4354-3890-6

The Instructor Resources is a robust computerized tool for all instructional needs! A must-have for all instructors, this comprehensive and convenient CD-ROM contains the following:

- **The Instructor's Manual** features a correlation guide from the ninth to tenth edition, sample syllabi for 10-week and 16-week courses, quizzes for each unit, midterm exam, and comprehensive final exam. In addition, suggestions for course design, class activities, games, and unit word part lists are also included.
- **ExamView® Computerized Testbank** contains over 1,400 questions with answers organized according to the fifteen units in the textbook. This CD-ROM testbank assists in creating personalized unit, midterm, and final examinations.
  Features include:
  - An interview mode or wizard, to guide instructors through the steps of creating a test in less than 5 minutes
  - The capability to edit questions or to add an unlimited number of questions
  - Online (Internet-based) testing capability
  - Online (computer-based) testing capability
  - A sophisticated word processor
  - Numerous test layout and printing options
  - Link groups of questions to common narratives
- **Instructor slides** created in PowerPoint® include images and animations and are designed to aid in planning class lectures.

WebTUTOR™ Advantage

Designed to complement the text, WebTUTOR™ is a content-rich, Web-based teaching and learning aid that reinforces and clarifies complex concepts. Animations enhance learning and retention of material. The WebCT™ and Blackboard™ platforms also provide rich communication tools to instructors and learners, including a course calendar, chat, email, and threaded discussions.

WebTUTOR™ Advantage on WebCT™ (ISBN: 1-4354-3892-2)

Text Bundled with WebTUTOR™ Advantage on WebCT™ (ISBN: 1-4354-3089-1)

Text Bundled with WebTUTOR™ Advantage on WebCT™ and Audio CDs
    (ISBN: 1-1110-8038-0)

WebTUTOR™ Advantage on Blackboard™ (ISBN: 1-4354-3891-4)

Text Bundled with WebTUTOR™ Advantage on Blackboard™ (ISBN: 1-4354-3097-2)

Text Bundled with WebTUTOR™ Advantage on Blackboard™ and Audio CDs
    (ISBN: 1-1110-8037-2)

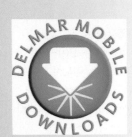

Mobile Downloads

Expand your knowledge with Delmar/Cengage Learning mobile downloads including
audio for iPods, MP3 players, and cell phones! Now you can study anywhere, anytime
and make learning fun! Visit http://www.podcasts.cengage.com/healthcare.

ADDITIONAL RESOURCES

Delmar/Cengage Learning's Medical Terminology Audio Library

This extensive audio library of medical terminology includes four audio CDs with
over 3,600 terms pronounced, and a software CD-ROM. The CD-ROM presents terms
organized by body system, medical specialty, and general medical term categories. The
user can search for a specific term by typing in the term or key words, or clicking on a
category to view an alphabetical list of all terms within the category. Hear the correct
pronunciation of one term or listen to each term on the list pronounced automatically.
Definitions can be viewed after hearing the pronunciation of terms.

   Institutional Version ISBN: 1-4018-3223-7
   Individual Version ISBN: 1-4018-3222-9

Complete Medical Terminology Online Course

Designed as a stand-alone course, there is no need for a separate book. Everything
is online! Content is presented in four major sections: study, practice, tests, and
reports.

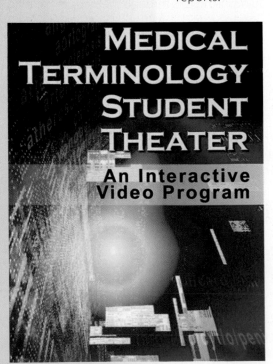

The study section includes the content from the text, along with
graphics and audio links. The practice section includes exercises and
games to reinforce learning. The test section includes tests with a
variety of question types for each unit. A midterm and final exam
are also available. The report section features student and instructor
reports.

   Individual Course ISBN: 0-7668-2754-2
   Educational Course ISBN: 0-7668-2753-4

Delmar/Cengage Learning's Medical Terminology Student Theater:
An Interactive Video Program ISBN: 1-4283-1863-1

Organized by body system, this CD-ROM is invaluable to learners
trying to master the complex world of medical terminology. The
program is designed for allied health and nursing students who
are enrolled in medical terminology courses. A series of video
clips leads learners through the various concepts, interspersing
lectures with illustrations to emphasize key points. Quizzes and
games allow learners to assess their understanding of the video
content.

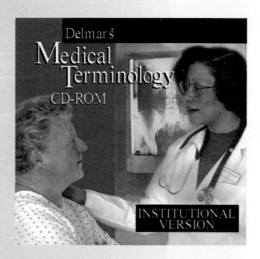

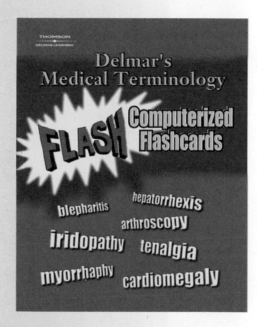

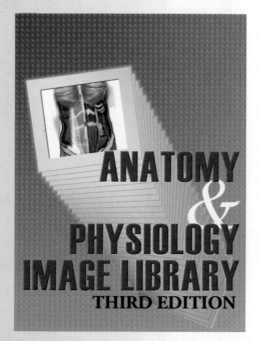

Delmar/Cengage Learning's Medical Terminology CD-ROM Institutional Version ISBN: 0-7668-0979-X

This exciting interactive reference, practice, and assessment tool is designed to complement any medical terminology program. Features include the extensive use of multimedia—animations, video, graphics, and activities—to present terms and word-building features. The difficult functions, processes, and procedures help learners to more effectively learn from a textbook.

Delmar/Cengage Learning's Medical Terminology Video Series

This series of fourteen medical terminology videotapes is designed for allied health and nursing students who are enrolled in medical terminology courses. The videos may be used in class to supplement a lecture or in a resource lab by users who want additional reinforcement. The series can also be used in distance learning programs as a telecourse. The videos simulate a typical medical terminology class, and are organized by body system. The on-camera "instructor" leads students through the various concepts, interspersing lectures with graphics, video clips, and illustrations to emphasize points. This comprehensive series is invaluable to students trying to master the complex world of medical terminology.

> Complete Set of Videos ISBN 0-7668-0976-5 (Videos can also be purchased individually.)

Delmar/Cengage Learning's Medical Terminology Flash!: Computerized Flashcards ISBN: 0-7668-4320-3

Learn and review over 1,500 medical terms using this unique electronic flashcard program. Flash! is a computerized flashcard-type question and answer association program designed to provide learners with correct spellings, definitions, and pronunciations. The use of graphics and audio clips make it a fun and easy way for users to learn and test their knowledge of medical terminology.

Delmar/Cengage Learning's Anatomy and Physiology Image Library CD-ROM, Third Edition ISBN: 1-4180-3928-4

This CD-ROM includes over 1,050 graphic files. These files can be incorporated into a PowerPoint®, Microsoft® Word presentation, used directly from the CD-ROM in a classroom presentation, or used to make color transparencies. The Image Library is organized around body systems and medical specialties. The library includes various anatomy, physiology, and pathology graphics of different levels of complexity. Instructors can search and select the graphics that best apply to their teaching situation. This is an ideal resource to enhance your teaching presentation of medical terminology or anatomy and physiology.

It is our intent that *Medical Terminology: A Programmed Systems Approach*, Tenth Edition, Delmar/Cengage Learning, be the best edition yet and continues to serve the needs of the learners and teachers who use it. We maintain our commitment to the original philosophy and integrity of this classic textbook.

ACKNOWLEDGMENTS

Medical Terminology: A Programmed Systems Approach, Tenth Edition, would not have been possible without many people contributing their expert observations, testing, evaluation, and skills. I would like to first thank the following team members from Delmar/Cengage Learning whose dedicated professional publishing skills maintain the quality and integrity of this work.

Acquisitions Editor: Matthew Seeley
Senior Product Manager: Debra Myette-Flis
Editorial Assistant: Samantha Zullo
Content Project Manager: Thomas Heffernan
Senior Art Director: Jack Pendleton
Technology Project Manager: Patricia Allen

For many years I have been able to count on a number of healthcare practitioners and experienced medical terminology instructors in the community of Jackson, Michigan, who have made content contributions to this and previous editions. I extend my continued thanks to:

Billie Jean Buda, CMA, Medical Assistant Instructor
Lynne Schreiber MA, RT(R), RDMS
Ann Wentworth, BS, RT(R), RDMS, Medical Terminology Instructor
Marina Martinez-Kratz, MSN, Nursing Instructor
Grant Brown, Pharm D, Brown's Option Care
Andrew J. Krapohl, MD, Retired Obstetrician and Gynecologist
Patricia Krapohl, RN, MPH
Chip Smith, EMT-P
Denise Brzozowski, AAS, COT
Ann Blaxton, CCC-A, Professional Hearing Services
Sharon Rooney-Gandy, DO, General Surgery Board Certified
Paul H. Ernest, MD, TLC Eye Care PC
Shawn McKinney, COMT, American College of Ophthalmic Technology
Noreen Calus, MS, RHIA (posthumous)
Allegiance Healthcare, Jackson, MI
Faculty and staff of Jackson Community College, Jackson, MI

I would like to express thanks to the reviewers who continue to be a valuable resource through their comments, suggestions, and attention to detail.

Dominica Austin
Academic Dean, Lincoln College of Technology, Marietta, Georgia

Bradley S. Bowden, PhD
Professor of Biology Emeritus, Alfred University, Alfred, New York

Leah A. Grebner, MS, RHIA, CCS, FAHIMA
Director of Health Information Technology, Midstate College, Peoria, Illinois

Anne M. Loochtan, PhD, RRT
Associate Dean of Health and Public Safety, Adjunct Faculty Member, Cincinnati State Technical and Community College, Cincinnati, Ohio

Additionally, I am particularly grateful to the following technical accuracy reviewers who were instrumental in assisting in my commitment to creating quality materials for learners and instructors.

Ellen Anderson, MAdEd, RHIA, CCS
Associate Professor, College of Lake County, Grayslake, Illinois

Bradley S. Bowden, PhD
Professor of Biology Emeritus, Alfred University, Alfred, New York

Lisa M. Carrigan, RN
Instructor, Health Sciences, Medical Terminology, Applied Technology Center and
    South Carolina Virtual School Program, Rock Hill, South Carolina

Anne M. Loochtan, PhD, RRT
Associate Dean of Health and Public Safety, Adjunct Faculty Member, Cincinnati
    State Technical and Community College, Cincinnati, Ohio

Susan L. Nawrot, MT, CSR
Instructor, Jackson Community College, Allied Health Department, Adrian,
    Michigan

Karen R. Smith, RN, BSN
Health Science Consultant, Kentucky Department of Education, Division of Career
    and Technical Education, Frankfort, Kentucky

I would also like to acknowledge the contribution that 30 years of medical terminology students have made at Jackson Community College in Jackson, Michigan, and other students from around the world. Through direct comments, letters, and emails, they remind me what it is like to be a beginning medical terminology student, what improvements are needed in the textbook to enhance learning, and what details must be addressed.

Finally, I am grateful for the continued support and understanding of my husband and computer technician, Timothy J. Dennerll, PhD; my daughter, Diane; my son, Raymond; and my mother, Helen Stamcos Tannis. You are my inspiration.

Sincerely,
Jean M. Tannis Dennerll BS CMA (AAMA)

LIST OF ILLUSTRATIONS

ABOUT THIS PROGRAMMED SYSTEM

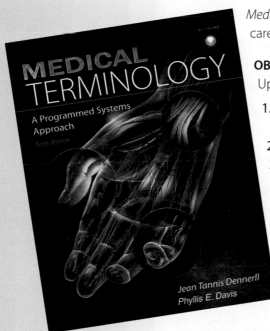

Medical Terminology: A Programmed Systems Approach, Tenth Edition, is carefully designed to help you learn medical terminology.

OBJECTIVES OF THE LEARNING SYSTEM

Upon completion of this system, the learner should be able to:

1. Build literally thousands of medical words from Greek and Latin prefixes, suffixes, word roots, and combining forms.
2. Define medical words by analyzing their Greek and Latin parts.
3. Spell medical words correctly.
4. Use a medical dictionary.
5. Pronounce medical words correctly.
6. Recall acceptable medical abbreviations that represent phrases and terms.

To maximize the benefits of this learning system, familiarize yourself with the following features.

PROGRAMMED LEARNING FORMAT

Information is presented and learned in small numbered sections called frames. You will have an active part in learning medical terminology using this successful programmed approach. The right column contains a statement and an answer blank; the left column provides the answer. Cover the answer column with a bookmark (two are provided as part of the back cover). Read the right column of the frame and write your answer in the blank. Pull down the bookmark to reveal the answer and confirm your response. Then move on to the next frame. Learning one bit of information

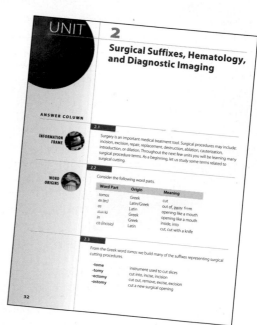

at a time is part of programmed learning. Another part is continual reinforcement of word parts and terms throughout the book.

WORD-BUILDING SYSTEM AND WORD PARTS

Word roots, combining forms, prefixes, and suffixes are important building blocks in the

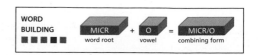

word-building system. **Combining forms** are highlighted in bold, **prefixes** in blue with a hyphen after each, and **suffixes** in pink with a hyphen preceding each.

	1.9
INFORMATION FRAME	Adding a vowel (a, e, i, o, u, or y) to a word root to create a combining form allows two or more word roots to be joined to form a compound word. It also allows a word root to be joined with a suffix (ending of a word) to form a word. In addition, the vowel assists by making the term easier to pronounce. "O" is the most commonly used combining vowel.

FEATURES FRAMES

Information—present interesting facts to help retention

	4.117
SPELL CHECK	In the spelling of the combining form for abdomen, the "e" changes to "i"—**abdomin/o**. EXAMPLE: The abdominal incision was made in the RLQ of the abdomen.

	4.118
TAKE A CLOSER LOOK	Abdomin/al is an adjective that means _____ NOTE: For descriptive reference the abdomen may be divided into four quadrants including the right upper quadrant (RUQ), the left upper quadrant (LUQ), the right lower quadrant (RLQ), and the left lower quadrant (LLQ).
pertaining to the abdomen	

Spell Check—clues and special notes on troublesome spelling

Take a Closer Look—analyzes similar terms

	5.151
WORD ORIGINS	**drom/o** comes from the Greek word for run. A hippodrome was an open air stadium built for racing horses or chariots in ancient Greece. Drom/o/mania is an insane impulse to wander or roam. You usually use drom with the prefixes syn- and pro-.

Word Origins—encourages memory retention through fascinating references using Greek and Roman mythology, legends, and etymology

	4.21
DICTIONARY EXERCISE	Find the word myeloblast in your dictionary. Write the meaning here. * _____
bone marrow germ cell myel/o	The combining form of myel is _____/_____

Dictionary Exercise—provides learners with practice using a medical dictionary

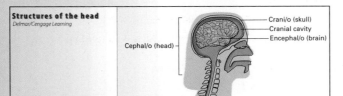

Structures of the head
Delmar/Cengage Learning

Crani/o (skull)
Cranial cavity
Encephal/o (brain)
Cephal/o (head)

FULL-COLOR ART

Even more full-color illustrations and photos are included in this edition. Art and photos are placed near their reference—not in a separate color section. A complete list of all art is on pages xv–xvi.

PROFESSIONAL PROFILE

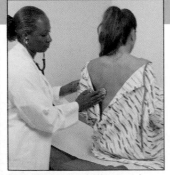

Doctor of Osteopathy (DO): Osteopathic physicians are fully licensed to practice medicine, performing the same duties as a medical doctor (MD, allopathic doctor). Because of the original philosophy of osteopathic medicine, founded by Dr. Andrew Still in 1874, they identify the musculoskeletal framework as a key element to health. They also believe that the body has a natural ability to heal itself given a favorable environment and good nutrition and so act as teachers to help patients take a responsible role in their own well-being and to change unhealthy patterns. In addition, osteopathic manipulative therapy (OMT) is incorporated in the training and practice of osteopathic physicians. Although 60% practice primary care, osteopathic physicians may specialize in surgery,

Osteopathic physican performing an exam *Delmar/Cengage Learning*

PROFESSIONAL PROFILES

Vignettes and photos describing the function and credentials of many allied health professions are placed throughout the text. These profiles give information about various professions and possible career paths as well as reinforce the importance of medical terminology for all health professionals.

CASE STUDY INVESTIGATION (CSI)

Spleen
Pathology Report: Gross examination of a spleen

An entire spleen, weighing 127 grams and measuring 13.0 × 4.1 × 9.2 **cm**. The **external** surface is smooth, leathery, **homogeneous**, and dark purplish-brown. There are no defects in the capsule. The blood vessels of the hilum of the spleen are **patent**, with no **thrombi** or other **abnormalities**. The hilar soft tissues contain a single, **ovoid**, 1.2-cm lymph node with a dark grey cut surface and no focal **lesions**.

Source: By Edward O. Uthman, MD. (uthman@neosoft.com). Diplomate, American Board of Pathology.

CASE STUDY INVESTIGATION (CSI)

The Case Study Investigation (CSI) features excerpts from actual medical records and a vocabulary challenge that encourages you to apply what you've learned in the chapter through analyzing medical terms from the case study, breaking down terms into their respective word parts, defining word parts, and defining abbreviations.

Abbreviation	Meaning
AAD	American Academy of Dermatology
ALL	acute lymphocytic leukemia
ARDMS	American Registry for Diagnostic Medical Sonography
ARRT	American Registry of Radiologic Technologists
ASRT	American Society of Radiologic Technologists
CABG	coronary artery bypass graft
CAT Scan	computed axial tomography
CBC	complete blood count
CCU	cardiac care unit (critical care unit)
CE	cardiac enlargement (cardiomegaly)
CT	Computed Tomography
cTnI and cTnT	Troponin I and Troponin T (serum cardiac proteins indicating myocardial injury)
Diff	differential white blood cell count
DMS	diagnostic medical sonography

ABBREVIATIONS

Abbreviations are covered many ways. Several frames work abbreviations, a list of abbreviations and meanings is included in each unit, and activities specifically identify and test abbreviations. Appendix B includes a comprehensive list of abbreviations.

To complete your study of this unit, work the **Review Activities** on the following pages. Also, listen to the Audio CD that accompanies *Medical Terminology: A Programmed Systems Approach*, 10th edition, and practice your pronunciation.

AUDIO CDS

After completing each unit, you may want to listen to the Audio CDs that accompany the text. You can use the Audio CDs to listen to each term and repeat the term aloud for pronunciation practice. You may also write the term and its definition to check spelling and meaning comprehension.

GLOSSARY

blastocyte	immature cell	etiology	the study of the origin of the cause of disease
cardialgia	heart pain	gastralgia	stomach pain
cardiologist	physician specialist in heart disease	gastrectomy	excision of the stomach
cardiomegaly	enlarged heart	gastric	pertaining to the stomach (adj.)
cyanoderma	blueness of the skin	gastroduodenostomy	making a new opening between the stomach and duodenum
cyanosis	condition of blueness		
cytologist	a technologist who studies cellular disease	gastromegaly	enlarged stomach
cytology	the science of studying cells	gastrostomy	making a new opening in the stomach
cytometer	instrument used to count cells	histoblast	immature tissue cells
cytometry	process of using a cytometer	histology	the science of studying tissues
dermatology	the science of studying the skin	hypodermic	pertaining to below the dermis

GLOSSARY

Unit end glossaries summarize terms and definitions in a frame-type format for easy study and review.

REVIEW ACTIVITIES

SELECT AND CONSTRUCT

Select the correct word parts (some may be used more than once) from the following list and construct medical terms that represent the given meaning.

-ac	acro	-al	-algia	-blast	cardi(o)
chlor	cyano	cyt(e)(o)	derm(a)o	dermato	duodeno
echo	ectomy	electro	-emia	-er	erythro
gastr/o(ia)	-gram	-graph	-graphy	-ia	-ic
-itis	leuko	-logy	mania	megal(o)(y)	melano
osis	-ostomy	paralysis	-pathy	penia	radio
sono	thrombo	tom(e)(o)	-tomy	um	xantho

1. excision of the stomach _____

2. make a new opening (connection) between the stomach and the duodenum _____

3. blueness of the skin _____

4. disease condition of the skin _____

5. red blood cell _____

6. embryonic dark pigmented cell _____

REVIEW ACTIVITIES

Activities include a variety of exercises to reinforce terms learned within the frames. Also included are *case study* excerpts from actual medical records featuring medical terms in context along with questions to test and reinforce spelling and definitions. *Crossword puzzles* provide definition to term review in an easy, fun format.

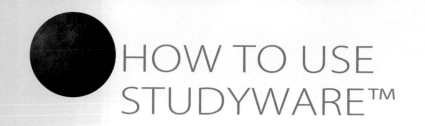

HOW TO USE STUDYWARE™

to Accompany *Medical Terminology: A Programmed Systems Approach,* **Tenth Edition**

MINIMUM SYSTEM REQUIREMENTS

Operating systems: Windows XP w/SP 3, Windows Vista w/ SP 1

Processor: Minimum required by Operating System

Memory: Minimum required by Operating System

Hard Drive Space: 200 MB

Screen resolution: 1024 × 768 pixels

CD-ROM drive

Sound card and listening device required for audio features

Flash Player 10. The Adobe Flash Player is free, and can be downloaded from http://www.adobe.com/products/flashplayer/.

Adobe Reader

SETUP INSTRUCTIONS

1. Insert disc into CD-ROM drive. The StudyWARE™ installation program should start automatically. If it does not, go to step 2.
2. From My Computer, double-click the icon for the CD drive.
3. Double-click the setup.exe file to start the program.

TECHNICAL SUPPORT

Telephone: 1-800-648-7450
Monday–Friday
8:30 A.M.–6:30 P.M. EST
E-mail: delmar.help@cengage.com
StudyWARE™ is a trademark used herein under license.
Microsoft® and Windows® are registered trademarks of the Microsoft Corporation.

Pentium® is a registered trademark of the Intel Corporation.

GETTING STARTED

The StudyWARE™ software helps you learn terms and concepts in *Medical Terminology: A Programmed Systems Approach,* Tenth Edition. As you study each chapter in the text, be sure to explore the activities in the corresponding chapter in the software. Use StudyWARE™ as your own private tutor to help you learn the material in your *Medical Terminology: A Programmed Systems Approach,* Tenth Edition textbook.

Getting started is easy. Install the software by inserting the CD-ROM into your computer's CD-ROM drive and following the on-screen instructions. When you open the software, enter your first and last name so the software can store your quiz results. Then choose a chapter from the menu to take a quiz or explore one of the activities.

MENUS

You can access the menus from wherever you are in the program. The menus include Quizzes and other Activities.

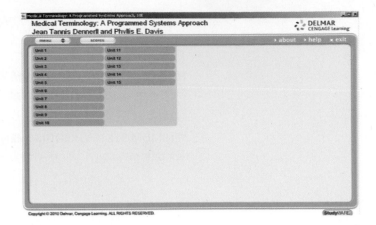

Quizzes. Quizzes include multiple choice and fill-in questions. You can take the quizzes in both practice mode and quiz mode. Use practice mode to improve your mastery of the material. You have multiple tries to get the answers correct. Instant feedback tells you whether you're right or wrong and helps you learn quickly by explaining why an answer was correct or incorrect. Use quiz mode when you are ready to test yourself and keep a record of your scores. In quiz mode, you have one try to get the answers right, but you can take each quiz as many times as you want.

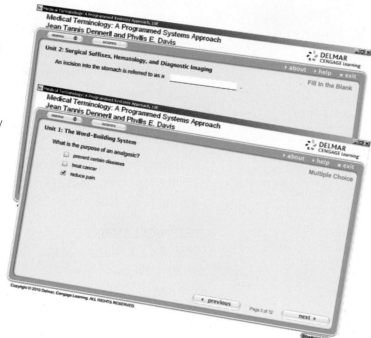

Scores. You can view your last scores for each quiz and print your results to hand in to your instructor.

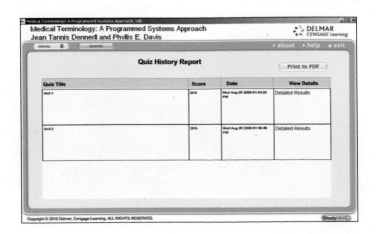

Activities. Activities include image labeling, hangman, concentration, crossword puzzle, spelling bee, and championship. Have fun while increasing your knowledge!

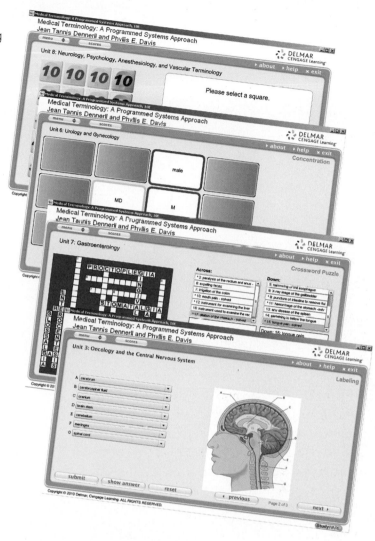

Animations. Animations expand your learning by helping you visualize concepts related to anatomy and physiology.

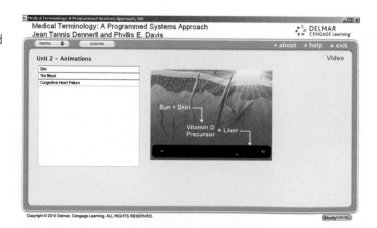

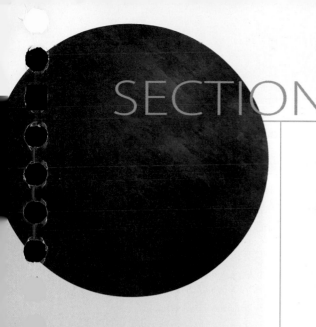

SECTION A

How to Work the Program—Directions for Use of Programmed Learning

frame
Now go on to Frame A.2

A.1

Directions: Tear off the bookmark from the back cover and use it to cover the answer column.

A frame is a piece of information, plus a blank (_____) in which you write. All this material following the number A.1 is a _____.

Check your answer by sliding down your bookmark.

correct
Now go on to Frame A.3

A.2

By checking your answer immediately, you know if you are correct. This immediate knowledge helps you to learn only what is (choose one) _____ (correct/incorrect).

Check your answer by sliding down your bookmark.

program

A.3

Programmed learning is a way of learning that gives you immediate feedback and allows you to work at your own speed. When you work a series of frames and are certain that you know the terms, you are learning using a _____.

Check your answer by sliding down your bookmark.

check
Write

A.4

Always _____ your answers immediately. _____ your answers in the blank or on a separate paper.

The first time you read the frames you may want to just think of the answer. Then read the frames a second time and write the answer on the blank provided or on a separate sheet of paper and check your answer again.

ANSWER COLUMN

INFORMATION
FRAME

A.5

When you write a new word and check your answer, you will usually find the pronunciation given. Pronounce the word aloud and listen to what you are saying. Practice proper pronunciation by listening to the Audio CDs prepared to accompany *Medical Terminology: A Programmed Systems Approach,* Tenth Edition. Pronouncing words correctly assists in spelling correctly, speaking medical phrases correctly, and understanding medical terms when you hear them pronounced (as in dictation).

A.6

pró nun sē ǎ´ shun

The front inside cover presents a pronunciation key to vowel and consonant sounds and the phonetic system used in this text. The syllable with the major accent is highlighted in bold print.

A.7

aloud

Practice saying each new medical word _____ several times. Practicing pronunciation helps you to focus on each syllable so you do not miss any part of the word as you read. Pronunciation will also help you see each letter of the word and improve your spelling.

A.8

medical
one

When you see a blank space (_____) your answer will need only one word. In the sentence, "This is a program in _____ terminology," you know to use _____ word.

A.9

long

A single blank (_____) contains a clue. It is proportional to the length of the word needed. A short blank (_____) means one short word.
A long blank (_____) means one _____ word.

A.10

medical terminology
more than one word

When you see an asterisk and a blank (*_____), your answer will require more than one word. In the sentence, "This is a programmed course in
*_____,"
your answer requires *_____.

A.11

more than one word

When you see (*_____) there is no clue to the length of the words. The important thing to remember is that an asterisk and a blank means
*_____.

A.12

aloud

Use the pronunciation key on the inside front cover to aid in proper practice when saying words _____.

A.13

spelling

Saying each term aloud will also improve your _____.

ANSWER COLUMN

A.14

anything from interesting
to dull (if you did not
answer this one,
it doesn't matter)
use your own words

When you see a double asterisk and a blank (**_____),
use your own words. In the sentence, "I think a programmed course in
medical terminology will be **_____," you are expected to
**_____.

A.15

never look ahead

When working a program, *never look ahead*. The information presented in the
frames is in a special order, so do not skip around and

*_____.

A.16

one
length
more than one
use your own
aloud
never look ahead

Now summarize what you have learned so far.
A single blank means _____ word.
A single blank gives a clue about the _____ of the word.
A single asterisk means *_____ word.
A double asterisk means *_____ words.
Practice saying each term _____.
The frames are in a special order so *_____.

A.17

Saying, listening, seeing, writing, and *thinking* will do much for your learning. On
the following drawing, find the parts of the brain used when saying, listening,
seeing, writing, and thinking.

1. thinking area
2. hearing area
3. saying area
4. seeing area
5. writing area

A.18

**INFORMATION
FRAME**

If you have five parts of the brain working for you at the same time, you will learn
much faster. This is efficient learning. It makes sense to say a word, listen to it, look
at it, write it, and think about it in one operation.

A.19

five

This programmed learning, word-building system encourages you to *read* (look
and understand) about medical terms, *say* them aloud correctly, *listen* to them on
Audio CD, *write* the terms as answers in the blanks and review activities, and *think*
about the terms as you use them to complete statements. Doing this uses at least
_____ areas of your brain and helps you learn more efficiently.

See how efficiently you
are learning!

You are now ready to move on to an introduction of the word-building system
and learning your first medical terms.

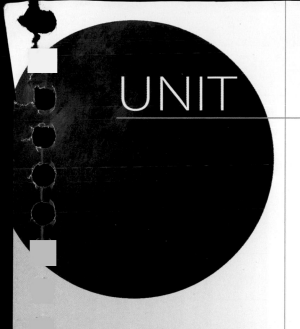

UNIT 1

The Word-Building System— Introduction to Word Parts Including Word Roots, Suffixes, Prefixes, Parts of Speech, and Plural Formation

1.1

Welcome to your study of medical terminology using both this unique method of programmed learning and the word-building system. By combining programmed learning and the word-building system, you will soon be learning hundreds, even

medical

thousands, of _____ terms.

1.2

It would be impossible to simply memorize thousands of medical terms and remember them for very long. The word-building system teaches word parts including word roots, combining forms, prefixes, and suffixes as well as rules about grammar usage and spelling. In a short time you will be easily using the

word-building system

* _____.

1.3

All words are built using word roots. Word roots come from their language of origin. In English medical terminology most word roots originate from Greek and Latin. Greek and Roman physicians studied anatomy and were responsible for naming body structures and identifying early diseases. This formed the basis for the development of western medical language. Medical terms are built

word roots

using * _____.

1.4

The word root is the foundation of a word. Trans/port, ex/port, im/port, and

word root

sup/port have **port** as their * _____.

1.5

word root

Suf/fix, pre/fix, af/fix, and fix/ation have **fix** as their * _____.

1

ANSWER COLUMN

1.6

gastr

The word root for stomach in **gastr**/itis, **gastr**/ectomy, and **gastr**/ic is

_____.

NOTE: Notice that when a combining form is presented by itself it is printed in bold text.

EXAMPLE: **gastr/o** is the combining form meaning stomach.

1.7

word root

The foundation of the word is the * _____.

NOTE: A slash mark (diagonal) "/" is used to divide words into their word parts.

EXAMPLE:

gastr/	**o**/	**duoden**/	**-ostomy**
word root	combining vowel	word root	suffix

1.8

combining form

A *combining form* is a word root plus a vowel. In the word therm/o/meter,

therm/o is the * _____.

WORD BUILDING
■ ■ ■ ■ ■

MICR — word root + O — vowel = MICR/O — combining form

1.9

INFORMATION FRAME

Adding a vowel (a, e, i, o, u, or y) to a word root to create a combining form allows two or more word roots to be joined to form a compound word. It also allows a word root to be joined with a suffix (ending of a word) to form a word. In addition, the vowel assists by making the term easier to pronounce. "O" is the most commonly used combining vowel.

1.10

vowel or letter o

In the word cyt/o/meter (instrument used to measure [count] cells), the

* _____ allows **cyt** to be joined to meter.

1.11

combining form
word root

In the words micr/o/scope, micr/o/film, and micr/o/be, **micr/o** is a

* _____ and **micr** is a * _____.

ANSWER COLUMN

SPELL CHECK

1.12

COMBINING FORM RULE: Use a combining form when adding a word root to another word root or suffix that begins with a *consonant* (for example b, d, m, p, s, t, v). When building a word from "acr" and the suffix "-megaly", use the combining form "acr/o" to form the correctly spelled term "acromegaly". Try this for yourself.

Build words from the following parts:

gastr and **duoden** and **–scopy**

gastr/o/duoden/o/scopy
gas' trō doo' ō den **os**' ko pē

_____/_____/_____/_____/_____

micr and **-scope**

micr/o/scope
mī' krō skōp

_____/_____/_____

WORD BUILDING

■ ■ ■ ■ ■

 GASTR/O + 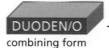 **DUODEN/O** + **SCOPY** = 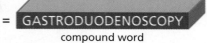 **GASTRODUODENOSCOPY**

combining form + combining form + suffix = compound word

Compound microscope
Delmar/Cengage Learning

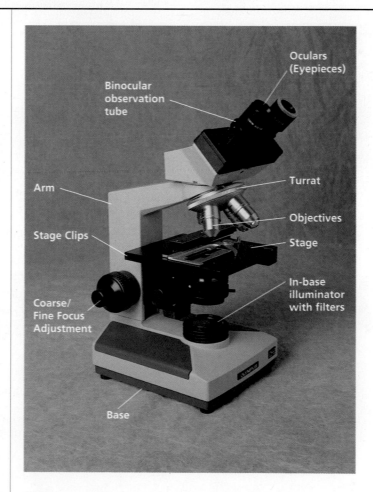

Oculars (Eyepieces)

Binocular observation tube

Arm

Turrat

Objectives

Stage Clips

Stage

Coarse/ Fine Focus Adjustment

In-base illuminator with filters

Base

ANSWER COLUMN

1.13

would
neur/o/spasm

You (choose one) _____ (would/would not) use a combining form to join the word roots **neur** and **spasm** to form

_____ / _____ / _____ .

1.14

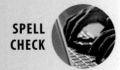

SPELL CHECK

WORD ROOT RULE: Use a word root when joining a word root to another word root or suffix that begins with a vowel (a, e, i, o, u, y). When building a word using "aden" and "-itis" use the word root "aden" to create aden/itis. *Aden(o)itis* is an incorrect spelling. Try this for yourself.
Build a word using:
lymph and **–oma** (lymphatic tumor)

lymph/oma
limf ō′ mə

_____ / _____

ot and **–algia** (ear pain)

ot/algia
ō **tal′** gē ə

_____ / _____

Good job.

WORD BUILDING
■ ■ ■ ■ ■

 DERMAT
word root
+
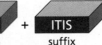 ITIS
suffix
=
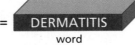 DERMATITIS
word

1.15

would not

lymph/aden/o/pathy
limf ad en **op′** ə thē

You (choose one) _____ (would/would not) use a combining form to join the words "lymph" and "adenopathy" to form

_____ / _____ / _____ / _____ .

1.16

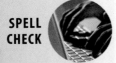

SPELL CHECK

Combining forms are never used as a suffix. They require an ending to complete a word. There are many exceptions to the rules about combining form usage stated above. Always consult your medical dictionary for correct spelling of new terms. That way you will know if the new word you created is actually a medical word.

1.17

compound words

Compound words can be formed when two or more word roots are used to build the word. Even in ordinary English, two or more word roots are used to form

* _____ (for example, shorthand or download).

ANSWER COLUMN

1.18

Sometimes word roots are whole words. Two or more words combined form a compound word. Chickenpox is a * _____ .

compound word

 WORD BUILDING 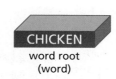 CHICKEN + 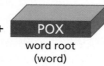 POX = 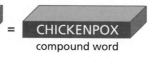 CHICKENPOX

WORD BUILDING ■ ■ ■ ■ ■   CHICKEN word root (word)   +   POX word root (word)   =   CHICKENPOX compound word

---

1.19

Form a compound word using the word roots under and age.

underage   _____

1.20

Form a compound word from the words "brain" and "stem."

brainstem   _____ .

1.21

Because they are formed by joining two or more word roots, therm/o/meter, cyt/o/meter, micr/o/scope, and micr/o/surgery are all ·

compound words   * _____ .

1.22

Compound words can also be formed from a combining form and a whole word. Thermometer is a compound word built from a combining form and a word. In

combining form   the word therm/o/meter, **therm/o** is the * _____ ,

whole word (suffix)   meter is the * _____ .

1.23

Micr/o means small.
Build a compound word using the combining form **micr/o** plus
-scope

micr/o/scope   micr/o/ _____ (instrument used to see small things);
mī' krō skōp

-surgery

micr/o/surgery   micr/o/ _____ (surgery using a microscope);
mī krō **ser'** jer ē

-meter

micr/o/meter   micr/o _____ (device used to measure small things).
mī **krō'** me ter

Remember to practice pronouncing the terms aloud as well.

CASE STUDY INVESTIGATION (CSI)

Shingles. Varicella zoster virus (VZV). Herpes zoster. Postherpetic neuralgia.

Mrs. S, a 75-year-old female, presented with a herpetic blister-like rash on the face and back. She stated that the rash areas burned and were very painful. The shooting pain followed nerve lines and **postherpetic neuralgia** was suspected. The pain was level 8 "very painful and difficult to tolerate." Mrs. S has a history of childhood **chickenpox** and had not received a herpes zoster **immunization** (Zostervax). She was diagnosed with breast cancer two months ago and recently completed radiation therapy and **chemotherapy** treatments. The blisters were examined and a viral culture ordered. The culture results confirmed that varicella zoster **virus** (VZV) was responsible for the lesions and the patient had shingles. An anti-viral medication and cream were prescribed along with an **analgesic** medication. Mrs. S experienced remission and recurrence of symptoms for about four months before finally being rash- and pain-free.

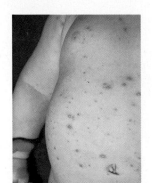

Herpes zoster *Courtesy of Robert A. Silverman, MD, Pediatric Dermatology, Georgetown University*

CSI Vocabulary Challenge

From what you have learned about the word building system and with assistance from your medical dictionary, answer questions about the following terms taken from the case.

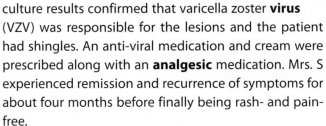

Varicella—chickenpox *Courtesy of Robert A. Silverman, MD, Pediatric Dermatology, Georgetown University*

1. A herpetic lesion is a herpes viral blister. In the term post/herpet/ic **post-** is a _____ (word part) indicating pertaining to after the development of herpetic lesions.

2. **Chickenpox** is a _____ word for the disease also known as Varicella.

3. Zostervax is a type of _____ that may help prevent those with a history of childhood chickenpox from developing shingles after age 60.

4. The combining form **chem/o** was used to build the term chem/o/therapy because the word therapy begins with a _____.

5. Indicate the part of speech of the term **analgesic** as used in this case study.

    _____

6. Write the term that means: condition of nerve pain. _____

7. The adjective viral means pertaining to a _____.

ANSWER COLUMN

1.24

Hydr/o means water.
Build a compound word using the combining form **hydr/o** plus
-phobia

hydr/o/phobia
hī drō **fō'** bē ə

hydr/o/_____(fear of water);

-cele

hydr/o/cele
hī' drō sēl

hydr/o/ _____ (water a saclike cavity);

-therapy

hydr/o/therapy
hī drō **thair'** ə pē

hydr/o/ _____ (treatment using water).

1.25

-ic is an adjective suffix. In medical terminology, compound words are usually built from a combining form, a word root, and a suffix. In the word micr/o/scop/ic, **micr/o** is the combining form;
scop is the word root;

suffix

-ic is the _____.

1.26

In medical terminology, compound words are usually built in the following order: combining form + word root + suffix. The word part coming first

combining form

is usually a * _____. The word part that comes last

suffix

is the _____.

NOTE: The suffixes are highlighted in **[pink]** print throughout this textbook for easy identification.

1.27

In the word therm/o/metr/ic,
therm/o is the combining form;

word root

metr is the * _____;

suffix

-ic is the _____.

1.28

Build a word from the combining form **radi/o** and the suffix

radi/o/grapher
rā dē **og'** raf er

-grapher. _____/_____/_____

1.29

Build a word from the combining form **acr/o**; the word root dermat; and the

acr/o/dermat/itis
a' krō der' ma **ti'** tis

suffix **-itis**. _____/_____/_____/_____

ANSWER COLUMN

1.30

**SPELL
CHECK**
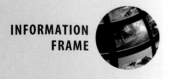

When a definition is stated, the suffix is usually described first, for example:
(1) Definition: pertaining to electricity
   suffix (**–ic**), word root (electr) — electr/ic
(2) Definition: inflammation of the bladder
   suffix (**-itis**), word root (cyst) = cyst/itis

1.31

The ending that follows a word root or combining form is called a **suffix**. You can change the meaning of a word by putting another part after it. This other part is

suffix   called a _____ (highlighted in **pink**).

1.32

The suffix **-er** means one who or one which. The word root **port** (to carry) is changed by putting **-er** after it. In the word port/er (one who carries), **-er** is a

suffix   _____.

1.33

one who   A medical practition/er is * _____ practices medicine.

1.34

In the word inject/able, **-able** changes the meaning of inject.

suffix   **-able** is a _____.

**WORD
BUILDING**
■ ■ ■ ■ ■

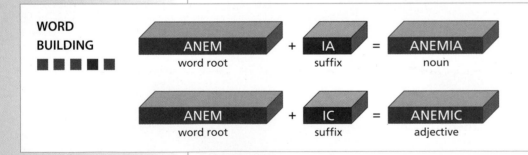

1.35

**INFORMATION
FRAME**

Let's review some basic grammar. Suffixes may change the part of speech of a word. A *noun* is a word that names or labels a person, place, or thing. In medical terms a person's name may become the name of a disease and would be a *proper noun*. Here are some examples of proper noun diagnoses: Down syndrome; West Nile virus. Names of diseases that are not capitalized, such as appendicitis or carcinoma, are *common nouns*. In medical terminology nouns are also labels or names for body parts, instruments, and medical procedures.

ANSWER COLUMN

1.36

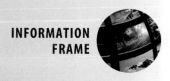

INFORMATION FRAME

Adjectives describe or modify the meaning of a *noun*. In the phrase "small cell," small is an adjective describing the size of the cell (noun). In a medical phrase an *adjective* may describe size, amount, shape, color, level of severity, and quality. In the following phrases the *adjectives* are underlined:

<u>chronic</u> cough
<u>reddened</u> skin
<u>duodenal</u> ulcer
<u>triple</u> bypass

1.37

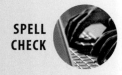

SPELL CHECK

A *noun* may become an *adjective* by changing the suffix. Each noun form has a specific adjectival form that comes from the language of origin of the word. You cannot just switch adjective suffixes to make any noun an adjective. Study the following table showing *nouns* and their suffixes and how they are changed into *adjectives*.

Noun	Suffix	Adjective	Suffix
cyanosis	**-osis**	cyanotic	**-otic**
anemia	**-ia**	anemic	**-ic**
mucus	**-us**	mucous	**-ous**
ilium	**-um**	iliac	**-ac**
condyle	**-e**	condylar	**-ar**
carpus	**-us**	carpal	**-al**
emesis	**-sis**	emetic	**-tic**

1.38

-osis

-ia

-um

In the words cyan/osis, anem/ia, and ili/um, the *noun* suffixes

are _____,

_____,

and _____.

1.39

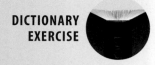

DICTIONARY EXERCISE

By now you may be curious about the meanings of several of these medical terms. Look up the following words in your medical dictionary, then write the meaning below.

Word	Meaning
<u>cyanosis</u>	_____
<u>condyle</u>	_____
<u>anemia</u>	_____
<u>emetic</u>	_____

Good work.

1.40

List the suffixes that make the following nouns adjectives.

-ac
-otic
-ic
-al
-ous
-ar
-iac
-itic
-tic

Adjective	Nouns
ili/ac	ilium
cyan/otic	cyanosis
anem/ic	anemia
duoden/al	duodenum
vomit/ous	vomit
condyl/ar	condyle
man/iac	mania
arthr/itic	arthritis
eme/tic	emesis

Read and study this table. Then move on to the next frame.

Noun Suffixes	Examples
-ism—condition, state, or theory	hyperthyroidism
-tion—condition	contraction, relaxation
-ist—specialist	psychiatrist
-er—one who	radiographer
-ity—quality	sensitivity

Adjectival Suffixes	Examples
-ous—possessing, having, full of	nervous, mucous
-able ⎫	injectable
-ible ⎭ —ability	edible

1.41

condition or state

Hyper/thyroid/ism is a _____ of too much secretion by the thyroid gland.

1.42

theory

Darwin/ism presents a theory of evolution. Mendel/ism presents a _____ of heredity.

1.43

condition

condition

Contrac/tion is a _____ of muscle shortening. Relax/a/tion is the _____ of diminished tension.

1.44

nouns

Contrac/tion and relax/a/tion are (choose one) _____ (nouns/adjectives) because they name a condition.

ANSWER COLUMN

1.45

a specialist

A psychiatr/ist is * _____ who practices psychiatry.

one who

A medical practition/er is * _____ practices medicine.

1.46

noun

The word practitioner is a (choose one) _____ (noun/adjective).

1.47

quality

-ity indicates a quality. Conductiv/ity expresses the _____
of conducting nerve and muscle impulses. Sensitiv/ity expresses the

quality

_____ of nervous tissue excitability related to receiving stimuli.

1.48

noun

Irritabil/ity is a (choose one) _____ (noun/adjective).

1.49

having a material
(substance)

Mucus, a noun, is a watery secretion. Muc/ous, an adjective, refers to the nature
of * _____ secreted by
the mucous membrane.

having, possessing

Ser/ous refers to the nature of _____ material lining
closed body cavities such as the abdomen.

1.50

having, possessing

Nerv/ous refers to _____ too much stress, or

nerve

having a type of tissue made of _____ cells.

1.51

adjectives

Words ending in **-ous** are (choose one) _____ (nouns/adjectives).

1.52

-ible and **-able** indicate ability. To say a food is digestible is to say it has the

ability

_____ to be digested. To say a fracture is reducible is to say that it

ability

has the _____ to be reduced.

STUDY WARE™ CONNECTION

After completing this unit, you can play a hangman or other interactive game on your
StudyWARE™ CD-ROM that will help you learn the content in this chapter.

1.53

ability

To say that lungs are inflatable is to say that they have the _____ to inflate.

1.54

adjectives

Words ending in **-ible** or **-able** are (choose one) _____ (nouns/adjectives).

1.55

INFORMATION FRAME

Verbs are words that represent action or a state of being.

EXAMPLE: incise, ambulate, love.
Verbs also have "tense," which tells you when the action is happening: past, present or future.

1.56

vomited

vomiting

The suffixes **-ed** or **-ing** added to the verb vomit alter the tense of this word (when the action takes place). Create the past tense by adding **-ed** to

vomit: _____, and the present participle by adding **-ing** to

vomit: _____.

1.57

injected

injecting

Use the suffixes **-ed** and **-ing** with the word inject.

_____ past tense;

_____ present participle.

Injectable forms of medication:
(A) ampule,
(B) cartridge,
(C) multidose vial
Delmar/Cengage Learning

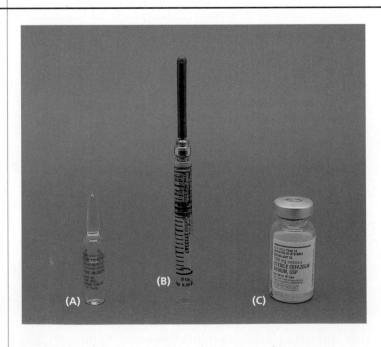

ANSWER COLUMN

INFORMATION FRAME

1.58

Helping verbs are also used to indicate the tense of a verb. The helping verbs and verbs are identified in the following phrases below.
Future tense:
The nurse *will* (helping verb) *inject* (verb) the medication.
Present tense:
Dr. Jones *is* (helping verb) *performing* (verb) the biopsy today.
Past tense:
Sam *was* (helping verb) *transferred* (verb) from the ER to CCU.

WORD ORIGINS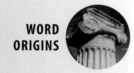

1.59

Since most medical terms in English come from Greek or Latin words, the rules for forming plurals from singular nouns also often come from the Greek and Latin languages. We typically use "s" and "es" added to a singular noun to make it plural (e.g., chair [chairs], box [boxes]). Study the table indicating the proper plural ending associated with each singular noun ending.

Singular Suffixes	Plural Suffixes
Greek	
-on	-a
-ma	-mata
-sis	-es
-nx	-ges
Latin	
-a	-ae
-us	-i
-um	-a
-is	-es
-ex	-ices
-ix	-ices
-ax	-aces

1.60

Now see if you are able to recognize the suffix patterns and write them in the blanks provided. Check your answers. Then look up each word in the medical dictionary.

Greek Singular Noun	Greek Plural Form
spermatozoon	spermatozoa
ganglion	ganglia

-on, -a

suffix _____   suffix _____

carcinoma	carcinomata
lipoma	lipomata

-ma, -mata

suffix _____   suffix _____

(continued)

ANSWER COLUMN

crisis	crises
prognosis	prognoses

-is, -es

suffix _____   suffix _____

larynx (**laryng/o**)   larynges
pharynx (**pharyng/o**)   pharynges

-nx, -ges

suffix _____   suffix _____

1.61

Use what you just learned about Greek to form the plurals for the following terms.

protozoa   prō tō **zō′** ə   protozoan (protozoon)   _____

sarcomata   sär **kō′** ma tə   sarcoma   _____

diagnoses   dī əg **nō′** sēs   diagnosis   _____

phalanges   fə **lan′** jēz   phalanx (**phalang/o**)   _____

Great! Now go on to the Latin forms.

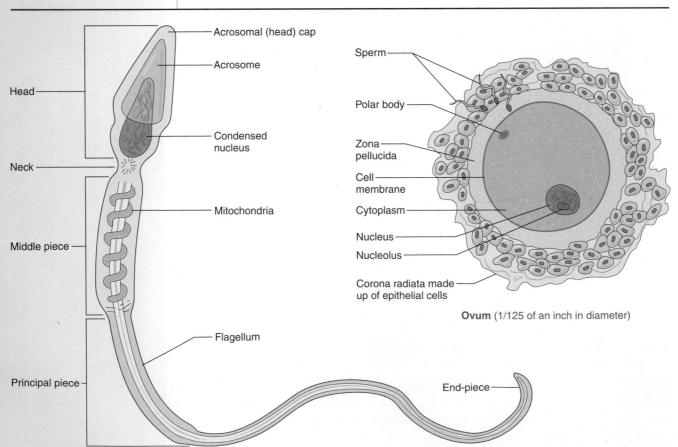

Head

— Acrosomal (head) cap

— Acrosome

Neck

— Condensed
nucleus

Middle piece

— Mitochondria

Principal piece

— Flagellum

Sperm —

Polar body —

Zona
pellucida —

Cell
membrane —

Cytoplasm —

Nucleus —

Nucleolus —

Corona radiata made
up of epithelial cells —

End-piece —

Ovum (1/125 of an inch in diameter)

Sperm and ovum (*Note:* Actual size comparison of sperm entering ovum) *Delmar/Cengage Learning*

ANSWER COLUMN

1.62

Latin Singular Noun	Latin Plural Form
vertebra	vertebrae
conjunctiva (kon **junk**′ tiv ə)	conjunctivae (kon **junk**′ ti vē)

-a, -ae

suffix _____   suffix _____

bacillus (ba **sil**′ us)   bacilli (ba **sil**′ ī)
bronchus (**bron**′ kus)   bronchi (**bron** kī)

-us, -i

suffix _____   suffix _____

testis (**test**′ is)   testes (**test**′ ēz)

-is, -es

suffix _____   suffix _____

ilium (**il**′ ē um)   ilia (**il**′ ē ə)
bacterium (bak **tear**′ ē um)   bacteria (bak **tear**′ ē ə)

-um, -a

suffix _____   suffix _____

cortex (**kor**′ tex)   cortices (**kor**′ ti sēz)

-ex, -ices

suffix _____   suffix _____

appendix (a **pen**′ dix)   appendices (a **pen**′ di sēz)

-ix, -ices

suffix _____   suffix _____

thorax (**thor**′ aks)   thoraces (**thor**′ ə sēz)

-ax, -aces

suffix _____   suffix _____

1.63

Use what you just learned about Latin to form the plurals for the following terms.

cocci   **kok**′ sī   coccus   _____

calcanea   kal **kā**′ nē ə   calcaneum   _____

vertices   **ver**′ ti sēz   vertex (**vertic/o**)   _____

cervices   **ser**′ vi sēz   cervix (**cervic/o**)   _____

thoraces   **thôr**′ ə sēz   thorax (**thorac/o**)   _____

Great work! As you continue through the text, you may wish to refer back to this section to review the rules for plural formation. Plural forms will be included with many of the frames as you learn the singular noun form. When in doubt, consult your dictionary.

1.64

A **prefix** is a word part that goes in front of a word root. You can change the meaning of the word by putting another word part in front of it. This other part is

prefix

a _____.

NOTE: Notice in this book the prefixes are highlighted in **blue** and are followed by a hyphen.

(continued)

ANSWER COLUMN

Prefix	Word	New Word
ex-	tension	extension
ex-	press	express
dis-	please	displease
dis-	ease	disease
post-	after	postherpetic

1.65

The prefix **ex-** means either from or out from. The word press means to squeeze or push on. Placing **ex-** in front of press changes its meaning to "squeeze out." In the word ex/press, **ex-** is a _____.

prefix

1.66

In the word dis/ease, **dis-** changes the meaning of ease. **dis-** is a

_____.

prefix

1.67

In the words im/plant, sup/plant, and trans/plant, the prefixes are _____,

_____, and _____.

im-

sup-, trans-

1.68

Before learning more, review what you have learned. The foundation of a word is a

* _____.

word root

1.69

The word part that is placed in front of a word root to change its meaning is a

_____. In a later unit, you will learn many prefixes.

prefix

1.70

The word part that follows a word root is a _____.

suffix

1.71

A suffix may change a noun to an _____ or change the tense

of a _____.
Good!

adjective

verb

1.72

When a vowel is added to a word root, the word part that results is a

* _____.

combining form

ANSWER COLUMN

1.73

compound word

When two or more word roots are used to form a word, the word formed is called a * _____.

PRONUNCIATION NOTE

1.74

Pronunciation symbols, descriptions, and rules are described on the inside front cover. They will also appear through the text below new terms and at other appropriate times. Refer to this Pronunciation Key or your medical dictionary when in doubt about how to say a word. Also, listen to the Audio CD that accompanies *Medical Terminology: A Programmed Systems Approach,* 10th edition.

Notice the diagrammed sentence below, which illustrates the use of adjectives, nouns, and verbs.

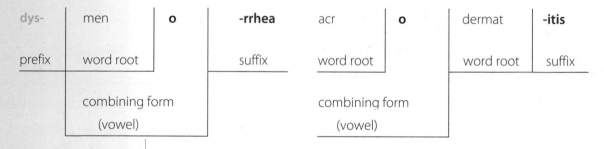

Notice the diagrammed words below indicating their word parts.

dysmenorrhea   **acrodermatitis**

dys-	men	o	-rrhea	acr	o	dermat	-itis
prefix	word root		suffix	word root		word root	suffix
	combining form (vowel)				combining form (vowel)		

1.75

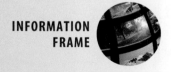

INFORMATION FRAME

How do you know what to put where? The following material will assist you with word building. This is a system that you may have already figured out. If not, study these rules.

RULE I: Most of the time the definitions indicate the last part of the word first. The descriptive phrases usually start with the suffix and then indicate the body part.

EXAMPLES

1. Inflammation (1) of the bladder (2)

    inflammation   _____ / **itis**

    (of the) bladder   cyst/_____

                                                        cyst/itis

                                                        (2) (1)

(continued)

2. One who specializes (1) in skin disorders (2)

    one who specializes (studies)

    _____/ /logist

    (in) skin (disorders)

    dermat/o/_____

    dermat/o/logist

    (2)   (1)

3. Pertaining to the abdomen (1) and bladder (2)

    pertaining to

    _____/ / /ic

    (the) abdomen

    abdomin/o/_____/___

    (and) bladder

    _____/ /cyst/___

    abdomin/o/cyst/ic

    (2)   (1)

RULE II: Where body systems are involved, words are usually built in the order that organs are studied in the system.

EXAMPLES

1. Inflammation of the stomach and small intestine

    inflammation

    _____/ /itis

    (of the) stomach

    gastr/o/_____/___

    (and) small intestine

    _____/ /enter/___

    gastr/o/enter/itis

2. Removal of the uterus, fallopian tubes, and ovaries

    removal of

    _____/ / / /ectomy

    (the) uterus

    hyster/o/_____/ / /___

    fallopian tubes

    _____/ /salping/o/___/___

    (and) ovaries

    _____/ / / /-oophor/___

    hyster/o/salping/o/-oophor/ectomy

RULE III: The body part usually comes first and the condition or procedure is the ending.

EXAMPLES

1. dermat/o/mycosis
    (skin) (fungal condition)
2. cyst/o/scopy
    (bladder) (process of examining the urinary bladder with a scope)

1.76

In this learning program, the word root is followed by a slash and a vowel to make a combining form. In **acr/o**, **acr** is the * _____;

word root

o is the _____;

vowel

and **acr/o** is the * _____.

combining form

ANSWER COLUMN	
	1.77
acr/o *or* acr	**acr/o** is used to build words that refer to the *extremities*. To refer to extremities, physicians use these word parts _____.
	1.78
acr/o	**acr/o** is found in words concerning the extremities, which in the human body are the arms and legs. To build words about the arms use _____/_____. NOTE: Think of an acrobat.
	1.79
acr/o	To build words about the legs, use _____/_____.
	1.80
extremities	**acr/o** any place in a word should make you think of the extremities. When you read a word containing acr or **acr/o**, you think of _____.
	1.81
extremities	In the word acr/o/paralysis (acroparalysis), **acr/o** refers to _____.
	1.82
word root vowel combining form	In **megal/o** (enlarged, large), **megal** is the * _____; **o** is the _____; and **megal/o** is the * _____.
	1.83
extremities	**-megaly** is used as a suffix for enlarged. The words acr/o/megaly (acromegaly), acr/o/cyan/osis (acrocyanosis), and acr/o/dermat/itis (acrodermatitis) refer to the _____.
	1.84
enlarged	A word containing **megal/o** or **-megaly** will mean something is _____.
	1.85
acr/o/megaly ak rō **meg′** ə lē	Acr/o/megaly means enlargement of the extremities. The word that means a person has either enlarged arms and legs or hands and feet is _____/_____/_____.
	1.86
acromegaly	Acr/o/megal/ic gigantism is a specific disorder of the body. The signs are enlargement of the bones of the hands and feet as well as some of the bones of the head. The term describing these signs is _____.

ANSWER COLUMN

Acromegaly *Delmar/ Cengage Learning*

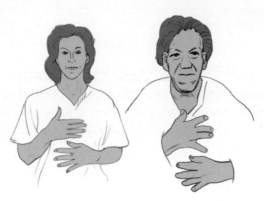

Normal proportion   Acromegaly

STUDY WARE™ CONNECTION

When you complete this unit, remember to go to your **StudyWARE™ CD-ROM** and take a practice quiz.

	1.87
noun	**-y** is a suffix meaning the process or condition that makes a word a noun. Acromegaly is a _____.
	1.88
skin	**dermat/o** refers to the skin. When you see dermat or **dermat/o**, think immediately of _____.
	1.89
	-logy and **-logist** are suffixes.
	-logos is Greek for study
	-logy—noun, study of
	-logist—noun, one who studies
	A dermat/o/logist (dermatologist) is a specialist studying diseases of
skin	the _____. The study of skin is
dermat/o/logy	_____ /_____ /_____.
dûr mə **tol'** ō gē	
	1.90
	Acr/o/dermat/itis (acrodermatitis) is a word that means inflammation of the skin of the extremities. A person with inflamed hands has
acr/o/dermat/itis	_____ /_____ /_____ /_____.
ak' rō dûr mə **tī'** tis	

PROFESSIONAL PROFILE

A **dermatologist** is a physician specialist in the study of skin, hair, and nail disorders. Dermatologists provide diagnoses and treatments for skin cancer, infections, contact dermatitis, allergies, lesion removal, burns, injuries, and cosmetic procedures. They are part of a team including other physicians and surgeons, physician assistants (PA), nurse practitioners, and medical aestheticians who perform skin treatments and promote healthy skin.

ANSWER COLUMN

1.91

inflammation

Remembering the word acrodermatitis, which means inflammation of the skin of the extremities, draw a conclusion. **-itis** is a suffix that means _____.

1.92

acr/o/paralysis
ak′ rō pə **ral′** ə sis

Paralysis is a word that means loss of movement. Form a compound word meaning paralysis of the extremities: _____ / _____ / _____.

1.93

word root

vowel

combining form

In **dermat/o**, dermat (skin) is the * _____ ;

o is the _____ ;

and **dermat/o** is the * _____ .

**Contact dermatitis—
poison ivy** *Photo by Timothy J. Dennerll, RT(R), Ph.D.*

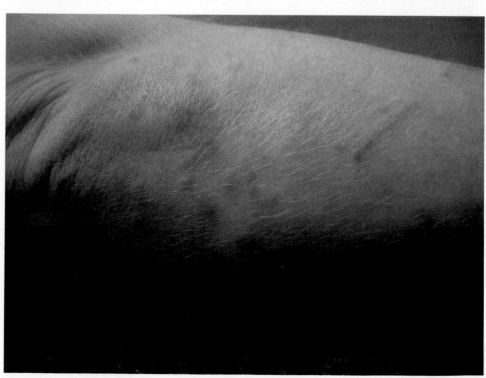

ANSWER COLUMN

SURFACE LESIONS

A.

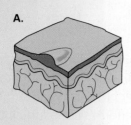

Papule
Solid, elevated lesion less
than 0.5 cm in diameter
Example
Warts, elevated nevi

B.

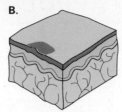

Macule
Localized changes in skin
color of less than 1 cm
in diameter
Example
Freckle

C.

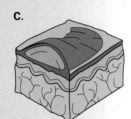

Wheal
Localized edema in the
epidermis causing irregular
elevation that may be red
or pale
Example
Insect bite or a hive

D.

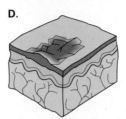

Crust
Dried serum, blood, or pus
on the surface of the skin
Example
Impetigo

FLUID FILLED

E.

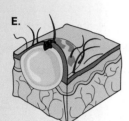

Boil (Furuncle)
Skin infection originating
in gland or hair follicle
Example
Furunculosis

F.

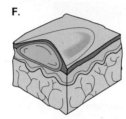

Bullae
Same as a vesicle only
greater than 0.5 cm
Example
Contact dermatitis, large
second-degree burns,
bulbous impetigo, pemphigus

G.

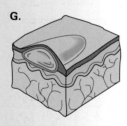

Pustule
Vesicles or bullae that
become filled with pus,
usually described as less
than 0.5 cm in diameter
Example
Acne, impetigo, furuncles,
carbuncles, folliculitis

H.

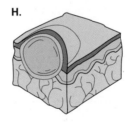

Cyst
Encapsulated fluid-filled or
a semi-solid mass in the
subcutaneous tissue or
dermis
Example
Sebaceous cyst, epidermoid
cyst

Lesions *Delmar/Cengage Learning*

1.94

Analyze the word dermat/itis. **-itis** means inflammation; dermat means of

skin

the _____.

1.95

Dermat/osis means any skin condition. This word denotes an abnormal
skin condition. The suffix that means condition, status, or process is

-osis

_____.

CASE STUDY INVESTIGATION (CSI)

Dermatitis

A 45-year-old white male presents with hand **dermatitis exacerbated** by use of hand soap. Physical examination revealed **erythema** and scaling on both hands. Fissures and **hypopigmentation** was seen on the fingers. Allergy tests including a scratch test for scented soaps revealing a ++ reaction at 48 hours indicating the dermatitis resulted from an **allergy** to perfume scents in the soap. The patient was advised to use unscented soaps and hand moisturizers and avoid other scented products on his skin.

CSI Vocabulary Challenge

Use a medical dictionary to help you analyze the terms listed from the case study. Divide the term into word parts by drawing in the slashes. Then, write the definition in the space provided.

dermatitis _____

exacerbated _____

erythema _____

fissures _____

hypopigmentation _____

allergy _____

1.96

acrodermatitis

Signs of inflammation include redness, swelling, pain, and heat. Acrodermatitis could result from stepping in a patch of poison ivy. A person with red, inflamed skin on his or her feet has _____.

1.97

-itis

Dermat/itis means inflammation of the skin. There are many causes of inflammation, including infection, allergic reaction, and trauma. The suffix that means inflammation is _____.

1.98

dermat/itis
dûr mə **tī'** tis

Bacterial, fungal, or parasitic infections may cause red, inflamed skin called _____/_____.

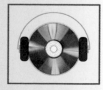

To complete your study of this unit, work the **Review Activities** on the following pages. Also, listen to the Audio CD that accompanies *Medical Terminology: A Programmed Systems Approach*, 10th edition, and practice your pronunciation.

ANSWER COLUMN

STUDY WARE™ CONNECTION

To help you learn the content in this chapter, take a practice quiz or play an interactive game on your **StudyWARE™ CD-ROM**.

Take five minutes and study the abbreviations listed below that were presented in Unit 1.

Abbreviation	Meaning
adj	adjective
ccu	critical care unit
ER	emergency room
Gr	Greek
HSV-1, HSV-I	herpes simplex virus 1
HSV-2, HSV-II	herpes simplex virus 2
L	Latin
n	noun
PA	Physician Assistant
pl	plural
s	singular
v	verb
VAR	varicella zoster vaccine (chickenpox vaccine)
VZV	varicella zoster virus

REVIEW ACTIVITIES

CIRCLE AND CORRECT

Circle the correct answer for each question. Then check your answers in Appendix E.

1. The base of the word is the
   a. prefix
   b. combining form
   c. ending
   d. word root

2. A _____ comes in front of a word root to change its meaning.
   a. prefix
   b. combining form
   c. suffix
   d. pronoun

3. A suffix may change the
   a. part of speech
   b. meaning
   c. plural/singular form
   d. all of these

4. If two or more word roots are combined to build a word, this is a _____ word.
   a. combining form
   b. complex
   c. compound
   d. plural

5. When joining two word roots together you may need to use a(n)
   a. combining form
   b. consonant
   c. adjective
   d. prefix

6. Which word part would indicate inflammation when building a word meaning inflammation of the stomach?
   a. prefix
   b. word root
   c. compound word
   d. suffix

7. When building words about conditions of body parts, the word root for the body part usually comes
   a. first
   b. last
   c. the suffix comes first
   d. the condition comes first

REVIEW ACTIVITIES

8. –y is a suffix that usually makes a word a(n)

   _____.

   a. adjective   b. verb
   c. noun   d. plural

9. When building words with a suffix that begins with a vowel, for example, -itis, you would
   a. put the suffix first   b. use a combining
   c. use a word root   form in front
      in front   d. all of these

10. The correct plural form for thorax is
    a. thoraces   b. thoraxes
    c. thora   d. thoranges

11. The part of speech that indicates action or state of being is a(n)
    a. noun   b. adjective
    c. verb   d. plural

12. –ity is a suffix that indicates
    a. a condition   b. quantity
    c. lack of   d. quality

13. –ism is a suffix that indicates
    a. condition or theory   b. inflammation
    c. adjective   d. lack of

14. –ed and –ing are usually suffixes used to make a word a(n)
    a. noun   b. adjective
    c. verb   d. plural

15. The suffix indicating a condition is
    a. –tic   b. –itis
    c. –tion   d. –er

16. The suffix indicating being full (i.e., full of a substance) is
    a. –ist   b. –ous
    c. –er   d. –tion

SELECT AND CONSTRUCT

Select the correct word parts (some may be used more than once) from the following list and construct medical terms that represent the given meaning.

acr/o	an-	cyt/o	dermat/o	duoden/o	-emia
-er	gastr/o	-graph	hydr/o	-ic	-itis
-megal/y	-meter	micr/o	-phobia	radi/o	-scope
-scopy	surgery	therm/o	-emic		

1. enlargement of the extremities _____

2. instrument used to look at small things _____

3. pertaining to lack of blood _____

4. one who makes x-ray images _____

5. inflammation of the skin on the extremities _____

6. fear of water _____

7. instrument used to measure heat _____

8. surgery using a microscope _____

9. looking into the stomach and duodenum with a scope _____

10. instrument used to measure (count) cells _____

REVIEW ACTIVITIES

PLURAL/SINGULAR FORMS

Using the rules you have learned, form the plural for each of these singular terms.

1. bursa _____

2. coccus _____

3. carcinoma _____

4. protozoan _____

5. crisis _____

6. appendix _____

7. ovum _____

8. phalanx _____

DEFINE AND DISSECT

Give a brief definition and dissect each listed term into its word parts in the space provided. Check your answers by referring to the frame listed in parentheses and to your medical dictionary. Then listen to the Audio CD to practice pronunciation.

Key: rt (word root), v (vowel)

1. gastritis (1.6)   _____/_____
                                                              rt   suffix

   meaning _____

2. practitioner (1.32)   _____/_____/_____/_____
                                      rt   v   suffix   suffix

   _____

3. cytometer (1.10)   _____/_____/_____
                                                    rt   v   suffix (word)

   _____

4. micrometer (1.23)   _____/_____/_____
                                                    rt   v   suffix (word)

   _____

5. gastroduodenoscopy (1.12)   _____/_____/_____/_____/_____
                                          rt   v   rt   v   suffix

   _____

6. lymphadenopathy (1.15)   _____/_____/_____/_____/_____
                                          rt   rt   v   suffix

   _____

7. chickenpox (1.19)   _____/_____
                                                 rt (word)   rt (word)

   _____

REVIEW ACTIVITIES

8. hydrocele (1.24)

_____/_____/_____
          rt   v   suffix

_____

9. hyperthyroidism (1.41)

_____/_____/_____
          pre   rt   suffix

_____

10. psychiatrist (1.45)

_____/_____
          rt   suffix

_____

11. acromegaly (1.85)

_____/_____/_____
          rt   v   suffix

_____

12. neurospasm (1.13)

_____/_____/_____
          rt   v   suffix

_____

13. radiographer (1.28)

_____/_____/_____/_____
          rt   v   rt   suffix

_____

14. dermatologist (1.89)

_____/_____/_____
          rt   v   suffix

_____

15. microscope (1.23)

_____/_____/_____
          rt   v   suffix

_____

16. thermometer (1.22)

_____/_____/_____
          rt   v   suffix

_____

17. irritability (1.48)

_____/_____
          rt   suffix

_____

18. mucous (1.49)

_____/_____
          rt   suffix

_____

REVIEW ACTIVITIES

ADJECTIVE FORMS

Write the adjective for each of the following nouns.

1. cyanosis   _____

2. anemia   _____

3. duodenum   _____

4. mucus   _____

5. arthritis   _____

6. inject   _____

7. emesis   _____

8. condyle   _____

MATCHING

Match the abbreviation on the left with the meaning on the right.

_____ 1. adj

_____ 2. Gr

_____ 3. HSV-1, HSV-I

_____ 4. L

_____ 5. n

_____ 6. VAR

_____ 7. VZV

a. Greek

b. Latin

c. Varicella zoster vaccine (chickenpox vaccine)

d. adjective

e. noun

f. herpes simplex virus 1

g. varicella zoster virus

REVIEW ACTIVITIES

CROSSWORD PUZZLE

Check your answers by going back through the frames or checking the solution in Appendix F.

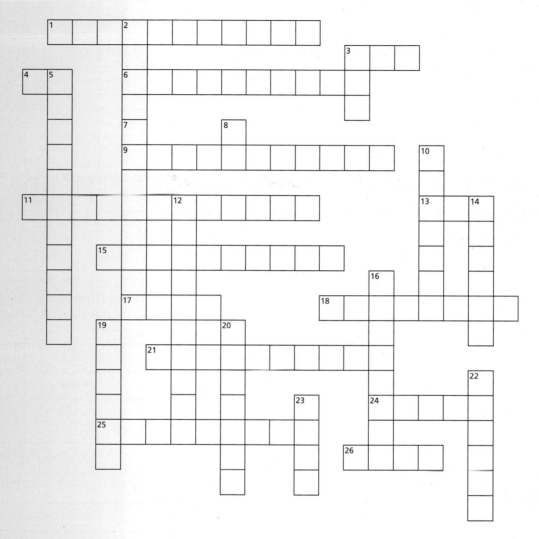

Across

1. instrument: used to measure temperature
3. suffix; quality
4. adjective suffix: pertaining to
6. inflammation of the skin
7. combining vowel
9. excision of the stomach
11. redness, swelling, pain, warmth
13. adjective suffix: full of, possessing
15. compound word for Varicella infection
17. The word _____ is the base of a word.
18. condition of blueness
21. enlarged extremities
24. word root for stomach
25. part of speech: describes a noun
26. suffix: condition

Down

2. one who makes radiographic images
3. suffix: specialist
5. plural of carcinoma
8. suffix: one who
10. combining form for duodenum
12. instrument: looks at very small things
14. placed at the end of a word
16. plural of larynx
19. singular of thoraces
20. past tense verb: vomit
22. placed in front of the word root
23. part of speech: shows action or a state of being

REVIEW ACTIVITIES

GLOSSARY

acrodermatitis	inflammation of the skin extremities	disease	abnormal function or condition
acromegaly	enlarged extremities	extension	stretching or elongation
acroparalysis	paralysis of the extremities	gastrectomy	excision of the stomach
adjective	descriptor, modifies nouns	gastric	stomach (adjectival form)
anemia/anemic	lack of blood, noun/adjective	gastritis	inflammation of the stomach
appendix/appendices	glandular structure below the cecum, singular/plural	gastroduodenoscopy	examination by looking into the stomach and the duodenum with a scope
bacillus/bacilli	rod-shaped bacteria, singular/plural	gastroduodenostomy	make a new surgical opening between the stomach and duodenum
bacterium/bacteria	microorganism group, singular/plural	hydrocele	herniation or sac containing water (fluid)
brainstem	brain structure that includes: midbrain, pons, medulla oblongata	hydrophobia	abnormal fear of water
		hydrotherapy	therapy using water
carcinoma/carcinomata	cancerous tumor (epithelial origin), singular/plural	hyperthyroidism	overactive thyroid condition
carpus, carpal, carpi	wrist bone(s), (noun/ adjective/plural)	ilium/iliac	upper pelvic bone, noun/ adjective
chickenpox	viral infection with Varicella zoster	inflammation	condition defined by redness, swelling, pain, and warmth
combining form	word root plus a vowel		
compound word	word made of two or more word roots	inject, injected, injecting	put in using a needle, verbs
		injectable	able to be injected (adjective)
condyle/condylar	rounded bony process (noun/adjective)	larynx/larynges	voice box (singular/plural)
contraction	condition of shortening a body part, tension, muscle function	lymphadenopathy	disease of a lymph gland
		microbe	very small organism
crisis/crises	acute (severe) situation (singular/plural)	microfilm	image reduced to small size on film
cyanosis/cyanotic	condition of blueness (noun/adjective)	micrometer	one millionth of a meter
cytometer	instrument that measures (counts) cells	microscope	instrument used to look at small structures
		microsurgery	surgery using a microscope
dermatitis	inflammation of the skin	mucus/mucous	watery substance produced by a membrane, (noun/ adjective)
dermatology	the study of the skin, medical specialty		

REVIEW ACTIVITIES

neurospasm	nerve spasm (twitching)	suffix	follows a word root to change its meaning or part of speech
noun	name of a person, place, or thing	thermometer	instrument that measures temperature
practitioner	one who practices	transport	carry across
prefix	placed before a word root to change its meaning	verb	action or state of being word
psychiatrist	specialist in treating mental disorders	vertebra/vertebrae	spinal bones (singular/plural)
radiographer	one who makes x-ray images	vomit, vomited, vomiting	evacuate stomach contents (verbs)
sensitivity	quality of being sensitive	word root	base of a word
spermatozoon	sperm (pl. spermatozoa)		

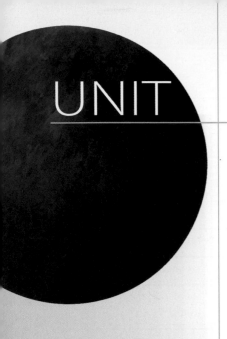

UNIT 2

Surgical Suffixes, Hematology, and Diagnostic Imaging

2.1

INFORMATION FRAME

Surgery is an important medical treatment tool. Surgical procedures may include: incision, excision, repair, replacement, destruction, ablation, cauterization, introduction, or dilation. Throughout the next few units you will be learning many surgical procedure terms. As a beginning, let us study some terms related to surgical cutting.

2.2

WORD ORIGINS

Consider the following word parts.

Word Part	Origin	Meaning
tomos	Greek	cut
ex (ec)	Latin/Greek	out of, away, from
os	Latin	opening like a mouth
stoma	Greek	opening like a mouth
in	Greek	inside, into
cis (incisio)	Latin	cut, cut with a knife

2.3

From the Greek word *tomos* we build many of the suffixes representing surgical cutting procedures.

-tome   instrument used to cut slices

-tomy   cut into, incise, incision

-ectomy   cut out, remove, excise, excision

-ostomy   cut a new surgical opening

ANSWER COLUMN

DICTIONARY EXERCISE

derma/<u>tome</u>
dûr′ mə tōm

gastro/<u>tomy</u>
gas **trot**′ ō mē

duoden/<u>ectomy</u>
dōō′ ō də **nek**′ tō mē

col/<u>ostomy</u>
co **los**′ tō mē

cut

gastr/ectomy
gas **trek**′ tō mē

gastr/o/tomy
gas **trot**′ ō mē

gastr/ostomy
gas **tros**′ tō mē

2.4

Underline the surgical suffix in the following terms. Then, use your dictionary to help you write the meaning of each type of surgical procedure.

dermatome _____

gastrotomy _____

duodenectomy _____

colostomy _____

2.5

Remember to associate *tom* (**-tome, -ectomy, -ostomy,** and **-tomy**) with cutting.

A **-tome** is a surgical instrument used to _____ slices.

2.6

gastr/o is the combining form for stomach. Remembering the rule about when to use a combining form and when to use a word root, build a word that means

ex/cision of the stomach _____/_____;

in/cision into the stomach _____/_____/_____;

make a surgical opening in the stomach _____/_____.

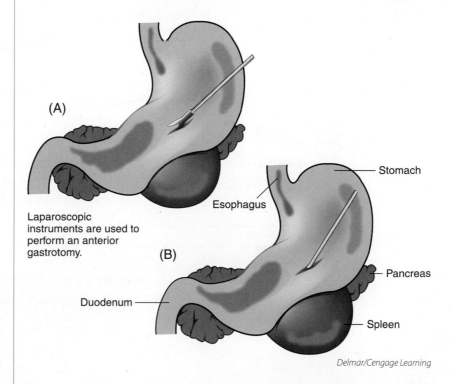

(A)

Laparoscopic instruments are used to perform an anterior gastrotomy.

(B)

Esophagus

Stomach

Pancreas

Duodenum

Spleen

Delmar/Cengage Learning

2.7

A derm/a/tome is an instrument that cuts thin slices of skin. When a surgeon needs to excise a thin slice of skin for examination or skin grafting, s/he may use

a _____/_____/_____.

derm/a/tome
dûr′ mə tōm

2.8

Recall that **-tome** referred to cutting or a cutting instrument. Gastr/ectomy means excision (removal) of all or part of the stomach. **-ectomy** is a suffix

excision or removal

meaning _____. (Refer to Frame 2.9.)

2.9

**INFORMATION
FRAME**

This is a free frame for those who are interested. Others may go on.

		meaning
ect/o	combining form	outside
tom/o	combining form	cut
-y	noun suffix	

Add **ect + om + y** = ectomy means excision

NOTE: One "t" is dropped when **-tome** is preceded by "ect."

2.10

**INFORMATION
FRAME**

Here's another free frame for those interested in **-ostomy**.

		meaning
os	combining form	mouth, opening
tom/o	combining form	cut
-y	noun suffix	

Add **os + tom + y** = ostomy means opening by cutting

2.11

gastr/o means stomach.
If a person is unable to swallow and a tube feeding directly into the stomach is necessary, a new opening may be made through the stomach, called

gastr/ostomy
gas **tros′** tō mē

a _____/_____.

2.12

duoden/o is the combining form for the duodenum, which is the first section of the small intestine. Build a word that means excision (removal) of the

duoden/ectomy
dōō ō dən **ek′** tō mē

duodenum. _____/_____

ANSWER COLUMN

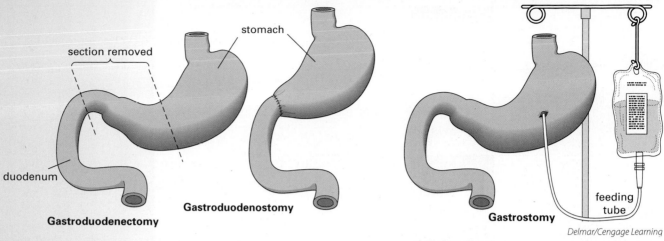

stomach

section removed

duodenum

Gastroduodenectomy

Gastroduodenostomy

Gastrostomy

feeding tube

Delmar/Cengage Learning

2.13	
gastr/o/duoden/ostomy gas′ trō dōō′ ō də **nos**′ tə mē	Gastr/o/duoden/o/stomy means forming a new surgical opening between the stomach and duodenum. A surgeon who removes the natural connection between the duodenum and stomach and then forms a new connection is performing a _____/_____/_____/_____.
2.14	
gastroduodenostomy	A gastroduodenostomy is a surgical procedure. When the pyloric sphincter (a valve that controls the amount of food going from the stomach to the duodenum) no longer functions, a _____ may be necessary.
2.15	
gastroduodenostomy	When a portion of the first part of the small intestine is removed because of cancer, a new artificial surgical opening is created by performing a _____.

WORD BUILDING ■■■■■ | GASTR *word root* + O *vowel* + DUODEN *word root* + OSTOMY *suffix*

2.16	
duoden/um dōō ō **dē**′ nəm dōō **od**′ ə nəm	**-tomy** is a suffix meaning incision into. A duoden/o/tomy is an incision into the _____/_____.
2.17	
duoden/o/tomy dōō ō də **not**′ ə mē	An incision into the duodenum is a _____/_____/_____.

ANSWER COLUMN

gastr/ectomy
gas **trek**′ tə mē

2.18

A gastr/ectomy is a surgical procedure. When a gastr/ic ulcer has perforated, a partial _____/_____ may be indicated to remove part of the stomach.

NOTE: Remember, the combining form is not used when the suffix begins with a vowel.

gastrectomy

2.19

Cancer of the stomach may also be treated by removal of the stomach,

called _____.

gastr/itis
gas **trī**′ tis

2.20

-itis is the suffix used for inflammation. A word that means inflammation of the stomach is _____/_____.

stomach

2.21

-megaly is a suffix meaning *enlarged* or *enlargement*. Gastromegaly is one word for enlarged stomach. **gastr/o** is the combining form for _____.

SPELL CHECK

2.22

Some medical terms use combining forms at the beginning of the word that may be changed to suffixes and then used at the end of a word. For example **megal/o** is a combining form that may be changed to **–megaly** and used as a suffix. There is usually a conventional order of word parts in compound words. Medical terms usually begin with the body part and end with the condition or procedure suffix. However, some terms have word parts that are able to be flipped. Here are some examples.
gastromegaly, megalogastria
cardiomegaly, megalocardia
salpingo-oophoritis, oophorosalpingitis
Always check with your medical dictionary to confirm correct spellings.

gastr/o/megaly
gas trō **meg**′ ə lē

megal/o/gastria
meg ə lō **gas**′ trē ə

2.23

Two words that mean enlargement of the stomach

are _____/_____/_____

and _____/_____/_____.

duodenotomy

2.24

A surgeon who makes an incision into the duodenum is performing

a _____.

ANSWER COLUMN

2.25

Inflammation is a tissue and blood vessel response to injury. It is characterized by redness and swelling of a body part. **-itis** is a suffix for inflammation. When physicians are listing conditions of the duodenum and they want to say it is

duodenitis

inflamed, they use the word _____.

2.26

An inflammatory response may be triggered by allergies, physical injury, chemical irritants, or infection caused by pathogenic organisms. When you see the terms sinus/itis, dermat/itis, and oste/itis, the cause is not known, but, the suffix **–itis**

in/flamma/tion
in flə **mā**′ shun

tells you the condition is _____/_____/_____.

2.27

SPELL CHECK

Watch the spelling on the variations of terms related to *inflammation*. The condition of redness and swelling may make you think of "flames." The noun and adjective forms are spelled with two "m"s and the verb forms are spelled with one. Study the list below.

inflammation	(noun)	in flə **mā**′ shun
inflammatory	(adjective)	in **fla**′ ma tôr ē
inflame	(verb)	in **flām**′
inflamed	(past tense verb)	in **flām′d**′
inflaming	(present participle verb)	in **flām**′ ing

2.28

-itis

duoden/itis
dōō ō də **nī**′ tis
dōō od′ e **nī**′ tis

The suffix for inflammation is _____. The word for inflammation of the duodenum is _____/_____

2.29

-**al** *or* -**ic**

Gastric and duoden/al are adjectives. **-al** and **-ic** are adjectival suffixes meaning pertaining to (whatever the adjective modifies). One adjectival suffix is _____.

2.30

duoden/al
dōō ō **dē**′ nəl
dōō **od**′ ə nəl
ulcer **ul**′ ser
lesion **lē**′ zhun

In duoden/al ulcer and duoden/al lesion, the adjective

is _____/_____, and the nouns modified

are _____.

2.31

duodenal

In the phrase, "Duodenal carcinoma was present," the adjective meaning that pertains to the duodenum is _____.

ANSWER COLUMN

(A) Computed tomography and (B) conventional x-ray procedure
Delmar/Cengage Learning

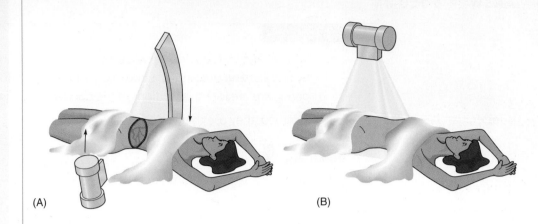

(A)   (B)

2.32

Recall that **-ostomy** means making a new surgical opening. The word to form a new opening into the duodenum is _____/_____.

duoden/ostomy
dōō ō də **nos**′ tə mē

2.33

A duodenostomy can be formed in more than one manner. If it is formed with the stomach, it is called a

gastr/o/duoden/ostomy
gas′ trō dōō ō dēn **os**′ tō mē

_____/_____/_____/_____.

2.34

The suffix for excision is _____.

-ectomy

The suffix for incision is _____.

-tomy

The suffix for forming a new opening is _____.

-ostomy

2.35

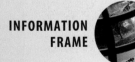

INFORMATION FRAME

Diagnostic imaging has emerged as an important assessment tool in medicine today. It includes any modality that creates a graph, picture, or other visual representation of body structures and/or their function. Cardi/o/pulmon/ary, radi/o/logy, neur/o/logy, and information processing departments have been responsible for the development and study of most imaging systems used today.

2.36

-graph is a suffix taken from the Greek verb *graphein*, meaning to write or record. In medical words, **-graph** refers to an instrument used to record data. A tom/o/graph is an x-ray instrument used to show tissue or organs in one plane (slice, so to speak). To obtain an x-ray of a slice of an organ, the radiographer would use

tom/o/graph
tō′ mō graf

a _____/_____/_____.

NOTE: The word root for to cut is tom; the combining form is **tom/o**.

ANSWER COLUMN

| 2.37 |

tom/o/graphy
tō **mog'** raf ē

tomograph
tom/o/gram
tō mō gram

-gram indicates a picture or record.

Adding a **-y** to **-graph** (as in biography) creates a suffix indicating the process of making a recording of data. The process of using a tomograph is called _____/_____/_____.

Computed tomography (CT) allows the radiologist to obtain a three-dimensional view of internal structures. A CT (or CAT) scanner is a type of _____.

The CT image is a _____/_____/_____.

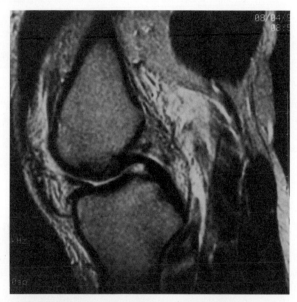

(A) MRI (magnetic resonance imaging) of the knee acquired in the sagittal plane *Delmar/Cengage Learning*

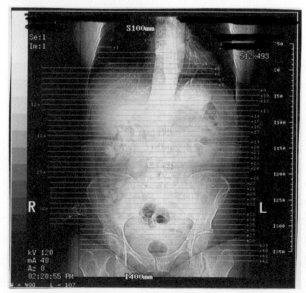

(B) This scout view of the abdomen helps localize the scan parameters of a CT (computed tomography) scan. Each horizontal line indicates the level of one slice. *Delmar/Cengage Learning*

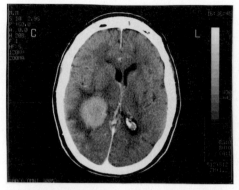

(C) CAT (computed axial tomography) scan demonstrates a meningioma surrounded by edema *Delmar/Cengage Learning*

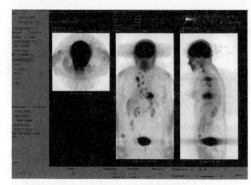

(D) PET (positron emission tomography) scan demonstrating tumor in right lung *Delmar/Cengage Learning*

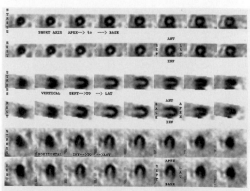

(E) SPECT (single photon emission computed tomography) *Delmar/Cengage Learning*

ANSWER COLUMN

2.38

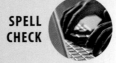

INFORMATION FRAME

Tom/o/graphy is a radi/o/graphic procedure that uses x-rays to produce images of a slice or plane of the body. Each of the following imaging procedures is a type of tomography.

MRI	magnetic resonance imaging
CT	computed tomography (CAT scan)
PET	positron emission tomography
SPECT	single photon emission computed tomography

For more information use your medical dictionary or perform a library or Internet search of these topics.

2.39

tomography

MRI, CT, PET, and SPECT are all types of _____.

2.40

cardi/algia
kär′ de **al**′ jē ə

-algia is one suffix that means pain. Form a word that means heart pain. (Clue: **-algia** is a suffix that begins with a vowel, you will use the word root rather than the combining form.) _____/_____

2.41

cardialgia

Gastr/algia means pain in the stomach. When a patient complains of pain in the heart, this symptom is known medically as _____.

2.42

-algia
gastr/algia
gas **tral**′ jē ə

One suffix for pain is _____. Stomach pain is _____/_____.

2.43

SPELL CHECK

cardi/o (**card/o**) is used in building words that refer to the heart. Card/itis is inflammation of the heart.

When using a suffix that begins with a vowel (i.e., **-itis, -ectomy**), use the word root. When using a suffix that begins with a consonant (i.e., **-dynia, -logy**), you will need a combining form. Examples are card/itis, cardi/ectomy, cardi/o/dynia, and cardi/o/logy.

2.44

cardiologist
kär dē **ol**′ ō jist

A cardi/o/logist discovers irregularities in the flow of the blood in the heart. The physician catheterizes the heart to view blood flow through the vessels of the heart. This heart specialist is a _____.

ANSWER COLUMN

Computed tomography (CT) planes of the body are imaged
Delmar/Cengage Learning

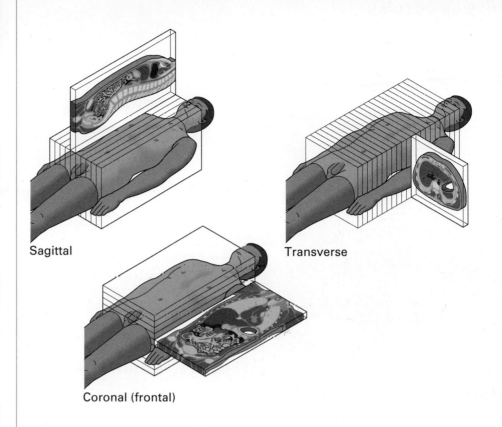

Sagittal

Transverse

Coronal (frontal)

2.45

A person who reads electr/o/cardi/o/grams (records of electrical impulses given off by the heart) is also a _____.

cardiologist
kär dē **ol′** ō jist

2.46

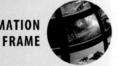

INFORMATION FRAME

When hospitalized, a patient with a severe heart condition is usually treated in a cardiac care unit (CCU). An electr/o/cardi/o/gram (EKG or ECG) may be performed to assess heart function.

2.47

an image, picture, or record of electrical activity of the heart

-gram is the suffix meaning record, image, or picture. **electr/o** is the combining form for *electrical*. Give the meaning of electr/o/cardi/o/gram. ** _____
_____.

2.48

electr/o/cardi/o/gram
e lek′ trō **kär′** dē ō gram

-graph is a suffix indicating an instrument used to make a recording or any imaging device. An electr/o/cardi/o/gram is the record produced. The electr/o/cardi/o/graph is the instrument used to record the picture, called an _____/_____/_____/_____/_____.

ANSWER COLUMN

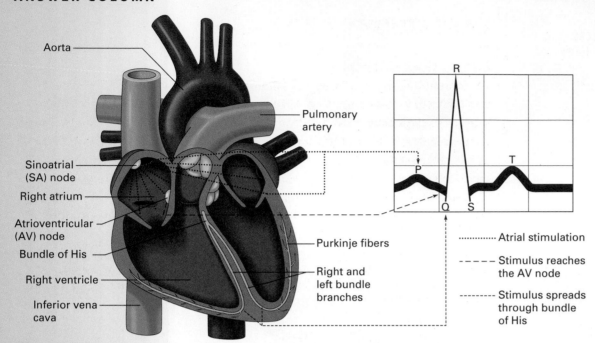

Conduction system of the heart showing the source of electrical impulses produced on an ECG (EKG) *Delmar/Cengage Learning*

2.49

-graphy is a suffix for the *process* of making a recording or image (EKG or ECG). The electr/o/cardi/o/gram is a record obtained by the process of electr/o/cardi/o/graphy. A technologist can learn electrocardiography, but it takes a cardiologist to

electrocardiogram

read the _____.

NOTE: The suffix **-gram** refers to the actual paper readout or picture on a computer screen. Think of obtaining a telegram from a telegraph.

2.50

A physician can read a tracing that looks like this,

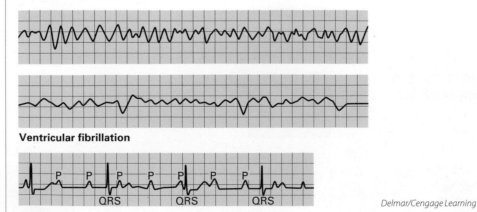

Ventricular fibrillation

Atrial tachycardia (atrial rate, 107; ventricular rate, 43)

Delmar/Cengage Learning

cardiologist
electrocardiogram

and learn something about a person's heart. The physician is a _____

and is reading an _____.

CASE STUDY INVESTIGATION (CSI)

Castleman's Disease

We present the case of a 74-year-old man with Castleman's disease. The disease was detected with a contrast-enhanced computed **tomography** (**CT**) scan and a **fluorodeoxyglucose** (**FDG**)-positron emission tomography (**PET**)/**CT** study; diagnosis was made with **histopathology**. After treatment with surgical **excision** followed by **chemotherapy**, the disease response was evaluated using both **diagnostic** techniques. However, only the PET study was able to identify the spread of the disease to the **abdominal** lymph nodes (**lymphadenopathy**), which were both enlarged and normal size, and, after treatment, to evaluate the disease response.

Source: Reprinted with permission by Ettore Pelosi[1], Andrea Skanjeti[*2], Angelina Cistaro[*1], and Vincenzo Arena[*1]. [1]IRMET PET Center, Via Onorato Vigliani, 10138 Turin, Italy[2] Nuclear Medicine Unit, University of Turin, Corso Bramante, 10126 Turin, Italy. "Fluorodeoxyglucose-positron emission tomography/computed tomography in the staging and evaluation of treatment response in a patient with Castleman's disease: a case report."

CSI Vocabulary Challenge

Use a medical dictionary to help you analyze the term listed from the case study. Divide the term into word parts by drawing in the slashes. Then, write the definition in the space provided.

tomography   _____

fluorodeoxyglucose   _____

histopathology   _____

excision   _____

chemotherapy   _____

diagnostic   _____

abdominal   _____

lymphadenopathy   _____

CT   _____

PET   _____

FDG   _____

ANSWER COLUMN

2.51

son/o is a combining form taken from the Latin word *sonus,* meaning sound. A supersonic transport travels above the speed of sound. A son/o/gram is a picture made by a sonograph. The process of obtaining the sonogram is

son/o/graphy
son **og'** ra fē

called _____/_____/_____ (ultrasonography).

2.52

Recall that the suffix **-er** means one who. The person who (one who) performs

son/o/graph/er
son **og'** ra fer

sonography is called a _____/_____/_____/_____.

ANSWER COLUMN

2.53

ech/o/cardi/o/gram
ek′ ō **kär′** dē ō gram

ech/o is a combining form meaning sound made by *reflected sound* waves. A record of sound waves reflected through the heart is an

_____/_____/_____/_____/_____.

2.54

ech/o/cardi/o/graphy
ek′ ō kär dē **og′** ra fē

The process of making the ech/o/cardi/o/gram is

called _____/_____/_____/_____/_____.

NOTE: *Echo*cardiography uses sound waves; *electro*cardiography uses electricity.

2.55

radi/o/gram
rād′ ē ō gram

radi/o is a combining form from the Latin word *radius*, meaning a ray coming from a central point. **radi/o** is used to refer to radiation such as that used in x-rays. A picture made by using x-rays (XR) is called

a _____/_____/_____.

NOTE: In practice, this is usually called a radiograph.

12 Lead Electrocardiogram ECG tracing or recording
Delmar/Cengage Learning

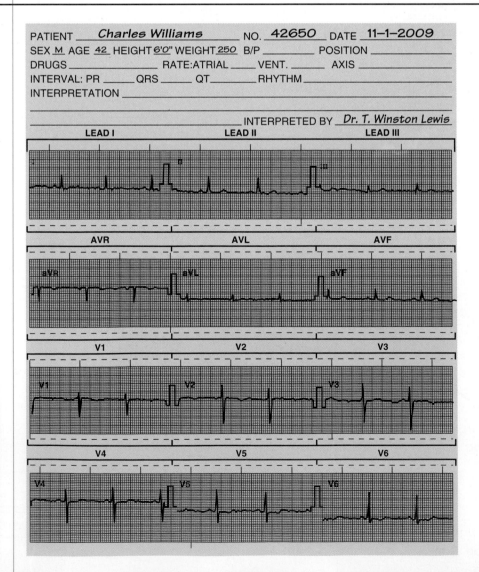

PATIENT ___*Charles Williams*___ NO. _42650_ DATE _11–1–2009_
SEX _M_ AGE _42_ HEIGHT _6′0″_ WEIGHT _250_ B/P _____ POSITION _____
DRUGS _____ RATE:ATRIAL ____ VENT. _____ AXIS _____
INTERVAL: PR _____ QRS _____ QT_____ RHYTHM_____
INTERPRETATION _____
_____
_____ INTERPRETED BY _Dr. T. Winston Lewis_

ANSWER COLUMN

**Electrocardiograph—
This EKG (ECG) machine
is used to record 12 Lead
EKGs** *Photo by Timothy J.
Dennerll, RT(R), Ph.D.*

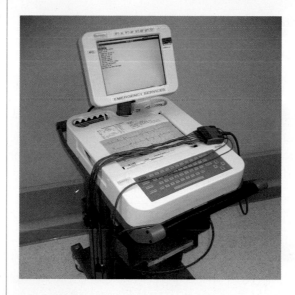

2.56

radi/o/grapher
rād' ē **og**' ra fer

radi/o/logist
rād ē **ol**' ō jist

Build words for the following meanings:

one who takes x-rays _____/_____/_____;

a physician specialist who studies (interprets)

x-rays _____/_____/_____.

2.57

radiologist

Radiation therapists (RATx) use x-rays to irradiate a cancerous area. These

treatments would be supervised by a physician specialist called a _____.

**Radiogram (radiograph):
fractured femur**
Delmar/Cengage Learning

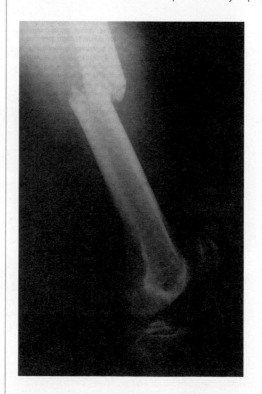

ANSWER COLUMN

2.58

skin

-**pathy** is a suffix meaning disease. Dermat/o/pathy means a disease condition of the _____.

2.59

path/o/logy
path **ol'** ō gē

Great! Now try this: **path/o** is a combining form meaning disease. Path/o/logy is the study of disease. A path/o/logist is a physician specializing in diagnosing (discovering) diseases. A pathologist usually works in the hospital laboratory department called clinical _____/_____/_____.

2.60

INFORMATION FRAME

Color is used in labeling cell and tissue types as well as describing observable signs such as skin color changes. Skin might appear pale yellow, pink, reddened, blue, darkened, or blotchy. These observations assist in making a correct assessment of the patient's condition.

2.61

jaundice
jawn' dis
hyper/bilirubin/emia
hī' per bil'ē rū bin ē' mē ə

Jaundice is not a color change of the actual skin pigment, but a reflection through the skin of bright yellow in the blood plasma. When a person has a high blood bilirubin level, hyper/bilirubin/emia, it gives the plasma a bright yellow color. This occurs, for example, as hepatitis B affects the liver. The patient's eyes, skin, and nailbeds appear yellow. This type of yellow look to the patient is called _____. The high bilirubin level in the blood is _____/_____/_____.

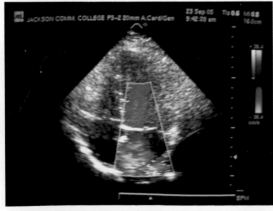

Echocardiogram *Image prepared by Carol Hoch, RDMS, courtesy of Jackson Community College, Jackson, MI. Photo by Timothy J. Dennerll, RT(R), Ph.D.*

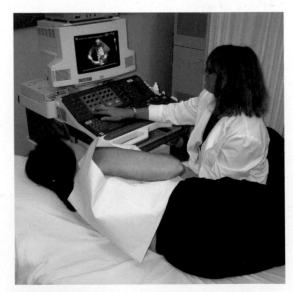

Echocardiograph *Image prepared by Carol Hoch, RDMS, courtesy of Jackson Community College, Jackson, MI. Photo by Timothy J. Dennerll, RT(R), Ph.D.*

PROFESSIONAL PROFILE

Registered radiologic technologists (RT[R]) use ionizing radiation (x-rays) to create images for diagnostic interpretation by physicians called radiologists. Knowledge of positioning patients for exposure, operation of the x-ray equipment and developers, anatomy, pathology, and human relations is essential. Education may be hospital or college based ranging from certificates to advanced degrees. The American Society of Radiologic Technologists (ASRT) and the American Registry of Radiologic Technologists (ARRT) monitor education standards and registration in this profession.

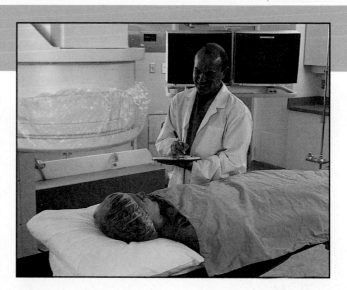

A radiologic technologist interviews a patient prior to an imaging procedure
Delmar/Cengage Learning

ANSWER COLUMN

2.62

jaundiced

Other liver conditions such as cancer or cirrhosis also cause a yellow or

_____ appearance to the skin.

2.63

blue skin or bluish
   discoloration of the skin
   (due to low O₂ levels)
noun

Derma is a word itself. It is a noun meaning skin. Cyan/o/derma is a compound word. It means ** _____

and is a (choose one) _____ (noun/adjective).

NOTE: **-derma** is often used as a suffix meaning condition of the skin.

2.64

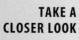

**TAKE A
CLOSER LOOK**

Most of these word parts are used as prefixes (e.g., leukocyte). An exception is **cyan/o**, which may be used either as a prefix (cyanoderma) or as a word root within a word (acrocyanosis).
Use this information for building words involving color:
(Frames 2.69–2.106)

leuk/o	white
melan/o	black (dark pigment)
erythr/o	red
cyan/o	blue
chlor/o	green
xanth/o	yellow

**Structures of the
skin** *Delmar/Cengage Learning*

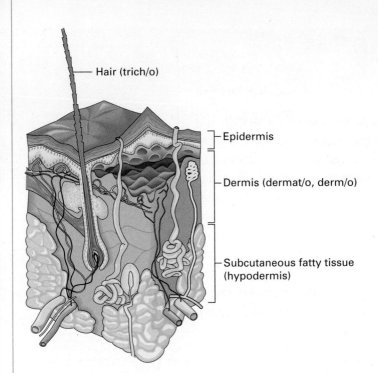

— Hair (trich/o)

⌐ Epidermis

— Dermis (dermat/o, derm/o)

— Subcutaneous fatty tissue
(hypodermis)

Structures of the Skin

2.65

cyan/o is used in words to mean blue or blueness. When photographers
want to say something about how a film reproduces the color blue, they

cyan/o *or* cyan   use _____.

2.66

-osis is a suffix,
forms a noun, and
means disease, condition, status, or process.
Build a word that means

cyan/osis
sī ə **nō′** sis   condition of blueness _____/_____

dermat/osis
dûr mə **tō′** sis   condition of the skin _____/_____

cyan/o/derma *or*
sī′ ən ō **dûr′** mə   condition of blueness of the skin _____/_____/_____
dermat/o/cyan/osis
dûr **mat′** ō sī ən ō′sis

2.67

-tic changes **-osis** from a noun to an adjective. Build the term that means
cyan/otic   pertaining to a condition of blueness: _____/_____.
sī ə **no′** tik

ANSWER COLUMN

2.68

Acr/o/cyan/osis means blueness of the extremities. The part of the word that tells

cyan

you that the color blue is involved is _____.

-osis

The part of the word that tells you this is a condition is _____.

2.69

Cyan/o/derma means blue skin. Build a word meaning red

erythr/o/derma

skin _____/_____/_____

e rith′ rō **der**′ mə

leuk/o/derma

white skin (vitiligo) _____/_____/_____

lōō kō **der**′ mə

xanth/o/derma

yellow skin _____/_____/_____

zan′ thō′ **der**′ mə

melan/o/derma

abnormally dark pigmented skin _____/_____/_____

mel′ an ō **der**′ mə

2.70

Eczema is a scaly reddened condition of the skin.

This reddened inflamed skin condition is a type of

erythr/o/derma

_____/_____/_____ or

e rith rō **derm**′ ə

erythr/o/derma/titis

_____/_____/_____/_____.

e rith′ rō derm ə **tī**′ tis

2.71

Look at the diagram of a section of skin. There are three main layers of tissues: the epi/**derm**/is, **derm**/is, and the hypo/**derm**/is (subcutaneous fatty tissue). Notice that all three of these names for the layers of the skin are built from the word

derm

root _____.

2.72

The outermost layer of the skin, which is upon the the dermis, is

epi/derm/is

the _____/_____/_____.

ep ə **derm**′ is

The layer of the skin below the dermis is

hypo/derm/is

the _____/_____/_____.

hī pō **derm**′ is

2.73

The suffix **-cyte** means cell. A chlor/o/cyte is a green cell (in plants). Build a word

melan/o/cyte

meaning black cell (dark pigmented) _____/_____/_____

mel′ an ō sīt

leuk/o/cyte

white (blood) cell _____/_____/_____

lōō′ kō sīt

erythr/o/cyte

red (blood) cell _____/_____/_____

e **rith**′ rō sīt

STUDY**WARE**™ C O N N E C T I O N

When you complete this unit, remember to go to your **StudyWARE™ CD-ROM** for additional activities that will help you learn the content in this chapter.

ANSWER COLUMN

Acrocyanosis (*blueness of the extremities*)
Delmar/Cengage Learning

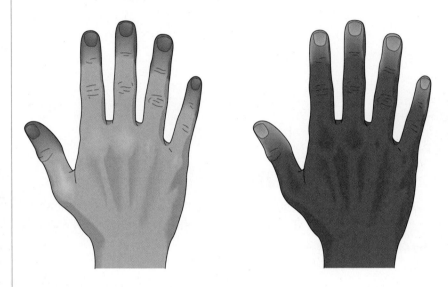

2.74

The suffix **-blast** means embryonic or immature cell. A leuk/o/blast is an embryonic white cell. Build a word meaning an embryonic cell of the following colors.

melan/o/blast

black (dark pigment) _____/_____/_____

erythr/o/blast
(You pronounce)

red _____/_____/_____

2.75

-emia is a suffix from the Greek word *hema*, for blood. **-emia** means blood condition. An/emia is a condition of lack of blood cells or hemoglobin. Build words involving the following colors referring to blood conditions.

xanth/emia
zan **thē**′ mē ə

yellow (jaundice) _____/_____

erythr/emia
e rith **rē**′ mē ə

red (polycythemia) _____/_____

chlor/emia
klor ē′ mē ə

green (increased chlorine in the blood) _____/_____

NOTE: Chlorosis is a condition in which the skin takes on a greenish tinge due to anemia.

ANSWER COLUMN

**TAKE A
CLOSER LOOK**

2.76

Look at the following terms. Now look up each term in the dictionary. You will find that they are similar in spelling but different in meaning and use. Write the definitions below.

eryth/ema _____

erythr/emia _____

erythr/o/derma _____

From the word parts you have learned so far, see if you can analyze them without looking up the answers. Which one

is a blood condition? _____;

is a skin condition? _____.

erythr/emia
er ə **thrē'** mē ə

erythr/o/derma
er ə thrō **dûr'** mə

2.77

A condition of "red" blood caused by the production of too many red cells is called erythr/emia (syn. polycythemia). If a person has a persistent high erythrocyte count (erythr/o/cyt/osis), they may be diagnosed with _____/_____.

erythr/emia

2.78

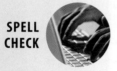

**SPELL
CHECK**

Erythr/emia is different from erythr/o/derma because erythremia is a condition of too many red blood cells and erythroderma is a condition of skin that is red. Just to add to the confusion, let us consider the term eryth/ema (adj. eryth/ema/tous) meaning reddened skin. All three of these conditions include the word roots **eryth** or **erythr,** which indicate the color red. Watch the spelling **e-r-y-t-h-r.** In Greek-based words it is common to use the "y" like an "i."

2.79

green	**chlor/o**	means _____.
yellow	**xanth/o**	means _____.
red	**erythr/o**	means _____.
white	**leuk/o**	means _____.
black	**melan/o**	means _____.

2.80

Cyanoderma sometimes occurs when children swim too long in cold water. A person who has a bluish discoloration of the skin is described as having _____/_____/_____.

cyan/o/derma
sī' ə nō **dûr'** mə
or dermat/o/cyanosis

2.81

leuk/o means *white*. Pay attention to the "eu" spelling. There are many words in medicine that refer to white. To say something is white, use _____.

leuk/o or leuk

ANSWER COLUMN

2.82

white skin, abnormally
white skin, lack of
pigment of the skin,
vitiligo

Leuk/o/derma means* _____

_____

2.83

A disease in which people have patchy white areas on their skin is called
vitiligo (vit i **lī'** gō). Sometimes these white areas are also called

leuk/o/derma

_____/_____/_____.

2.84

**SPELL
CHECK**

You may notice that some medical terms are particularly unusual and difficult to
spell correctly. From time to time in this program you will be given a Spell Check
frame which includes spelling hints that may be of assistance. Notice the unusual
diphthong (two vowels together) in the combining form **leuk/o**. The "eu" is
pronounced like a long "u" sound, but do not forget the e first, even though it is
silent. The correct spelling is l-e-u-k-o, as in leukocyte and leukoderma.

2.85

**WORD
ORIGINS**

As a general rule in Greek origin medical words, when two vowels are together,
the second vowel's long sound is used, as in these examples:
ea says ā;
ae says ē;
ie says ē;
ei says ī.

2.86

cyt/o

cyt/o refers to cells. A cell is the smallest structural unit of all living things. To refer
to this smallest part of the body, the combining form _____/_____ is used.

2.87

cyt/o

cells

Cytology is the study of cells. The part of cyt/o/logy that means cells

is _____/_____.

A cyt/o/lo/gist studies _____.

2.88

cyt/o/logy

-logy is a suffix that means the study of. Build a word that means the study of

cells. _____/_____/_____

2.89

path/o/logy *or*
path **ol'** ō gē
eti/o/logy
e tē **ol'** ō jē

Cyt/o/logists study the cause of diseases of the cell, like leukemia. The study of

the cause of disease is _____/_____/_____.

CASE STUDY INVESTIGATION (CSI)

Spleen

Pathology Report: Gross examination of a spleen

An entire spleen, weighing 127 grams and measuring 13.0 × 4.1 × 9.2 **cm**. The **external** surface is smooth, leathery, **homogeneous**, and dark purplish-brown. There are no defects in the capsule. The blood vessels of the hilum of the spleen are **patent**, with no **thrombi** or other **abnormalities**. The hilar soft tissues contain a single, **ovoid**, 1.2-cm lymph node with a dark grey cut surface and no focal **lesions**.

Source: By Edward O. Uthman, MD. (uthman@neosoft.com). Diplomate, American Board of Pathology.

CSI Vocabulary Challenge

cm _____

external _____

homogeneous _____

patent _____

thrombi _____

abnormalities _____

ovoid _____

lesions _____

ANSWER COLUMN

2.90

cyt/o/meter
sīt om' et er
cyt/o/metry
sīt om' et rē

-meter is a suffix meaning an instrument used to measure or count something. The instrument used to count cells is called a _____/_____.
-metry is a suffix meaning the process of measuring or counting something. The process of counting cells is called _____/_____/_____.

2.91

instrument

process

The word cyt/o/meter refers to the _____ used to measure or count.
The word cyt/o/metry refers to the _____ of measuring or counting.

2.92

cyt/o/techn/o/logist
sī tō tek **nol** ō jist

A technician that prepares and screens slides is

a _____/_____/_____/_____/_____.

ANSWER COLUMN

cell
sel

2.93

Of the several types of cells in blood, one is a leuk/o/cyte (refer to illustration). A leukocyte is a white blood _____ (WBC).

leuk/o/cyte
lōō′ kō sīt

2.94

When physicians want to know how many leukocytes there are, they ask for a _____/_____/_____ count.

leuk/o/cyte

2.95

There are several kinds of leukocytes in the blood. When physicians want to know how many of each type of leukocyte, they ask for a differential _____/_____/_____ count.

NOTE: Be aware there are many English words with acceptable alternative spellings used in different English-speaking countries. If you see an unusual spelling, look it up in your dictionary for verification. You may be surprised that it is correct. An example is the term "leukocyte." It may also be spelled "leucocyte."

leuk/o/cyt/o/penia
lōō′ kō sī′ tō pē′ nē ə

2.96

-penia is the Greek word (suffix) for poverty. The word that means decrease in or not enough white blood cells is

_____/_____/_____/_____/_____.

PROFESSIONAL PROFILE

Cytotechnologists prepare and screen tissue (cell) slides to detect abnormalities. They may issue results on normal tissues and work with pathologists to conclude final analysis of abnormal findings. A baccalaureate degree and clinical training will qualify the individual to take the Board of Registry of the American Society of Clinical Pathology (ASCP) certification exam to become a certified cytotechnologist, or CT (ASCP).

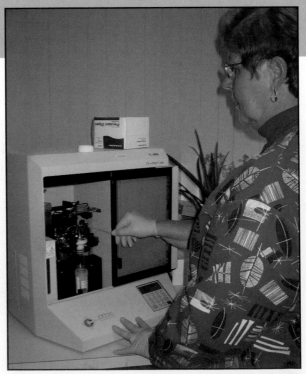

Delmar/Cengage Learning

ANSWER COLUMN

-penia

2.97

Leuk/o/cyt/o/penia (leukopenia) means a decrease in white blood cells. The part of the word that means decrease in is _____.

2.98

leukocytopenia

If the body does not produce enough white blood cells, the patient suffers from _____.

Blood cells (*leukocytes, erythrocytes, and thrombocytes*)
Delmar/Cengage Learning

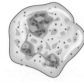

Erythrocytes (red blood cells)   Eosinophils   Neutrophils   Basophils

Leukocytes (white blood cells)

Monocytes   Small T   Small B   Plasma cell   Thrombocytes (Platelets)

Lymphocytes

Leukocytes (white blood cells)

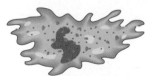

Wandering macrophage

Wright's stained blood smear *Delmar/Cengage Learning*

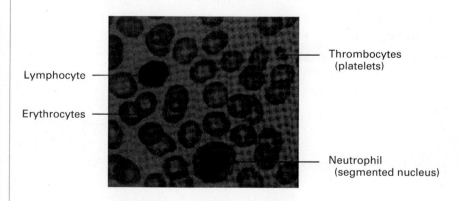

Lymphocyte

Erythrocytes

Thrombocytes (platelets)

Neutrophil (segmented nucleus)

ANSWER COLUMN

2.99

You have heard of leuk/emia, popularly called "blood cancer." **-ia** is a noun suffix meaning condition. **-em** comes from the Greek word *hema*, meaning blood. A noun meaning, literally, a condition of white blood is _____/_____.

leuk/emia
lōō **kē**′ mē ə

2.100

In leukemia the blood is not really white. A laboratory finding of this disease is the presence of too many immature white cells (leukocytes) in the blood. This finding was used to name the disease _____.

leukemia

2.101

Look at the table of values that follows. A WBC of 25,000 would be abnormally high. **-osis** may be used to indicate an increase in numbers of blood cells. Build a word that means an increase in

white blood cells _____/_____/_____/_____;

leuk/o/cyt/osis
lōō′ kō sī **tō**′ sis
erythr/o/cyt/osis
e rith′ rō sī **tō**′ sis

red blood cells _____/_____/_____/_____.

Complete Blood Count (CBC) Specimen: Whole Blood	
Test	**Normal Average Values**
Hgb (Hb)—hemoglobin	12–16 grams/100 milliliters
Hct—hematocrit	36–48% formed elements
RBC—red blood cell count	4.2–6.2 million/mm^3
WBC—white blood cell count	5,000–10,000/mm^3
Platelet (thrombocyte) count	350,000–450,000/mm^3

Diff—white blood cell differential count—Wright's stained smear analysis based on 100 WBCs:

Neutrophil (bands): 3–5%	Neutrophil (segs): 54–62%
Lymphocytes: 25–33%	Monocytes: 3–7%
Eosinophils: 1–3%	Basophils: 0–1%

2.102

lymph/o, from the Latin word *lympha*, meaning water or liquid, is used to refer to lymph/atic system structures. A lymph/o/cyte is a type of WBC produced by the _____/_____ system.

lymph/atic
lim **fa**′ tik

2.103

Edema is a condition of fluid accumulation in the tissues causing swelling or puffiness. Poor circulation in the extremities caused by blockages in the lymphatic vessels may cause _____/_____.

lymph/edema
limf ə **dē**′ mə

ANSWER COLUMN

Lymphatic system
Delmar/Cengage Learning

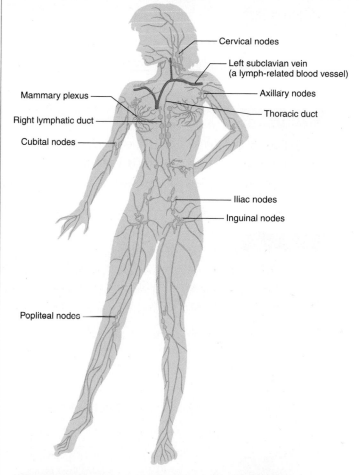

- Cervical nodes
- Left subclavian vein (a lymph-related blood vessel)
- Mammary plexus
- Axillary nodes
- Right lymphatic duct
- Thoracic duct
- Cubital nodes
- Iliac nodes
- Inguinal nodes
- Popliteal nodes

Cytometer—Automated instrument for analysis and counting blood cells
Delmar/Cengage Learning

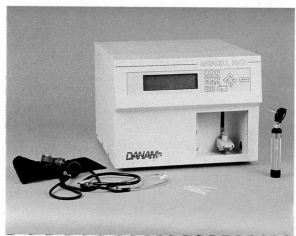

2.104

A type of leukocyte produced by the lymphatic system is

a _____/_____/_____.

lymph/o/cyte
lim' fō sīt

2.105

Acute lymphocytic leukemia (ALL) is a disease involving

the _____/_____/_____.

lymph/o/cytes

ANSWER COLUMN

2.106

erythr/o/cytes
e rith′ rō sīts

erythr/o means red. Cells that contain a red substance (hemoglobin) are called red blood cells (RBCs) or _____/_____/_____.

2.107

erythr/o/cyt/o/penia
e rith′ rō sīt′ ō **pē**′ nē ə

Look at the CBC values in the table on page 56. An RBC count of 2 million would be abnormally low. **-penia** is a suffix indicating deficiency in number. A patient who lacks red blood cells suffers from

_____/_____/_____/_____/_____.

2.108

thromb/o/cyt/o/penia
thromb′ ō sīt′ ō **pē**′ nē ə

Another type of blood cell is the thromb/o/cyte. Thrombocytes prevent excessive bleeding by allowing the blood to clot. An abnormal decrease in the number of these clot-forming cells

is _____/_____/_____/_____/_____.

2.109

thrombocytes

Blood-clotting cells (thrombocytes) are also called platelets. A platelet count would be done to obtain the number of _____.

2.110

thromb/o/cytes *or*
throm′ bō sīts
platelets
plāt′ lets

thromb/o means blood clot. A thromb/us is a blood clot. The blood cells that help form thromb/i are _____/_____/_____.

NOTE: Thrombus is singular, thrombi is plural.

2.111

thromb/o/cyt/osis
thromb′ ō sī **tō**′ sis

erythr/o/cyt/osis
e rith′ rō sī **tō**′ sis

-osis, used as a suffix with blood cells, indicates a condition characterized by increase in number. Build a term meaning increase in number of

platelets (thrombocytes) _____/_____/_____/_____;

red blood cells (erythrocytes) _____/_____/_____/_____.

2.112

blast/o

A blast/o/cyte is an embryonic or immature cell. The combining form for embryonic or immature is _____/_____.
Think of this…when you have a "blast," you may act immature!

ANSWER COLUMN

2.113

blast

A cell in its embryonic stage is called a _____.

2.114

cell
sel

-cyte may be used as a suffix to indicate a type of cell. A leuk/o/cyte is a term referring to a type of white blood _____.

2.115

immature or embryonic

-blast may be used at the end of a word to indicate an immature or embryonic cell. A hist/o/blast is a group of tissue cells that are * _____.

2.116

hist/o/blast
his′ tō blast
hist/o/logy
his **tol**′ ō jē
hist/ ō/logist
his **tol**′ ō jist
hist/ ō /cyte
his′ tō sīt

Hist/o means tissues. Build a word that means:

immature tissue _____/_____/_____;

the study of tissues _____/_____/_____;

one who studies tissues _____/_____/_____;

a tissue cell _____/_____/_____.

2.117

**DICTIONARY
EXERCISE**

Remember, your best friend is your medical dictionary. Look up the new terms you have learned for in-depth definitions. Look up words that begin with **histo** and make a list.

2.118

megaly

In the word acr/o/megaly, the suffix for enlarged is _____.

2.119

megal/o

The combining form for enlarged is _____/_____.

2.120

enlarged heart or
enlargement of the heart

cardi/o is the combining form for words about the heart. Cardi/o/megaly is a noun that means * _____

_____.

2.121

megal/o/cardia
meg′ ə lō **kär**′ dē ə

Megal/o/cardia also means enlargement or overdevelopment of the heart. When something causes an increase in the size of the

heart, _____/_____/_____ exists.

ANSWER COLUMN

2.122

megal/o/cardia *or*
meg' ə lō **kär**' dē ə

cardi/o/megaly
kär' dē ō **meg**' ə lē

Megalocardia refers to heart muscle. When any muscle exercises, it gets larger. If the heart muscle has to overexercise, _____/_____/_____ will probably occur.

2.123

megalocardia

Cardiac enlargement (CE) may be caused by prolonged, severe asthma that can reduce the supply of oxygen to the body and make the heart work harder. Another word for CE is _____.

2.124

gastr

Megal/o/gastria means large or enlarged stomach. The word root for stomach is _____.

2.125

megal/o/gastria
meg' ə lō **gas**' trē ə

megal/o means large; **gastr**, from the Greek *gaster*, is the word root for stomach, and **-ia** is a noun suffix. Form a noun that means large or enlargement of the stomach: _____/_____/_____.

2.126

gastr/o/megaly
gas' trō **meg**' ə lē
megal/o/gastria
meg' ə lō **gas**' trē ə

Another word for enlargement of the stomach is gastr/o/megaly. When the stomach is so large that it crowds other organs, _____/_____/_____ or _____/_____/_____ exists.

2.127

gastromegaly

Enlargement of the stomach is called megalogastria or _____.

2.128

condition

-ia is a noun suffix for condition. When megalogastria occurs, an undesirable _____ exists.

STUDY WARE™ CONNECTION

Remember, after completing this unit, you can complete a crossword puzzle or other interactive game on your **StudyWARE™ CD-ROM** that will help you learn the content in this chapter.

ANSWER COLUMN

2.129

Mania is an English word that comes directly from the Greek word *mania*, which means madness. Many mental disorders are designated by compound words that end in this word, _____, meaning a condition of madness or excessive preoccupation.

mania
mā′ nē ə

2.130

Mania is a noun meaning a condition of madness characterized by rapid speech, hyperactivity, and irritability and is associated with bipolar disorder (manic-depressive). The suffix that tells you mania is a noun and shows a condition is _____.

The adjectival form of mania is _____/_____.

-ia
man/ic
man′ ik

2.131

DICTIONARY EXERCISE

Use your medical dictionary, thesaurus, or web browser to look up *mania* as a noun and **–mania** as a suffix. You may find it interesting and surprising just how many different "manias" there are. List a few here with their meanings.

_____

_____

_____

_____

2.132

Megal/o/mania is a symptom of a mental disorder in which the patient has delusions of grandeur. Patients who have greatly enlarged opinions of themselves suffer from _____/_____/_____.

megal/o/mania
meg′ ə lō mā′ nē ə

2.133

People with megalomania are often treated in mental health centers. Many such centers have a patient who claims to be a king or president. These patients are diagnosed with _____.

megalomania

2.134

Many people think Adolf Hitler suffered from delusions of grandeur or _____.

megalomania

2.135

Megal/o/cardia means * _____.

cardi is the word root for _____.

enlargement of the heart
heart

ANSWER COLUMN

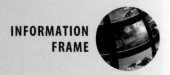

**INFORMATION
FRAME**

2.136

Recall that **-ic** and **-ac** are adjective suffixes that mean pertaining to.
The following are adjectival forms of the words you have just learned:

leukemic	leukocytic
dermic	cyanotic
manic	melanic
gastric	xanthemic
cardiac	erythroblastic

For review use the material in the following chart to work the next frame.

> **Words Are Formed By**

I. Word root + suffix
   (a) dermat/itis
   (b) cyan/osis
   (c) duoden/al
II. Combining form + suffix
   (this can be a word itself)
   (a) acr/o/cyan/osis
   (b) leuk/o/cyte
III. Any number of combining forms + word root + suffix
   (a) leuk/o/cyt/o/pen/ia
   (b) electr/o/cardi/o/graphy

2.137

word root	In I(a), dermat is the * _____ ;
suffix	**-itis** is the _____ .
word root	In I(b), cyan is the * _____ ;
suffix	**-osis** is the _____ .
duoden	In I(c), the word root is _____ ;
-al	the suffix is _____ .
combining form	In II(a), **acr/o** is the * _____ ;
word root	cyan is the * _____ ;
suffix	**-osis** is the _____ .
combining form	In II(b), **leuk/o** is the * _____ ;
suffix	**-cyte** is the _____ .
combining form	In III(a), **leuk/o** is a * _____ ;
combining form	**cyt/o** is a * _____ ;
suffix	**-penia** is a _____ .
electr/o	In III(b), the first combining form is _____/_____ ;
cardi/o	the second combining form is _____/_____ ;
-graphy	the suffix is _____ .
	Good job!

ANSWER COLUMN

Take five minutes and study the list of abbreviations in the following table.

Abbreviation	Meaning
AAD	American Academy of Dermatology
ALL	acute lymphocytic leukemia
ARDMS	American Registry for Diagnostic Medical Sonography
ARRT	American Registry of Radiologic Technologists
ASRT	American Society of Radiologic Technologists
CABG	coronary artery bypass graft
CAT Scan	computed axial tomography
CBC	complete blood count
CCU	cardiac care unit (critical care unit)
CE	cardiac enlargement (cardiomegaly)
CT	Computed Tomography
cTnI and cTnT	Troponin I and Troponin T (serum cardiac proteins indicating myocardial injury)
Diff	differential white blood cell count
DMS	diagnostic medical sonography
ECG, EKG	electrocardiogram
ECHO	echocardiogram
FDG	fluorodeoxyglucose
GA	gastric analysis
GI	gastrointestinal
Hct	hematocrit
Hgb	hemoglobin
mm^3, cu mm	millimeter cubed, cubic millimeter
mmol/L	millimole per Liter
MRI	magnetic resonance imaging
ms	millisecond
PET	positron emission tomography
Ra	radium (element)
RBC	red blood cell (count)
RDCS	Registered Diagnostic Cardiac Sonographer
RDMS	Registered Diagnostic Medical Sonographer
RT	Registered Technologist
RT (MR)	Registered Technologist (Magnetic Resonance Imaging)
RT (N)	Registered Technologist (Nuclear Medicine)
RT (R)	Registered Technologist (Radiography)
RT (S)	Registered Technologist (Sonography)
RT (T)	Registered Technologist (Radiation Therapy)
RVT	Registered Vascular Technologist
SPECT	single photon emission computed tomography
WBC	white blood cell (count)
XR	x-ray

ANSWER COLUMN

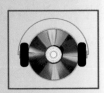

To complete your study of this unit, work the **Review Activities** on the following pages. Also, listen to the Audio CD that accompanies *Medical Terminology: A Programmed Systems Approach*, 10th edition, and practice your pronunciation.

STUDYWARE™ CONNECTION

To help you learn the content in this chapter, take a practice quiz or play an interactive game on your **StudyWARE™ CD-ROM**.

REVIEW ACTIVITIES

CIRCLE AND CORRECT

Circle the correct answer for each question. Then check your answers in Appendix E.

1. Combining form for extremities
   a. acr
   b. acro
   c. arc
   d. arco

2. Word root for stomach
   a. gastro
   b. gastric
   c. stomat
   d. gastr

3. Compound word
   a. duodenum
   b. microscope
   c. dermatitis
   d. subglossal

4. Suffix for incision
   a. -ex
   b. -de
   c. -tomy
   d. -ectomy

5. Suffix for enlarged
   a. -ex
   b. -sub
   c. -megaly
   d. -hyper

6. Noun for first part of the small intestine
   a. colon
   b. duodenal
   c. enteric
   d. duodenum

7. Verb for removed
   a. excision
   b. excised
   c. ectomy
   d. exeresis

8. Adjective for heart
   a. cardiac
   b. cardious
   c. cardium
   d. cranial

9. Suffix for condition
   a. -es
   b. -ia
   c. -itis
   d. -o

10. Pronunciation symbol for accent
    a. —
    b. ə
    c. ′
    d. ∧

11. Suffix meaning instrument used to cut slices
    a. -tome
    b. -tomy
    c. -meter
    d. -graph

12. Adjective for condition of blueness:
    a. cyanosis
    b. xanthotic
    c. cyanous
    d. cyanotic

13. Word root for x-ray
    a. tom
    b. graph
    c. echo
    d. radi

14. Suffix for making a new surgical opening
    a. -itis
    b. -ectomy
    c. -ostomy
    d. -tomy

15. Erythro means
    a. green
    b. red
    c. white
    d. blue

REVIEW ACTIVITIES

SELECT AND CONSTRUCT

Select the correct word parts (some may be used more than once) from the following list and construct medical terms that represent the given meaning.

-ac	acro	-al	-algia	-blast	cardi(o)
chlor	cyano	cyt(e)(o)	derm(a)o	dermato	duodeno
echo	ectomy	electro	-emia	-er	erythro
gastr/o(ia)	-gram	-graph	-graphy	-ia	-ic
-itis	leuko	-logy	mania	megal(o)(y)	melano
osis	-ostomy	paralysis	-pathy	penia	radio
sono	thrombo	tom(e)(o)	-tomy	um	xantho

1. excision of the stomach _____

2. make a new opening (connection) between the stomach and the duodenum _____

3. blueness of the skin _____

4. disease condition of the skin _____

5. red blood cell _____

6. embryonic dark pigmented cell _____

7. decrease in the number of platelets _____

8. enlargement of the stomach _____

9. overenlarged (delusional) opinion of self _____

10. instrument used to make a recording of heart activity _____

11. incision into the first part of the small intestine _____

12. adjectival form of the word for heart _____

13. the process of obtaining an image from reflected sound _____

14. the picture (record) of sound reflected through the heart _____

15. one who takes x-rays _____

16. increase in WBCs _____

17. enlarged extremities _____

18. x-ray picture made through slices of the body _____

19. condition of yellow skin _____

20. the study of cells _____

REVIEW ACTIVITIES

DEFINE AND DISSECT

Give a brief definition and dissect each listed term into its word parts in the space provided. Check your answers by referring to the frame listed in parentheses and to your medical dictionary. Then listen to the Audio CD to practice pronunciation.

Key: rt (word root), v (vowel)

1. duodenectomy (2.4)

                            _____/_____
                                  rt   suffix

    meaning _____

2. pathologist (2.59)

            _____/_____/_____
                 rt   v   suffix

_____

3. acrocyanosis (2.68)

     _____/_____/_____/_____
         rt   v   rt   suffix

_____

4. cyanotic (2.67)

            _____/_____/_____
                 rt   v   suffix

_____

5. dermatome (2.7)

            _____/_____/_____
                 rt   v   suffix

_____

6. erythroderma (2.69)

            _____/_____/_____
                 rt   v   suffix

_____

7. melanocyte (2.73)

            _____/_____/_____
                 rt   v   rt/suffix

_____

8. echocardiography (2.54)

   _____/_____/_____/_____/_____
       rt   v   rt   v   suffix

_____

9. leukocytopenia (2.96)

   _____/_____/_____/_____/_____
       rt   v   rt   v   suffix

_____

10. thrombocytes (2.110)

            _____/_____/_____
                 rt   v   suffix

_____

REVIEW ACTIVITIES

11. cardiomegaly (2.120)

_____/_____/_____
rt   v   suffix

_____

12. megalogastria (2.125)

_____/_____/_____
rt   v   rt/suffix

_____

13. electrocardiograph (2.48)

_____/_____/_____/_____/_____
rt   v   rt   v   suffix

_____

14. radiologist (2.57)

_____/_____/_____
rt   v   suffix

_____

15. gastrectomy (2.16)

_____/_____
rt   suffix

_____

16. gastroduodenostomy (2.12)

_____/_____/_____/_____/_____
rt   v   rt   v   suffix

_____

17. erythrocytosis (2.101)

_____/_____/_____/_____
rt   v   rt   suffix

_____

18. sonographer (2.52)

_____/_____/_____
rt   v   suffix

_____

19. radiographer (2.56)

_____/_____/_____
rt   v   suffix

_____

20. cytometer (2.90)

_____/_____/_____
rt   v   suffix

_____

21. erythremia (2.76)

_____/_____
rt   suffix

_____

22. cardialgia (2.40)

_____/_____
rt   suffix

_____

23. duodenotomy (2.17)

_____/_____/_____
rt   v   suffix

_____

REVIEW ACTIVITIES

24. tomography (2.37)

_____/_____/_____
rt   v   suffix

_____

25. cardiologist (2.44)

_____/_____/_____
rt   v   suffix

_____

26. inflammation (2.26)

_____/_____/_____
prefix   rt   suffix

_____

27. epidermis (2.72)

_____/_____/_____
prefix   rt   suffix

_____

28. hypodermis (2.72)

_____/_____/_____
prefix   rt   suffix

_____

29. echocardiography (2.54)

_____/_____/_____/_____/_____
rt   v   rt   v   suffix

_____

30. lymphedema (2.103)

_____/_____
word   word

_____

ABBREVIATION MATCHING

Match the following abbreviations with their definition.

_____ 1. ALL   a. registered technologist (radiographer)

_____ 2. EKG   b. cardiac care unit

_____ 3. CT   c. echocardiogram

_____ 4. CCU   d. computed tomography

_____ 5. DMS   e. cardiac telogram

_____ 6. GI   f. gastric contents

_____ 7. RT(R)   g. gastrointestinal

_____ 8. GA   h. diagnostic medical sonography

_____ 9. Ra   i. radium

_____ 10. ECHO   j. cardiac block catheter

                                   k. electrocardiogram

                                   l. acute lymphocytic leukemia

                             m. gastric analysis

REVIEW ACTIVITIES

ABBREVIATION FILL-IN

Complete the statements using only correct medical abbreviations.

11. A _____ blood test includes measuring hemoglobin and level of blood cells.

12. The hematocrit test measures the percentage of blood composed of _____.

13. The imaging modality that uses magnetic energy is an _____.

14. The _____ is a registered _____ technologist.

15. The cardiologist orders an _____ to assess electrical heart function.

16. A patient presenting with chest pain may be admitted to the _____.

17. Cardiac sonography is also called _____.

18. A severe acute form of leukemia is _____.

CASE STUDY

The following case study is taken from an actual patient record. This case and others throughout the text are presented to create contextual understanding of the use of medical terms. You may or may not have learned the key terms highlighted in the report. Write the correct term or abbreviation in the space provided next to its meaning given below. Use the text or your medical dictionary for assistance if needed.

CASE STUDY 2-1

Discharge Summary

DX: **acute** chest pain—**etiology** unknown

Mr. H is a 45-year-old male who is a heavy smoker and has a history of **hypertension**. He presented in the Emergency Department via ambulance with substernal pain on June 6. Mr. H was seen by Dr. C, the **cardiologist**, who ordered serial **EKG**s, an **ECHO**, and lab tests including a **CBC**, **cardiac** enzymes, **Troponins**, electrolytes, and a urinalysis. Dr. C's dictated consultation report is available in the record. The patient's vital signs were monitored and pain managed. The EKG and ECHO results were unremarkable. Lab tests were within normal limits except for slightly elevated **Triponins**. Mr. H was admitted to **CCU** on routine cardiac care orders, home meds, and continuous cardiac **telemetry**. Cardiac **angiography** was performed on June 7. The results showed only a slight blockage in one artery with no surgery recommended at this time. Mr. H became stable with rest and was discharged on June 10. A follow-up appointment is scheduled for June 14 with Dr. C.

1. severe and short term   _____

2. pertaining to the heart   _____

3. cardiac sonography   _____

4. electronic transmission of data   _____

5. complete blood count   _____

6. physician—heart specialist   _____

7. coronary care unit   _____

8. x-ray imaging of a vessel   _____

9. test for heart damage proteins   _____

10. high blood pressure   _____

REVIEW ACTIVITIES

CROSSWORD PUZZLE

Check your answers by going back through the frames or checking the solution in Appendix F.

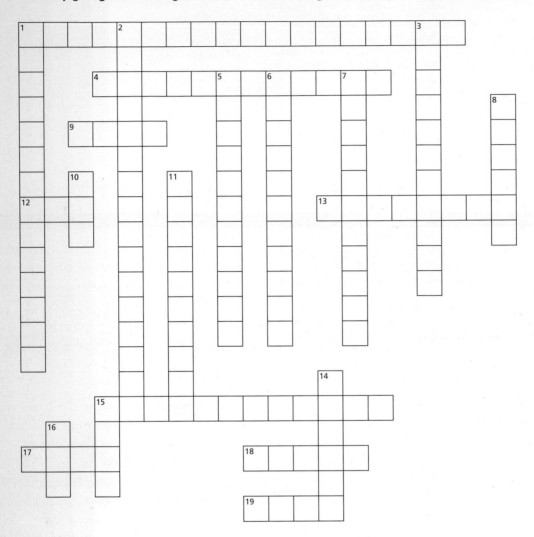

Across

1. instrument: makes an image (tracing) of heart activity (electrical)
4. red skin
9. suffix: incision into
12. complete blood count (abbr.)
13. image made using ultrasound
15. enlarged stomach
17. suffix: condition in the blood
18. combining form for tissue
19. _____cardiography

Down

1. increase number of red blood cells
2. low platelet count
3. physician specialist in study of disease
5. physician specialist in imaging (x-ray)
6. study of the skin
7. embryonic pigment cells
8. suffix: new surgical opening
10. cardiac care unit (abbr.)
11. technologist who studies cells
14. combining form for yellow
15. suffix: image or picture
16. diagnostic medical sonography (abbr.)

REVIEW ACTIVITIES

GLOSSARY

blastocyte	immature cell		etiology	the study of the origin of the cause of disease
cardialgia	heart pain		gastralgia	stomach pain
cardiologist	physician specialist in heart disease		gastrectomy	excision of the stomach
cardiomegaly	enlarged heart		gastric	pertaining to the stomach (adj.)
cyanoderma	blueness of the skin		gastroduodenostomy	making a new opening between the stomach and duodenum
cyanosis	condition of blueness			
cytologist	a technologist who studies cellular disease		gastromegaly	enlarged stomach
			gastrostomy	making a new opening in the stomach
cytology	the science of studying cells		histoblast	immature tissue cells
cytometer	instrument used to count cells		histology	the science of studying tissues
cytometry	process of using a cytometer		hypodermic	pertaining to below the dermis
dermatology	the science of studying the skin		inflamed	verb form for inflammation
dermatome	instrument used to cut slices of skin tissue		inflammation	tissue condition of redness, swelling, heat
duodenal	pertaining to the duodenum (adj.)		jaundice	yellow appearance due to high bilirubin level in the blood
duodenotomy	incision into the duodenum		leukemia	blood cancer involving leukocytes and bone marrow
duodenum	first part of the small intestine			
echocardiography	sonography of the heart		leukocyte	white blood cell
electrocardiogram	picture (tracing) representing the electrical activity of the heart during the cardiac cycle		leukocytopenia	low numbers of leukocytes
			leukocytosis	high numbers of leukocytes
			leukoderma	abnormally white skin (vitiligo)
electrocardiograph	instrument that produces the electrocardiogram		lymphatic	pertaining to the lymph system
electrocardiography	process of using the electrocardiograph		lymphedema	obstructed lymph vessels causing fluid buildup in tissues (swelling)
erythema	reddened skin (erythroderma)			
erythremia	abnormally red blood due to too many erythrocytes		lymphocyte	lymphatic system white blood cell
erythroblast	immature red blood cell		megalomania	abnormally enlarged self-image
erythrocytes	red blood cells		melanoblast	immature melanocyte
erythrocytopenia	low numbers of erythrocytes		melanocyte	pigment cell
erythrocytosis	high numbers of erythrocytes		melanoderma	dark patches of skin
erythroderma	redness of the skin			

REVIEW ACTIVITIES

pathologist	physician specialist in the study of disease
pathology	the science of studying disease
radiogram	x-ray picture (film) (radiograph)
radiograph	instrument used to produce the radiogram or the x-ray film
radiography	process of producing radiograms (radiographs)
radiologist	physician specialist in the interpretation of radiograms and other diagnostic imaging modalities
sonogram	image of the body produced by computerized reflected sound
sonograph	instrument that reflects sound waves through the body, picks them up with a transducer, and uses a computer to create an image of body structures

sonographer	technologist who performs sonography
sonography	process of using a sonograph (ultrasonography)
thrombocytes	platelets, blood-clotting cell fragments
thrombocytopenia	low numbers of thrombocytes
thrombocytosis	high numbers of thrombocytes
tomogram	picture made by a tomograph
tomograph	instrument that uses x-ray to produce images through planes (slices) of the body
tomography	the process of using a tomograph
xanthemia	yellow condition of the blood (carotenemia)

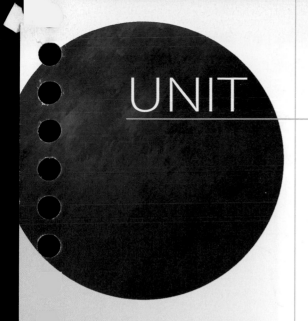

UNIT 3

Oncology and the Central Nervous System

3.1

INFORMATION
FRAME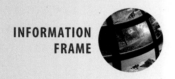

Cell, tissue, and organ growth, development, and repair are a part of a healthy functioning body. The following **specialties** are dedicated to the study of healthy and diseased tissues:
path/o/logy—study of disease
cyt/o/logy—study of cells
hist/o/logy—study of tissues
onc/o/logy—study of abnormal growths, tumors, and cancer

3.2

Cyt/o/log/ists study morph/o/logy or the structure of cells, becoming experts able to distinguish normal cell structures from diseased cell structures. This is important in the diagnosis of cancer.
The cell specialist is a

cyt/o/log/ist
sī **to'** lō jist

_____/_____/_____/_____.

3.3

tissue

The combining form that refers to tissue is **hist/o**. Hist/o/lysis is the destruction of _____.

3.4

tissue

A hist/o/genous substance is a substance that is made of _____.

ANSWER COLUMN

3.5

Build words meaning

the study of tissue

hist/o/logy
his **tol′** ə jē

_____/_____/_____;

one who studies tissues

hist/o/log/ist
his **tol′** əjist

_____/_____/_____/_____.

3.6

Build words meaning

an embryonic tissue (cell)

hist/o/blast
his′ tō blast

_____/_____/_____;

a tissue cell

hist/o/cyte
his′ tō sīt

_____/_____/_____;

resembling tissue

hist/oid
his′ toid

_____/_____.

3.7

morph/o is a combining form meaning form, shape, or structure.

morph/o/logy
môr **fo′** lō jē

The study of form or structure is _____/_____/_____.

3.8

WORD ORIGINS

Morpheus in Greek mythology was a god able to enter into a person's dreams. Once there, he would change into different forms and shapes of humans, thus influencing the dream experience.

3.9

Meta/morph/osis is a process of changing from one form into another. Normal cells that change their shape or form to become abnormal have undergone

meta/morph/osis
met ə **mor′** fə sis

_____/_____/_____.

NOTE: Think of the caterpillar changing into a butterfly.

3.10

DICTIONARY EXERCISE

-trophy, **-plasia**, and **–genesis** are all suffixes meaning development and growth. Each of these suffixes is used in a unique way and is not interchangeable when forming medical terms. Look up the following terms in your medical dictionary. Write the definitions below and compare.

(continued)

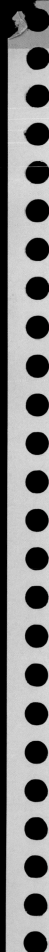

ANSWER COLUMN

hypertrophy _____

hyperplasia _____

hypergenesis _____

3.11

A prefix goes in front of a word to change its meaning. In the words hyper/trophy, hyper/emia, and hyper/emesis, **hyper-** changes the meaning of **-trophy**, **-emia**, and emesis. **hyper-** is a _____.

prefix

3.12

hyper- is a prefix that means above or more than normal. In common slang, someone who is overactive is hyper. To say that a person is overly critical, you would use the word _____/critic/al.

hyper-

Four types of tissue and their function
Delmar/Cengage Learning

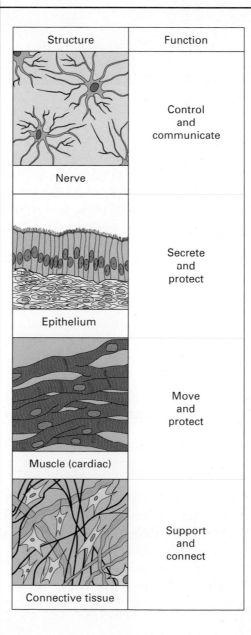

Structure	Function
Nerve	Control and communicate
Epithelium	Secrete and protect
Muscle (cardiac)	Move and protect
Connective tissue	Support and connect

Tissue specimen ready for examination by the pathologist *Photo by Timothy J. Dennerll, RT(R) Ph.D.*

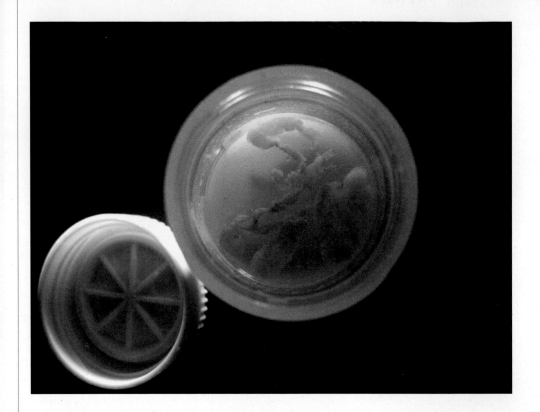

3.13

DICTIONARY EXERCISE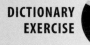

Our bodies do not work well when imbalanced by excesses. Look up the following conditions that are all caused by excesses. Write the substance or nature of the excess next to the term.

hypercholesterolemia _____

hypertoxicity _____

hyperkalemia _____

hyperactivity _____

hyperlipidemia _____

hyperproteinuria _____

3.14

hypo-

hypo- is a prefix that is just the opposite of **hyper-**. The prefix for below or less than normal is _____.

3.15

DICTIONARY EXERCISE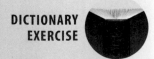

Below normal levels of substances, sizes, or activity may also produce critical imbalance. Use your dictionary to discover the nature of each condition and write your answer next to the term.

hypocalcemia _____

hypodactylia _____

hyposensitive _____

(continued)

ANSWER COLUMN

hypothermia _____

hypokalemia _____

hypothyroidism _____

hypodermic _____

3.16

Hypo/trophy (atrophy) means progressive degeneration. When an organ or tissue that has developed properly wastes away or decreases in size, it is

hypo/trophy *or*
hí **pot**′ rə fē
a/trophy
a trō fē

undergoing _____/_____.

3.17

Hyper/emesis gravidarum is a complication of pregnancy that can require hospitalization. The part of the disorder that tells you excessive vomiting occurs

hyper/emesis
hī pur **em**′ ə sis

is _____.

3.18

Gallbladder attacks can cause excessive vomiting. This, too, is

hyperemesis

called _____.

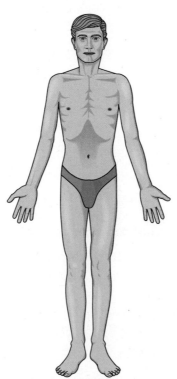

Hypotrophy

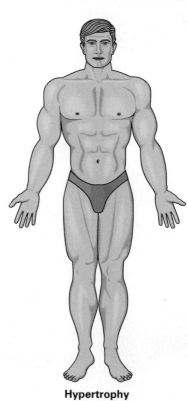

Hypertrophy

Delmar/Cengage Learning

Blood pressure is measured using a sphygmomanometer
Delmar/Cengage Learning

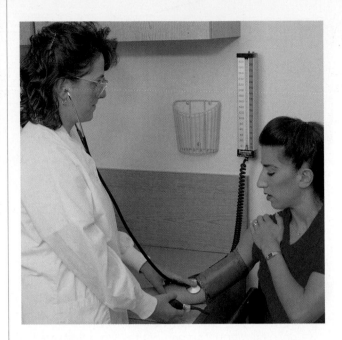

3.19

Hypertrophy means overdevelopment. **-trophy** comes from the Greek word *trophe*, for nourishment. See the connection between nourishment and development? Overdevelopment is called _____/_____.

hyper/trophy
hī **pûr'** trə fē

3.20

The liver, spleen, and heart may all become enlarged. If the heart overdevelops, the condition is _____ of the heart, also known as cardiomegaly.

hypertrophy

3.21

Abnormally high blood pressure (BP) is called _____/tension.

hyper

3.22

Essential hypertension (hī pûr **ten'** shən) and nonessential hypertension are both conditions of * _____.

high blood pressure

3.23

If hyper/tension is elevated BP, then hypo/tension indicates lowered BP. A blood pressure of 120/80 mmHg is a normal average. A BP of 90/50 mmHg may indicate _____/_____.

NOTE: mmHg means millimeters of mercury.

hypo/tension
hī pō **ten'** shun

3.24

Diuretic medications, which cause excretion of excess water, may be prescribed to lower the blood pressure in patients with _____.

hypertension

STUDY WARE™ CONNECTION

You can listen to the pronunciation of terms presented in this unit or play interactive games on your **StudyWARE™ CD-ROM** that will help you learn the content in this chapter.

ANSWER COLUMN

3.25

aden

aden/o

aden/o is used in words that refer to glands. The word root is _____.

The combining form is _____/_____.

3.26

aden/itis

ad ə nī′ tis

Build a word that means inflammation of a gland (word root + suffix rule):

_____/_____.

3.27

-ectomy

aden-

aden/ectomy

ad ə **nek′** tə mē

Aden/ectomy means excision or removal of a gland. The part that means excision

is _____. The part that means gland is _____. The word for

removal of a gland is _____/_____.

3.28

adenectomy

An adenectomy is a surgical procedure. If a gland is tumor/ous (full of tumors),

part or all of it can be excised. This operation is an _____.

3.29

aden/oma

ad ə **nō′** mə

A tumor is an abnormal growth of cells, also referred to as a neo/plasm

(new growth). **-oma** is the suffix for tumor. Form a word that means tumor of a

gland: _____/_____.

NOTE: Not all tumors are cancerous.

3.30

adenoma

Sometimes the thyroid gland develops an aden/oma. In this case, a patient's

history might read, " . . . hyperthyroidism noted—due to presence of a

thyroid _____ ".

3.31

adenoma

adenectomy

or thyroidectomy

thī roid **ek′** tō mē

When a thyroid _____ (tumor of a gland) is found, an

_____ (excision of gland) may be

performed.

ANSWER COLUMN

3.32

word root
vowel
aden/o/pathy
ad ə **nop'** ə thē

Recall **-pathy** is a suffix meaning disease. Aden/o/pathy means any disease of a gland. In this word you have a *_____ plus a _____ and suffix to form the word _____/_____/_____.

3.33

adenopathy

Adenopathy means glandular disease in general. When the diagnosis is made of a diseased gland but the disease is not specifically known or stated, the word used is _____.

3.34

Adenopathy
adenoma
adenectomy

_____ (glandular disease) could be diagnosed as an _____ (glandular tumor). If so, the surgeon may advise that an _____ (excision of a gland) be performed.

3.35

lymph/aden/o/pathy
limf ad' ə **nop'** ə thē

Recall **lymph/o** refers to lymphatic tissue. Any disease of the lymph glands could be called _____/_____/_____/_____.

3.36

adenitis
adenectomy

When a gland is found to have a mild _____ (inflammation), no _____ (surgery) is indicated.

3.37

tumor
tōō mer
fat

An adenoma is a glandular tumor. **-oma** is the suffix for _____.
A lip/oma is a tumor containing fat. **lip/o** is the combining form for _____.

3.38

lip/oma
lip ō' mə

A lip/oma is usually benign (noncancerous). A fatty tumor is called a _____/_____.

3.39

lymph/oma
lim fō' mə

A tumor composed of lymph tissue is called a _____/_____.

ANSWER COLUMN

Malignant melanoma
Courtesy of Robert A. Silverman, MD, Pediatric Dermatology, Georgetown University

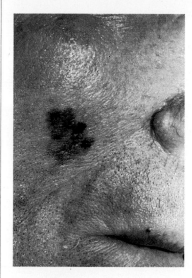

TAKE A CLOSER LOOK

lesion
lē′ zhun
ulcer
ul′ ser
tumor
too′ mer

3.40

Lesion, ulcer, tumor, and growth. We often hear these terms used, but are they the same? How do we know when and how to use them?
A **lesion** may be one of many possible types of abnormal tissue conditions including macules, vesicles, papules, ulcers, abscesses, and tumors, just to name a few.
Ulcers are a more specific type of lesion. They are open sores on the skin or mucous membranes.
A **tumor** is an abnormal growth in numbers and/or types of cells and may be cancerous.
The term "**growth**" is a common term that is nonspecific and used less often in formal diagnosis. Look up these terms in your dictionary and you will find several pages of interesting information.

3.41

cancerous tumor or
malignant tumor

carcin/o, from the Greek word *carcinos*, meaning crab, is the combining form for cancer (CA). A carcin/oma is a * _____.

3.42

carcinoma

A carcin/oma may occur in almost any part of the body and is composed of abnormal epithelial tissue. A stomach cancer is called gastric _____.

3.43

SPELL CHECK
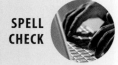

Make sure you use and say the correct form:

metastasis	singular noun	me **ta′** sta sis
metastases	plural noun	me **ta′** sta sēs
metastatic	adjective	me ta **sta′** tik
metastasize(d)	verb	me **ta′** sta sīzd

ANSWER COLUMN

3.44

Meta/stasis is the transfer of a disease from one organ to another not connected to it. Carcinoma may meta/stasize (spread to other parts of the body) through the lymphatic system. The intestine has a rich blood supply. For this reason,

carcin/oma
kär sin ō′ mə

intestinal _____/_____ is extremely dangerous, as it may metastasize to the liver.

NOTE: **meta-** means beyond and **-stasis** means in one place (staying). Metastasis (met., metas., mets.) means spreading beyond the original place.

3.45

A carcinoma may spread to another body part. The portion that grows in a new

meta/stasis
me **ta′** sta sis

location is called a _____/_____.

3.46

Carcinoma may be confined to the site (from the Latin *situs*; think of *situ*ation) of

carcinoma

its origin. In this case, it is called _____ in situ.

3.47

Form a word that means cancer of glandular

aden/o/carcin/oma
ad′ ə nō kär sin ō′ mə

tissue: _____/_____/_____.

3.48

Carcinoma indicates the cancer originated from epithelial tissue. When cancer of connective tissue is found, it is called sarc/oma. Bone cancer

sarc/oma
sär **kō′** mə
sarcoma

is a type of _____/_____. Cancer of bone tissue is

oste/o/ _____.

3.49

From what you have just learned, draw a conclusion about this. Kaposi's sarcoma is a condition many people with acquired immunodeficiency syndrome (AIDS) develop. Sarcoma indicates this is a cancerous condition of

connective

_____ tissue.

3.50

black

melan/oma
mel ə **nō′** mə

melan/o means _____. Melan/osis means black pigmentation. A word

that means black tumor is _____/_____.

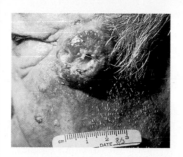

CASE STUDY INVESTIGATION (CSI)

Malignant Melanoma

Miss M, a 36-year old-woman with a history of seasonal tanning, was referred by her family physician for a raised **lesion** on the upper right shoulder. She stated that the pale brown to light gray color of the lesion had changed, grown, and was irritating. Upon examination, the **dermatologist** reported the lesion was a rough and coarsely granular oval lesion with an irregular border, measuring 2.0 cm × 1.0 **cm**. Clinically, this lesion was thought to resemble an irritated **seborrheic keratosis** and was biopsied. The **pathologist** reported examination of the deep shave **biopsy** showed the silhouette of a seborrheic keratosis but was confirmed as a **malignant melanoma**, Clark's level III, Breslow 1.34 **mm**. Routine complete surgical excision of the legion was performed with re-excision of border tissue. **Histological** exam reported no malignant melanoma. At the one year follow-up exam the patient shows no evidence of **metastasis**.

CSI Vocabulary Challenge

Use a medical dictionary to analyze the term or abbreviation listed from the case study. Divide the term into word parts by drawing in the slashes. Then, write the definition in the space provided.

lesion   _____

dermatologist   _____

cm   _____

seborrheic keratosis   _____

pathologist   _____

biopsy   _____

malignant melanoma   _____

mm   _____

histological   _____

metastasis   _____

TUMOR TERMINOLOGY

Combining Form	Meaning	Tumor
Epithelial Tissue		
Benign		
aden/o	gland	adenoma
melan/o	dark pigmented	melanoma
papill/o	small elevation of tissue	papilloma
fibr/o	fibrous tissue	fibroadenoma
Malignant		
aden/o	gland, glandular tissue	adenocarcinoma
melan/o	dark pigmented	melanocarcinoma (malignant melanoma)
carcin/o	squamous cell (skin)	squamous cell carcinoma
carcin/o	basal cell (skin)	basal cell carcinoma
Connective-Hematopoietic-Nerve Tissue		
Benign		
oste/o	bone	osteoma
chondr/o	cartilage	chondroma
leiomy/o	smooth muscle	leiomyoma
lip/o	fat	lipoma
ather/o	fatty, porridgelike	atheroma
hem/angi/o	blood vessel	hemangioma
neur/o	nerve	neuroma
Malignant		
oste/o	bone	osteosarcoma
chondr/o	cartilage	chondrosarcoma
leiomy/o	smooth muscle	leiomyosarcoma
lip/o	fat	liposarcoma
angi/o	vessel	angiosarcoma
leuk/o	white	leukemia
myel/o	bone marrow	myeloma
lymph/o	lymphatic	lymphosarcoma
neur/o	nerve	neurosarcoma

3.51

Melan/in is the pigment that gives dark color to the hair, skin, and choroid (dark pigmented area) of the eye. A black pigmented cell is

a _____/_____/_____.

melan/o/cyte
mel′ ə nō sı̄t
mə **lan′** ə sı̄t

3.52

Melanoderma means * _____.

black or dark skin
coloring (pigmentation)
(literally, black skin)

ANSWER COLUMN

Kaposi's sarcoma
Courtesy of Robert A. Silverman, MD, Pediatric Dermatology, Georgetown University

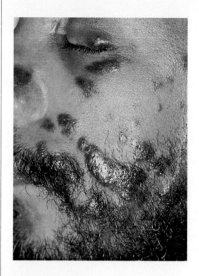

3.53

You have already learned that a carcin/oma is a form of cancer. A darkly pigmented cancer is _____/_____/_____/_____.

melan/o/carcin/oma
mel′ ə nō kär si **nō**′ mə

3.54

When a dark hairless mole on the skin grows or changes, a physician should be consulted for there is the possibility of black-mole cancer or _____.

melanocarcinoma

3.55

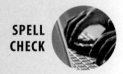

SPELL CHECK

Recall from the word-building section in Unit 1 that medical words often have special suffixes for plural formation. Words that end in **-oma** form a plural by using **-mata** as the suffix. In the list below, the first plural is done for you; *you* form the rest.

Plural Formation

Singular	Plural
carcinoma	carcinomata
lipoma	_____
sarcoma	_____
atheroma	_____
adenoma	_____
melanoma	_____

lipomata
sarcomata
atheromata
adenomata
melanomata

NOTE: Although these plural forms are proper medical terminology, you will see (and hear dictated) carcinomas, lipomas, melanomas, and so on. These have become accepted forms in many places.

3.56

onc/o from the Greek word *oncos,* meaning mass, is a combining form meaning tumor. The study of tumors is onc/o/logy. A specialist who studies tumors is called an _____/_____/_____.

onc/o/logist
on **kol**′ ō jist

ANSWER COLUMN

3.57

onc/o/logy
on **kol'** ō jē

A hospitalized patient with a disease caused by a malignant tumor might be

treated in the _____/_____/_____ unit.

3.58

lip/o

The combining form for fat is _____/_____. **-oid** is a suffix that

means like or resembling. Build a word that means fatlike or resembling

lip/oid
lip' oid

fat: _____/_____.

3.59

fat

The word lipoid is used in both chemistry and pathology. It describes a substance

that looks like fat, dissolves like fat, but is not _____. A word that

lipoid

means resembling fat is _____.

3.60

In proper amounts cholesterol is essential to health, but too much may cause

atherosclerosis (hardening of blood vessels due to fatty deposits). Cholesterol is

lipoid

an alcohol that resembles fat; therefore, it is _____.

3.61

ather/o is the combining form for fatty or porridgelike. A tumorlike thickening

and degeneration of the blood vessel walls that is caused by fatty deposits is

ather/oma
ather ō' me
ather/o/scler/osis
a' ther ō skler ō' sis

called an _____/_____. Hardening of vessel walls due to

fatty deposits is called

_____/_____/_____/_____.

NOTE: Ather/omata are different than lipo/mata. Atheromata are found in large

blood vessels and lipomata are found in body fat.

3.62

**SPELL
CHECK**

Watch out for these similar combining forms:
ather/o—porridgelike, fatty;
arteri/o—arteries;
arthr/o—joint.

3.63

neo- from the Greek *neos* means new. Neo/genesis means generation of

new

_____ tissue.

3.64

new

Neo/natal refers to the _____ born. A neo/plasm is a tumor or

new

_____ growth (formation—plasm/o).

ANSWER COLUMN

3.65

neo/natal
nē ō **nāt′** əl

A special unit for the newborn is the _____/_____ intensive care unit.

3.66

Neo/plasm refers to any kind of tumor or abnormal growth of cells.

neo/plasm
nē′ ō plaz əm

A nonmalignant tumor is called a benign _____/_____.

3.67

A neoplasm may be a malignant tumor. Carcinoma is a malignant

neoplasm

_____. A melanoma can be a malignant

neoplasm

_____. An onc/ologist is a physician who studies

neoplasms

_____ (plural).

3.68

neoplasm

A sarcoma is a malignant _____ of connective tissue.

neoplasm

Oste/o/sarcoma is a malignant _____ of the bone.

3.69

anti- is a prefix meaning against. **–plast/ic** is an adjective suffix for abnormal growth. A therapeutic agent that works against cancerous neoplasms is called

anti/neo/plastic
an′ ti nē ō **plas′** tik

an _____/_____/_____ agent.

-genesis refers to development. An agent that inhibits the development

anti/tumor/i/genic
an′ ti tōō/môr ə **jen′** ik

of tumors is an _____/_____/_____/_____ _____ (adjective) agent.

The process of inhibiting development of a tumor

anti/tumor/i/genesis
an′ ti tōō/môr ə **jen′** ə sis

is _____/_____/_____/_____ (noun).

3.70

About half of the patients with cancer are treated with radi/o/therapy as a primary treatment or in combination with chem/o/therapy and surgery. Radi/o/therap/eutics have been improved through careful planning and precision techniques used in the administering of ionizing radiation. Whether it is an internal or external application, use of radiation for cancer treatment is

radi/o/therapy
rā dē ō **thair′** ə pē

called _____/_____/_____.

3.71

If anti/neo/plastic chemical or drug agents are used for cancer treatment, this is

chem/o/therapy
kē mō **thair′** ə pē

called _____/_____/_____.

PROFESSIONAL PROFILE

Medical technologists (MTs [ASCP]), medical laboratory technicians (MLTs), and **certified laboratory assistants (CLAs)** physically and chemically analyze and culture urine, blood, and other body fluids and tissues to determine the presence of all types of diseases. They work closely with physician specialists such as oncologists, pathologists, and hematologists. Knowledge of specimen collection, anatomy and physiology, biochemistry, laboratory equipment, asepsis, and quality control is essential. The American Society of Clinical Pathology (ASCP) is a professional organization that oversees credentialing and education in the medical laboratory professions.

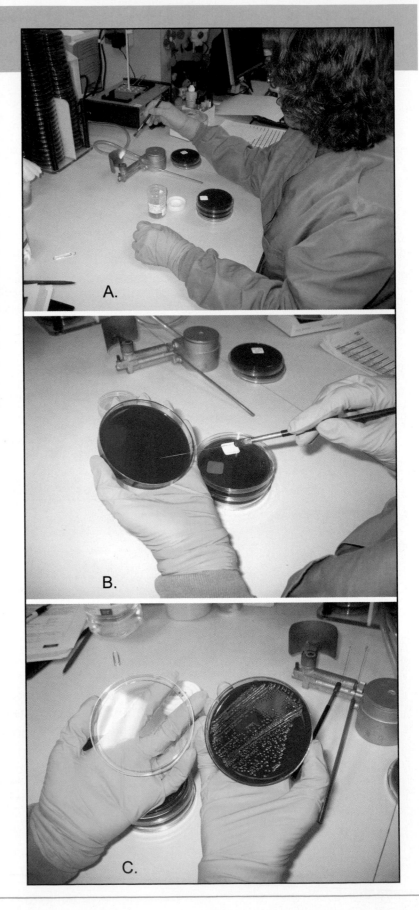

A.

B.

C.

Microbiologist frame sterilizing culture plating loop (A). Plating urine culture on a blood agar plate (B). Bacterial colonies grown from urine culture (C).
Photos by Timothy J. Dennerll, RT(R), Ph.D., courtesy of Allegiance Health, Jackson, MI

ANSWER COLUMN

3.72

From what you have just learned list three treatments for cancer.

surgery

chemotherapy

radiotherapy

_____

_____

_____

Good job!

3.73

Muc/oid means resembling mucus. **-oid** is a suffix meaning

like or resembling

muc

muc/o

* _____. The word root for mucus is

_____ and its combining form is _____/_____.

CASE STUDY INVESTIGATION (CSI)

Ovarian Cancer

Mrs. P, a 32-year-old woman, is diagnosed with small cell **carcinoma** of the ovary, FIGO III C. **Diagnosis** occurred during a Cesarean section. A complete total abdominal **hysterectomy** and **lymphadenectomy** was performed. The **histology** exam reported that she had **lymphatic metastasis** in 20 of 70 removed pelvic and para-aortic lymph nodes. She was treated with three cycles of **chemotherapy** followed by whole abdomen **radiotherapy (RT)**. Mrs. P is an unusually successful long-term survivor of five years.

CSI Vocabulary Challenge

Use a medical dictionary to analyze the term or abbreviation listed from the case study. Divide the terms into word parts by drawing in the slashes. Then, write the definition in the space provided. Write the meaning of the abbreviation.

diagnosis _____

carcinoma _____

hysterectomy _____

lymphadenectomy _____

lymphatic _____

metastasis _____

chemotherapy _____

radiotherapy _____

histology _____

RT _____

PROFESSIONAL PROFILE

Radiation therapists (RT[T]) are specialists in the administration of radiation therapy for the purpose of treating cancer. They begin their careers as registered radiographic technologists (RT[R]), and through advanced study become certified to administer radiation treatments. They work closely with radiologists, who are physicians specialized in the use of radiation for diagnosis and treatment, as well as oncologists, who are experts in the diagnosis and treatment of tumor disorders. The department in which they work is called radiation oncology.

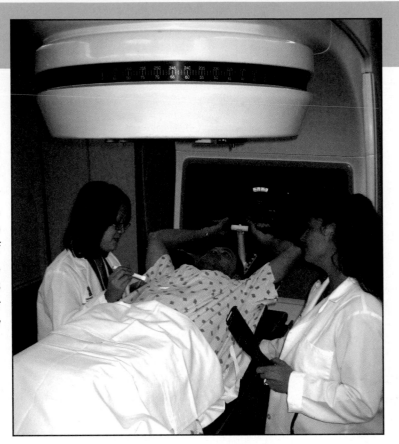

Two radiation therapists preparing patient for treatment
Photo by Timothy J. Dennerll, RT(R), Ph.D., courtesy of Allegiance Health, Jackson, MI

ANSWER COLUMN

Anterior view of ventral cavities
Delmar/Cengage Learning

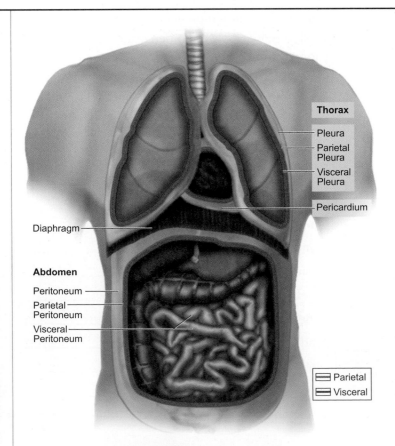

Thorax
- Pleura
- Parietal Pleura
- Visceral Pleura
- Pericardium

Diaphragm

Abdomen
- Peritoneum
- Parietal Peritoneum
- Visceral Peritoneum

Parietal
Visceral

ANSWER COLUMN

3.74

muc/oid
myoō koid

Mucoid is an adjective that means resembling or like mucus. There is a substance in connective tissue that resembles mucus. This is a _____/_____ substance.

3.75

muc/us
myoō kəs

Muc/us is a secretion of the muc/ous membrane. **-us** is a noun suffix. **-ous** is an adjectival suffix. The muc/ous membrane secretes _____/_____.

3.76

mucus

Mucus is secreted by cells in the nose. It traps dust and bacteria from the air. One of the body's protective devices is _____.

3.77

mucus
muc/ous
myoō′ kəs

The muc/ous membrane secretes _____. The tissue that secretes mucus is the _____/ _____ membrane or muc/osa.

3.78

mucus
mucous

The noun (the secretion) built from **muc/o** is _____. The adjective (pertaining to) built from **muc/o** is _____.

3.79

muc/osa
myoō **kō′** sə

The mucous membrane or mucosa is found lining the open body cavities. This protective, mucous membrane can also be called the _____/ _____.

NOTE: The digestive system is considered an open body cavity because it is essentially open from mouth to anus.

3.80

mucosa

The stomach lining is the gastric _____.

3.81

mucus
mucoid
mucosa or
mucous membrane

The mucosa secretes _____. Anything that resembles mucus is _____. Mucoid substances are not mucus; therefore, they are not secreted by the * _____.

ANSWER COLUMN

3.82

The serous membranes line the closed body cavities and cover the outside of organs such as the intestines. Serosa is the noun form. The intestinal

ser/osa
se **rō'** sə

_____/ _____ is a membrane that covers the intestine.

3.83

ser/ous
ser' us

The mucous membranes line the open body cavities and the _____/_____ (adjective) membranes line the closed cavities.

3.84

You can form words without even knowing their meaning. In the next three frames use what is needed from **encephal/o + -itis** to form a

encephal/itis

word: _____/ _____.

3.85

Use what is needed from **encephal/o**,
                          malac/o, and
                          -ia

encephal/o/malac/ia
en sef' ə lō mal **ā'** shə

_____/ _____/ _____/ _____.

3.86

Use what is needed from **encephal/o**,
                          mening/o, and
                          -itis

encephal/o/mening/itis
en sef' ə lō men' in **jī** tis

_____/ _____/ _____/ _____.

3.87

Use what is needed from **encephal/o**,
                          myel/o, and
                          -pathy

encephal/o/myel/o/pathy
en sef' ə lō mi' əl **op'** ə thē

_____/ _____/ _____/ _____/ _____.

3.88

At this stage of word building, learners sometimes find that they have one big pain in the head. The word for pain in the head is cephal/algia (often shortened

cephal

to cephalgia). The word root for head is _____.

3.89

-algia

One suffix for pain is _____.

ANSWER COLUMN

Structures of the head
Delmar/Cengage Learning

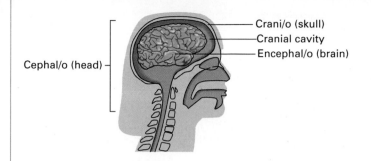

Cephal/o (head)

Crani/o (skull)
Cranial cavity
Encephal/o (brain)

3.90

cephal/algia
sef ə **lal'** jē ə

If you are suffering from cephal/algia, persevere, for later this gets to be fun. Any pain in the head may be called _____ / _____.

3.91

cephalalgia

The combining form for head is **cephal/o**. The word for pain in the head is _____.

3.92

cephal/o/dynia
sef ə lō **din'** ē ə
cephal/algia

Odyne is a Greek word for pain. Another word for pain in the head is cephal/o/ dynia. This word shows the combining form plus a suffix. If this seems a headache, relax. Either word, _____ / _____ / _____ or _____ / _____, will do for headache.

NOTE: Cephalgia is also correct spelling.

3.93

word root

combining form

Recall the suffixes **-algia** and **-dynia**. They are usually interchangeable.

When **-algia** is used as a suffix it is preceded by a (choose one) * _____ (combining form/word root). When **-dynia** is used, it is preceded by a (choose one) * _____ (combining form/word root).

3.94

cephal/o/dynic
sef ə lō **din'** ik

-dynia can take the adjectival form **-dynic**. An adjective that means pertaining to head pain is _____ / _____ / _____.

STUDYWARE™ CONNECTION

Remember, after completing this unit, you can play a concentration or other interactive game on your **StudyWARE™ CD-ROM** that will help you learn the content in this chapter.

ANSWER COLUMN

3.95

To say medically that headache (HA) discomfort exists, use the adjective

cephalodynic

_____ for headache.

3.96

cephalalgia
cephalodynia
cephalodynic

Two nouns for head pain are _____ and _____.
The adjective used for head pain is _____.

3.97

adjective

-ic

Cephal/ic means pertaining to or toward the head. Cephal/ic is a(n) _____
(noun/adjective). This is evident because cephalic ends in _____.

3.98

cephal/ic
sə **fal'** ik

Cephalic is an adjective. A case history reporting head cuts due to an accident
might read, "_____ / _____ lacerations present."

3.99

cephalic

In the phrase "lack of cephalic orientation," the adjective is _____.

3.100

encephal/itis
en sef' ə **lī'** tis

_In_side the head, _en_closed in bone, is the brain; **encephal/o** is used in
words pertaining to the brain. Build a word meaning inflammation of the
brain: _____ / _____.

3.101

-oma

encephal/oma
en sef ə **lō'** mə

The suffix for tumor is _____. Use what is necessary from encephal/o to
build a word for brain tumor: _____ / _____.

3.102

**WORD
ORIGIN**

The Greek word _kele_ means an abnormal protrusion, swelling, or a herniation.
Think of a keel on a sailboat. It is a protrusion from the bottom of the boat that is
used to stabilize and guide the boat. The suffix **–cele** originates from _kele_ and is
used in medical terms indicating herniation.

3.103

hernia/tion
her nē **ā'** shun

encephal/o/cele
en **sef'** əl ō sēl

Encephal/o/cele is a _____ of the brain. When brain tissue
protrudes through a cranial fissure (see illustration on p. 95), this is an

_____ / _____ / _____.

ANSWER COLUMN

Encephalocele
Delmar/Cengage Learning

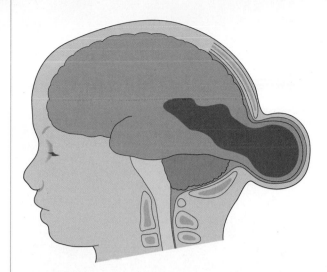

3.104

-cele

encephalocele

Any hernia is a projection of a part from its natural cavity. Herniation is indicated by the suffix _____. A projection of brain tissue from its natural cavity is an _____.

3.105

encephalocele

Brain herniation is sometimes a finding in hydrocephaly. This condition, in medical language, is called an _____.

3.106

softening of brain tissue

Malacia is a word meaning softening of a tissue. Encephal/o/malac/ia means

* _____.

3.107

encephal/o/tomy
en sef′ ə **lot′** ō mē

-tomy is used as a suffix for making an *incision* or temporary opening. An incision into the brain is an _____/ _____/ _____.

3.108

malac/o/tomy
mal ə **kot′** ə mé

Using what is necessary from malac/o with the suffix **-tomy**, form a word that means incision of soft areas: _____/ _____/ _____.

3.109

encephal/o/malac/ia
en sef′ ə lō mə **lā′** shə

Encephal/o/malac/ia ends in **-ia**, which is a suffix that forms a noun and indicates a condition. A noun meaning softening of brain tissue is

_____/ _____/ _____/ _____.

Sagittal section of the brain *Delmar/Cengage Learning*

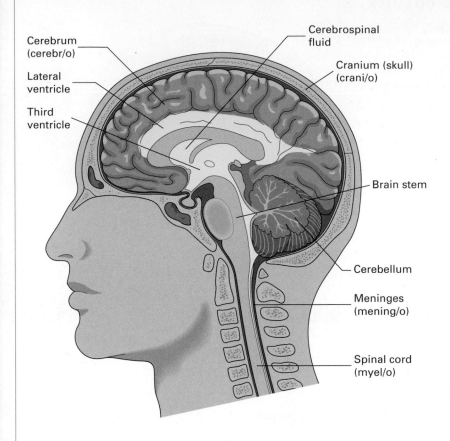

- Cerebrum (cerebr/o)
- Cerebrospinal fluid
- Cranium (skull) (crani/o)
- Lateral ventricle
- Third ventricle
- Brain stem
- Cerebellum
- Meninges (mening/o)
- Spinal cord (myel/o)

3.110

An accident causing brain injury could result in the softening of some brain tissue,

encephalomalacia

or _____ .

3.111

From your knowledge of word building, use **electr/o**, **encephal/o**, and **-gram** to build a term meaning picture of the electrical activity of the brain:

electr/o/encephal/o/gram
e lek′ trō en **sef′** ə lō gram

_____ / _____ / _____ / _____ / _____ (EEG).

3.112

The process of recording electrical brain activity is called

electr/o/encephal/o/graphy
e lek′ trō en sef ə **log′** ra fē

_____ / _____ / _____ / _____ / _____ .
The instrument used to record the EEG is

electr/o/encephal/o/graph
e lek′ trō en **sef′** ə lō graf

an _____ / _____ / _____ / _____ / _____ .

3.113

The study of brain wave activity, whether awake or asleep, is the work of physicians assisted by the

electr/o/neur/o/diagnos/tic
ē lek′ trō nōō′ rō dī əg
nos′ tik

_____ / _____ / _____ / _____ / _____ / _____
(END) technologist.

PROFESSIONAL PROFILE

Electroneurodiagnostic (END) technologists are allied health professionals who perform electroencephalography (EEG), evoked potentials (EP), polysomnography (PSG), nerve conduction studies (NCS), and electronystagmography (ENG). The END technologist works under the supervision of a physician who is responsible for interpretation and clinical correlation of the results. Individuals entering the END profession may be graduates of a Committee on Accreditation of Allied Health Education Programs (CAAHEP) accredited associate degree program and may take a national certification exam in electroneurodiagnostic technology developed by the American Board of Registration of EEG and EP Technologists.

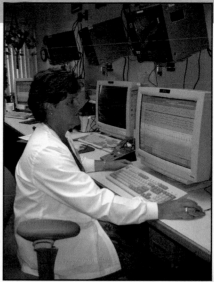

Photo by Timothy J. Dennerll, RT(R), Ph.D., courtesy of Allegiance Health, Jackson, MI

ANSWER COLUMN

3.114

surgical repair of
the skull or cranium

crani/o is used in words referring to the crani/um or skull. **-plasty** is the suffix for surgical repair. Crani/o/plasty means * _____

_____ .

3.115

The word for softening of the bones of the skull is

crani/o/malac/ia
krā′ nē ō mə **lā′** shə

_____ / _____ / _____ / _____ .

**Right lateral view
of the cranium**
Delmar/Cengage Learning

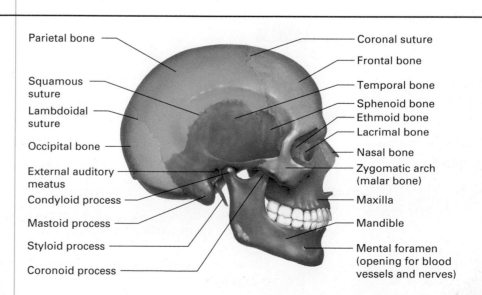

Parietal bone

Squamous
suture

Lambdoidal
suture

Occipital bone

External auditory
meatus

Condyloid process

Mastoid process

Styloid process

Coronoid process

Coronal suture

Frontal bone

Temporal bone

Sphenoid bone

Ethmoid bone

Lacrimal bone

Nasal bone

Zygomatic arch
(malar bone)

Maxilla

Mandible

Mental foramen
(opening for blood
vessels and nerves)

ANSWER COLUMN

3.116

The word meaning excision of part of the cranium is

crani/ectomy
krā′ nē **ek′** tə mē

_____/_____.

3.117

crani/o/tomy
krā nē **ot′** ə mē

The word for incision into the skull is _____/ _____/ _____.

3.118

-meter is the suffix for instrument used to measure. An instrument used to

crani/o/meter
krā′ nē **om′** ə tər

measure the cranium is the _____/ _____/ _____.

3.119

cranial

cranial

There are cranial bones. There are also _____ nerves. There are

grooves and furrows called _____ fissures.

3.120

adjectival

Crani/al is the (choose one) _____ (noun/adjectival) form of cranium.

3.121

cerebr/um
ser′ ə brəm, sə **rē′** brəm

Crani/o/cerebr/al refers to the skull and the cerebr/um. The cerebr/um is a part of

the brain. **Cerebr/o** is used to build words about the _____/ _____.

3.122

cerebrum

The cerebrum is the part of the brain in which thought occurs. When you think,

you are using your _____.

3.123

cerebrum

Feeling (sensation) is interpreted in the cerebrum. Motor (movement) impulses

also arise in the _____.

3.124

cerebrum

Thinking, feeling, and movement are controlled by the gray matter of

the _____. (Were you ever told to use your gray matter? This is why.)

3.125

cerebr/al
ser′ ə brəl, sə **rē′** brəl

The adjectival form of cerebrum is _____/ _____.

ANSWER COLUMN

3.126

cerebral

There is a cerebral reflex. There are cerebral fissures. You have probably heard of _____ hemorrhage (bleeding).

3.127

inflammation of
the cerebrum

Cerebr/itis means * _____

_____.

3.128

a cerebral tumor

A cerebr/oma is * _____.

3.129

cerebr/o/tomy
ser ə **brot'** ə mē

An incision into the cerebrum to drain an abscess is

a _____/ _____/ _____.

3.130

cerebrum (brain)

The vascular system refers to the blood vessels. A cerebr/o/vascular accident (CVA; stroke) occurs because a vascular lesion within the

_____ either blocks blood flow or causes a hemorrhage.

3.131

cerebr/o/vascul/ar
ser ē' brō **vas'** kū lär

People with hypertension are at high risk for a CVA or

_____/ _____/ _____/ _____ accident.

**Exterior left lateral
view of the brain**
Delmar/Cengage Learning

Cerebral cortex

Frontal lobe

Parietal lobe

Occipital lobe

Temporal lobe

Brain stem

Cerebellum

ANSWER COLUMN

3.132

Use what you have learned to analyze the following condition by writing its meaning in the blank.

high blood pressure

hyper/tensive * _____

vessels of the heart

cardi/o/vascul/ar * _____

abnormal function

dis/ease* _____

Abbreviation: HCVD

3.133

Cerebr/o/spin/al refers to the brain and spinal cord. There is fluid that bathes the

cerebr/o/spin/al

cerebrum and spinal cord. It is _____ / _____ / _____ /_____

ser ē′ brō **spī**′ nəl

fluid (CSF).

3.134

cerebrospinal

A spin/al puncture is sometimes done to remove _____ fluid.

3.135

cerebrospinal

There is even a disease called _____ meningitis.

3.136

Meninx is a Greek word for membrane. **mening/o** is the combining form for the meninges, a three-layered membrane that covers the brain and spinal cord. These three layers include the pia mater, arachnoid, and dura mater. The protective

mening/es

covering of the brain and spinal cord is the _____ / _____.

me **nin**′ jēz

3.137

mening/o/cele

A herniation of the meninges is a _____ / _____ / _____.

me **nin**′ gō sēl

3.138

meninges

A mening/o/cele is a herniation of the _____.

3.139

meninges

Mening/o/malac/ia means softening of

the _____.

3.140

Mening/itis can occur as cerebr/al meningitis, spin/al meningitis, or cerebr/o/

mening/itis

spin/al _____ / _____.

men in **ji**′ tis

ANSWER COLUMN

Meningocele and myelomeningocele
Delmar/Cengage Learning

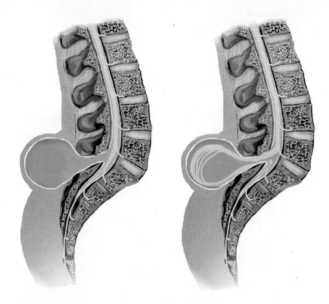

(A) Meningocele   **(B) Myelomeningocele**

3.141

meningitis

There are many kinds of meningitis. The tubercle bacillus can cause tuberculous meningitis. Mening/o/cocci are bacteria that cause epidemic _____.

3.142

When g is followed by e, i, y it is usually pronounced like a "j" (soft g) as in ginger. When g is followed by a, o, u it is pronounced like a hard "g" sound as in goat, gate, and gut. Practice saying: meningitis, meningocele j (soft g) (hard g).

Abbreviation	Meaning
AIDS	acquired immunodeficiency syndrome
ASCP	American Society of Clinical Pathology
BX, Bx	Biopsy
BCC	basal cell carcinoma
BP	blood pressure
Ca	calcium
CA	cancer
CIS	carcinoma in situ
CLA	certified laboratory assistant
CM, cm	centimeter
CP	cerebral palsy
CSF	cerebrospinal fluid
CV	cardiovascular
CVA	cerebrovascular accident (stroke)
EEG	electroencephalography, electroencephalogram
END	electroneurodiagnostic
ENG	electronystagmography
EP	evoked potential

(continued)

ANSWER COLUMN

Abbreviation	Meaning
HA	headache
HCVD	hypertensive cardiovascular disease
HTN	hypertension
MBD	minimal brain dysfunction
met., metas., mets.	metastasis/metastases
MLT	medical laboratory technician
mm	millimeter
mmHg	millimeters of mercury (pressure)
MT	medical technologist
NCS	nerve conduction studies
PSG	polysomnography
RT	radiotherapy
TIA	transient ischemic attack

3.143

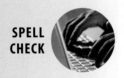

**SPELL
CHECK**

"**nx**" is not a typical consonant blend found in English words. It is typical of Greek terms like: pharynx, larynx, phalanx. Meninx is the singular form of the name of the membrane that surrounds the brain and spinal cord usually referred to as the meninges (plural). The combining form mening/o is used to build words about the

mening/es
men **in'** jez

_____ (plural) or the

meninx
men' inks

_____ (singular).

A myel/o/mening/o/cele is a herniation of the meninges and the

spinal cord

* _____.

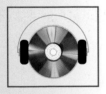

To complete your study of this unit, work the **Review Activities** on the following pages. Also, listen to the Audio CD that accompanies *Medical Terminology: A Programmed Systems Approach,* 10th edition, and practice your pronunciation.

STUDYWARE™ CONNECTION

To help you learn the content in this chapter, take a practice quiz or play an interactive game on your **StudyWARE™ CD-ROM.**

REVIEW ACTIVITIES

CIRCLE AND CORRECT

Circle the correct answer for each question. Then check your answers in Appendix E.

1. Word root for development
   a. troph
   b. tropic
   c. tome
   d. path

2. Combining form for gland
   a. glandul
   b. adreno
   c. adeno
   d. glando

3. Prefix for below or less than normal
   a. hyper-
   b. hypo-
   c. ology-
   d. en-

4. Suffix for disease condition
   a. -pathy
   b. -patho
   c. -tropho
   d. -ic

5. Combining form for cancer
   a. cancerous
   b. situ
   c. carcino
   d. neoplasm

6. Suffix for one who studies
   a. -logy
   b. -ist
   c. -logist
   d. -er

7. Suffix for instrument that records
   a. -phonogram
   b. -graph
   c. -gram
   d. -graphy

8. Word root for head
   a. myel
   b. cephal
   c. encephal
   d. crani

9. Suffix for herniation
   a. -itis
   b. -malacia
   c. -cytes
   d. -cele

10. Combining form for brain
    a. myelo
    b. encephalo
    c. cerebr
    d. meningo

11. The membrane surrounding the closed cavities
    a. mucosa
    b. dermal
    c. serosa
    d. meninges

12. Suffix for like or resembling
    a. -oid
    b. -oma
    c. -ous
    d. -ible

13. Combining form for skull
    a. cephal/o
    b. occipital
    c. crani/o
    d. oste/o

14. Word root for tumor
    a. oma
    b. onc
    c. sarc/o
    d. carcin

15. Suffix for pain
    a. -cele
    b. -oid
    c. -alic
    d. -dynia

16. Combining form for tissue
    a. cyt/o
    b. hyper
    c. neo
    d. hist/o

SELECT AND CONSTRUCT

Select the correct word parts from the following list and construct medical terms that represent the given meaning.

aden(o)	anti	blast	carcin(o)	cele
cephal(o)	cerebr(o)	crani(o)	cyte	ectomy
electr(o)	encephal(o)	epitheli(o)	genesis	graph
graphy	histo	hyper	hypo	itis
lip(o)	logist	logy	lymph(o)	malac(ia)
mening(o)	muc(o)	mucosa	neo	nat/al
oid	oma	onc(o)	pathy	plasm (plastic)
plasty	sarc(o)	spinal	tension	tomy
trophy				

REVIEW ACTIVITIES

1. herniation of the brain _____

2. instrument for recording brain function _____

3. surgical repair of the skull _____

4. brain and spinal cord (adjective) _____

5. malignant tumor of a gland _____

6. resembling mucus _____

7. fatty tumor _____

8. softening of the skull _____

9. incision into the cerebrum _____

10. inflammation of the meninges _____

11. one who studies tumors _____

12. connective tissue tumor _____

13. tumor involving lymph glands _____

14. overdevelopment _____

15. low blood pressure _____

16. specialist in study of tissues _____

17. new growths (tumors) _____

18. agent that works against tumors _____

19. immature tissue cell _____

20. pertaining to the newborn _____

TUMOR TERMINOLOGY MATCHING

Match the term on the left with the definition on the right.

_____ 1. lesion

_____ 2. malignant

_____ 3. sarcoma

_____ 4. carcinoma

_____ 5. morphology

_____ 6. chemotherapy

_____ 7. biopsy

_____ 8. radiotherapy

_____ 9. pathology

_____ 10. antitumorigenic

a. study of disease

b. treatment using chemicals or drugs

c. cancerous growth of epithelial tissue

d. study of form or development

e. excision of tissue for study

f. agent that prevents tumor growth

g. bad, worsening, may result in death

h. cancer of connective tissue origin

i. treatment using ionizing radiation

j. wound or tissue pathology

REVIEW ACTIVITIES

DEFINE AND DISSECT

Give a brief definition and dissect each listed term into its word parts in the space provided. Check your answers by referring to the frame listed in parentheses and to your medical dictionary. Then listen to the Audio CD to practice pronunciation.

1. encephalomalacia (3.85)

   _____/_____/_____/_____

   rt　　　　　　v　　　　rt　　　　　suffix

   meaning _____

2. hypotrophy (3.16)

   _____/_____

   pre　　　　　suffix

   _____

3. hyperemesis (3.17)

   _____/_____

   pre　　　　rt/suffix

   _____

4. adenectomy (3.27)

   _____/_____

   rt　　　　　suffix

   _____

5. hypertension (3.21)

   _____/_____

   pre　　　　rt/suffix

   _____

6. carcinoma (3.41)

   _____/_____

   rt　　　　　suffix

   _____

7. lipoid (3.58)

   _____/_____

   rt　　　　　suffix

   _____

8. oncology (3.57)

   _____/_____/_____

   rt　　　　v　　　　suffix

   _____

9. mucosa (3.79)

   _____/_____

   rt　　　　　suffix

   _____

10. cephalalgia (3.90)

    _____/_____

    rt　　　　　suffix

    _____

REVIEW ACTIVITIES

11. encephalocele (3.104)

_____/_____/_____
 rt   v   suffix

_____

12. electroencephalogram (3.111)

_____/_____/_____/_____/_____
 rt   v   rt   v   suffix

_____

13. craniomalacia (3.115)

_____/_____/_____
 rt   v   rt/suffix

_____

14. cerebrotomy (3.117)

_____/_____/_____
 rt   v   suffix

_____

15. meningitis (3.140)

_____/_____
 rt   suffix

_____

16. cerebrospinal (3.133)

_____/_____/_____/_____
 rt   v   rt   suffix

_____

17. histology (3.5)

_____/_____/_____
 pre   v   suffix

_____

18. atheroma (3.131)

_____/_____
 rt   suffix

_____

19. cerebrovascular (3.131)

_____/_____/_____/_____
 rt   v   rt   suffix

_____

20. metastasis (3.45)

_____/_____
 pre   suffix

_____

21. serous (3.83)

_____/_____
 rt   suffix

_____

REVIEW ACTIVITIES

22. craniometer (3.118)

_____/_____/_____
rt   v   suffix

_____

23. neoplasm (3.66)

_____/_____
pre   suffix

_____

24. electroneurodiagnostic (3.113)

_____/_____/_____/_____/_____/____
rt   v   rt   v   rt   suffix

_____

25. melanocarcinoma (3.53)

_____/_____/_____/_____
rt   v   rt   suffix

_____

26. morphology (3.7)

_____/_____/_____
rt   v   suffix

_____

27. chemotherapy (3.72)

_____/_____/_____/_____
rt   v   rt   suffix

_____

28. radiotherapeutics (3.70)

_____/_____/_____/_____
rt   v   rt   suffix

_____

29. hyperkalemia (3.13)

_____/_____/_____
pre   v   suffix

_____

30. osteosarcoma (3.48)

_____/_____/_____/_____
rt   v   rt   suffix

_____

31. atheromata (3.61)

_____/_____/_____
rt   v   suffix

_____

32. antineoplastic (3.69)

_____/_____/_____/_____
pre   rt   v   suffix

_____

REVIEW ACTIVITIES

IMAGE LABELING

Label the following structures of the head and neck by placing the number in front of the correct combining form below.

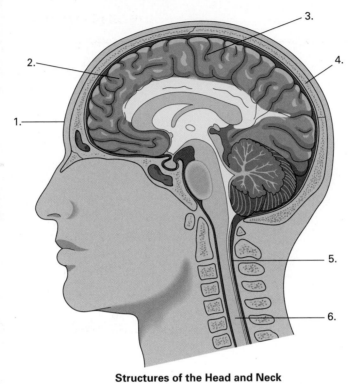

Structures of the Head and Neck
Delmar/Cengage Learning

Write the body part represented by

_____ myel/o   _____

_____ crani/o   _____

_____ mening/o   _____

_____ cerebr/o   _____

_____ encephal/o   _____

_____ cephal/o   _____

REVIEW ACTIVITIES

ABBREVIATION MATCHING

Match the following abbreviations with their definition.

_____ 1. RT

_____ 2. EEG

_____ 3. MBD

_____ 4. met., metas., mets.

_____ 5. TIA

_____ 6. CP

_____ 7. CSF

_____ 8. CIS

_____ 9. HA

_____ 10. CA

a. basal cell carcinoma

b. cancer

c. metastasis/metastases

d. radiotherapy

e. electrocardiogram

f. heart and chronic venereal disease

g. minimal brain dysfunction

h. cerebrospinal fluid

i. carcinoma in situ

j. myocardial infarction

k. cerebral palsy

l. electroencephalogram

m. headache

n. transient ischemia attack

ABBREVIATION FILL-IN

Fill in the blanks with the correct abbreviations.

11. The medical laboratory technician (_____) prepared the blood sample for testing.

12. Having blood pressure (_____) that is abnormally high (200/100 _____) and blood vessel disease is serious for the patient with _____.

13. The patient has experienced several episodes of blurred vision, dizziness, and fatigue brought on by a loss of blood flow to the brain. A _____ could be a precursor to a stroke or _____, which is followed by paralysis, loss of consciousness, and possibly death.

14. The biopsy indicated a basal cell carcinoma (_____).

REVIEW ACTIVITIES

CASE STUDY INVESTIGATION (CSI)

West Nile Virus

A 68-year-old woman had fever, **myalgia**, progressive weakness, and **respiratory** insufficiency. In 9 days, flaccid areflexic quadriparesis and bulbar palsy developed. She died 26 days after the onset of her illness. Serum and **cerebrospinal** fluid serology were positive for West Nile virus. **Neuropathological** study showed changes consistent with a viral encephalomyelitis similar to **polio-myelitis**. The brainstem showed neuronal loss and multiple foci of **necrosis**. The spinal cord showed severe loss of **anterior** and **posterior** horn neurons. **Immunohistochemistry** identified West Nile virus antigens in the brainstem and spinal cord. Paralysis in West Nile virus **encephalitis** is caused by destruction of motor **neurons**.

Author(s)

AGAMANOLIS Dimitri P.[1] ; LESLIE Michael J.[2] ; CAVENY Elizabeth A.[3] ; GUARNER Jeannette[4] ; SHIEH Wun-Ju[4] ; ZAKI Sherif R.[4] ;" Neuropathological findings in West Nile virus encephalitis: A case report" *Annals of Neurology* **ISSN** 0364-5134 **CODEN** ANNED3. 2003.

CSI Vocabulary Challenge

Analyze the following terms from the case study by drawing slashes to identify the word parts if possible. Use your medical dictionary to help you write out the definitions.

1. myalgia   _____

2. respiratory   _____

3. cerebrospinal   _____

4. neuropathological   _____

5. poliomyelitis   _____

6. necrosis   _____

7. anterior   _____

8. posterior   _____

9. encephalitis   _____

10. immunohistochemistry   _____

11. neurons   _____

REVIEW ACTIVITIES

CROSSWORD PUZZLE

Check your answers by going back through the frames or checking the solution in Appendix F.

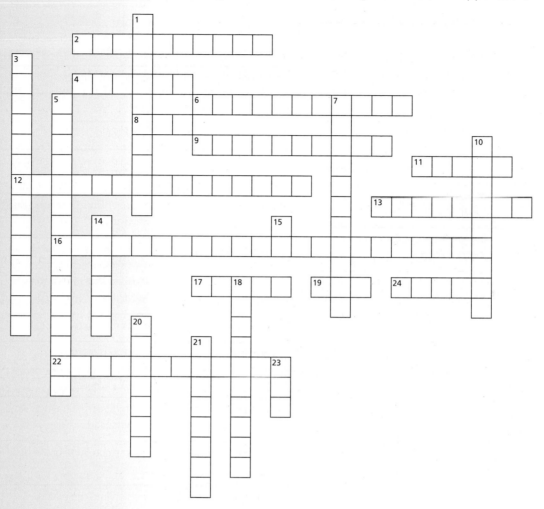

Across

2. remove a gland
4. usually benign fat tumor
6. hernia of the meninges
8. suffix for tumor
9. loss in structure size
11. suffix for instrument used to measure
12. hardening of a vessel caused by fat
13. tumor of melanocytes
16. process of producing EEG
17. watery substance produced by mucosa
19. carcinoma in situ (abbr.)
22. high blood pressure
24. a new growth is a neo_____.

Down

1. cancer specialist
3. glandular cancer
5. disease of lymph glands
7. synonym cephalodynia
10. muscle tissue tumor (fibroid)
14. membrane covering closed cavities (noun)
15. blood pressure (abbr.)
18. incision into the skull
20. connective tissue cancer
21. inside the head, brain (word root)
23. a newborn is a _____nate.

REVIEW ACTIVITIES

GLOSSARY

adenectomy	excision of a gland
adenitis	inflammation of a gland
adenoma	tumor of a gland or glandular tissue
adenopathy	disease condition of a gland or glandular tissue
antineoplastic	agent that works against tumor growth
antitumorigenic	agent that prevents tumor growth
atheroma pl. atheromata	fatty (porridgelike) tissue tumor found in blood vessels
atherosclerosis	hardening of blood vessels caused by fatty growths
biopsy	excision of live tissue for examination
carcinoma	cancer of epithelial tissue
cephalalgia	head pain (synonym for cephalodynia)
cephalic	pertaining to the head
cephalodynic	pertaining to head pain (adjective)
cerebral	pertaining to the cerebrum (adjective)
cerebritis	inflammation of the cerebrum
cerebroma	tumor of the cerebrum
cerebrospinal	pertaining to the cerebrum and spine
cerebrovascular	pertaining to the cerebrum and blood vessels
cerebrum	largest part of the brain includes the frontal, temporal, and occipital lobes
chemotherapy	treatment using chemicals or drugs
craniectomy	excision of part of the skull
craniomalacia	softening of the skull

craniometer	instrument used to measure the size of the skull
cranioplasty	surgical repair of the skull
craniotomy	incision into the skull
cranium	skull
cytologist	specialist in study of cells
cytotechnologist	specialized technician that tests cells
electroencephalogram	tracing (picture) showing brain wave activity
electroencephalograph	instrument used to turn brain waves into electrical patterns showing a picture of changes in activity
encephalitis	inflammation of the brain
encephalocele	herniation of brain tissue
encephalomalacia	softening of brain tissue
encephalomeningitis	inflammation of the brain and meninges
encephalomyelopathy	disease condition of the brain and spinal cord
encephalotomy	incision into the brain
electroneurodiagnostic	electrical diagnostic testing (imaging) of nervous system function
glandular	pertaining to a gland
herniation	abnormal protrusion of an organ or other body structure through a defect or natural opening
histoblast	immature tissue
histology	study of tissues
hyperemesis	excessive vomiting
hypertension	high blood pressure
hypertrophy	overdevelopment, increase in size
hypotension	low blood pressure

REVIEW ACTIVITIES

hypotrophy	underdevelopment, decrease in size	metastatic	pertaining to a metastasis or metastases
lesion	wound, injury, or pathologic tissue	morphology	study of form or development
lipoid	resembling fat	mucoid	resembles mucus
lipoma	fatty tissue tumor	mucosa	mucous membrane (noun)
lymphadenopathy	disease condition of the lymph glands	mucus	watery substance secreted by mucous membranes
lymphoma	lymph tissue tumor	neonatal	pertaining to newborn
malacotomy	incision into soft tissue	neoplasm	new growth (tumor)
malignant	bad, worsening, or leading to death	neurodiagnostic	pertaining to diagnostic studies performed to examine the nervous system by detecting electrical changes
melanocarcinoma	malignant (cancerous) melanoma		
melanocyte	dark pigmented cell (contains melanin)	oncologist	physician specialist in diseases involving tumors
melanoma	tumor involving growth of melanocytes	oncology	the science that studies tumors
meninges	three-layered membrane surrounding the brain and spinal cord	pathology	study of disease
		sarcoma	cancer of connective tissue
meningitis	inflammation of the meninges	serosa	serous membrane
meningocele	herniation of the meninges	tumor	abnormal growth of tissue
metastasis	tumor that spreads beyond its origin (noun) pl. metastases	ulcer	crater-like sore
metastasize	to spread beyond its origin (verb)	vascular	pertaining to vessels (i.e blood vessels)

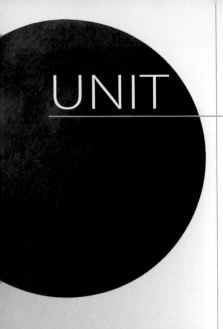

UNIT 4

Orthopedics, Osteopathy, and Body Regions

4.1

TAKE A CLOSER LOOK

Now that you are learning more complex terms, it is time to focus on some of the commonly mispronounced words. Begin with the suffixes **-scope** and **-scopy**. The suffix **-scope** is pronounced just as it looks (skōp) as in arthroscope (**är′** thrō skōp), endoscope (**en′** dō skōp).

But **-scopy** is not pronounced as it looks. The "o" from the combining form blends with the suffix and is a short "o" sound as in os′ trich or op′era. The accent is also placed on this vowel-suffix blend (**os′** kō pē) as in arthroscopy (arthr **os′** kō pē) and endoscopy (end **os′** kō pē).

Many other suffixes follow a similar pronunciation pattern.

Try the first few familiar terms and apply the pattern to the rest.

Suffix	Pronunciation	Example
o/graphy	**og′** ra fē	photography
o/meter	**om′** ə ter	thermometer
o/metry	**om′** ə trē	geometry
o/logy	**ol′** ə gē	biology
o/stomy	**os′** tō mē	colostomy
o/pathy	**op′** ə thē	dermatopathy
o/lysis	**ol′** ə sis	cytolysis
o/stasis	**os′** st ə sis	hemostasis
o/trophy	**ot′** trō fē	hypotrophy
o/clysis	**ok′** lə sis	rectoclysis
o/tomy	**ot′** ə mē	gastrotomy

Refer back to this list as you learn these suffixes.

ANSWER COLUMN

4.2

Osteon is a Greek word meaning bone. Oste/o/pathy means disease of the bones. From this word, identify the combining form for bone:

oste/o

_____/_____.

4.3

oste/itis
os tē ī' tis

A word meaning inflammation of the bone is _____/_____.

NOTE: The "e" in oste is part of the word root.

4.4

Oste/o/malac/ia means softening of the bones. To say that bones have lost a detectable amount of their hardness, use the noun

oste/o/malac/ia
os' tē ō mə **lā'** shə

_____/_____/_____/_____.

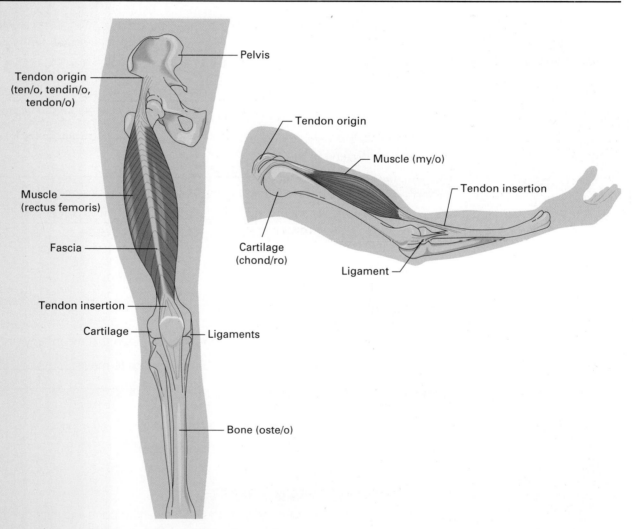

Connective tissue structures of the leg and arm *Delmar/Cengage Learning*

ANSWER COLUMN

4.5

The eti/o/logy of oste/o/malacia (adult rickets) includes vitamin D deficiency, phosphate deficiency, and abnormal excretion of calcium by the kidneys. A contributing factor is use of tobacco products. Whatever the cause, softening of the bone is called _____/_____/_____/_____.

oste/o/malac/ia

The study of the cause of a disease is _____/_____/_____.

eti/o/logy
et ē **ol′** ə gē

4.6

A disorder of the parathyroid glands (hyper/parathyroid/ism) can cause calcium to be withdrawn from the bones. When this occurs, _____ may develop.

osteomalacia

4.7

Recall **-pathy** means any disease. Form a word that means disease of bone: _____/_____/_____.

oste/o/pathy
os′ tē **op′** ə thē

4.8

A doctor of osteopathy (DO) receives special training about the skeleton and its relationship to disease. Using the adjectival form, we call this special type of doctor an _____/_____/_____/_____ physician.

oste/o/path/ic
os tē ō **path′** ik

4.9

A hard growth on a bone may be a bone tumor or _____/_____.

oste/oma
os tē **ō′** mə

Build the plural form: _____/_____/_____.

oste/o/mata
os′ tē **ō′** mə ta

4.10

-pathy means disease. Oste/o/arthr/o/pathy is a noun that means any disease involving bones and joints. **arthr/o** is used in words to mean _____.

joint

4.11

Oste/o/arthr/o/pathy is a compound noun. Analyze it:

_____/_____ bone (combining form);

oste/o

_____/_____ joint (combining form);

arthr/o

_____ disease (suffix).

pathy

Now put these together and form the term meaning bone and joint disease.

_____/_____/_____/_____/_____

oste/o/arthr/o/pathy
os′ tē ō är **throp′** ə thē

ANSWER COLUMN

**Structural changes
due to osteoporosis**
Delmar/Cengage Learning

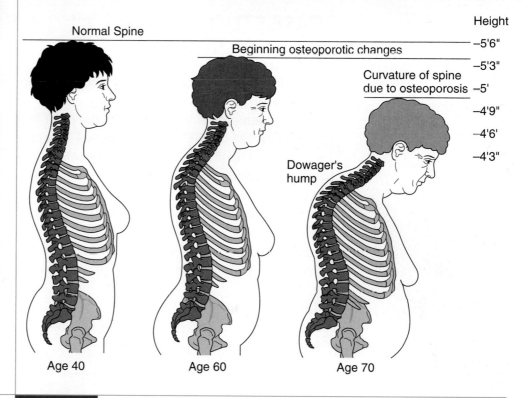

Normal Spine

Beginning osteoporotic changes

Curvature of spine
due to osteoporosis

Dowager's
hump

Age 40   Age 60   Age 70

Height
–5'6"
–5'3"
–5'
–4'9"
–4'6'
–4'3"

4.12

Poros is a Greek word meaning passageway. Oste/o/por/osis is a disease condition of the bone in which there is deterioration of the bone matrix causing pores and weakness. Calcium deficiency and hormone changes associated with menopause in women along with a hereditary predisposition can lead to

oste/o/por/osis
os' tē ō por **ō**' sis

_____/_____/_____/_____.

4.13

Recall that **-penia** is a suffix meaning low number or loss. Bone loss may occur do to the aging process and osteoporosis. Loss of bone is called oste/o/penia. Red blood cell loss is erythr/o/cyt/o/penia. The suffix that indicates loss

-penia

is _____.

4.14

A proper diet that includes adequate calcium in addition to weight-bearing exercise such as walking may help to prevent porosity of the bones, called

osteoporosis
oste/o/penia
os' tē ō **pē**' nē ə

_____. Bone loss is called _____/_____/_____.

4.15

Recall *sarcoma* is used to indicate cancer of connective tissue. Bone is connective

oste/o/sarc/oma
os' tē ō sar **cō**' mə

tissue; therefore, bone cancer is called _____/_____/_____/_____.

CASE STUDY INVESTIGATION (CSI)

Osteoporosis

Mrs. O is a 62-year-old Caucasian woman who is a retired school secretary. She presents with concerns about remaining on **hormone** replacement therapy **(HT)** with estrogen/progestin. She is not on any other medication at this time. Mrs. O is 5'8", weighs 125 lbs, BP 118/82, P 80, R 14, T 98, smokes one pack of cigarettes per day, drinks at least 1–2 glasses of wine per night and does not exercise other than housework. At age 48 she began HT for **menopause symptoms** and prevention of **osteoporosis**. She has a mother who experienced hip fracture at age 70 due to osteoporosis and a sister, age 68, who has been diagnosed with **osteopenia** and **kyphosis**. Mrs. O's bone mass density test (BMD) results showed a T score −1.5 on the right hip indicating slightly low **BMD**. The low BMD, low weight, smoking, and lack of exercise indicate that she is at risk of **osteoporotic fracture**.

CSI Vocabulary Challenge

Use a medical dictionary to analyze each term and abbreviation and write the definition in the space provided.

hormone   _____

HT   _____

menopause   _____

symptoms   _____

osteoporosis   _____

osteopenia   _____

osteoporotic   _____

kyphosis   _____

BMD   _____

fracture   _____

ANSWER COLUMN

4.16

myel/o is a combining form used to mean either the bone marrow or the spinal cord. A condition characterized by increased and abnormal bone marrow or spinal cord development is myel/o/dys/plasia:
myel/o—bone marrow or spinal cord
dys-—prefix for difficult or poor
-plasia—suffix for growth and development
When you see **myel/o**, read further to see whether it

spinal cord,   refers to *_____

bone marrow   or *_____

PROFESSIONAL PROFILE

Doctor of Osteopathy (DO): Osteopathic physicians are fully licensed to practice medicine, performing the same duties as a medical doctor (MD, allopathic doctor). Because of the original philosophy of osteopathic medicine, founded by Dr. Andrew Still in 1874, they identify the musculoskeletal framework as a key element to health. They also believe that the body has a natural ability to heal itself given a favorable environment and good nutrition and so act as teachers to help patients take a responsible role in their own well-being and to change unhealthy patterns. In addition, osteopathic manipulative therapy (OMT) is incorporated in the training and practice of osteopathic physicians. Although 60% practice primary care, osteopathic physicians may specialize in surgery,

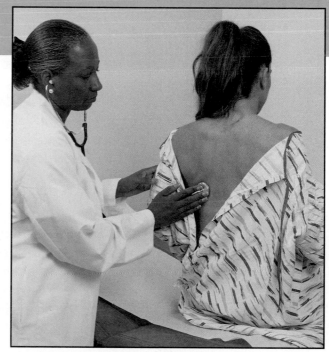

Osteopathic physican performing an exam *Delmar/Cengage Learning*

obstetrics, anesthesiology, internal medicine, psychiatry, and other medical specialties. The American Osteopathic Association (AOA) is the national professional organization that oversees education and licensure of Doctors of Osteopathy.

ANSWER COLUMN

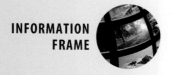

INFORMATION FRAME

4.17

poli/o is a combining form meaning gray and referring to the gray matter of the nervous system. White matter is made of myelinated nerve fibers that appear white. The nerve cell bodies are not myelinated and appear gray. The brain and part of the spinal cord that is made up of mostly nerve cell bodies is called gray matter.

4.18

Poli/o/myel/itis an inflammation of the gray matter of the spinal cord caused by a viral infection. This disease may cause paralysis of the limbs and muscle hypotrophy. Inactivated poliovirus vaccine (IPV) is given to produce an immune

poli/o/myel/itis
pō′ lē ō mī ə lī′ tis

response to prevent _____/_____/_____/_____.

CASE STUDY INVESTIGATION (CSI)

Post-Polio Syndrome

A 57-year-old woman presented via wheelchair in the office with leg weakness and progressive difficulty walking, joint and muscle pain. Upon examination, bilateral **atrophy** was seen in her legs. **Cranial** nerve examination was normal. The right triceps and supinator reflexes were absent but other reflexes preserved. Lower extremities were areflexic with plantar flexion of the left foot. Limited **electromyographic** studies showed partial denervation in keeping with a history of childhood **polio** and **median** nerve delay indicating **carpal** tunnel syndrome. She was diagnosed with **poliomyelitis** by age 6 and had several foot and ankle surgeries, used **prosthetics** to assist ankle and leg strength as well as crutches until age around 13, when she improved and was able to walk unassisted for many years and became an excellent swimmer. Beginning at age 40 she experienced right arm pain and **dysfunction** and progressive weakness in her legs, falling several times and requiring walking assistance. She recently developed **paresthesia** in the right arm with difficulty using her right hand in the mornings. A diagnosis of post-polio syndrome **(PPS)** and **osteoarthritis** was made.

CSI Vocabulary Challenge

Analyze the terms by dividing them into their word parts and writing the definition. Use your dictionary if needed for assistance.

atrophy _____

cranial _____

extremities _____

electromyographic _____

polio _____

median _____

carpal _____

poliomyelitis _____

prosthetics _____

paresthesia _____

osteoarthritis _____

PPS _____

ANSWER COLUMN

encephal/o/myel/o/pathy
en sef′ ə lō mī el **op′** ə thē

oste/o/myel/itis
os′ tē ō mī′ ə **li′** tis

myel/o/dys/plasia
mī′ el ō dis **plā′** zha

4.19

Any disease of the brain and spinal cord is called

_____/_____/_____/_____/_____.

Inflammation of the bone and marrow is called

_____/_____/_____/_____.

Defective formation of the spinal cord is called

_____/_____/_____/_____.

ANSWER COLUMN

	4.20

arthr/o is the combining form for joint. An instrument used to look at something is a **-scope**. An instrument used to look into a joint is an

arthr/o/scope
är′ thrō skōp

_____/_____/_____.

	4.21

DICTIONARY EXERCISE

Find the word myeloblast in your dictionary. Write the meaning here.

* _____

bone marrow germ cell
myel/o

The combining form of myel is _____/_____.

	4.22

DICTIONARY EXERCISE

Use your dictionary to help build a word meaning
pertaining to myelocytes

_____/_____/_____/_____;

myel/o/cyt/ic
mī′ el ō **sit′** ik
myel/o/cele
mī′ el ō sēl
mening/o/myel/o/cele
menin′ gō **mī′** el ō sēle

herniation of the spinal cord

_____/_____/_____;

herniation of the spinal cord and meninges

_____/_____/ _____/_____/_____.

Meningomyelocele
Delmar/Cengage Learning

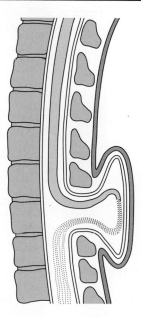

ANSWER COLUMN

4.23

-plasia means development or formation. This kind of formation occurs naturally instead of being done by a plastic surgeon. Hyper/plasia is an increase in the number of cells in a tissue (i.e., tumor). **dys-** means defective.

defective (poor or
abnormal) formation
defective formation
of a joint

Dys/plasia means *_____.
Arthr/o/dys/plasia means

*_____.

4.24

Build a term that means defective (abnormal) formation of the spinal cord:

myel/o/dys/plasia
mī′ ə lō dis **plā′** zhə

_____/_____/_____/_____
(body part + disorder).

oste/o/dys/plasia
os′ tē ō dis **plā′** zhə

Defective bone development is _____/_____/_____/_____.

4.25

hyper/plasia
hī per **plā′** zhə

a/plasia means failure of an organ to develop. A word that means overgrowth or too much development is _____/_____.

Arthoplasty: (A) total
hip replacement;
(B) total knee
replacement. A strong
polyethylene plastic
replaces the articular
(joint) cartilage and
a metal-like stainless
steel or titanium
is used to replace
bone. *Delmar/Cengage Learning*

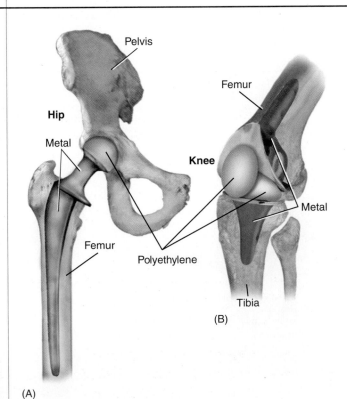

ANSWER COLUMN

Internal view of knee through arthroscope
Delmar/Cengage Learning

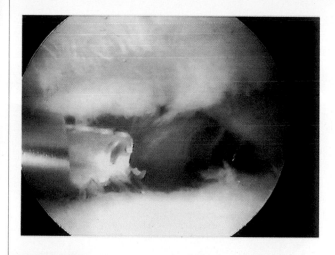

4.26

Hypo- is the opposite of **hyper-**. If excessive development is hyperplasia,

deficient development is expressed as _____/_____.

Complete lack of development is _____/_____.

hypo/plasia
hī pō **plā′** zhə
a/plasia
ā **plā′** zhə

4.27

arthr/o is the combining form for joint. The name of the procedure for examining the joints by looking with an arthroscope is called

_____ /_____/_____.

arthr/o/scopy
är **thros′** kō pē

4.28

SPELL CHECK

As you learn the medical terms about joints, watch the spelling of the word root arthr and combing form **arthr/o** for joint. They are easily confused with two other word parts that look similar but have quite different meanings.

arthr/o	joint (an "r" before the "t" and no "e")
ather/o	fatty or porridgelike (no "r" before the "t" and an "e" after the "h")
arteri/o	artery (no "h" following the "t")

4.29

_____/_____/_____ means surgical repair of a joint.
-plasty means surgical repair.

Arthr/o/plasty
är′ thrō plas′ tē

4.30

TAKE A CLOSER LOOK

Plastic surgery has nothing to do with plastic (the material). The word root plast means form, mold, or rebuild. Think of a plast/ic surgeon building a new nose or molding a face. This is surgical reconstruction. The suffix **-plasty** or means

*_____.

surgical repair or
reconstruction

ANSWER COLUMN

Arthroscope in use
Delmar/Cengage Learning

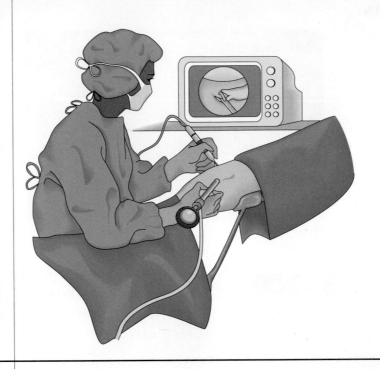

Use the following table to make a distinction between various terms related to development and growth.

-plasia	refers to changes in number and form of cells
a/plasia, a/plastic	lack of or decreased cell growth (syn: hypoplasia)
ana/plasia	abnormal growth of undifferentiated cells
dys/plasia	production of abnormally formed cells or tissues
hyper/plasia	abnormal increase in number of cells
hypo/plasia	abnormal decrease in number of cells or tissues
-trophy	refers to changes in size of cells and organs
a/trophy	decrease in size of tissues, wasting
hyper/trophy	increase in size of cells, tissues, or organs
hypo/trophy	progressive degeneration (syn: atrophy)
-genesis	refers to original growth of cells and organs
a/genesis	absence of original development
hyper/genesis	repeated creation of body parts or organs (extra organs)
hypo/genesis	congenital underdevelopment of organs

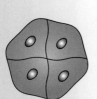
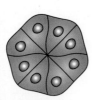
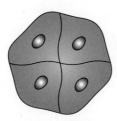
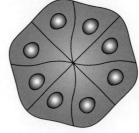
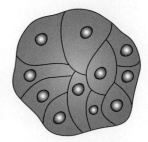

Normal (size and number normal)   Hyperplasia (increased numbers)   Hypertrophy (increased size)   Hypertrophy and hyperplasia (increase in size and number)   Dysplasia (abnormal cells and increase in numbers)

Hyperplasia, hypertrophy, dysplasia *Delmar/Cengage Learning*

ANSWER COLUMN

4.31

Arthr/o/plasty may take many forms. When a joint has lost its ability to move,

arthroplasty
        movement can sometimes be restored by an _____.

4.32

Arthr/itic means pertaining to a joint. Form a word that means inflammation of a

arthr/itis
är **thrī′** tis
arthr/itic
är **thrī′** tik
    joint: _____/_____. A medication used to treat arthritis is

an anti /_____/_____ agent.

4.33

Arthritis characterized by inflammation and destruction of bone and joint tissue is

oste/o/arthr/itis
os′ tē ō är **thrī′** tis
    called _____/_____/_____/_____(OA).

4.34

Rheumatoid is Greek for resembling discharge or fluid. Rheumatoid arthritis (RA)
affects the softer tissues of the joint often accompanied by fluid in the joints.

arthritis
    RA still causes inflammation of the joint or _____.

4.35

You're getting to be pretty good at this, aren't you? Form a word that means

arthr/o/tomy
är **throt′** ə mē
    incision into a joint: _____/_____/_____.

4.36

INFORMATION FRAME

Rheumat/o/logy is a medical specialty that studies, diagnoses, and treats
rheumatic conditions. *Rheum* is a Greek word root that means flux (body fluids).
Patients with rheumatoid arthritis develop changes in joint structures, an increase
in synovial (joint) fluid, inflammation, pain, and joint deformity. This type of
arthritis is caused by a systemic autoimmune response.

4.37

Build a term that means:
the study of rheumatic disorders

rheumat/o/logy
rōō mə **tol′** ō jē

rheumat/o/logist
rōō mə **tol′** ō jist
    _____/_____/_____;

the physician specialist who treats rheumatic conditions

_____/_____/_____.

4.38

INFORMATION FRAME

In Latin *tendo* means to stretch. **Tendons** are made of connective tissue and
attach muscle to bone. **Ligaments** attach bone to bone and **fascia** attaches
muscle to muscle.

ANSWER COLUMN

A bone density scan is performed to determine a baseline and a client's fracture risk. The patient is positioned, the scanner aligned, and a computer image created. A physician then interprets the results. *Delmar/Cengage Learning*

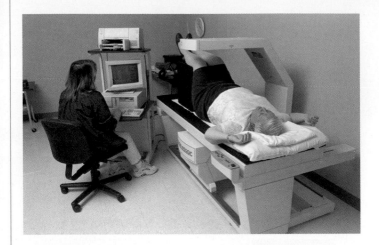

4.39

ten/o, **tend/o**, and **tendin/o** are all combining forms for tendon. Use your dictionary to help you. Build three terms meaning repair of the tendons:

tend/o/plasty
ten′ dō plas tē

_____/_____/_____,

ten/o/plasty
ten′ ō plas tē

_____/_____/_____, and

tendin/o/plasty
ten′ din ō plas tē

_____/_____/_____.

4.40

tendin/o is used to build words about inflammation of the tendons.

tendin/itis
ten′ din ī′ tis

Inflammation of a tendon is _____/_____.

NOTE: Tendinitis is the proper term, but tendonitis is accepted.

4.41

ten/o is used to build the terms for pain in a tendon. Two terms for tendon pain are

ten/algia
ten **al′** jē ə

_____/_____ and

ten/o/dynia
ten′ ō **din′** ē ə

_____/_____/_____.

4.42

Bursa in Latin means purse or bag. A bursa is a small serous sac between a tendon and a bone. **burs/o** refers to the *bursae* (plural) of the body. Build words meaning:

burs/itis
bûr **sī′** tis

inflammation of a bursa _____/_____;

(continued)

ANSWER COLUMN

burs/ectomy
bûr **sek′** tə mē

excision of a bursa _____/_____;

burs/ae
bûr′ sē

more than one bursa _____/_____.

4.43

The word oste/o/chondr/itis means inflammation of bone and cartilage.

chondr/o

The combining form for cartilage is _____/_____.

4.44

Cartilage is a tough, elastic connective tissue found in the ear, nose tip, and

cartilage
kär′ ti lədj

rib ends. The lining of joints also contain _____.

4.45

Form two words meaning pain in or around cartilage:

chondr/algia
kon **dral′** gē ə

_____/_____

   (word root)   (suffix)

chondr/o/dynia
kon′ drō **din′** ē ə

_____/_____/_____.

   (combining form)   (suffix)

4.46

Use **ten/o** to build words meaning:

ten/o/plasty
ten′ ō plast tē

repair of tendons _____/_____/_____;

ten/o/dynia
ten′ ō **din′** ē ə

pain in tendons _____/_____/_____.

4.47

excision of cartilage

Chondr/ectomy means * _____.

Rib cage and shoulder joint Delmar/Cengage Learning

Clavicle
Manubrium
Bursa (burs/o)
Ribs (cost/o)
Scapula
Intercostal muscle
Humerus
Sternum (stern/o)
Costal cartilage (chondr/o)
False ribs
Xiphoid process (xiph/o)
Floating ribs

ANSWER COLUMN

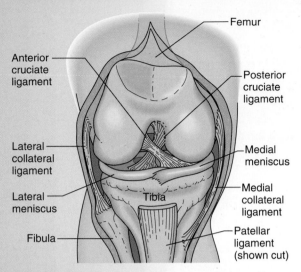

Major ligaments of the knee, anterior view
Delmar/Cengage Learning

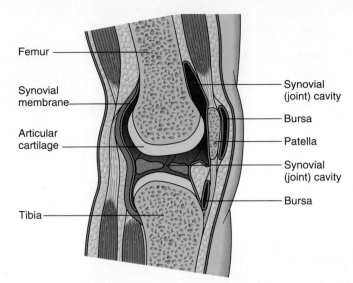

Synovial joint and bursa, right lateral view
Delmar/Cengage Learning

	4.48
ribs	Chondr/o/cost/al means pertaining to ribs and cartilage. **cost/o** is used in words about the _____.

	4.49
cost/ectomy kos **tek'** tə mē	Form a word that means excision of a rib or ribs: _____/_____.

	4.50
adjective	Chondr/o/cost/al is an adjective. This is evident because **-al** is the ending for an _____.

	4.51
chondr/o cost al chondr/o/cost/al kon' drō **kos'** təl pertaining to cartilage and ribs	Analyze chondr/o/cost/al: _____/_____ cartilage; _____ rib; _____ suffix. Now put them together: _____/_____/_____/_____. This means * _____.

ANSWER COLUMN

	4.52
	Meniskos is a Greek term meaning crescent shaped. In the knee joint there is a crescent-shaped cartilage structure that is called the meniscus. The lateral menisc/us is on the outer portion of the knee and the medial
menisc/us me **nis'** cus	_____ is located toward the inner part of the knee joint. **NOTE:** The "c" is followed by a "u" so it is pronounced like a "k."
	4.53
menisc/itis me ni **sī'** tis	Inflammation of the meniscus is _____/_____. **NOTE:** The "c" is followed by an "i so it is pronounced like an "s."
	4.54
menisc/ectomy me ni **sek'** to mē	Injury to the knee may produce a tear in the meniscus, requiring surgery. Excision of the torn meniscus is called a _____/_____.
	4.55
cost/al **kos'** təl	Form a word that means pertaining to the ribs: _____/_____.
	4.56
inter-	Inter/cost/al means between the ribs. The prefix for between is _____. **EXAMPLE:** International means between nations.
	4.57
	Hypo/chondr/iac means below the cartilage, referring to the region below the rib cage cartilage. Form an adjective that means between cartilages:
inter/chondr/al in' t ə r **kon'** drəl	_____/_____/ al.
	4.58
between	Inter/cost/al means between the ribs. **inter-** is the prefix that means _____.
	4.59
inter/cost/al inter **kos'** təl	Inter/cost/al may refer to the muscles between the ribs. The muscles that move the ribs when breathing are the _____/_____/_____ muscles.
	4.60
intercostal	The external intercostal muscles assist with inhalation by enlarging the rib cage. The internal intercostal muscles assist with breathing out by decreasing the size of the rib cage. Breathing is assisted by the _____ muscles.

ANSWER COLUMN

4.61

dent

Inter/dent/al means between the teeth. The word root for tooth is _____.

4.62

dent/al
den′ təl

Combining forms for tooth or teeth are dent/o and dent/i.

Form an adjective that means pertaining to the teeth: _____/_____.

4.63

dent/algia
den **tal′** jē ə

Pain in the teeth, or a toothache, is called _____/_____.

(A) Maxillary arch
(B) Mandibular arch
Delmar/Cengage Learning

Upper jaw (maxilla)   Lower jaw (mandible)

Incisors
Incisors
Canines
Premolars
Molars

A   B

i-CAT three-dimensional CAT scan of the mouth for the purpose of studying tooth and jaw structure for implants, extractions, and other dental procedures
Courtesy of Cynthia A. Rider, DMD, Maxillofacial Surgeon, Jackson, MI

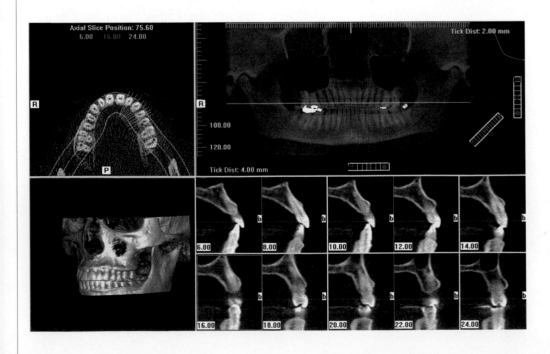

ANSWER COLUMN

4.64

dent/oid
den' toid

Great! Try this: **-oid** is the suffix that means like or resembling. Form a word that means tooth shaped or resembling a tooth: _____/_____.

4.65

teeth

teeth

A dent/ist (Doctor of Dental Surgery DDS) takes care of _____.

A dent/ifrice is used for cleaning _____.

4.66

orth/odont/ist
ôr' thŏ **don'** tist

orth/o is a combining form taken from the Greek word *orthos*, meaning straight. **odont/o** means shaped like a tooth. A dentist who specializes in straightening abnormally positioned teeth is called an _____/_____/_____.

4.67

around or near

peri- is a prefix meaning around or near. Peri/odont/al disease is diseased tissue * _____ the teeth.

Orthodontists use braces to straighten teeth *Photo by Timothy J. Dennerll, RT(R), Ph.D.*

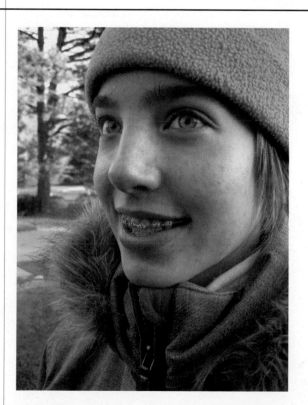

ANSWER COLUMN

4.68

A periodontist may perform surgery of the gums or tissues around the teeth.

peri/odont/al
pair′ ē ō **don′** tal

This is _____/_____/_____ surgery.

4.69

Build terms meaning the membrane around the bone:

peri/oste/um
pair′ ē **os′** tē əm

_____/_____/um;

the membrane around the cartilage:

peri/chondr/ium
pair′ ē **kon′** drē əm

_____/_____/ium;

the membrane around the heart:

peri/cardi/um
pair′ ē **kar′** dē əm

_____/_____/um.

4.70

An orth/o/ped/ist (ōr thō **pēd′** ist) is a physician who specializes in the prevention and treatment of musculoskeletal disorders. The combining form indicating that

orth/o

"straightening" may be done is _____/_____.

4.71

A broken bone is called a fracture (Fx). Often the fracture must be manipulated so

orth/o/ped/ist
ôr thō **pēd′** ist

that the bone will heal straight. An _____/_____/_____/_____ is the specialist who treats fractures.

4.72

TAKE A CLOSER LOOK

Orth/o/tics is the science that studies and develops mechanical appliances used as supportive devices. The specialist who designs and fits these devices is called an orth/o/tist. This practice is closely related to the prosthet/ists who work with patients in need of replacing an amputated limb. The appliance the prosthet/ist produces is called a prosthesis. Look in the "ortho" and "prosth" sections of your dictionary to find the word that means

orth/o/sis
ôr thō′ sis

condition of straightening or supporting: _____/_____/_____;

devices used to stabilize or prevent deformity: _____/_____/_____;

orth/o/tic
ôr tho′ tik

specialist in making artificial body parts: _____/_____/_____;

prosthet/ist
pros′ the tist

pertaining to (adjective) a prosthesis: _____/_____.

prosthet/ic
pros **the′** tik

ANSWER COLUMN

Orthotic device used to straighten the wrist, holding it firmly *Delmar/ Cengage Learning*

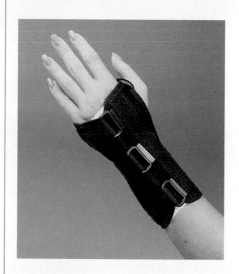

4.73

Splints and casts are orth/o/tic devices that are used to support and protect injured bones and soft tissue. Immobilizing and supporting an injury reduces pain, swelling, and muscle spasm. Because a cast supports a body part it is a(n)

orth/o/tic
ôr **tha′** tik
_____/_____/_____ (noun).

4.74

lumb/o builds words about the lower back. Lumb/ar is the adjectival form.

lumb/ar
lum′ b ər, **lum′** bär
An adjective meaning pertaining to the lower back is _____/_____.

4.75

lumbar
There are five lumbar vertebrae. Low back pain is called _____ pain.

4.76

lumbar
L_1, L_2, L_3, L_4, and L_5 are the five _____ vertebrae.

4.77

adjective

pertaining to the chest and lower back or something near these areas
thorac/o is the combining form for chest or thorax. Thorac/o/lumb/ar is a(n)

(choose one) _____

(noun/adjective) meaning ** _____.

NOTE: T_1–T_{12} are the twelve thoracic vertebrae.

4.78

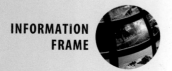

INFORMATION FRAME

supra- is a prefix that means on, higher in position, over, or above.

Thorax and regions of the abdomen *Delmar/Cengage Learning*

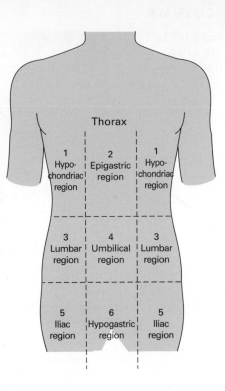

Direction	Prefix	Word root/ Suffix
below	hypo	chondr/iac
upon	epi	gastr/ic
above	supra	lumb/ar
below	hypo	gastr/ic

4.79

Supra/lumb/ar means above the lumbar region. A prefix that means above

supra

is _____.

4.80

above the lumbar region
or above the lower back

Supra/lumb/ar means * _____.

4.81

above the ribs

Supra/cost/al means * _____.

4.82

on top of

Supra/crani/al refers to the surface of the head * _____ the skull.

4.83

noun

The pubis is a bone of the pelvis. Pub/is is a (choose one) _____ (noun/adjective).

4.84

pubis
pyoo′ bis
pubic
pyoo′ bik

From **pub/o** form a noun _____; an adjective _____.

(See the illustration of the pelvic bones in Unit 14.)

ANSWER COLUMN

4.85

pub/is
pyoo′ bis

The pub/ic bone is also called the _____/_____.

4.86

pubis

Supra/pub/ic means above the pubis. **pub/o** is used in words about

the _____.

4.87

supra/pub/ic
soo prə **pyoo′** bik

The suprapubic region is above the arch of the pub/is. When the urinary bladder is incised above the pubis, an incision is made in the

_____/_____/_____ region.

4.88

suprapubic

incision

region

"The incision is made in the suprapubic region." From this sentence pick out

the adjective _____;

two nouns _____ .

4.89

anything close to incision

of bladder from the

suprapubic region

Try to figure out what surgery is done in a supra/pub/ic cyst/o/tomy

* _____

_____.

4.90

pelv/is
pel′ vis

pelves
pel′ vēs

The pelv/is is formed by the pelv/ic bones. **pelv/i** refers to the

_____/_____ (noun).

The plural of pelvis is _____.

4.91

pelv/i/metry
pel **vim′** ə trē

Pelv/i/metry is done during pregnancy to determine the measurements of the pelvis. To find a woman's pelvic size, the physician does

_____/_____/_____.

4.92

pelvimetry

Look up pelvimetry or pelvis in your dictionary. Taking pelvic measurements

is called _____.

ANSWER COLUMN

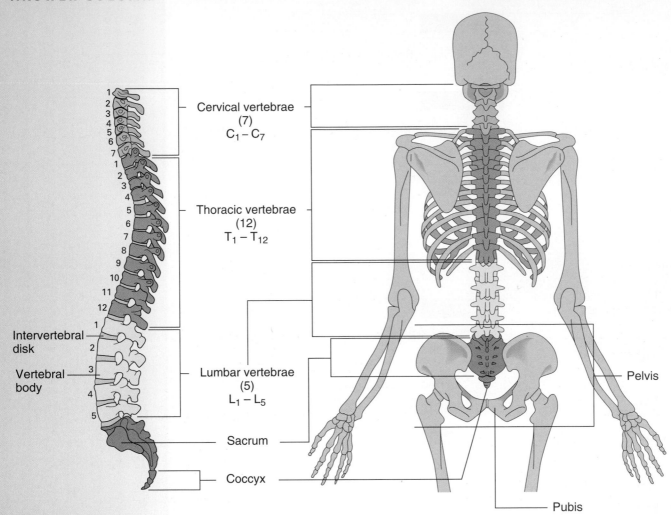

Divisions of the vertebral column *Delmar/Cengage Learning*

Labels on the diagram:

Cervical vertebrae (7) C₁ – C₇

Thoracic vertebrae (12) T₁ – T₁₂

Intervertebral disk

Vertebral body

Lumbar vertebrae (5) L₁ – L₅

Sacrum

Coccyx

Pelvis

Pubis

	4.93
	Cephal/o/pelvic disproportion (CPD) can lead to serious complications during delivery. A physician may determine whether a woman will have trouble during
pelvimetry	labor by doing _____.
	4.94
	Look in the dictionary for a word that names the device used for pelvimetry.
pelv/i/meter	It is a _____/_____/_____.
pel **vim'** ə tər	
	4.95
	A pelvimeter measures the diameter of the pelvis. When the head (**cephal/o**) of the fetus is larger than the diameter of the mother's pelvis (**pelv/o**), this is
cephal/o/pelv/ic	called _____/_____/_____/_____
cef' əl ō **pel'** vik	disproportion (CPD).

ANSWER COLUMN

4.96

supra/pelv/ic
sōō pr ə **pel'** vik

The adjective meaning *above* the pelvis is _____/_____/_____.

4.97

instrument
instrument

-meter is a suffix meaning an instrument used to measure. A speed/o/meter is an _____ to measure speed. A pelv/i/meter is an _____ to measure the pelvis.

4.98

measures (counts)

measures

thorac/o/meter
thôr' ə **kom'** ə tər

cardi/o/meter
kär' dē **om'** ə tər

A cyt/o/meter _____ cells.

A cephal/o/meter _____ the head.

A thorac/o/_____ measures the chest.

A cardi/o/_____ measures the heart.

4.99

pre

Ab/norm/al is a word that means deviating (turning away) from what is normal.
ab- is a _____/ fix that means from or away from.

4.100

away from
or not

Abnormal is used as an ordinary English word. Abnormal means
* _____ normal.

4.101

from or away from

ab- is a prefix that means * _____.

4.102

wandering from (the
normal course of events)

Ab/errant uses the prefix **ab-** before the English word (errant) for wandering.
Ab/errant means * _____.
NOTE: Think of an error or something gone wrong.

4.103

ab/errant
ab **air'** ənt *or*
ab' air ənt

Ab/errant is used in medicine as a term to describe a structure that wanders from the normal path. When some nerve fibers follow an unusual route, they form an _____/_____ nerve.

ANSWER COLUMN

	4.104
aberrant	Aberrant nerves wander from the normal nerve track. Blood vessels that follow a path of their own are _____ vessels.
	4.105
aberrant	Lymph vessels may be found in unexpected areas of the body. They follow an _____ course.
	4.106
ab/duct/ion ab **duk′** shən	In Latin *ducere* (word root: duct) means to lead or move. Ab/duct/ion means movement away from a midline. When the arm is raised away from the side of the body, _____/_____/_____ has occurred.
	4.107
abduction	Abduction can occur from any midline. When the fingers of the hand are spread apart, _____ has occurred in four fingers.
	4.108
abducted ab **duk′** td	A child who has been kidnapped and taken away from home has been _____ (past tense verb).
	4.109
ad/duct/ion ə **duk′** shən ad/duct a **dukt′**	**ad-** is a prefix meaning toward. Movement toward a midline is _____/_____/_____ (noun). When a patient is asked to move his arm toward his body, he is asked to _____/_____ (verb) his arm. **NOTE:** In medical dictation, the physician may emphasize a-b duct (abduct) or a-b duction (abduction) and a-d duct (adduct) or a-d duction (adduction), to avoid misunderstanding. This would be a good time for you to make a note of the difference as well.
	4.110
ad/dict/ion ə **dik′** shən	Ad/diction means being drawn toward some habit. The person who takes drugs habitually suffers from drug _____/_____/_____.
	4.111
addiction	Addiction implies habit. Alcoholism is an _____ to alcohol.

ANSWER COLUMN

Abduction/Adduction
Delmar/Cengage Learning

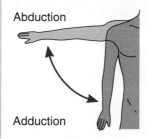

Abduction

Adduction

4.112

A person addicted to drugs is a drug addict. A person addicted to cocaine is a

addict   cocaine _____.

4.113

An ad/hes/ion is formed when two normally separate tissues join together.
They adhere to each other. Adhering to another part forms an

ad/hes/ion   _____/_____/_____.
ad **hē′** zhən

4.114

Patients are usually encouraged to ambulate soon after surgery to help prevent

adhesions   postoperative _____.

4.115

adhesions   Pain or intestinal obstruction may be caused by abdominal _____.

4.116

abdomin/o is used to form words about the abdomen. When you see **abdomin/o**

ab/domen   any place in a word, you think about the _____/_____.
ab′ də mən

4.117

**SPELL
CHECK**

In the spelling of the combining form for abdomen, the "e" changes to
"i"—**abdomin/o**.

EXAMPLE: The abdominal incision was made in the RLQ of the abdomen.

4.118

**TAKE A
CLOSER LOOK**

Abdomin/al is an adjective that means

*_____.

NOTE: For descriptive reference the abdomen may be divided into four quadrants
including the right upper quadrant (RUQ), the left upper quadrant (LUQ), the right
lower quadrant (RLQ), and the left lower quadrant (LLQ).

pertaining to the
abdomen

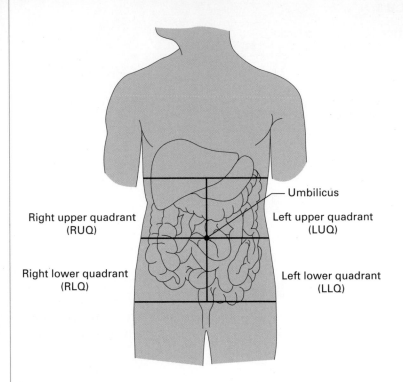

4.119

the insertion of a needle into a body cavity for the purpose of aspirating fluid

Look up the words *paracentesis* and *centesis* in your dictionary. Write the definition here: ** _____

_____.

NOTE: p. abdominal is paracentesis of the abdomen or abdominocentesis.

4.120

Abdomin/o/centesis means tapping or puncturing of the abdomen for the removal of fluid. The word for surgical puncture of the abdomen is

_____/_____/_____.

abdomin/o/centesis
ab dom′ i nō sen **tē′** sis

4.121

Centesis (surgical puncture) is a word in itself used as a suffix. Build a word meaning surgical puncture, or tapping of the abdomen: _____.

abdominocentesis

4.122

amni/o refers to the amnion, the protective sac that surrounds the fetus. Tapping or puncturing this sac to remove cells for genetic testing is called

_____/_____/_____.

amni/o/centesis
am′ nē ō sen **tē′** sis

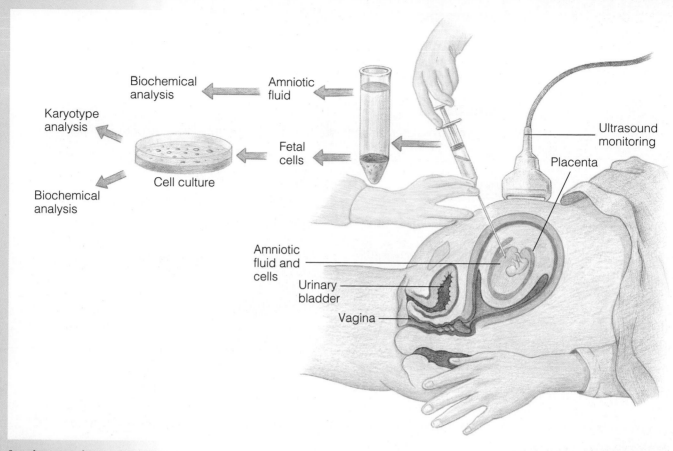

Amniocentesis *Delmar/Cengage Learning*

ANSWER COLUMN

4.123

During genetic amniocentesis, fluid and cells are removed from the amnion.

amniocentesis

Surgical puncture of the amnion is called _____.

4.124

cardi/o/centesis
kär′ dē ō sen **tē**′ sis

The word for surgical puncture into the heart chambers is

_____/_____/_____, used for diagnosis and treatment.

4.125

Abdomin/o/cyst/ic means pertaining to the abdomen and urinary bladder.
Analyze abdominocystic:

abdomin/o

_____/_____ combining form;

cyst

_____ word root;

ic
abdomin/o/cyst/ic
ab dom′ i nō **sis**′ tik

_____ suffix.
Now put them together to form the word

_____/_____/_____/_____.

ANSWER COLUMN

	4.126
cyst	From abdomin/o/cyst/ic you see that the word root for urinary bladder is _____.
	4.127
bladder	**cyst/o** is used to form words that refer to a fluid-filled sac or the urinary _____.
	4.128
cyst/o/tomy sis **tot′** ə mē	The word for incision into the urinary bladder is _____/_____/_____.
	4.129
cyst/ectomy sis **tek′** t ə mē	The word for excision of the urinary bladder is _____/_____.
	4.130
cyst/o/scopy sis **tos′** cō pē	Recall that **-scopy** is a suffix for the procedure used to look into an organ or body cavity with a scope. The process of examining by looking with an instrument into the urinary bladder is _____/_____/_____.

Cystoscopy *Delmar/Cengage Learning*

Cystoscope

Urethra

Bladder

Prostate gland

ANSWER COLUMN

	4.131
urinary bladder	A cyst/o/scop/ic exam (cysto) is used to look inside the * _____.
	4.132
cyst/o/plasty **sis'** tō plas' tē	Surgical repair of the bladder is _____/_____/_____.
	4.133
cystocele	When the bladder wall weakens and forms a hernia into the vagina, a _____ is formed.
	4.134
thorac/ic thô **ras'** ik	**thorac/o** is used to form words about the thorax or chest. A word that means pertaining to the chest is _____/_____. See the illustration of body cavities.

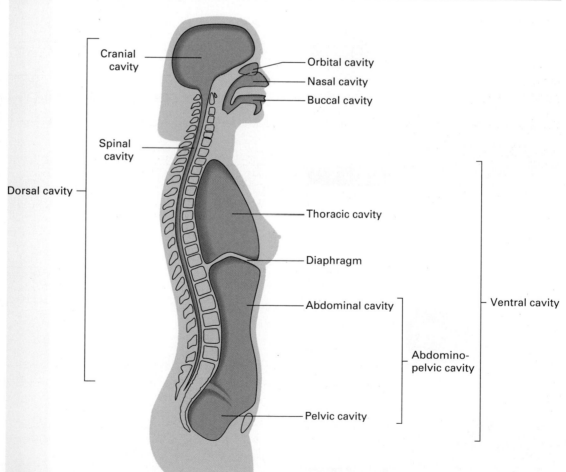

Body cavities *Delmar/Cengage Learning*

Cranial cavity

Orbital cavity

Nasal cavity

Buccal cavity

Spinal cavity

Dorsal cavity

Thoracic cavity

Diaphragm

Abdominal cavity

Ventral cavity

Abdomino-pelvic cavity

Pelvic cavity

ANSWER COLUMN

4.135

thoraces
thôr′ ə sēs

The plural form of thorax is _____.

4.136

Abdomin/o/thorac/ic means pertaining to the abdomen and thorax. The thorax is

the chest. Supply the word parts for _____/_____ abdomen;

abdomin/o

thorac

_____ thorax;

ic

_____ suffix—pertaining to.
Now put them together to form

abdomin/o/thorac/ic
ab dom′ i nō thô **ras′** ik

_____/_____/_____/_____.

4.137

Abdomin/o/thorac/ic pain means, literally, pain in the abdomen and chest.
A physician who describes lesions in these areas could call them

abdominothoracic

_____ lesions.

4.138

An incision may be made into the chest to insert a chest tube for the purpose
of draining blood and fluid from the lung. A word that means incision of the

thorac/o/tomy
thôr′ ə **kot′** ə mē

chest is _____/_____/_____.

4.139

A word that means surgical tapping (puncture) of the chest to remove fluids

thorac/o/centesis
thôr′ ə kō sen **tē′** sis

is _____/_____/_____.

4.140

**SPELL
CHECK**

Usually, thoracocentesis is shortened to thoracentesis (thôr′ ə sen **tē′** sis). Find
out which form is used by your local hospital.

4.141

thorac/o/pathy
thôr′ ə **kop′** ə thē

A word that means any chest disease is _____/_____/_____.

4.142

Build a term meaning pertaining to the thoracic and lumbar vertebrae:

thorac/o/lumbar
thôr′ ak ō **lum′** bar

_____/_____/_____.

ANSWER COLUMN

**TAKE A
CLOSER LOOK**

4.143

Take a closer look at terms referring to cysts and bladders. The terms cyst and bladder both refer to any fluid-filled, saclike structure and describe the urinary bladder, the gallbladder, or an abnormality such as an ovarian cyst. A cyst (**-cyst**) may be used as a word or as a suffix. If **cyst/o** is used at the beginning of a word, it usually refers to the urinary bladder, i.e., cyst/o/scopy. If **-cyst** is used as a suffix, it indicates a less specific fluid-filled saclike structure, i.e., hydrocyst. To indicate the gallbladder, use the word root cholecyst/, e.g., cholecyst/itis.

4.144

water or fluid or
watery fluid

A hydro/cyst is a sac (or bladder) filled with watery fluid. **hydro-** is used as a prefix in words to mean * _____ .

NOTE: Think of a fire hydrant.

4.145

hydro/cele
hī′ drō sēl

An accumulation of fluid in a saclike cavity, especially in the scrotum, is called a hydro/cele. Two- to five-year-old boys often develop this fluid-filled saclike swelling in the scrotum called a _____ / _____ .

4.146

hydrocele

A hydrocyst and a hydrocele are both fluid-filled sacs. The more specific term used to name the condition often found in infant and young boys is _____ .

Hydrocele Delmar/Cengage
Learning

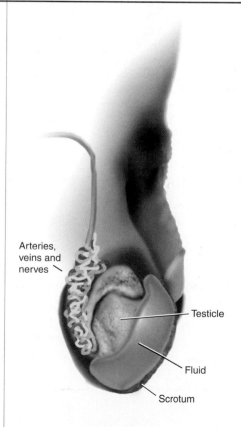

Arteries,
veins and
nerves

Testicle

Fluid

Scrotum

ANSWER COLUMN

SPELL CHECK

4.147

It is easy to get confused when terms seem to have the same meaning, are spelled similar, but have quite different practical uses. Look up the following terms in your medical dictionary to be sure of their use.

cyst/o/cele—urinary bladder herniation, most common in women; a cystocele is usually a weakened anterior vaginal wall with the urinary bladder bulging into the vagina

hydr/o/cyst—a sacklike structure with watery contents; may be found almost anywhere in the body

hydr/o/cele—collection of fluid in a herniated cavity, most often related to a congenital condition; fluid-filled peritoneum herniated into the scrotum

---

4.148

hydro/cephal/us
hī′ drō **sef′** ə ləs

Hydro/cephalus is characterized by an enlarged head due to increased amount of fluid in the skull. A collection of fluid in the head is called

_____/_____/_____.

4.149

Hydrocephalus

Hydrocephalus, unless arrested, results in deformity. The face seems small. The eyes are abnormal. The head is large. _____ also causes brain damage.

4.150

hydrocephalus

Because of the damage to the brain, children with _____ are usually mentally challenged.

4.151

Hydro/cephal/ic
hī′ dro se **fal′** ik

Hydrocephalus is the noun. The adjectival suffix is **-ic**.

_____/_____/_____ children may attend schools for the mentally impaired.

4.152

abnormal fear
hydrophobia

-phobia, from the Greek word for fear, is used as a suffix meaning any

* _____. Build a word meaning abnormal fear of

water: _____.

DICTIONARY EXERCISE

4.153

Find the word **phobia** in a dictionary or thesaurus. It may list more than 100 types of phobias. How many phobias do you recognize already? ** _____.

An abnormal fear of water is _____/_____.

between three and twelve
hydro/phobia
hī′ drō **fō′** bē ə

ANSWER COLUMN

DICTIONARY EXERCISE

4.154

Cover the answer column. Look up the following **phobias** or make an intelligent guess at their meaning using what you have learned already from the word building system. Then check your answer.

fear of heights (extremely high places)	acrophobia
fear of men	androphobia
fear of being by one's self	autophobia
fear of bacteria	bacteriophobia
fear of cancer	carcinophobia
fear of hands	chirophobia
fear of confined spaces	claustrophobia
fear of deformity	dysmorphophobia
fear of women	gynephobia or gynophobia
fear of the color white	leukophobia

4.155

hydrophobia

If a person is bitten by a dog with rabies, he or she may contract rabies, which is also called _____ (so named because rabid animals are afraid of choking while drinking and will not drink water).

4.156

hydro/therapy

hī′ drō **ther′** ə pē

Therapy means treatment. Treatment by water (H_2O) is

_____/_____.

4.157

hydrotherapy

Physical therapists (PT) use swirling water baths to increase ease of movement. This is called _____.

Abbreviation	Meaning
AOA	American Osteopathic Association
C_1–C_7	cervical vertebrae 1–7
CPD	cephalopelvic disproportion
CXR	chest x-ray
cysto	cystoscopy
DDS	doctor of dental surgery (dentist)
DO	doctor of osteopathy
DTs	delirium tremens
FAS	fetal alcohol syndrome
Fx	fracture
H_2O	water
IPV	inactivated polio vaccine
L_1–L_5	lumbar vertebrae 1–5
LLQ	left lower quadrant (abdomen)

(continued)

ANSWER COLUMN

Abbreviation	Meaning
LUQ	left upper quadrant (abdomen)
OA	osteoarthritis
OMT	osteopathic manipulative therapy
ORTHO (ORTH)	orthopedics (orthopedist)
PPS	post-polio syndrome
PT	physical therapy (therapist)
RA	rheumatoid arthritis
RLQ	right lower quadrant (abdomen)
RUQ	right upper quadrant (abdomen)
T_1–T_{12}	thoracic vertebrae 1–12

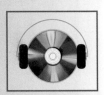

To complete your study of this unit, work the **Review Activities** on the following pages. Also, listen to the Audio CD that accompanies *Medical Terminology: A Programmed Systems Approach,* 10th edition, and practice your pronunciation.

STUDY**WARE**™ CONNECTION

To help you learn the content in this chapter, take a practice quiz or play an interactive game on your **StudyWARE™ CD-ROM**.

REVIEW ACTIVITIES

CIRCLE AND CORRECT

Circle the correct answer for each question. Then check your answers in Appendix E.

1. Word root for bone
   a. calci
   b. ortho
   c. oste
   d. osteo

2. Combining form for joint
   a. arther
   b. artero
   c. arthero
   d. arthro

3. Suffix for instrument used to look
   a. -scope
   b. -scopy
   c. -graph
   d. -scopic

4. Combining form for tendon
   a. chondro
   b. teno
   c. tendonitis
   d. tendon

5. Word root for rib
   a. costal
   b. chondr
   c. cost
   d. ribo

6. Prefix for between
   a. inter-
   b. intra-
   c. peri-
   d. endo-

7. Combining form for tooth
   a. toid
   b. dentin
   c. dontia
   d. dento

8. Combining form for straight
   a. oto
   b. ortho
   c. donto
   d. oligo

9. Prefix for above
   a. inter-
   b. hypo-
   c. supra-
   d. infra-

10. Suffix for the process of measuring
    a. -metro
    b. -meter
    c. -metr
    d. -metry

REVIEW ACTIVITIES

11. Prefix meaning toward

    a. ab-   c. in-

    b. hyper-   d. ad-

12. Adjective for bladder or sac

    a. cystosis   c. cytic

    b. cystic   d. cystal

13. Word root for move or lead

    a. mor   c. duct

    b. domin   d. go

14. Adjective suffix

    a. -ous   c. -us

    b. -ia   d. -sis

15. Combining form for abdomen

    a. abdomen/o   c. stomach/o

    b. stomat/o   d. abdomin/o

SELECT AND CONSTRUCT

Select the correct word parts from the following list and construct medical terms that represent the given meaning.

a (an)	ab	abdomin(o)	ad	al
amni/o	arthr(o)	cele	centesis	cephal(ic)(o)
chondr(o)	cost(o)	cyst	dent(o)	dont(o)
duct	dys	errant	hydro	hyper
hypo(o)	inter	ist	itis	lumb(o)(ar)
malacia	metr/o(y)(ic)(er)	oma	orth(o)	oste(o)
osteo	pathy	ped	pelv/i(o)	peri
phobia	plasia	plasty	pubo(is)(ic)	sarc(o)
scope(y)(ic)	supra	tendin(o)	tendon	tendin/o
ten/o, tend/o	therapy	thorac(o)(ic)	(t)ion	troph/y/ic

1. softening of the bone _____

2. movement away from the body _____

3. water-filled sac _____

4. water on the brain (adjective) _____

5. above the pubic bone _____

6. between the ribs _____

7. surgical puncture of the abdomen _____

8. process of looking into a joint _____

9. wandering in an abnormal path _____

10. specialist in straightening teeth _____

11. inflammation of the cord that connects

    muscle to bone _____

12. instrument to measure the pelvis _____

13. pertaining to the head and pelvis _____

REVIEW ACTIVITIES

14. bone and joint specialist _____

15. bone cancer _____

16. increase in size of tissues or an organ _____

17. abnormally formed cells _____

18. defective development of cartilage _____

19. surgical puncture for removal of cells

     from the amniotic sac _____

20. just above the lower back _____

DEFINE AND DISSECT

Give a brief definition and dissect each term listed into its word parts in the space provided. Check your answers by referring to the frame listed in parentheses and to your medical dictionary. Then listen to the Audio CD to practice pronunciation.

1. osteomalacia (4.4)   _____ / _____ / _____ / _____
                                      rt   v   rt   suffix

     meaning _____

2. osteoarthropathy (4.11)   _____ / _____ / _____ / _____ / _____
                                     rt   v   rt   v   suffix

_____

3. arthroscopy (4.27)   _____ / _____ / _____
                                     rt   v   suffix

_____

4. tendoplasty (4.39)   _____ / _____ / _____
                                     rt   v   suffix

_____

5. chondralgia (4.45)   _____ / _____
                                     rt   suffix

_____

6. intercostal (4.56)   _____ / _____ / _____
                                     rt   rt   suffix

_____

7. orthodontist (4.66)   _____ / _____ / _____
                                     rt   rt   suffix

_____

REVIEW ACTIVITIES

8. suprapubic (4.88)

_____/_____/_____
       pre   rt   suffix

_____

9. thoracolumbar (4.77)

_____/_____/_____/_____
     rt   v   rt   suffix

_____

10. pelvimetry (4.91)

_____/_____/_____
       rt   v   suffix

_____

11. aberrant (4.103)

_____/_____
       pre   rt

_____

12. adduction (4.106)

_____/_____/_____
       pre   rt   suffix

_____

13. myelodysplasia (4.24)

_____/_____/_____/_____
     rt   v   pre   suffix

_____

14. abdominocentesis (4.120)

_____/_____/_____
       rt   v   suffix

_____

15. thoracotomy (4.138)

_____   _____/_____/_____
       rt   v   suffix

_____

16. periosteum (4.69)

_____/_____
       pre   rt/suffix

_____

17. hydrophobia (4.152)

_____/_____
       pre   rt/suffix

_____

18. orthopedist (4.71)

_____/_____/_____/_____
     rt   v   rt   suffix

_____

REVIEW ACTIVITIES

19. hypochondriac (4.57)

_____/_____/_____
pre   rt   suffix

_____

20. cephalopelvic (4.95)

_____/_____/_____/_____
rt   v   rt   suffix

_____

21. cystoscopy (4.130)

_____/_____/_____
rt   v   suffix

_____

22. adhesion (4.114)

_____/_____/_____
pre   rt   suffix

_____

23. bursectomy (4.42)

_____/_____
rt   suffix

_____

24. tendinitis (4.40)

_____/_____
rt   suffix

_____

25. osteosarcoma (4.15)

_____/_____/_____/_____
rt   v   rt   suffix

_____

26. orthotic (4.72)

_____/_____/_____
rt   v   suffix

_____

27. prosthetist (4.72)

_____/_____
rt   suffix

_____

28. hydrocele (4.146)

_____/_____
pre   suffix

_____

29. poliomyelitis (4.18)

_____/_____/_____/_____
rt   v   rt   suffix

_____

30. osteopenia (4.13)

_____/_____/_____
rt   v   suffix

_____

REVIEW ACTIVITIES

31. rheumatology (4.37)

_____/_____/_____
    rt   v   suffix

_____

32. meniscectomy (4.54)

_____/_____
    rt   suffix

_____

33. osteoarthritis (4.33)

_____/_____/_____/_____
    rt   v   rt   suffix

_____

34. dentoid (4.64)

_____/_____
    rt   suffix

_____

IMAGE LABELING 1

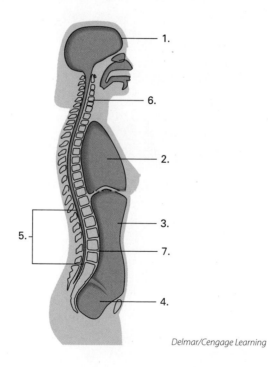

Delmar/Cengage Learning

Label the diagram by placing the number in front of the correct combining form.

Write the body part name.

_____ pelv/o/i   _____

_____ crani/o   _____

_____ thorac/o   _____

_____ abdomin/o   _____

REVIEW ACTIVITIES

_____ lumb/o   _____

_____ oste/o   _____

_____ arthr/o   _____

IMAGE LABELING 2

Label the diagram by placing the number in front of the combining form or structure name.

Label Number	Combining Form	Structure Name

Label Number   **Combining Form**   **Structure Name**

_____ tendin/o   _____

_____ chondr/o   _____

_____ my/o   _____

_____ arthr/o   _____

_____ oste/o   _____

_____ _____   fascia

_____ _____   ligament

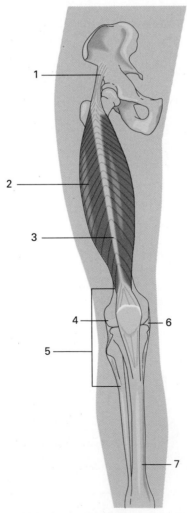

Delmar/Cengage Learning

REVIEW ACTIVITIES

IMAGE LABELING 3

Label each region of the abdomen.

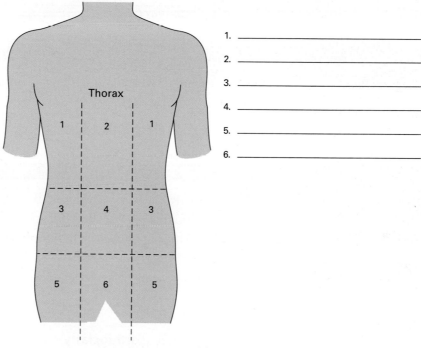

1. _____
2. _____
3. _____
4. _____
5. _____
6. _____

Delmar/Cengage Learning

ABBREVIATION MATCHING

Match the following abbreviations with their definition.

_____ 1. CPD

_____ 2. LLQ

_____ 3. OA

_____ 4. H_2O

_____ 5. PPS

_____ 6. Fx

_____ 7. cysto

_____ 8. RA

_____ 9. PT

_____ 10. FAS

a. cerebropulmonary disease

b. fracture

c. fetal alcohol syndrome

d. cephalopelvic disproportion

e. left upper quadrant

f. hydrogen

g. orthopedist

h. osteoarthritis

i. right abdomen

j. bladder

k. rheumatoid arthritis

l. physician therapist

m. cystoscopy

n. left lower quadrant

o. physical therapist

p. water

q. doctor of dental surgery

r. post-polio syndrome

REVIEW ACTIVITIES

ABBREVIATION FILL-IN

Fill in the blanks with the correct abbreviations.

11. An alcoholic experiencing withdrawal symptoms may get the _____.

12. The liver is located in the _____ of the abdomen.

13. DOs may use _____ as treatment to relieve back pain.

14. A dentist is indicated by the abbreviation _____.

15. The department that cares for patients with bone fractures is _____.

CASE STUDY

Write the term next to its meaning given below. Then draw slashes to analyze the word parts. Note the use of medical abbreviations. Look these up in your dictionary or find them in Appendix B. If you have any questions about the answers, refer to your medical dictionary or check with your instructor for the answers in Appendix E.

CASE STUDY 4-1

Report Summary

Preoperative diagnosis: Septic **arthritis** of the left knee

Orthopedic procedure: **Arthroscopic** examination, culture, **arthroplasty** left knee

A large bore cannula was introduced from the upper and **medial** quadrant of the knee joint through a stab **incision** (**arthrotomy**). The trocar was removed and **pyorrhea** was observed. A swab was sent for culture. All pus was aspirated and the knee joint irrigated then inflated with 3 L of saline. The **arthroscope** was introduced through the inferior lateral quadrant of the knee through a similar stab incision. The knee was inspected and the entire field looked inflamed. The **patella** showed grade 2 **chondromalacia**, and the patella was tilted only in contact with the lateral condyle at about 30 degrees suggesting chronic patellar malalignment. The medial meniscus showed evidence of much more **inflammation** than the condyle, the margins thick, and fraying. . . . The scope was moved to the **mediolateral** side and inspected. . . . A motorized synovial cutter was introduced, and a partial synovectomy was performed; the soft cartilage of the patellar facets were shaved. The ends of the meniscus were trimmed (**meniscectomy**). The wound was irrigated with saline, Maracaine instilled, and a hemovac drain inserted through one of the cannulas before the instruments were removed. A padded dressing and knee immobilizer was applied and hemovac attached to its bag. The patient was transferred to the recovery room in excellent condition.

1. reddened and swollen _____

2. instrument used to look into a joint _____

3. pertaining to the middle and side _____

4. excision of the meniscus _____

5. softening of the cartilage _____

6. inflammation of a joint _____

7. pertaining to the use of an arthroscope _____

8. kneecap _____

9. pertaining to bone specialty _____

10. middle _____

REVIEW ACTIVITIES

11. discharge of pus   _____

12. cut into   _____

13. incision into a joint   _____

14. surgical repair of a joint _____

CROSSWORD PUZZLE

Check your answers by going back through the frames or checking the solution in Appendix F.

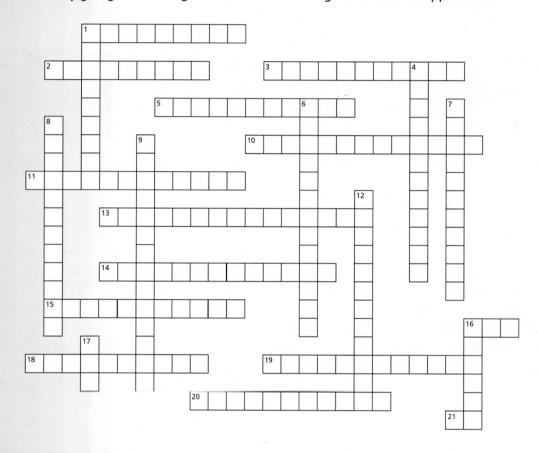

Across

1. tissues growing together that normally do not
2. pertaining to the abdomen
3. tissue around the teeth
5. physician (DO)
10. synonym for tenoplasty
11. excision of cartilage
13. surgical puncture to remove fluid from chest
14. pertaining to ribs and cartilage
15. area above the lower back or waist
16. post-polio syndrome (abbr.)
18. inflamed tendon
19. bone cancer
20. person who develops artificial limbs
21. rheumatoid arthritis (abbr.)

Down

1. raising arm to the side away from the middle
4. used to measure chest circumference
6. enlarged head due to fluid (congenital)
7. process of examining a joint with a scope
8. specialist in straightening teeth
9. defective development of bone marrow
12. condition of porous bones
16. suffix for development
17. dentist (abbr.)

REVIEW ACTIVITIES

GLOSSARY

abdomen	belly area, cavity below the thorax		cystoplasty	surgical repair of the urinary bladder
abdominocentesis	surgical puncture of the abdomen to remove fluid		cystoscopy	process of examining the bladder using a scope
abduct	move away from the midline (verb)		cystotomy	incision into the urinary bladder
abduction	movement away from the midline, e.g., arm abducted from side		dentalgia	tooth pain
			dentist	specialist in care of teeth
aberrant	wandering from normal location, process, or behavior		dentoid	resembling a tooth
abnormal	deviating from the average or expected		dysplasia	poor or defective development
			etiology	study of the origin of a disease
addiction	habitual attraction, may include physical dependence		fascia	tissue that connects muscle to muscle
adhesions	tissues grown together that are normally separate		fracture	break or crack
			hydrocele	serous fluid accumulation in a saclike cavity (Example: testicular hernia)
amniocentesis	surgical puncture of the amnion to obtain cells for testing		hydrocephalus	fluid in the skull causing deformity and brain damage
arthritis	inflammation of a joint		hydrocyst	fluid-filled sac
arthroplasty	surgical repair or reconstruction of a joint		hydrophobia	abnormal fear of water, rabies
arthroscope	instrument used to look into a joint		hydrotherapy	therapy using water
arthroscopy	process of using an arthroscope to examine a joint		hyperplasia	abnormally increased development referring to quantity of cells
arthrotomy	incision into a joint		interchondral	pertaining to between the cartilage (intercartilaginous)
bursa	serous sac between a tendon and bone (pl. bursae)		intercostal	pertaining to between the ribs
bursectomy	excision of a bursa		interdental	pertaining to between the teeth
bursitis	inflammation of a bursa		kyphosis	(hunch back) posterior thoracic curvature
cardiocentesis	surgical puncture of the heart to remove fluid		ligament	tissue that connects bone to bone and supports visceral organs
chondralgia, chondrodynia	cartilage pain		lumbar	pertaining to the lower back, between the thorax and sacrum
chondrectomy	excision of cartilage		meniscitis	inflammation of the meniscus
chondrocostal, costochondral	pertaining to cartilage and rib		meniscectomy	excision of the meniscus of the knee
costectomy	excision of a rib		myelocytes	bone marrow cells
cystocele	herniation of the urinary bladder (into the vagina)		myelodysplasia	defective development of the bone marrow or spinal cord

REVIEW ACTIVITIES

orthodontics	dental practice of straightening teeth	periodontist	dentist specializing in treatment of diseased tissue around the teeth
orthodontist	dentist specializing in straightening teeth	periosteum	around the bone (membrane)
orthopedist	physician specialist in treatment of skeletal and joint disorders	poliomyelitis	inflammation of gray matter of the spinal cord
orthotics	pertaining to appliances used to support muscoloskeletal system	prosthesis	artificial limb or other body part replacement
orthotist	specialist who develops and assists patients with orthotics	prosthetics	pertaining to prostheses
osteitis	inflammation of the bone	prosthetist	specialist who develops and assists patients with prostheses
osteoarthritis	inflammation of the bone and joint	pubic	pertaining to the pubis, bone in the lower anterior pelvis
osteoarthropathy	disease of bone and joint	rheumatology	study of rhematic disease
osteochondritis	inflammation of the bone and cartilage	supracostal	above the ribs
osteoma	bone tumor	supracranial	above or on top of the skull
osteomalacia	softening of the bone	supralumbar	above the lumbar spine
osteomyelitis	inflammation of the bone and bone marrow	suprapubic	above the pubis
osteopathic	pertaining to the practice of osteopathic physicians or bone disease	tenalgia, tenodynia	tendon pain
		tendinitis	inflammation of a tendon
osteopathy	disease of the bones	tendon	tissue that connects muscle to bone
osteopenia	loss of bone	tendinoplasty, tenoplasty, tendoplasty	surgical repair of a tendon
osteoporosis	porous condition of the bone due to deterioration of bone matrix		
osteosarcoma	cancer of the bone	thoracocentesis, thoracentesis	surgical puncture of the thorax to remove fluid
pelvis	the bony structure including the ilium, ischium, pubis, sacrum, and coccyx	thoracolumbar	pertaining to the chest and lower spine
		thoracometer	instrument used to measure the chest
pericardium	around the heart (membrane)	thoracopathy	disease of the chest
perichondrium	around the cartilage (membrane)	thoracotomy	incision into the thorax
periodontal	around the tooth	thorax	chest, area of the back posterior to the chest (pl. thoraces)

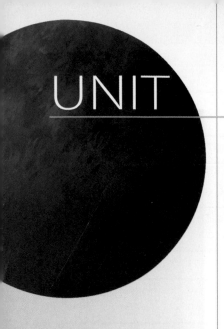

5

Pathology, Otorhinolaryngology, and Prefixes dys-, brady-, tachy-, poly-, syn-

ANSWER COLUMN

5.1

INFORMATION FRAME

Path/o/logy is the specialty that studies diseases and is especially concerned about infectious disease. Infections may be caused by many different kinds of path/o/genic organisms including micro-organisms. Bacteria, viruses, fungi, and parasites all have pathogenic forms that may cause infection or infestation. Pronouncing their names is a challenge and takes practice.

5.2

TAKE A CLOSER LOOK

In words such as carcinoma and coccus, the first "c" is pronounced as a hard "c" with a "k" sound. When followed by o, u, a, or a consonant, "c" is pronounced with a "k" sound, e.g., coat, cut, cake, cluck.

In the words colon and cardiac, the "c" is pronounced with a

* _____ sound.

NOTE: Listen to the Audio CD that accompanies this text for coaching on pronunciation.

hard "c" or "k"
(pronounce them aloud)
kō' lən
kär' dē ək

5.3

TAKE A CLOSER LOOK

In the words cerebrum and incision, the "c" is pronounced with a soft "c" or "s" sound. When "c" is followed by i, e, or y, it is pronounced with a soft "c" or "s" sound, e.g., city, cereal, cycle.

5.4

According to the "c" rule, in the words cystocele and encephalitis each "c" is

pronounced with a * _____ sound.
Remember the "c" rule for those terms that follow.

soft "c" or "s"

ANSWER COLUMN

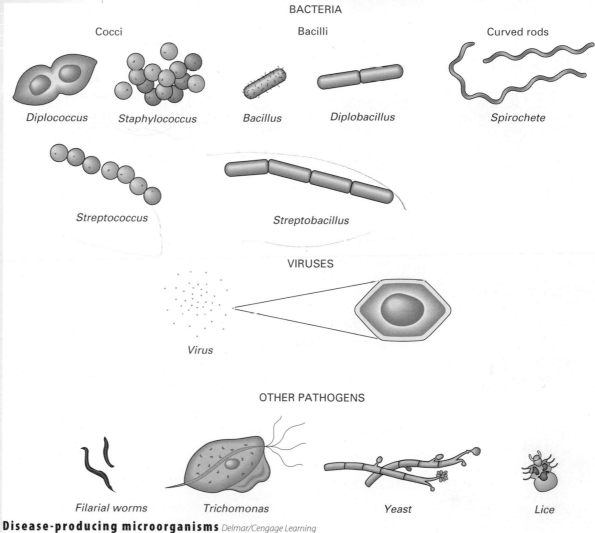

BACTERIA

Cocci

Diplococcus   Staphylococcus

Streptococcus

Bacilli

Bacillus   Diplobacillus

Streptobacillus

Curved rods

Spirochete

VIRUSES

Virus

OTHER PATHOGENS

Filarial worms   Trichomonas   Yeast   Lice

Disease-producing microorganisms *Delmar/Cengage Learning*

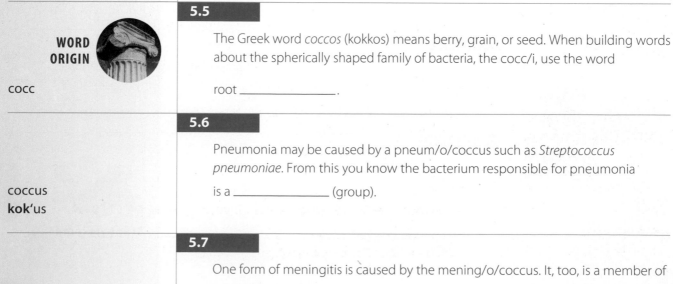

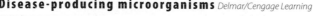

5.5

WORD
ORIGIN

cocc

The Greek word *coccos* (kokkos) means berry, grain, or seed. When building words about the spherically shaped family of bacteria, the cocc/i, use the word

root _____.

5.6

coccus
kok′us

Pneumonia may be caused by a pneum/o/coccus such as *Streptococcus pneumoniae*. From this you know the bacterium responsible for pneumonia

is a _____ (group).

5.7

cocci
kok′ sī

One form of meningitis is caused by the mening/o/coccus. It, too, is a member of

the (plural group) _____.

5.8

There are three main types of cocci: diplococci, streptococci, and staphylococci.

cocci
kok′ si

Cocci growing in pairs are diplo/ _____.

5.9

Gon/o/rrhea is a sexually transmitted bacterial infection caused by *Neisseria gonorrhoeae*. This gon/o/coccus grows in pairs, so it is a

dipl/o/cocc/us
dip′lō **kok′** us

_____/_____/_____.

5.10

cocci

Cocci growing in twisted chains are strept/o/ _____.

cocci

Cocci growing in clusters are staphyl/o/_____.

5.11

strept/o means twisted chains or strips. Streptococci (strep) grow in twisted chains as shown here. If you should see a chain of cocci when examining a slide under the microscope, you would say they were

strept/o/cocc/i
strep′ tō **kok′** sī

_____/_____/_____/_____.

Streptococcus *Delmar/ Cengage Learning*

5.12

Name the type of coccus in the following statements. Sore throat may be caused by a spherical bacteria growing in twisted chains called

strept/o/cocc/us
Strept/o/cocc/us

_____/_____/_____/_____. A pus-forming bacteria

is _____/_____/_____/_____ *pyogenes*.

5.13

Staphyle is the Greek word for bunch of grapes. **staphyl/o** is used to build words that suggest growing in bunches like grapes. Staphylococci (staph)

grapes

grow in clusters like a bunch of _____.

5.14

Staphylococci grow in clusters like grapes. If you should see a cluster of cocci when using the microscope, you would say they were

staphyl/o/cocc/i
staf i lō **kok′** sī

_____/_____/_____/_____.

Staphylococcus *Delmar/ Cengage Learning*

ANSWER COLUMN

Impetigo pustules caused by either streptococcus or staphylococcus *Courtesy of Robert A. Silverman, MD, Pediatric Dermatology, Georgetown University*

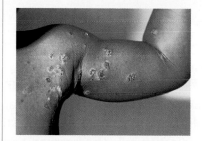

5.15

Methicillin-resistant *Staphylococcus aureas* (MRSA) is a bacterium that causes a serious infection that is difficult to treat because it is resistant to many different antibiotics. This type of infection is most common in the elderly and those with poor immune systems. Healthcare workers wear gloves and wash their hands when caring for these at-risk patients to help prevent the spread of Methicillin-

Staphylococcus
staf ə lō **kok'**us

resistant _____ aureas.

5.16

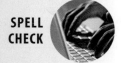

SPELL CHECK

Proper genus and species names are used to identify bacteria and parasites. They are italicized with the genus name capitalized, for example: *Staphylococcus aureus*, *Escherichia coli*. When abbreviating, you may use the genus initial and the species name. The genus initial is capitalized but the phrase is not italicized, for example: S. aureus, E. coli.

5.17

dipl/o/bacill/us
dip' lō ba **sil'** us

strept/o/bacill/us
strep' tō ba **sil'** us

In Latin *baculus* means staff or rod. A *bacillus* (plural *bacilli*) is a rod-shaped bacterium (plural *bacteria*). Use bacillus to form a term that means a rod-shaped double bacillus

_____/_____/_____/_____;
a rod-shaped bacillus growing in twisted chains

_____/_____/_____/_____.
Now, you've got it!

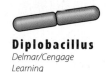

Diplobacillus
Delmar/Cengage Learning

5.18

bacill/i
bə **sil'** ī

Klebsiella pneumoniae, a pneum/o/bacill/us, is a common cause of pneumonia. These rod-shaped bacteria are _____/_____ .

HINT: The word bacteria is plural, so the plural form is needed to complete this statement correctly. Bacterium is singular.

5.19

bacterium
bak **ter'** ē um
bacilli
bə **sil'** ī

The plural term bacteria is normally used because we rarely find one bacterium. Remember the plural rule: **-um** is singular, **-a** is plural.

The singular of bacteria is _____.
Now try this one: If the plural of coccus is cocci, the plural of bacillus

is _____.
Good.

CASE STUDY INVESTIGATION (CSI)

E. Coli Infection

Escherichia coli 0157:H7 (**enterohemorrhagic** E. coli) is a normal flora **bacillus** bacteria living in balance with other organisms inhabiting the intestine in humans and animals. When this **bacterium** is ingested in large amounts it can cause a food-borne infection called **hemorrhagic colitis**. Undercooked or raw ground beef, unpasteurized fruit juices and milk, dry-cured meats, game meat, and contaminated vegetables have been implicated in many of the documented outbreaks. Patients present with the following symptoms: severe abdominal pain and cramping, **diarrhea**, watery and/or bloody stool, low-grade or absent **fever,** and occasional vomiting. The illness lasts an average of eight days and is self-limiting in healthy individuals. Infants, young children, the elderly, and those with immune compromise may develop severe life-threatening conditions including kidney failure due to **hemolytic** uremic **syndrome** (HUS).

CSI Vocabulary Challenge

Use your dictionary if necessary to look up the following terms presented in this case study and write their definition in the space provided. Analyze terms by dividing them into their word parts and drawing the slashes.

enterohemorrhagic _____

bacillus _____

bacterium _____

hemorrhagic _____

colitis _____

diarrhea _____

fever _____

hemolytic _____

syndrome _____

5.20

Most bacteria that form pus grow in a cluster.

staphylococci

They are _____ .

5.21

A common form of food poisoning is caused by fresh foods prepared

staphyl/o/cocc/i

with creamy dressing contaminated with

_____ / _____ / _____ / _____ .

5.22

staphyl/o/ cocc/us
staf′ ə lō **kok′** us

A common skin bacterium responsible for acne infections

is _____ / _____ / _____ / _____ .

ANSWER COLUMN

Acne pustule *Photo by Timothy J. Dennerll, RT(R), Ph.D.*

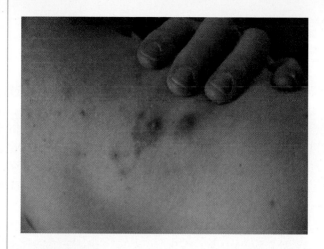

5.23

Staphyl/o is also used to represent the uvula. Surgical repair of the uvula

is _____/_____/_____ .

staphyl/o/plasty
staf′ i lō plas′ tē

Sexually Transmitted Diseases (STDs)	
Causative Agent	**Disease**
Bacteria	
Chlamydia trachomatis	Chlamydia, urogenital infection
Neisseria gonorrhoeae	gonorrhea (clap)
Treponema pallidum	syphilis
Viruses	
hepatitis B virus (HBV)	hepatitis
human immunodeficiency virus (HIV)	HIV infection, which converts to AIDS (acquired immunodeficiency syndrome)
human papilloma virus (HPV)	condylomata acuminata (venereal warts)
herpes simplex virus (HSV)	genital herpes lesions
Parasites	
Trichomonas vaginalis	trichomoniasis, urogenital infection
Phthirus pubis	lice, pediculosis pubis (crabs)
Sarcoptes scabiei	scabies (mites)
Fungi	
Candida albicans	candidiasis (yeast infection)

5.24

inflammation of the uvula

Staphyl/itis (uvul/itis) means *_____ .

5.25

excision of the uvula
yōō′ vyōō lə

Staphyl/ectomy (uvul/ectomy) means _____ .

ANSWER COLUMN

5.26

Staphyl/o, from the Greek, means cluster of grapes. **uvul/o**, from the Latin word meaning cluster of grapes, is also used when referring to the palatine uvula. Build words meaning inflammation of the uvula

_____/_____ or _____/_____;

removal of the uvula

_____/_____ or _____/_____.

staphyl/itis
staf' i **lī**' tis
uvul/itis
yōō' vyōō **lī**' tis
staphyl/ectomy
staf' i **lek**' tō mē
uvul/ectomy
yōō' vyōō **lek**' tō mē

5.27

py/o is the combining form used for words involving pus. A py/o/cele is a hernia containing _____.

pus

5.28

-**genic** is the adjectival form of the suffix -**genesis**, meaning producing or forming. Many staphylococci are pyogenic. Bacteria that produce pus are

_____/_____/_____/_____.

py/o/gen/ic
pī' ō **jen**' ik

5.29

Try this one. Remember that **onc/o** refers to tumors. If a condition or substance promotes tumor production, it is said to be

_____/_____/_____/_____.

If organisms produce disease, they are

_____/_____/_____/_____.

Good try.

onc/o/gen/ic
on' kō **jen**' ik
path/o/gen/ic
pa' thō **jen**' ik

5.30

Now build the noun form of the term that means:
producing cancer

_____/_____/_____;

producing pus

_____/_____/_____;

producing disease

_____/_____/_____.

onc/o/genesis
on kō **jen**' ə sis

py/o/genesis
pī ō **jen**' ə sis

path/o/genesis
path ō **jen**' ə sis

ANSWER COLUMN

5.31

py/o/thorax
pī′ ō **thôr′** aks

Py/o/thorax means an accumulation of pus in the thoracic cavity. When pus-forming bacteria invade the thoracic lining, _____/_____/_____ results.

5.32

pyothorax

Pneumonia (fluid and infection) and lung abcess are two other diseases causing

_____.

5.33

py/o/gen/ic
pī′ ō **jen′** ik

A py/o/gen/ic bacterium is one that forms pus. You may know the noun genesis, meaning creation or beginning, as in the words generate and generation. The adjective that means something that produces or forms pus is

_____/_____/_____/_____.

5.34

pyogenic

Pyogenic bacteria are found in boils. Boils become purulent (contain pus). This pus is formed by _____ bacteria.

5.35

pyogenic

Look up purulent in your medical dictionary. It means pus forming

or _____.

Structures of the mouth
Delmar/Cengage Learning

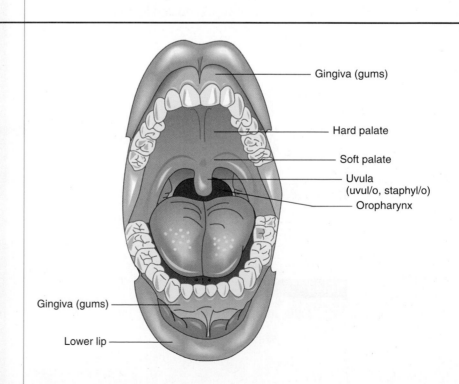

- Gingiva (gums)
- Hard palate
- Soft palate
- Uvula (uvul/o, staphyl/o)
- Oropharynx
- Gingiva (gums)
- Lower lip

ANSWER COLUMN

5.36

-rrhea is a suffix meaning flow or discharge. Think of dia/rrhea, which means to flow through.

flow or discharge of pus

Py/o/rrhea means * _____.

5.37

SPELL CHECK

The "rrh" in -rrhea is an unusual spelling for English words. It comes from the Greek language.

There will be three more suffixes with "rrh" in their spelling in future frames: **-rrhagia** (hemorrhage), **-rrhaphy** (suturing), and **-rrhexia** (rupture).

-rrhea

To indicate flow or discharge use the suffix _____.

5.38

py/o

Py/o/rrhea alveolaris is a disease of the teeth and gums. The part of this disease's name that tells you that pus is discharged is _____/_____.

5.39

py/o/rrhea
pī ō **rē′** ə

There is also a disease of a salivary gland for which there is a flow of pus.

This is _____/_____/_____ salivaris.

5.40

ear
ear
ear

ot is a Greek word root meaning ear. Ot/o/rrhea means a discharge from the ear.

ot/o is the combining form for _____.

An ot/o/scope is used to examine the _____.

An ot/ic solution is prepared for treatment of the _____.

5.41

ot/o/scopy
ō **tos′** kō pē

ot/ic
ō′ tik

The process of examining the ear using an otoscope is called

_____/_____/_____.

The term that means pertaining to the ear is _____/_____.

5.42

ot/o/rrhea
ō tō **rē′** ə

Ot/o/rrhea is both a sign and a disease. No matter which is meant, the word

_____/_____/_____ is used for a discharge from the ear(s).

5.43

otorrhea

Otitis media involves discharge, inflammation, and deafness. One of the signs of this disease is discharge or _____.

ANSWER COLUMN

**Otoscope with
different sized
reusable specula**
Delmar/Cengage Learning

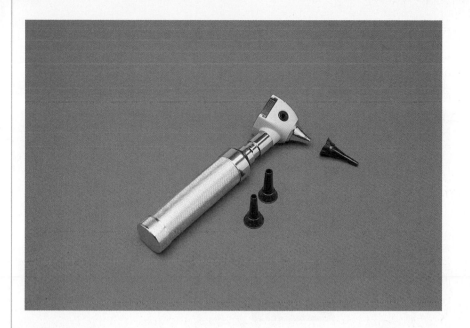

5.44

Otorrhea may be caused by ot/itis media (OM), an infection in the middle ear causing inflammation and discharge. Ot/itis means

inflammation of the ear

* _____ .

5.45

ot/algia
ō **tal'** jē ə
ot/o/dynia
ō tō **din'** ē ə

Auris sinistra (AS) refers to the left ear. Auris dextra (AD) refers to the right ear, and auris uterque (AU) to both ears. Ot/itis media causes pain in ears which are inflamed.

Ear pain is _____/_____ or _____/_____/_____ .

Structures of the ear
Delmar/Cengage Learning

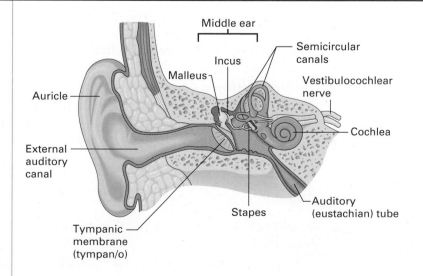

Middle ear

Auricle

Malleus

Incus

Semicircular
canals

Vestibulocochlear
nerve

Cochlea

External
auditory
canal

Stapes

Auditory
(eustachian) tube

Tympanic
membrane
(tympan/o)

STUDY**WARE**™ C O N N E C T I O N

View an animation about *How We Hear* on your **StudyWARE™ CD-ROM.**

ANSWER COLUMN	

5.46

otodynia *or* otalgia

When otitis media is prolonged, there has usually been enough destruction of the tissue that _____ (ear pain) no longer occurs.

5.47

otodynia *or* otalgia

Small children often complain of earache. Medically, this could be called _____.

5.48

eardrum

Recall that AS (auris sinistra) refers to the left ear and AD (auris dextra) refers to the right ear. Membrana tympani dextra (MTD) refers to the right eardrum. Membrana tympani sinistra (MTS) refers to the left _____.

CASE STUDY I N V E S T I G A T I O N (C S I)

Otitis Media
A 3-year-old girl is brought to the office by her mother reporting that her daughter is complaining of right ear **otalgia.** She has no significant medical history. The child is not happy to be in the office and is crying. Her mother explains that she developed a "cold" about two days ago with **rhinorrhea** and has been pulling on her right ear. Her temperature is 37.8°C (100°F), and the rest of the physical examination is completed. On examination the nose is full of thick green **mucus,** the **tympanic** membranes are red, and there is evidence of fluid in the middle ear. Treatment with **antibiotics** is recommended.

CSI Vocabulary Challenge
Use your dictionary if necessary to look up the following terms presented in this case study and write their definition in the space provided. Analyze terms by dividing them into their word parts and drawing the slashes.

otitis _____

otalgia _____

rhinorrhea _____

mucus _____

tympanic _____

antibiotics _____

ANSWER COLUMN

5.49

eardrum
tympan/o

Look up tympanum in your dictionary. The tympanum is the _____.

One combining form for tympanum is _____/_____.

5.50

Build a word meaning:

tympan/ic
tim **pan'** ik

pertaining to the eardrum _____/_____;

tympan/o/tomy
tim' pə **not'** ə mē

incision into the eardrum _____/_____/_____;

tympan/ectomy
tim' pə **nek'** tə mē

excision of the eardrum _____/_____.

NOTE: A common synonym for tympan/o/tomy is myring/o/tomy (mī rin **got'** ə mē). Both are incisions for the purpose of inserting tubes in the eadrum.

5.51

Recall that **metr** is the word root for measure. **-metry** indicates the process of measuring. The process of measuring the function of the eardrum is called

tympan/o/metry
tim' pə **nom'** ə trē

_____/_____/_____.

5.52

In your dictionary, using the word root tympan, find a word that means distended with gas—as tight as a drum. The word is

tympan/ites
tim' pə **nī'** tēz

_____/_____.

5.53

If a patient complains of a very bloated, gassy feeling and has a distended

tympanites

abdomen, the doctor may write _____ on the chart.

5.54

Study the following prefixes to be used to build words related to voice, speaking, breathing, heart rate, swallowing, and digestion.

Prefix	Meaning	Example
a-	not, lack of (before a consonant)	a/genesis
an-	not, lack of (before a vowel)	an/emia
brady-	abnormally slow	brady/phagia
dys-	difficult, abnormal, poor, painful	dys/pepsia
tachy-	abnormally fast	tachy/cardia

ANSWER COLUMN

5.55

audi/o is a combining form for hearing. The study of hearing is audi/o/logy. Build terms that mean an instrument used to measure hearing

audi/o/meter
aw' dē **om'** ət ər

_____/_____/_____;

the process of measuring hearing

audi/o/metry
aw' dē **om'** ə trē

_____/_____/_____;

a record made by the instrument used to test hearing

audi/o/gram
aw' dē ō gram

_____/_____/_____.

NOTE: An audi/ence listens in an audi/torium.

5.56

audi/o/log/ist
aw' dē **ol'** ō jist

A hearing specialist is called an _____/_____/_____/_____.

5.57

phon/o means voice or vocal sounds.
A/phonia means

unable to make sounds

*_____.

Dys/phonia means

weak voice (poor, etc.)

*_____.

PROFESSIONAL PROFILE

Audiologists are health professionals who promote healthy hearing, communication competency, and quality of life for persons of all ages through the prevention, identification, assessment, and rehabilitation of hearing, auditory function, balance, and other related systems. They facilitate prevention of hearing loss through providing the fitting of hearing protective devices, education programs for industry and the public, hearing screening/conservation programs, and research. Audiologists hold a master's or doctorate degree in audiology from a program accredited by the Council on Academic Accreditation in Audiology and Speech-Language Pathology (CAA) of the American Speech-Language-Hearing Association (ASHA). Professional certification (Certificate of Clinical Competency in Audiology (CCC-A)), licensure, or registration may also be required to pratice audiology.

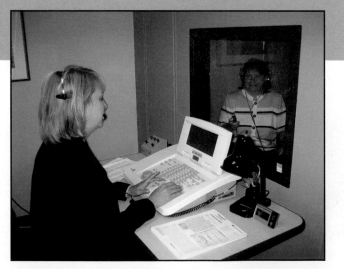

Audiologist performing audiometry *Photo by Timothy J. Dennerll, RT(R), Ph.D., courtesy of Allegiance Health, Jackson, MI*

ANSWER COLUMN

5.58

Brady/phasia means

slow speech

* _____.

A/phasia means

absence of speech

* _____.

Phon/ic means

pertaining to the voice

* _____.

A phon/o/meter is

an instrument for
measuring intensity
of vocal sounds

* _____.

_____.

5.59

Build terms that mean the study of:
voice or vocal sounds

phon/o/logy
fon **ol'** ō jē

_____/_____/_____;

hearing

audi/o/logy
aw de **ol'** ō jē

_____/_____/_____;

speech

phas/o/logy
fās **ol'** ō jē

_____/_____/_____.

5.60

-rrhea is a suffix meaning flow or discharge. Rhinorrhea means discharge from the

nose

nose. rhin/o is used in words about the _____. **-rrhea** is used to indicate

flow or discharge

* _____.

5.61

Rhinoceros is from the Greek word meaning nose-horn. Using what is necessary
from **rhin/o**, form a word that means inflammation of the nose:

rhin/itis
rī **nī'** tis

_____/_____.

5.62

Rhin/o/rrhea is a symptom. Drainage from the nose due to a head cold is a

rhin/o/rrhea
rī nō **rē'** ə

symptom called _____/_____/_____.

5.63

rhinorrhea

A discharge from the sinuses through the nose is a form of _____.

ANSWER COLUMN

Hearing aid *Delmar/Cengage Learning*

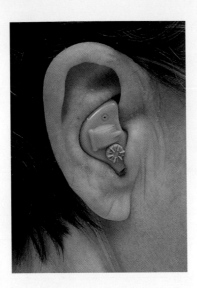

5.64

rhinorrhea

Nasal catarrh (ka tär′) is another source of _____.

5.65

rhin/o/plasty
rī′ nō plas′ tē

Build a word that means surgical repair of the nose. _____/_____/ _____

5.66

rhin/o/tomy
rī **not**′ ə mē

Form a word that means incision of the nose. _____/_____/_____

5.67

calculus or stone

A rhin/o/lith is a calculus or stone in the nose. **lith/o** is the combining form for

* _____.

5.68

calculi (calculus) or stones

lith/o/gen/ic
lith ō **jen**′ ik

-genesis is used as a noun suffix meaning generating, producing, or forming. Lith/o/genesis means producing or forming

* _____. The adjectival form of

lithogenesis is _____/_____/_____/_____.

5.69

WORD
ORIGIN

The word origin of **calculus** comes from the Latin meaning "pebble used in counting." From this ancient practice of counting stones evolved calculating and the mathmatical study of calculus. Because stones were used, the term calculus is also used to indicate a stone formed in the body. The heel bone is shaped like a stone and was named the calcaneus bone.

(continued)

ANSWER COLUMN

The word root **lith** comes from Greek for stone. A monolith is an ancient structure made of a column of one stone. Lith/iasis is the infestation of the body with stones. Lith/o/logy is the science of dealing with or studying

calculi or stones

* _____ .

5.70

Using what is necessary from **lith/o**, build a word meaning an incision for the removal of a stone _____/_____/_____ .

lith/o/tomy
li **thot′** ə mē

Name an instrument for measuring the size of calculi.

_____/_____/_____

lith/o/meter
li tho′ me ter

5.71

Calculi or stones can be formed in many places in the body. A chol/e/lith means a gallstone. **chol/e** is the combining form for * _____ .

gall or bile

5.72

Chol/e/lith means gallstone. One result of gallbladder disease is the presence of a gallstone or _____/_____/_____ .

chol/e/lith
kō′ lə lith

5.73

INFORMATION FRAME

-iasis is a suffix used to indicate a pathologic condition. **-iasis** may also be used when an infestation has occurred. Choledocholithiasis (ko led′ əko li thi″·əsis) is the presence of gallstones in the common bile duct (choledoch/o).

Cholelithiasis and ductal stones
Delmar/Cengage Learning

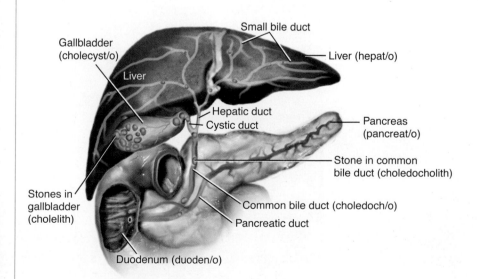

Small bile duct

Gallbladder (cholecyst/o)

Liver (hepat/o)

Liver

Hepatic duct

Cystic duct

Pancreas (pancreat/o)

Stone in common bile duct (choledocholith)

Common bile duct (choledoch/o)

Pancreatic duct

Stones in gallbladder (cholelith)

Duodenum (duoden/o)

ANSWER COLUMN

5.74

Lith/iasis is a disease condition characterized by the presence of stones (calculi). The presence of gallstones in the gallbladder is called

chol/e/lith/iasis
ko' lē lith ī' ə sis

_____/_____/_____/_____.

5.75

Look up the following terms in your medical dictionary. What is the "organism" that causes each infestation?

trichomonas

trichomoniasis _____

yeast (monilia)

moniliasis   _____

filarial worm or local inflammation of lymph nodes

elephantiasis * _____

_____

giardia lamblia

giardiasis * _____

INFORMATION FRAME

5.76

Trichomonas vaginalis is a protozoan parasite with a flagella. Trichomoniasis may infect the urinary and reproductive tracts and is considered an STD.

5.77

Bile (gall) is secreted by the gallbladder (GB). Chol/e/cyst is a medical name

gallbladder

for the _____.

Trichomonas vaginalis
Delmar/Cengage Learning

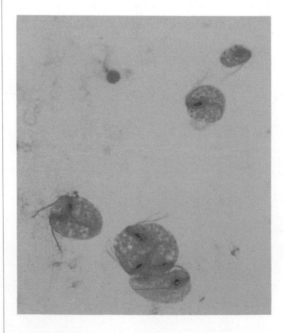

ANSWER COLUMN

5.78

Recall that **-gram** refers to a picture and **-graphy** refers to the process of taking the picture or recording. Build terms from the following meanings:

an x-ray of the gallbladder

chol/e/cyst/o/gram
kō′ lē **sist′** ō gram

_____/_____/_____/_____/_____;

chol/e/cyst/o/graphy
kō′ lē sist **og′** raf ē

the process of taking a gallbladder x-ray

_____/_____/_____/_____/_____.

5.79

Gallstones can result in inflammation of the gallbladder (chol/e/cyst). Medically,

chol/e/cyst/itis
kō′ lə sist ī′ tis

this is called _____/_____/_____/_____.

NOTE: Ultrasound (US) of the gallbladder (GB) is becoming a common procedure for diagnosing cholecystitis.

5.80

Cholecystitis is accompanied by pain and hyperemesis. Fatty foods aggravate

cholecystitis

these symptoms and should be avoided in cases of _____.

5.81

Butter, cream, and even whole milk contain fat and may have to be avoided by

cholecystitis

patients with _____.

5.82

When a cholelith causes cholecystitis, surgery may be needed. One surgical procedure is an incision into the gallbladder, called a

chol/e/cyst/o/tomy
kō′ lə sist **ot′** ə mē

_____/_____/_____/_____/_____.

5.83

Usually the presence of a gallstone calls for the excision of the gallbladder.

chol/e/cyst/ectomy
kō′ lə sist **ek′** tə mē

This is a _____/_____/_____/_____.

5.84

rhin/o/lith
rī′ nō lith

A calculus or stone in the nose is a _____/_____/_____.

5.85

slow

brady- is used in words to mean slow. Brady/cardia means _____ heart action.

ANSWER COLUMN

brady/phag/ia
brad ē **fā'** jē ə

5.86

Brady/phag/ia means slowness in eating. Abnormally slow swallowing is also called _____/_____/_____ .

bradyphagia

5.87

From brady/phagia you find the word root phag for eat. (More of phag/o later.) Slow eating is _____ .

bradyphagia

5.88

Elderly people who chew and swallow very slowly are exhibiting _____ .

brady/cardi/a
brad ē **kär'** dē ə

5.89

Abnormally slow heart action is _____/_____/_____ .

**Cholecystography
showing presence
of many gallstones**
Delmar/Cengage Learning

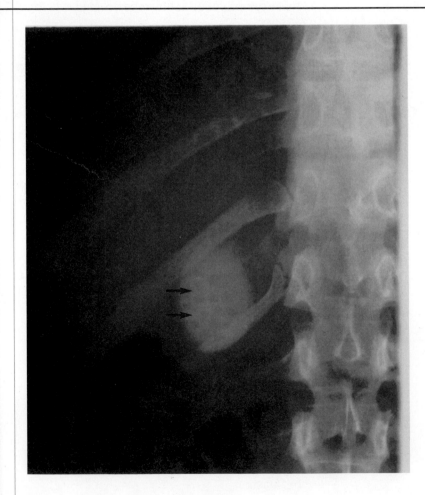

ANSWER COLUMN

5.90

tachy- is used in words to show the opposite of slow. tachy- means

fast or rapid

* _____.

5.91

rapid heart action

Tachy/cardia means * _____.

5.92

tachy/phagia
tak ē **fā'** jē ə

The word for fast eating is _____/_____ .

5.93

tach/o/gram
tak' ō gram

Tachos is a Greek word that means swiftness, as in tachometer. A record of the
velocity of the blood flow is a _____/_____/_____ .

5.94

tachy/cardi/a
tak ē **kär'** dē ə

An abnormally rapid heartbeat is called _____/_____/_____ .

5.95

respiration or breathing

pne/o comes from the Greek word *pneia*, meaning breath. **pne/o** any place
in a word means * _____.

5.96

silent

When **pne/o** begins a word, the "p" is silent. When **pne/o** occurs later in
a word, the "p" is pronounced. In pne/o/pne/ic, the first "p" is _____;
the second is pronounced (nē op' nē ik).

5.97

slow breathing

tachy/pnea
tak ip **nē'** ə *or*
tak **ip'** nē ə

-**pnea** is a suffix meaning breathing. Brady/pnea (brād ip nē' ə) means
* _____. A word for rapid breathing is
_____/_____ .

5.98

tachypnea

The rate of respiration (R) is controlled by the amount of carbon dioxide (CO_2) in the
blood. Increased carbon dioxide speeds up breathing and causes _____ .

5.99

tachypnea

Muscle exercise increases the amount of CO_2 in the blood. This speeds respiration
(R) and produces _____ .

ANSWER COLUMN

Paper speed is 25mm/sec.

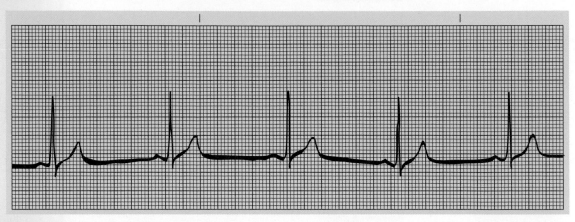

Bradycardia < 60 bpm *Delmar/Cengage Learning*

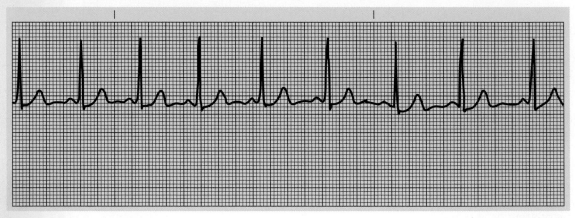

Tachycardia > 100 bpm *Delmar/Cengage Learning*

	5.100
tachypnea	Running a race causes _____ .
	5.101
without breathing	**a-** and **an-** are prefixes meaning without or lack of. A/pnea literally means * _____ .
	5.102
a/pnea ap **nē′** ə, **ap′** nē ə	Apnea means cessation of breathing. If the level of carbon dioxide in the blood falls very low, _____/_____ results.
	5.103
apnea brady/pnea brad ip **nē′** ə or brad **ip′** nē ə	When breathing ceases for a bit, _____ results. If breathing is merely very slow, it is called _____/_____ .

ANSWER COLUMN

5.104

a- and an-

The prefixes meaning without are *_____.

NOTE: **a-** and **an-** are prefixes meaning without or lack of. **a-** is used preceding a consonant. **an-** is used preceding a vowel.

5.105

without generation
(origin)

Genesis is both a Greek and an English word. It means generation (origin or beginning). A/gen/esis means *_____.

5.106

a/gen/esis
ə **jen'** ə sis

By extension, agenesis means failure to develop or lack of development. When an organ does not develop, physicians use the word

_____/_____/_____.

5.107

agenesis

Agenesis can refer to any part of the body. If a hand does not develop,

the condition is called _____ of the hand.

5.108

agenesis

When the stomach is not formed, _____ of the stomach results.

5.109

carcin/o/gen/esis
kär' si nō **jen'** ə sis

The development of cancer is called

_____/_____/_____/_____.

5.110

carcin/o/gen/ic
kär' si nō **jen'** ic

A term that means pertaining to the development of cancer is

_____/_____/_____/_____.

5.111

INFORMATION FRAME

dys- is the prefix for painful, faulty, diseased, bad, or difficult. **men/o** is the combining form for menstruation. **-rrhea** means flow or discharge.

5.112

dys/men/o/rrhea
dis' men ō **rē'** ə

Build words that mean
painful or difficult menstruation

_____/_____/_____/_____;

(continued)

ANSWER COLUMN

a/men/o/rrhea
ā′ men ō **rē**′ ə

absence of menstruation

_____/_____/_____/_____.

5.113

Dysphagia means difficult swallowing. Analyze dysphagia:

dys/phag/ia
dis **fā**′ jē ə

difficult

_____/_____/_____.

dys- in dysphagia means

_____.

5.114

Dys/trophy literally means poor development. The word for difficult breathing

dys/pnea
disp **nē**′ ə, **disp**′ nē ə

is _____/_____.

5.115

Pepsis is the Greek word for digestion. From this you get the combining form

digestion
dī **jest**′ shun

peps/o and the adjective pep/tic to use in words about _____.

5.116

digestion
dys/peps/ia
dis **pep**′ shə

Dys/peps/ia means poor _____. The result of food eaten too rapidly

may be _____/_____/_____.

5.117

dyspepsia

Dyspeps/ia is a noun. Eating under tension also may cause _____.

5.118

a/peps/ia
a **pep**′ shə
brady/peps/ia
brad i **pep**′ shə
pept/ic
pep′ tik

Cessation of digestion (without digestion) is _____/_____/_____,

while slow digestion is _____/_____/_____, and

stomach ulcers are _____/_____ ulcers.

5.119

a/rrhythm/ia
ā **rith**′ mē ə

a/rrhythm/ia is a condition in which there is loss of correct rhythm. If the heart

beat is too slow or too fast this would be an _____/_____/_____.

5.120

a/rrhythm/ias
ā **rith**′ mē əs

Tachycardia and bradycardia are types of _____/_____/_____.
(plural)

ANSWER COLUMN

5.121

SPELL CHECK

A synonym for arrhythmia is dys/rrhythm/ia. This also indicates an irregular or abnormal rhythm. Both of these terms are spelled with an "rrh"—pronounced like an "r," and a "y"—pronounced like an "i." These are typical of Greek origin words but not so familiar in English. For review recall the terms listed below with "rrh" in their spellings:

rhin/o/rrhea	rī nō **rē'** ə
ot/o/rrhea	ō tō **rē'** ə
a/rrhythm/ia	ā **rith'** mē ə
dys/rrhythm/ia	dis **rith'** mē ə

5.122

dys/lex/ia
dis **leks'** ē ə

Lexis is a Greek word meaning word or phrase. Students with normal to above level intelligence but who have difficulty recognizing words and may transpose letters or numbers may have a condition known as dys/lex/ia. Special learning skills may need to be used by students with _____/_____/_____.

5.123

dys/phag/ia

dys/phon/ia

dys/lex/ia

dys/phas/ia

Use what you have learned in the past few frames to build terms that mean a condition characterized by difficulty:

swallowing _____/_____/_____;

vocalizing _____/_____/_____;

reading and putting letters in order _____/_____/_____;

speaking _____/_____/_____.

5.124

therm/o/meter
thûr' **mom'** ə tər

Normal average body temperature is 37°C or 98.6°F. **therm/o**, from th Greek word *thermos*, is the combining form that means heat. An instrument to measure heat is a _____/_____/_____ which may be calibrated in Celsius or Fahrenheit.

Correlation between Celsius and Fahrenheit scales *Delmar/Cengage Learning*

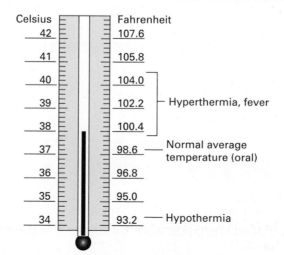

Celsius	Fahrenheit	
42	107.6	
41	105.8	
40	104.0	
39	102.2	Hyperthermia, fever
38	100.4	
37	98.6	Normal average temperature (oral)
36	96.8	
35	95.0	
34	93.2	Hypothermia

ANSWER COLUMN

5.125

Build words meaning
pertaining to heat

therm/al, therm/ic
thûr′ məl, **thur′** mik

_____/_____;

therm/o/esthesi/a
thûr′ mō es **thēs′** ē ə

oversensitivity to heat _____/_____/esthes/ia;

therm/o/algesia
thûr′ mō al **jēs′** ē ə

_____/_____/algesia

formation of (body) heat

therm/o/gen/esis
thûr′ mō **jen′** ə sis

_____/_____/gen/esis.

5.126

Build a word meaning abnormal fear of heat

therm/o/phobia
thûr′ mō **fō′** bē ə

_____/_____/_____;

heatstroke (paralysis)

therm/o/plegia
thûr′ mō **plē′** jē ə

_____/_____/plegia;

heating through tissue (treatment)

dia/therm/y
di′ ə thûr mē

dia/_____/_____.

5.127

Diarrhea literally means to flow through and refers to a watery bowel movement
(BM). Dia/therm/y means generating heat through (tissues).

through

dia- means _____;

heat

therm means _____;

suffix

-y is a noun _____.

5.128

**TAKE A
CLOSER LOOK**

Body temperature above 101°F can indicate fever. For information about
temperature scales or variations in body temperature, look in the dictionary
for words beginning with

therm or therm/o

* _____.

(Try it!)

STUDYWARE™ CONNECTION

Remember, after completing this unit, you can play a championship or other interactive game on
your **StudyWARE™ CD-ROM** that will help you learn the content in this chapter.

ANSWER COLUMN

5.129

hyper/therm/ia
hī' per **thûr'** mē ə
hypo/therm/ia
hī' pō **thûr'** mē ə

Using **hyper-** and **hypo-**, build a word that means

high body temperature (fever) _____/_____/_____ ;

low body temperature _____/_____/_____ .

Vital Signs Normal Values*				
	Infant	**6-Year-Old**	**14-Year-Old**	**Adult**
Blood pressure (BP)	65–122 / 30–84	85–115 / 48–64	99–120 / 50 70	100–120 / 60–80
Respirations (R)	30–50	16–22	14–20	12–20
Pulse (P)	100–170	70–115	60–110	60–100
All Ages				

Temperature (T)
Oral (PO)   98.6°F, 37°C
Rectal (R)   99°F, 37.7°C
Axillary (AX)   97.6°F, 36.4°C

*2009 update National Institutes of Health/U. S. Department of Health and Human Services.

5.130

micro- means small. Hydro/cephal/us is a condition involving fluid in the head. A condition of an abnormally small head is called

micro/cephal/us
mī' krō **sef'** ə ləs

_____/_____/_____ .

5.131

Microcephalus limits the size of the brain. Most microcephalic people are mentally impaired. Occasionally a baby is born with an unusually small head,

microcephalus

or _____ .

5.132

A cyst is a sac containing fluid.
A very small cyst is a

micro/cyst
mī' krō sist

_____/_____ .

A very small cell is a

micro/cyte
mī' krō sīt

_____/_____ .

A condition of having a small heart is

micro/cardi/a
mī' krō **kär'** dē ə

_____/_____/_____ .

(continued)

ANSWER COLUMN

micro/gram
mī′ krō gram

One thousandth of a milligram (0.001 mg) is a _____/_____ (mcg) (0.000001 g one millionth of a gram).

5.133

Surgery performed on minute structures using a microscope and small instruments is _____/_____.

micro/surgery
mī′ krō **sûr′** jər ē

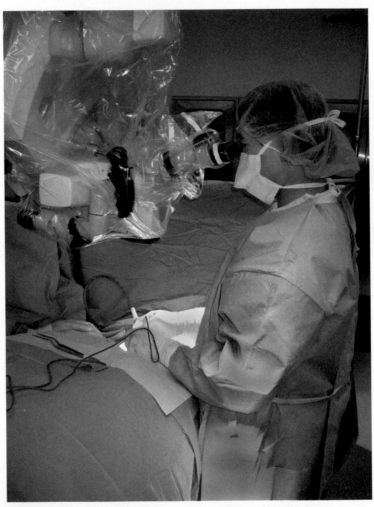

Stanley Lee, MD, Orthopedic Surgeon performing microsurgery *Photo by Timothy J. Dennerll, RT(R), Ph.D.*

5.134

macro- is the opposite of micro-. macro- is used in words to mean

large

_____.

NOTE: micro- and macro- are combining forms used as prefixes.

5.135

Things that are macro/scop/ic can be seen with the naked eye. Very large cells are

macro/cyte(s)
mak′ rō sīt(s)

called _____/_____.

ANSWER COLUMN

5.136

An abnormally large head is a

macro/cephal/us
ma′ krō **sef′** ə ləs

_____/_____/_____ .

A large embryonic (germ) cell is a

macro/blast
ma′ krō blast

_____/_____ .

A very large coccus is a

macro/cocc/us
ma′ krō **ko′** kus

_____/_____/_____ .

5.137

abnormally
large tongue

Use your dictionary to help you define the following conditions.

macro/gloss/ia   *_____

large ear(s)

macrot/ia   *_____

large nose

macro/rhin/ia   *_____

large lips

macro/cheil/ia   *_____

5.138

Dactylos is a Greek word meaning finger. Macro/dactyl/ia is a condition of abnormally large fingers or toes. The word root for fingers or toes

dactyl

is _____ .

5.139

Another way of saying large fingers or toes is dactyl/o/megal/y. The combining

dactyl/o

form for finger or toe is _____/_____ .

5.140

A finger or toe is also called a digit. (When you see digit, finger, or toe, use **dactyl/o**.) Build a word meaning
inflammation of a digit

dactyl/itis
dak ti **lī′** tis

_____/_____ ;

cramp or spasm of a digit

dactyl/o/spasm
dak ti lō spaz′ əm

_____/_____/_____ ;

a fingerprint

dactyl/o/gram
dak′ ti lō gram

_____/_____/_____ (picture).

5.141

condition of having
abnormally large
fingers or toes (digits)
fingers or toes (digits)

Macro/dactyl/ia means *_____

_____ .

Poly/dactyl/ism means too many *_____ .

ANSWER COLUMN

5.142

syn- is a prefix meaning with or together. Syn/dactyl/ism means a joining together of two or more digits. The prefix that means together or with

syn-

is _____.

5.143

A person with two or more fingers joined together has a condition called

syn/dactyl/ism

sin **dak'** til izm

_____/_____/_____.

**DICTIONARY
EXERCISE**

5.144

You may have noticed that some medical terms have several noun forms and it is confusing to know which ending to use when you are first learning the words. You will discover the term "polydactylism" has several noun forms that are correct including: polydactylia and polydactyl. See if you can find the following terms in your dictionary as alternative noun forms:

polydactyl, polydactylism, polydactylia

_____

hydrocephalus, hydrocephaly

_____

synergy, synergism

_____

5.145

Syn/erg/ism occurs when two or more drugs or organs working together produce an increased effect (**syn-**, join; erg, work; **-ism**, condition or state). Drugs that work together to increase each other's effects are

syn/erg/istic

sin er **jis'** tik

called _____/_____/_____ (adjective) drugs.

5.146

Syn/ergetic also means working (erg) together (**syn-**), but usually it refers to muscles that work together. The three muscles in the forearm that work together

syn/erg/etic

sin er **jet'**ik

are _____/_____/_____ muscles.

5.147

Tylenol tablets with codeine are frequently more effective for killing pain than

synergistic

Tylenol alone. This is because Tylenol and codeine are _____ drugs.

5.148

Alcohol intake is contraindicated (recommended against) when taking analgesics because the effects can multiply central nervous system depression. This is a

synergistic

dangerous _____ effect.

ANSWER COLUMN

Syndactylism *Delmar/ Cengage Learning*

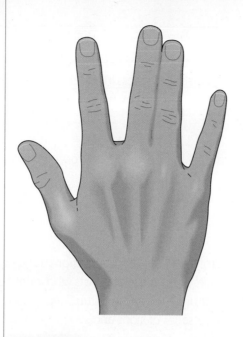

syn- arthr osis	**5.149** Analyze synarthrosis. prefix _____ word root (joint) _____ condition _____
syn/arthr/osis sin är **thrō′** sis	**5.150** Syn/arthr/osis indicates an immovable joint. The joined bones are fused together. When bones are fused at a joint so that there is no movement, _____/_____/_____ occurs. EXAMPLE: sacrum, pelvis, skull.

Cranial sutures— synarthrotic joints
Delmar/Cengage Learning

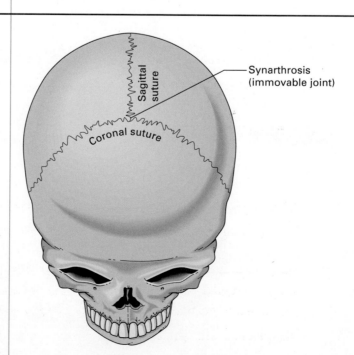

ANSWER COLUMN

WORD ORIGINS

5.151

drom/o comes from the Greek word for run. A hippodrome was an open air stadium built for racing horses or chariots in ancient Greece. Drom/o/mania is an insane impulse to wander or roam. You usually use drom with the prefixes **syn-** and **pro-**.

5.152

A syn/drome is a variety of symptoms occurring (running along) together.

The complete picture of a disease is its _____.

syndrome
sin′ drōm

INFORMATION FRAME

5.153

Look up syndrome in your medical dictionary. Read about the syndromes, many of which are named after the scientists who identified them.
Korsakoff's syndrome was named after Sergei S. Korsakoff, a Russian neurologist, who described a series of signs and symptoms brought on by alcoholism that pointed to evidence of organic brain damage.
Reye's syndrome was named in honor of Ralph Douglas Kenneth Reye, an Australian pathologist, who discovered postinfection encephalopathy in children linked to acute fever, influenza, or chickenpox, which could lead to death from cerebral edema.

5.154

Korsakoff's syndrome

A syndrome due to alcoholism is * _____.
Expectant mothers are warned not to drink alcohol during pregnancy to prevent

syndrome

deformities in the newborn, known as fetal alcohol _____ (FAS).

5.155

syndrome

Behavior changes and hyperemesis following a viral infection and fever are

symptoms occurring together that may indicate Reye's _____.

5.156

Pro/drome means running before (a disease). A symptom indicating an

pro/drome
prō′ drōm

approaching disease is a _____/_____.

5.157

prodromes

The sneezes that come before a common cold are the _____ (plural)
of the cold.

5.158

Chickenpox has a macular rash that precedes the papules. This is known as

pro/drom/al
prō **drō′** məl

a _____/_____/_____ (adjective) rash.

ANSWER COLUMN

5.159

dips

Dipsia is Greek for thirst. Poly/dips/ia means excessive thirst (desire for much fluid). The root word for thirst is _____.

5.160

poly/dips/ia
pol ē **dip'** sē ə

poly- is a prefix meaning too much or too many. Poly/dipsia can be caused by something as simple as eating too much salt. A highly salted meal may cause _____/_____/_____.

5.161

polydipsia

Polydipsia can be caused by something as complex as an upset in pituitary secretion. If the pituitary gland secretes too much of one hormone, salt is retained in the body, and _____ results.

5.162

polydipsia

High blood sugar levels and lack of insulin in patients with diabetes also cause _____ (excessive thirst).

5.163

dips/o/man/ia
dip sō **mā'** nē ə

Dips/o/mania is an old term for alcoholism. A person who drinks alcohol excessively and becomes physically and psychologically addicted suffers from _____/_____/_____/_____ or alcoholism.

5.164

alcohol/ism
al' kō hol izm

Korsakoff's syndrome characterized by nerve inflammation, insomnia, hallucinations, disorientation, and nerve pain is a sequel to chronic _____/_____.

5.165

TAKE A CLOSER LOOK

Alcoholism, a chronic physical and psychological disease, has grave consequences for the individuals who are afflicted as well as for the family members surrounding them. Read more about this disease in your dictionary or encyclopedia. Treatment of alcoholism includes carefully planned withdrawal from alcohol, nutrition, rest, and psychotherapy. Alcoholics Anonymous (AA) offers many support group programs for the alcoholic, spouses (Al-Anon), and children (Ala-Teen). There are even groups (ACOA*) for adults whose parents were alcoholic and who still suffer the effects of being raised in an alcoholic or dysfuntional home.
*Adult Children of Alcoholics

Abbreviation	Meaning
AA	Alcoholics Anonymous
ACOA	Adult Children of Alcoholics
AD**	right ear, *auris dextra* (Latin)
AFB	acid-fast bacillus (i.e., TB)
Al-Anon	AA support group for spouses of alcoholics
Ala-Teen	AA support group for children of alcoholics
AS**	left ear, *auris sinistra* (Latin)
AU**	both ears, *auris uterque* (Latin)
BP	Blood pressure
C°	Celsius degrees (metric temperature)
C&S	culture and sensitivity (antibiotic susceptibility)
CO_2	carbon dioxide
DM	diabetes mellitus
F°	Fahrenheit degrees
FAS	fetal alcohol syndrome
GB	gallbladder
GNID	gram-negative intracellular diplococcus
HBV	hepatitis B virus
HIV	human immunodeficiency virus
HPV	human papillomavirus
HSV	herpes simplex virus
Ht	height
HUS	hemorrhagic uremic syndrome
LMP	last menstrual period
mcg	microgram(s)*
mg	milligram(s)*
MRSA	Methicillin resistant *Staphylococcus aureas*
MTD	right eardrum (*membrana tympani dextra*)
MTS	left eardrum (*membrana tympani sinistra*)
NVS	neurologic vital signs
OM	otitis media
O&P	ova and parasites
P	pulse
PAR	perennial allergic rhinitis
R	respiration (rate)
RUQ	right upper quadrant
SIDS	sudden infant death syndrome
SOB	short (shortness) of breath
staph	staphylococcus
strep	streptococcus
T, temp	temperature
TB	tuberculosis
VS	vital signs (T, P, R, BP)
Wt	weight
°	degree symbol

*We do not pluralize abbreviations. Each stands for singular and plural.
**Abbreviation use warning. These abbreviations have been judged to be dangerous and should not be used.

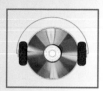

To complete your study of this unit, work the **Review Activities** on the following pages. Also, listen to the Audio CD that accompanies *Medical Terminology: A Programmed Systems Approach*, 10th edition, and practice your pronunciation.

STUDYWARE™ CONNECTION

To help you learn the content in this chapter, take a practice quiz or play an interactive game on your **StudyWARE™ CD-ROM**.

REVIEW ACTIVITIES

CIRCLE AND CORRECT

Circle the correct answer for each question. Then check your answers in Appendix E.

1. Sound made by c followed by an o, as in costal
   - a. s
   - b. k
   - c. j
   - d. x

2. Sound made by c followed by an i, as in cervicitis
   - a. s
   - b. k
   - c. j
   - d. x

3. Plural for round-shaped bacteria
   - a. bacilli
   - b. bacillus
   - c. coccus
   - d. cocci

4. Prefix for double
   - a. tri-
   - b. diplo-
   - c. daplo-
   - d. ex-

5. Combining form for twisted chains
   - a. strep
   - b. strepto
   - c. stretp
   - d. strept

6. Combining form for uvula
   - a. staphylo
   - b. strepto
   - c. vulvo
   - d. uvul

7. Suffix for flow or discharge
   - a. -itis
   - b. -rrhagia
   - c. -pnea
   - d. -rrhea

8. Combining form for ear
   - a. audio
   - b. tympano
   - c. oto
   - d. oculo

9. Suffix for surgical repair
   - a. -acopy
   - b. -tomy
   - c. -ectomy
   - d. -plasty

10. Combining form for bile (gall)
    - a. chole
    - b. calcul
    - c. lith
    - d. bil

11. Singular for rod-shaped bacteria
    - a. bacilla
    - b. bacillus
    - c. coccus
    - d. bacterium

12. Combining form for pus
    - a. genic
    - b. gen/o
    - c. staphyl/o
    - d. py/o

13. Word root for nose
    - a. ot
    - b. rhin
    - c. nas/o
    - d. lith

14. Suffix meaning infestation (condition)
    - a. -iasis
    - b. -pathy
    - c. -lith
    - d. -oid

15. Suffix for breathing
    - a. -pne
    - b. -pneo
    - c. -pnea
    - d. -pepsia

16. Combining form for heat
    - a. tempero
    - b. thermal
    - c. thermo
    - d. Fahrenheit

17. Prefix for small
    - a. incro-
    - b. macro-
    - c. micro-
    - d. hypo-

18. Prefix for large
    - a. macro-
    - b. megaly-
    - c. micro-
    - d. poly-

REVIEW ACTIVITIES

19. Prefix for join together
    a. inter-   b. intra-
    c. osis-   d. syn-

20. Suffix for thirst
    a. -hydro   b. -dipsia
    c. -mania   d. -poly

21. Word root for finger or toe (digits)
    a. acro   b. dactyl
    c. digit   d. phalang

22. Prefix for many or much
    a. poly-   b. olig-
    c. hyper-   d. sub-

SELECT AND CONSTRUCT

Select the correct word parts (some may be used more than once) from the following list and construct medical terms that represent the given meaning.

a	algia	audio	blast	brady	cardio(a)	cephalus
chole	cysto	cyte	dactylo(ia)	dia	dipso(ia)	drome(al)
dynia	dys	ectomy	ergetic(ergy)	geno(ic) esis	graphy(gram)	hemat
hyper	hypo	ia	iasis	ic	ism	ites
itis	lith(o)	macro	metry	micro	neur	osis
ot(o)(ia)	pepsia	phago(ia)	pnea	poly	pro	pyo
rhino	rrhea	spasm	staphyl	syn	tachy	therapy
therm(o)(al)(y)	tomy	tympan(o)	uvul(o)			

1. slow heart rate _____

2. fast eating (swallowing) _____

3. inflammation of the uvula _____

4. stones in the gallbladder _____

5. earache _____

6. process of measuring hearing _____

7. difficulty with digestion _____

8. pus-forming (adjective) _____

9. discharge from the nose _____

10. record of eardrum function _____

11. distended with gas (abdomen) _____

12. x-ray picture of gallbladder _____

13. absence of breathing _____

14. heat therapy (heating through) _____

15. excessive thirst _____

16. working together _____

17. abnormally small head _____

REVIEW ACTIVITIES

18. very large cell _____

19. before the onset of illness _____

20. low body temperature _____

MIX AND MATCH

Match the organism on the left with its description or disease name on the right.

_____ 1. streptococcus   a. double dot–shaped bacteria

_____ 2. staphylococci   b. HIV is a _____.

_____ 3. diplococcus   c. parasite protozoan with flagella

_____ 4. trichomonas   d. skin bacteria growing in bunches

_____ 5. virus   e. moniliasis

_____ 6. yeast   f. β hemolytic _____ causes throat infection.

_____ 7. filarial worm   g. elephantiasis

_____ 8. giardia   h. giardiasis

DEFINE AND DISSECT

Give a brief definition and dissect each term listed into its word parts in the space provided. Check your answers by referring to the frame listed in parentheses and to your medical dictionary. Then listen to the Audio CD to practice pronunciation.

1. diplococcus (5.9)   _____/_____/_____/_____
                                rt   v   rt   suffix

   meaning _____

2. staphylococcus (5.22)   _____/_____/_____/_____
                                rt   v   rt   suffix

   _____

3. uvulectomy (5.25)   _____/_____
                                                rt   suffix

   _____

4. pyocele (5.27)   _____/_____/_____
                                        rt   v   suffix

   _____

5. otorrhea (5.42)   _____/_____/_____
                                        rt   v   suffix

   _____

REVIEW ACTIVITIES

6. tympanotomy (5.50)

_____/_____/_____
rt   v   suffix

_____

7. audiogram (5.55)

_____/_____/_____
rt   v   suffix

_____

8. rhinolith (5.84)

_____/_____/_____
rt   v   rt

_____

9. cholecystitis (5.79)

_____/_____/_____/_____
rt   v   rt   suffix

_____

10. trichomoniasis (5.76)

_____/_____/_____/_____
rt   v   rt   suffix

_____

11. bradyphagia (5.86)

_____/_____/_____
pre   rt   suffix

_____

12. tachypnea (5.97)

_____/_____
pre   suffix

_____

13. dyspepsia (5.116)

_____/_____/_____
pre   rt   suffix

_____

14. cholecystography (5.78)

_____/_____/_____/_____/_____
rt   v   rt   v   suffix

_____

15. staphyloplasty (5.23)

_____/_____/_____
rt   v   suffix

_____

16. gonorrhea (5.9)

_____/_____/_____
rt   v   suffix

_____

17. diplobacillus (5.17)

_____/_____/_____/_____
rt   v   rt   suffix

_____

REVIEW ACTIVITIES

18. tympanometry (5.51)

_____/_____/_____
       rt   v   suffix

_____

19. audiologist (5.56)

_____/_____/_____
       rt   v   suffix

_____

20. aphasia (5.58)

_____/_____
      pre   suffix

_____

21. lithotomy (5.70)

_____/_____/_____
       rt   v   suffix

_____

22. cholelithiasis (5.74)

_____/_____/_____/_____
    rt   v   rt   suffix

_____

23. carcinogenesis (5.109)

_____/_____/_____
       rt   v   rt/suffix

_____

24. dyspnea (5.114)

_____/_____
      pre   suffix

_____

25. tympanites (5.52)

_____/_____
       rt   suffix

_____

26. thermometer (5.124)

_____/_____/_____
       rt   v   suffix

_____

27. microsurgery (5.133)

_____/_____
      pre   rt/suffix

_____

28. macrocephalus (5.136)

_____/_____
      pre   rt/suffix

_____

REVIEW ACTIVITIES

29. polydactylism (5.141)

_____/_____/_____
      pre   rt   suffix

_____

30. synergistic (5.145)

_____/_____/_____
      pre   rt   suffix

_____

31. synarthrosis (5.150)

_____/_____/_____
      pre   rt   suffix

_____

32. syndrome (5.152)

_____/_____
      pre   rt/suffix

_____

33. prodromal (5.158)

_____/_____/_____
      pre   rt   suffix

_____

34. polydipsia (5.160)

_____/_____/_____
      pre   rt   suffix

_____

35. dipsomania (5.163)

_____/_____/_____/_____
   rt   v   rt   suffix

_____

36. alcoholism (5.164)

_____/_____
      rt   suffix

_____

37. microgram (5.132)

_____/_____
      pre   suffix

_____

38. hyperthermia (5.129)

_____/_____/_____
      pre   rt   suffix

_____

39. syndactylism (5.143)

_____/_____/_____
      pre   rt   suffix

_____

REVIEW ACTIVITIES

40. dactylospasm (5.140)

_____/_____/_____
       rt   v   suffix

_____

41. diathermy (5.126)

_____/_____/_____
      pre   rt   suffix

_____

42. microcyst (5.132)

_____/_____
      pre   rt

_____

43. thermoalgesia (5.125)

_____/_____/_____/_____
    rt   v   rt   suffix

_____

44. pathogenesis (5.30)

_____/_____/_____
      rt   v   suffix

_____

45. dyslexia (5.122)

_____/_____/_____
    pre   v   suffix

_____

46. arrhythmia (5.119)

_____/_____/_____
    pre   rt   suffix

_____

ABBREVIATION MATCHING

Match the following abbreviations with their definition.

_____ 1. AA   a. Methicillin-resistant *Staphylococcus aureas*

_____ 2. T   b. milligram(s)

_____ 3. °F   c. degrees Celsius

_____ 4. MRSA   d. fetal alcohol syndrome

_____ 5. SIDS   e. oculomotor

_____ 6. VS   f. degrees Fahrenheit

_____ 7. FAS   g. acid-fast bacillus

_____ 8. GB   h. gonorrhea

_____ 9. MTD   i. left ear

(continued)

REVIEW ACTIVITIES

_____ 10.   HPV

_____ 11.   AS

_____ 12.   OM

j. Al-Anon

k. microscopic

l. temperature

m. otitis media

n. right eardrum

o. human papilloma virus

p. vital signs

q. sudden infant death syndrome

r. Alcoholics Anonymous

s. gallbladder

CASE STUDY

Write the term next to its meaning given below. Then draw slashes to analyze the word parts. Note the use of medical abbreviations. Look these up in your dictionary or find them in Appendix B. If you have any questions about the answers, refer to your medical dictionary or check with your instructor for the answers in Appendix E.

CASE STUDY 5-1

Operative Report—Cholecystectomy

Pt: Female, age 39, Ht 5'3", Wt 192 lb., BP 130/84, **T 99.6°F**, P 80, R 18

Summary: Ms. Colette Stone is a 39-year-old female who was seen in the office with complaints of repeated pain in the **epigastric** region and **RUQ** of the abdomen. The pain radiates to her shoulder and back. Ms. Stone states that the pain becomes aggravated with consumption of any kind of food, particularly greasy, fatty, or fried food. A complete workup was done, including **ultrasound** of the **gallbladder**. This revealed the presence of a **cholelith**.

Surgical Report Findings: The gallbladder was **edematous** and somewhat thick-walled. There was a stone impacted in the outlet of the gallbladder, measuring about 1 **cm** in diameter. Operative **cholangiograms** showed a small **ductal** system, but there were no filling defects, and there was good emptying of the contrast medium into the duodenum.

1. pertaining to a duct _____

2. swollen _____

3. cholecyst _____

4. gallstone _____

5. x-ray of bile ducts _____

6. centimeter _____

7. upon the stomach _____

8. right upper quadrant _____

9. excision of the gallbladder _____

10. use of high-frequency sound waves _____

11. temperature, 99.6 degrees Fahrenheit _____

REVIEW ACTIVITIES

Check your answers by going back through the frames or checking the solution in Appendix F.

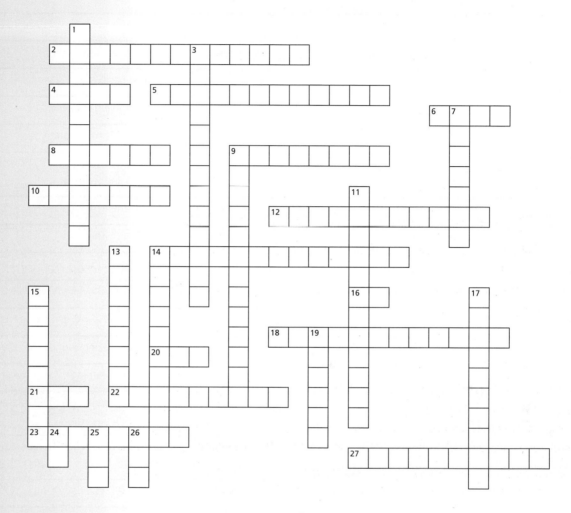

Across

2. inflamed gallbladder
4. suffix for breathing
5. promoting cancer growth (adj.)
6. prefix for many
8. suffix for paralysis
9. Korsakoff's _____
10. having trouble breathing
12. slow heart rate
14. enlarged fingers
16. tuberculosis (abbr.)
18. fever
20. culture and sensitivity (abbr.)
21. human immuno-deficiency virus (abbr.)
22. large cell
23. failure to develop
27. organism that produces disease (adj.)

Down

1. surgical repair of the nose
3. round bacteria in twisted chains
7. ear pain
9. excision of the uvula
11. fused joint with no movement
13. eardrum
14. gram-negative intracellular _____ (plural)
15. purulent discharge
17. runny nose
19. suffix for eating (swallowing)
24. gallbladder (abbr.)
25. neurologic vital signs (abbreviation)
26. prefix for joined

REVIEW ACTIVITIES

GLOSSARY

agenesis	lack of development	dactylitis	inflammation of the fingers and/or toes
alcoholism	chronic physical and psychological addiction to alcohol	dactylogram	fingerprint
		dactylospasm	spasm of a digit
amenorrhea	absence of menstruation	diplobacillus	double bacillus
apepsia	cessation of digestion	diplococci	cocci growing in pairs
aphasia	unable to speak	dipsomania	abnormal compulsion to drink
aphonia	no voice, unable to make sounds	dyslexia	condition characterized by difficulty reading and spelling
apnea	absence of breathing		
arrhythmia	loss of rhythm	dysmenorrhea	painful menstruation
audiogram	graphic record of hearing function	dysrrhythmia	irregular rhythm
audiologist	hearing specialist	dyspepsia	poor digestion
audiology	science that studies hearing	dysphagia	difficulty swallowing
audiometer	instrument to test hearing	dysphasia	difficulty speaking, garbled speech
audiometry	process of testing hearing	dysphonia	difficulty making sounds with the voice
bacillus	rod-shaped bacterium	dyspnea	difficulty breathing
bradycardia	slow heart rate	hydrocephalus	enlarged head due to fluid accumulation (congenital)
bradypepsia	slow digestion		
bradyphagia	slow eating (swallowing)	hyperthermia	abnormally high body temperature (synonym fever)
bradypnea	slow breathing		
calculi	small stones	hypothermia	abnormally low body temperature
carcinogenesis	formation of cancer	lithometer	instrument to measure stones
cholangiogram	x-ray of the bile ducts	lithotomy	incision for the removal of stones
cholecyst	gallbladder	macroblast	abnormally large immature cell
cholecystitis	inflammation of the gallbladder	macrocephalus	large head size
cholecystogram	x-ray of the gallbladder	macrocheilia	enlarged lips
cholecystography	process of obtaining x-ray of the gallbladder	macrococcus	large coccus
		macrocyte	large cell
cholecystotomy	incision into the gallbladder	macrodactylia	abnormally large digits
cholelith	gallstone	macroglossia	enlarged tongue
cholelithiasis	infestation with gallstones	macrorhinia	enlarged nose
coccus	sphere-shaped bacterium	microcardia	abnormally small-sized heart

REVIEW ACTIVITIES

microcephalus	abnormally small head		staphylectomy	excision of the uvula (synonym uvulectomy)
microcyst	a small cyst		staphylitis	inflammation of the uvula (synonym uvulitis)
microcyte	a small cell		staphylococci	bacteria growing in bunches (like grapes)
microgram	one millionth of a gram		staphyloplasty	surgical repair of the uvula
microsurgery	surgery performed using a microscope or other magnifying device		streptobacillus	bacillus growing in twisted chains
moniliasis	yeast infection		streptococci	round bacteria growing in twisted chains
oncogenesis	tumor forming		synarthrosis	joints that are fused and immovable
otic	pertaining to the ear		syndactylism	fingers or toes that are fused (congenital)
otodynia	earache (synonym otalgia)		syndrome	symptoms that occur together to characterize a disease
otorrhea	discharge from the ear		synergistic	works together
otoscope	instrument used to look into the ear		tachycardia	fast heart rate
paraphasia	abnormal speech		tachyphagia	fast eating
pathogenic	disease producing		tachypnea	fast breathing
pathology	study of disease		thermal	pertaining to heat (synonym thermic)
peptic	pertaining to digestion		thermoesthesia	oversensitivity to heat (synonym thermoalgesia)
phasology	science that studies speech		thermogenesis	generation of heat
phonic	pertaining to the voice		thermophobia	abnormal fear of heat
phonology	science that studies the voice sounds		thermoplegia	paralysis caused by a person being exposed to too high of a temperature (synonym heat stroke)
polydactylism	condition of having more than five digits on hands or feet		trichomoniasis	infestation with *Trichomonas*
polydipsia	condition of excessive thirst		tympanectomy	excision of the eardrum
prodrome	symptoms before the onset of a disease		tympanic	pertaining to the eardrum
pyogenic	pus forming (adj.)		tympanites	distended with gas (abdomen)
pyorrhea	flow or discharge of pus		tympanometry	process of measuring eardrum function
pyothorax	pus in the chest cavity		tympanotomy	incision into the eardrum (synonym myringotomy)
rhinitis	inflammation of the nose			
rhinolith	calculus in the nasal passages			
rhinoplasty	surgical repair of the nose			
rhinorrhea	runny nose			

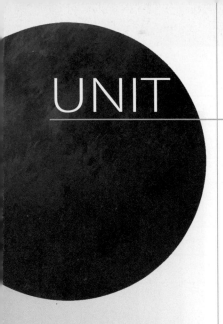

UNIT 6

Urology and Gynecology

Information for Frames 6.1–6.34

Word	Combining Form	New Suffix to Use When Needed
urine	**ur/o**	**-lith** (stone)
kidney	**nephr/o**	**-lysis** (destruction)
	ren/o	**-pexy** (surgical fixation)
renal pelvis	**pyel/o**	**-ptosis** (prolapse)
ureter	**ureter/o**	**-rrhagia** (hemorrhage or "bursting forth" of blood)
bladder	**cyst/o**	**-rrhaphy** (suturing or stitching)
urethra	**urethr/o**	**-uria** (condition of urine or urination)

6.1

Urology is the study of the urinary tract. The urinary tract is responsible for forming urine from excess water and waste materials in the blood and eliminating urine from the body. What would you guess to be the combining form for

urine? _____.

(See the illustration of a kidney on page 207.)

ur/o

STUDYWARE™ CONNECTION

View an animation about the *Formation of Urine* on your **StudyWARE™ CD-ROM**.

Urinalysis using a reagent strip (dipstick urine) to analyze chemical make up, pH, and specific gravity *Delmar/Cengage Learning*

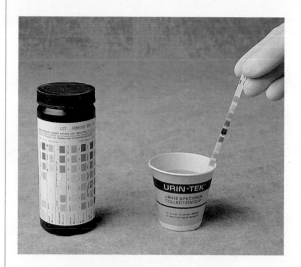

6.2

A ur/o/logist is a physician specialist with expertise in treating disorders of the male and female urinary system and male reproductive system. Men with concerns about infertility or impotence may consult

ur/o/logist
yōō **rol′** ō jist

a _____/_____/_____. The descriptor or adjective in this phrase

urin/ary
yōō′ rin air ē

"urinary system" is _____/_____ .

6.3

Build words meaning
pertaining to urinary tract and genitals

ur/o/genital
yōō rō **jen′** i tal

_____/_____/_____ or _____/_____/_____;

genit/o/urinary
jen′ ə tō **yōō′** rin air ē

ur/o/pathy
yōō **rop′** ə thē

any disease of the urinary tract

_____/_____/_____ .

6.4

poly- is a prefix that means many or much. **-uria** is a suffix meaning condition of the urine. Poly/uria means excessive amount of urine. When a person drinks too

poly/uria
pol ē **yōōr′** ē ə

much water, _____/_____ results. Another cause of

polyuria

_____ is diabetes mellitus.

Urinalysis performed by an automated strip reader *Photo by Timothy J. Dennerll, RT(R), Ph.D., courtesy of Jackson Community College, Jackson, MI*

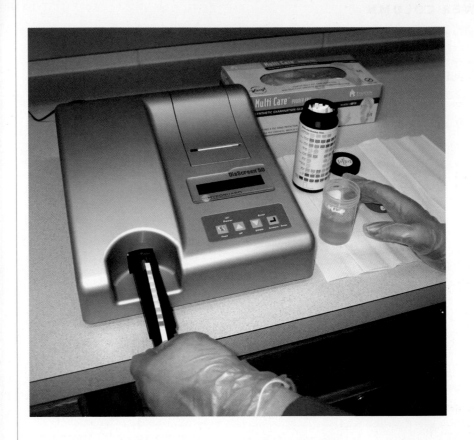

CONDITIONS INVOLVING URINATION

Condition	Description
poly/uria	too much (frequent) urination
noct/uria	excessive urination at night
an/uria	suppressed (lack of) urination
olig/uria	abnormally low amounts of urine
hemat/uria	blood in the urine
albumin/uria	protein (albumin) in the urine
glycos/uria	sugar in the urine
keton/uria	ketones in the urine
nocturn/al en/ur/esis	bed wetting
bacter/i/uria	bacteria in the urine
dys/uria	difficult or painful urination

6.5

Refer to the table listing conditions of urination. Build words meaning urinating at night

noct/uria
nok **tyoor′** ē ə

_____/_____;

frequent urination

poly/uria
pol ē **yoor′** ē ə

_____/_____;

(continued)

ANSWER COLUMN

hemat/uria
hem at **yōor′** ē ə

olig/uria
ō lig **yōor′** ē ə

dys/uria
dis **yōo′** rē ə

blood in the urine

_____/_____;

low (scant) amount of urine

_____/_____;

difficult or painful urination

_____/_____ .

6.6

Poly/neur/o/pathy means disease of many nerves. The word for inflammation

poly/neur/itis
pol ē nōo **rī′** tis

of many nerves is _____/_____/_____ .

6.7

Build words meaning
inflammation of many joints

poly/arthr/itis
pol ē är **thrī′** tis

poly/neur/algia
pol ē nōo **ral′** jē ə

poly/ot/ia
pol ē **ō′** shē ə

_____/_____/_____;

pain in many nerves

_____/_____/_____;

state of having too many or more than two ears

_____/_____/_____ .

**(A) Polycystic kidney
(B) Section through
kidney** *Delmar/Cengage Learning*

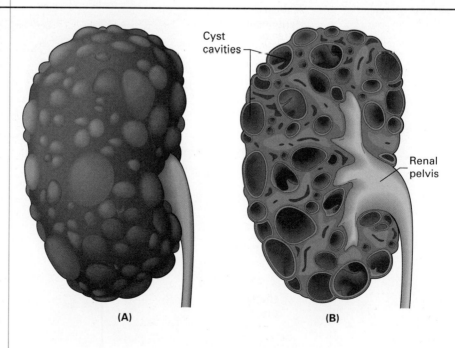

Cyst
cavities

Renal
pelvis

(A)   (B)

ANSWER COLUMN

	6.8
	Define the following terms
having many cysts	poly/cyst/ic * _____ ;
eating too much	poly/phagia * _____ ;
excessive fear of things (many phobias)	poly/phobia * _____ .

	6.9
ren/o	**ren** is one word root for kidney. The combining form for kidney is _____/_____ . Look up all the words that begin with **ren/o** in your dictionary.

	6.10
	Build words meaning pertaining to the kidney
ren/al **rē′** nəl	_____/_____ ; any kidney disease
ren/o/pathy re **nop′** ə thē	_____/_____/_____ ; record from an x-ray of the kidney
ren/o/gram **rē′** ō gram	_____/_____/_____ .
	NOTE: Ordering a KUB is ordering an x-ray of the kidneys, ureters, and bladder.

Urinary system *Delmar/ Cengage Learning*

- Adrenal (suprarenal glands) (adren/o)
- Cortex of the kidney
- Renal pelvis (pyel/o)
- Kidney (nephr/o, ren/o)
- Inferior vena cava
- Aorta
- Right ureter
- Left ureter (ureter/o)
- Urinary bladder (cyst/o)
- Prostate gland (males) (prostat/o)
- Urethra (urethr/o)
- Urinary meatus

ANSWER COLUMN

6.11

Renointestinal means

* _____ .

pertaining to the kidney
and intestine

Renogastric means

* _____ .

pertaining to the kidney
and stomach

6.12

nephr/itis
nef **rī'** tis

nephr/o is also used in words to refer to the kidney. A word that means

inflammation of the kidney is _____/_____ .

6.13

TAKE A
CLOSER LOOK

nephr/o comes from Greek, **ren/o** from Latin. Nephrons, the functional units of
the kidney, are tiny structures in the renal cortex. They filter blood to remove
waste and excess water to form urine. Look up **nephr/o** and **ren/o** in your
dictionary. Make a list of terms beginning with each and then compare them.

6.14

-ptosis is a suffix meaning condition of prolapse or displacement. Nephr/o/ptosis
can occur from a hard blow or jolt to the kidney. People who ride motorcycles
often wear special clothing or a kidney belt to protect against

nephr/o/ptosis
nef' rop **tō'** sis

_____/_____/_____ .

6.15

When nephroptosis occurs, one treament option could be to put the kidney back
in place using surgery. Nephr/o/pexy is fixation of a prolapsed kidney. The suffix

-pexy

for surgical fixation is _____ .

6.16

Nephr/o/plasty is also a repair of the kidney. The specific type of repair to treat

nephr/o/pexy
nef' rō pek sē

nephroptosis is _____/_____/_____ .

6.17

Recall the suffixes for stone, softening, enlargement, and destruction. Build words
meaning
stone in the kidney

nephr/o/lith
nef' rō lith

_____/_____/_____ ;

softening of kidney tissue

nephr/o/malac/ia
nef rō mə **lā'** shə

_____/_____/_____/_____ ;

(continued)

ANSWER COLUMN

nephr/o/megal/y
nef rō **meg'** ə lē

nephr/o/lysis
nef **rol'** ə sis

enlargement of the kidney

_____/_____/_____/_____;

destruction of kidney tissue

_____/_____/_____.

6.18

For review build terms that mean
gallstone

chol/e/lith

_____/_____/_____;

condition (infestation) of gallstones

chol/e/lith/iasis

_____/_____/_____/_____;

nasal stones

rhin/o/lith

_____/_____/_____.

Good. Now let's move on.

INFORMATION TABLE

Routine urinalysis includes the following tests using a color change reagent strip dipped into the urine sample to determine the following results.

Test	Normal Range
pH	5–8
protein	negative
glucose	negative
ketones	negative
bilirubin	negative
blood	negative
specific gravity	1.001–1.035

6.19

Locate the renal pelvis in the illustration of the kidney on page 207. The renal pelvis is formed at the juncture of the calyces. **pyel/o** refers to the

renal pelvis

* _____.

6.20

Using what you need from the combining form for renal pelvis, form words meaning
inflammation of the renal pelvis

pyel/itis
pī ə **lī'** tis

_____/_____;

surgical repair of the renal pelvis

pyel/o/plasty
pī' ə lō plas' tē

_____/_____/_____.

ANSWER COLUMN

6.21

condition of renal pelvis
and kidney

Pyel/o/nephr/osis means* _____

_____.

Form words that mean
inflammation of the renal pelvis and kidney

pyel/o/nephr/itis
pī′ ə lō nef **rī**′ tis

_____/_____/_____/_____;

x-ray of the renal pelvis

pyel/o/gram
pī′ ə lō gram

_____/_____/_____.

NOTE: An IVP is an intravenous pyelogram as shown in the following x-ray
illustration.

6.22

stone or calculus in the
ureter

Ureter/o/lith means * _____. Form words that mean
herniation of the ureter

ureter/o/cele
yōō **rē**′ tə rō sēl

_____/_____/_____;

any disease of the ureter

ureter/o/pathy
yōō rē′ tər **op**′ ə thē

_____/_____/_____.

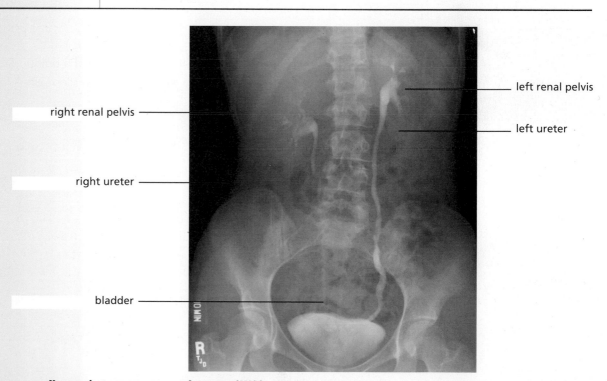

right renal pelvis ——

right ureter ——

bladder ——

—— left renal pelvis

—— left ureter

X-ray: intravenous pyelogram (IVP) *Delmar/Cangage Learning*

ANSWER COLUMN

6.23

plastic surgery of the
  ureter and renal pelvis

Ureter/o/pyel/o/plasty means* _____
_____ .

Form a word meaning inflammation of the ureter and renal pelvis

ureter/o/pyel/itis
yōō rē′ tə rō pī ə **lī**′ tis

_____/_____/_____/_____ .

6.24

Form words meaning
making a new opening between the ureter and bladder

ureter/o/cyst/o/stomy
yōō rē′ tə rō sis **tos**′ tə mē

_____/_____/_____/_____/_____ ;

a condition of the ureter involving pus

ureter/o/py/osis
yōō rē′ tə rō pī **ō**′ sis

_____/_____/_____/_____ .

6.25

Ureter/o/rrhaphy introduces a new word part: **-rrhaphy**. **-rrhaphy** means
suturing or stitching. Ureterorrhaphy means

suturing or stitching
  of the ureter

* _____ .

6.26

**SPELL
CHECK**

So far you have been introduced to three suffixes with the unique Greek spelling
"rrh": **-rrhea, -rrhagia**, and **-rrhaphy**. Although the h is silent, don't forget to
include it.
-rrhea (runny, flow, or discharge)
-rrhagia (hemorrhage, abnormal bleeding)
-rrhaphy (suturing or wound closure)

6.27

Form the word that means suturing of the ureter:

ureter/o/rrhaphy
yōō rē′ tər **ôr**′ ə fē

_____/_____/_____ ;

suturing of the skin

dermat/o/rrhaphy
dûr mə **tor**′ ə fē

_____/_____/_____ .

6.28

Form words meaning
suturing of a kidney

nephr/o/rrhaphy
nef **rôr**′ ə fē

_____/_____/_____ ;

suturing of the bladder

cyst/o/rrhaphy
sis **tôr**′ ə fē

_____/_____/_____ .

**Dermatorrhaphy:
(A) Interrupted
(individual) sutures
(B) Continuous sutures**
Delmar/Cengage Learning

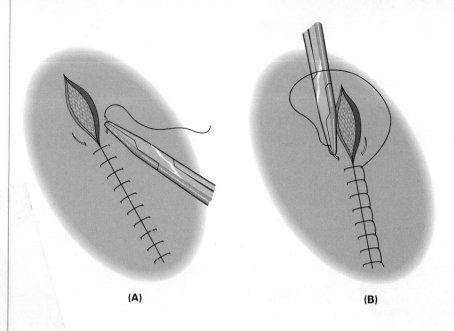

(A)   (B)

6.29

Use **neur/o** and **colp/o** to form words meaning
suturing of a nerve

neur/o/rrhaphy
noo **rôr'** ə fē

_____/_____/_____;

suturing of the vagina

colp/o/rrhaphy
kol **pôr'** ə fē

_____/_____/_____.

6.30

**SPELL
CHECK**

Normal anatomy includes two ureters and one urethra. Study these three
combining forms. Watch out! Their spellings are very close.

Combining Form	Word	Description
urethr/o	urethra	tube from urinary bladder to outside
ureter/o	ureters	tubes from each kidney to the bladder
uter/o	uterus	womb, female reproductive system

6.31

suturing of the urethra

urethr/o/rrhaphy means* _____.
Form words meaning
incision into the urethra

urethr/o/tomy
yōō rē **throt'** ə mē

_____/_____/_____;

urethr/o/spasm
yōō **rē'** thrō spaz əm

spasm of the urethra

_____/_____/_____.

ANSWER COLUMN

6.32

Urethr/o/rect/al means pertaining to the urethra and rectum.

urethra
yōō **rē′** thrə

Urethr/o/vagin/al means pertaining to the _____ and _____.

vagina

Form a word that means inflammation of urethra and bladder:

urethr/o/cyst/itis
yōō **rē′** thrō sis tī′ tis

_____/_____/_____/_____.

6.33

INFORMATION FRAME

-rrhagia is another complex word part that can be used as a suffix because it follows a word root and ends a word. **-rrhagia** means hemorrhage, or bursting forth of blood.

6.34

Gastr/o/rrhagia means stomach hemorrhage. Encephal/o/rrhagia means brain

hem/o/rrhage
hem′ ôr əg

_____/_____/_____.

A word that means hemorrhage of the urethra is

urethr/o/rrhagia
yōō rē′ thrō **rā′** jē ə

_____/_____/_____.

Excessive bleeding during menstruation is

men/o/rrhagia
men′ ō **rā′** jē ə

_____/_____/_____.

Hemorrhage of the bladder

cyst/o/rrhagia
sis tə **rā′** jē ə

_____/_____/_____;

Hemorrhage of the ureter

ureter/o/rrhagia
yōō rē′ tə rō **rā′** jē ə

_____/_____/_____.

Excellent!

6.35

Now turn your studies to a new body system. Look at the diagram of the male reproductive system on page 216. Sperma is the Greek word meaning seed. **spermat/o** and **sperm/o(i)** are two combining forms for *spermatozoa* or male germ cells (sperm).

formation of spermatozoa
   or formation of sperm
   or formation of male
   germ cells

Spermat/o/genesis means* _____

_____.

6.36

Build words meaning
the destruction of spermatozoa

sperm/o/lysis *or*
spûr′ **mol′** ə sis
spermat/o/lysis
spûr mə **tol′** ə sis

_____/_____/_____.

(continued)

ANSWER COLUMN

spermat/o/blast *or*
spûr **mat'** ō blast
sperm/o/blast
spûr' mō blast

an immature sperm cell

_____/_____/_____.

See illustration of sperm and ovum on p. 14.

6.37

A bladder or sac containing sperm is a

spermat/o/cyst
spûr **mat'** ō sist

_____/_____/_____.

A word for resembling sperm is

spermat/oid
spûr' mə toid

_____/_____.

A word for disease of the sperm is

spermat/o/pathy
spûr' mə **top'** ə thē

_____/_____/_____.

A herniated saclike structure containing sperm is

spermat /o/ cele
spûr **mat'** ō sēl

a _____/_____/_____.

**Internal structures
of the testes.
Spermatogenesis occurs
in the seminiferous
tubules of the testes;
sperm mature in the
epididymis and travel
to the vas deferens.**
Delmar/Cengage Learning

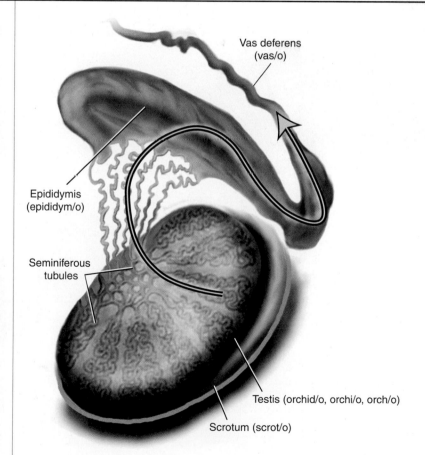

Vas deferens
(vas/o)

Epididymis
(epididym/o)

Seminiferous
tubules

Testis (orchid/o, orchi/o, orch/o)

Scrotum (scrot/o)

ANSWER COLUMN

	6.38
sperm/i/cide **spûr′** mə sīd	**-cide** is a Latin suffix meaning to kill or destroy. Think of suicide or genocide. An agent used to kill sperm is a _____ / _____ / _____ .
	6.39
spermicide	A condom (flexible sheath) placed over the erect penis provides a barrier to sperm. For contraceptive purposes condoms are used with creams and/or foams that contain a _____ .
	6.40
excision of the testicle	**orchid/o**, **orchi/o**, and **orch/o** are all Greek combining forms for testicle. Orchid/ectomy, orchi/ectomy, and orch/ectomy all mean * _____ . NOTE: Look up **orchid/o**, **orchi/o**, and **orch/o** to discover how each is used.

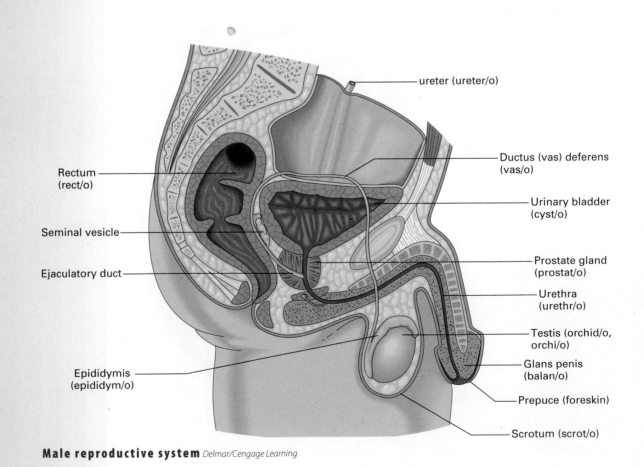

Male reproductive system *Delmar/Cengage Learning*

ureter (ureter/o)

Ductus (vas) deferens (vas/o)

Urinary bladder (cyst/o)

Prostate gland (prostat/o)

Urethra (urethr/o)

Testis (orchid/o, orchi/o)

Glans penis (balan/o)

Prepuce (foreskin)

Scrotum (scrot/o)

Rectum (rect/o)

Seminal vesicle

Ejaculatory duct

Epididymis (epididym/o)

ANSWER COLUMN

6.41

For this study use only **orchid/o** to build two terms that mean pain in the testes:

_____/_____ and _____/_____/_____.

orchid/algia
ôr′ kid **al′** gē ə
orchid/o/dynia
ôr′ kid ō **din′** ē ə

6.42

The Latin adjectival form for testicle is testicular. A person with orchidalgia is

experiencing _____/_____ pain.

testicul/ar
tes **ti′** kōō lar

6.43

**TAKE A
CLOSER LOOK**

Note that the following terms all refer to the testicles.

test/is	singular noun
test/es	plural noun
test/icle	singular noun
test/icles	plural noun
test/icular	adjectival form

6.44

Cancer of the testes, a very serious condition, occurs more frequently in males
between the ages of 18 and 35. Testicular self-exam (TSE) is recommended for

testicular

early detection of _____ cancer.

6.45

Around the time of birth, the testicles normally descend from the abdominal
cavity into the scrotum. Sometimes this fails to happen (crypt/orchid/ism).
Surgical repair may be indicated. The operation is called an

orchid/o/plasty
or′ kid ō plas tē

_____/_____/_____. This operation is also called

orchiopexy.

6.46

Build words meaning
herniation of a testicle

orchid/o/cele
ôr′ kid ō sēl

_____/_____/_____;

incision into a testicle

orchid/o/tomy
ôr′ kid **ot′** ə mē

_____/_____/_____.

ANSWER COLUMN

6.47

Crypt/orchid/ism means undescended testicle. crypt means hidden. When a testicle is hidden in the abdominal cavity, the condition is known as

crypt/orchid/ism
krip **tôr'** kid iz əm

_____/_____/_____.

6.48

A crypt/ic remark is one with a hidden meaning. A crypt/ic belief is one whose

hidden
hidden (undescended)

meaning is _____. Cryptorchidism refers to a _____ testicle.

6.49

prostat/o is used for words relating to the prostate gland. Prostat/ic is the adjectival form, as in the condition benign prostatic hyperplasia (BPH, enlargement of the prostate due to an increase in number of cells and aging). Build a term meaning inflammation of the prostate gland:

prostat/itis
pros tā **tī'** tis

_____/_____.

See the case study on transurethral resection (TUR) at the end of this unit.

6.50

The normal functioning prostate secretes a fluid that is added to sperm to create semen (**semin/o**). The combination of fluids and sperm is called

semin/al
sem' i nal
semin/al

_____/_____ (adjective) fluid. The _____/_____ vesical secretes fluid to lubricate and nurture sperm.

6.51

A semin/oma is a malignant neoplasm found most often in young men. It is a growth generated by the spermatoblast cells in a testis. A seminal tissue tumor

semin/oma
se mi **no'** mə

is called a _____/_____.

6.52

The seminal vesicles also secrete a fluid that combined with the prostatic fluid

semen
sē' men

and sperm is called _____.

STUDY WARE™ CONNECTION

Remember, after completing this unit you can complete a crossword puzzle or other interactive game on your **StudyWARE™ CD-ROM** that will help you learn the content in this chapter.

ANSWER COLUMN

(A) Normal prostate
(B) Benign prostatic
hypertrophy (BPH)
Delmar/Cengage Learning

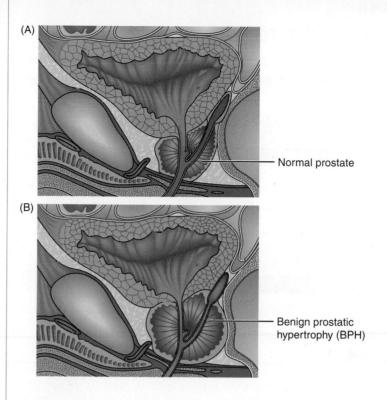

(A)

Normal prostate

(B)

Benign prostatic
hypertrophy (BPH)

6.53

prostat/o/rrhea
pros′ tā to **rē′** ə

An abnormal flow or discharge from the prostate gland is called

_____/_____/_____.

6.54

prostat/algia
pros′ tā **tal′** jē ə

Prostatic pain is called _____/_____.

prostat/ectomy
pros′ tāt **ek′** tō mē

Excision of the prostate is _____/_____.

6.55

balan/o/plasty
bal′ an ō plas tē

balan/o is the combining form for glans penis. Balan/itis is inflammation of the glans penis. Surgical repair of the glans penis is called

_____/_____/_____.

6.56

balan/o/rrhea
bal an ō **rē′** ə

An infection may cause a flow or discharge from the glans penis. This is called

_____/_____/_____.

6.57

pen/itis
pē **nī′** tis
scrot/um
skrō′ təm

The male external genitalia includes the scrotum and penis. **pen/o** is used to build words about the penis. Pen/ile is the adjectival form. Inflammation of

the penis is _____/_____. Scrot/al is the adjective

for _____/_____.

ANSWER COLUMN

6.58

pen/ile
pē′ nīl

Trauma, prostatectomy, or diabetes may cause impotence (the inability to have an erection). A device can be implanted into the penis that is filled with fluid to produce an erection. This is called a _____/_____ prosthesis (implant).

6.59

scrot/um
skrō′ təm

pen/o/scrot/al
pē′ nō **skrō′** təl

The saclike structure that contains the testes is the _____/_____. Build a term that means pertaining to the penis and scrotum:

_____/_____/_____/_____.

6.60

an embryonic egg cell
  (a cell that will become
  an ovum)

The Greek word for egg is *oon*. In scientific words, **o/o** (pronounce both *o*s) means egg or ovum. An o/o/blast is * _____

_____.

PRONUNCIATION NOTE

In the terms oogenesis and oophoritis the "oo" is pronounced as ō ə. Look at the pronunciation in Frames 6.61 and 6.67.

6.61

o/o/gen/esis
ō ə **jen′** ə sis

O/o/gen/esis is the formation and development of an ovum. The changes that occur in the cell from ooblast to mature ovum are called

_____/_____/_____/_____.

6.62

oogenesis

O/o/gen/esis must be complete for the ovum to be mature. It is impossible for a spermatozoon to fertilize an ovum until _____ is complete.

6.63

ovary

The combining form used in words that refer to the ovary is **oophor/o**. (This literally means egg bearing.) When you see oophor in a word, you think of the _____.

6.64

ovary

The ovary is the organ that is responsible for maturing and discharging the ovum (ovulation). About every 28 days an ovum (plural ova) is discharged from the _____.

ANSWER COLUMN

6.65

This frame shows the development of the word oophorectomy:

o/o	egg from Greek, *oon*
phor/o	bear from Greek, *phoros*
ect/o	out from Greek, *ektos*
-tomy	cut from Greek, *tomos*

Ovary comes from Latin. An ovarium is a place that holds eggs. Think of aquarium and solarium. Ovarian is the adjective derived from ovarium.

6.66

oophor/o is used in words to refer to the ovary. Oophorectomy means

excision of the ovary

* _____ .

6.67

Using what you need from **oophor/o**, build words that mean

inflammation of an ovary

oophor/itis
ō ə fôr ī′ tis

_____ / _____ ;

excision of an ovary

oophor/ectomy
ō ə fôr **ek**′ tə mē

_____ / _____ ;

tumor of an ovary (ovarian tumor)

oophor/oma
ō ə fôr **ō**′ mə

_____ / _____ .

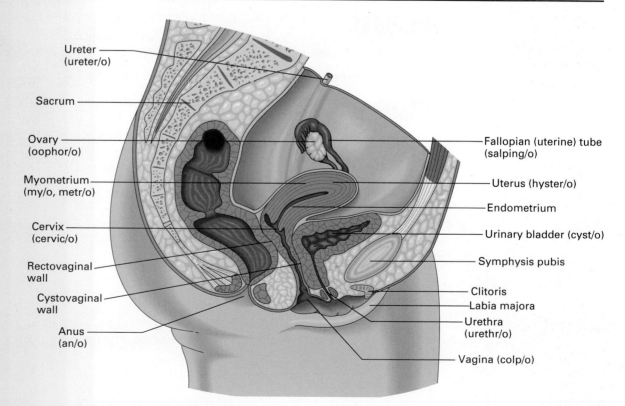

Ureter
(ureter/o)

Sacrum

Ovary
(oophor/o)

Myometrium
(my/o, metr/o)

Cervix
(cervic/o)

Rectovaginal
wall

Cystovaginal
wall

Anus
(an/o)

Fallopian (uterine) tube
(salping/o)

Uterus (hyster/o)

Endometrium

Urinary bladder (cyst/o)

Symphysis pubis

Clitoris

Labia majora

Urethra
(urethr/o)

Vagina (colp/o)

Female reproductive system *Delmar/Cengage Learning*

ANSWER COLUMN

6.68

Recall that **-pexy** is a suffix meaning fixation. Oophor/o/pexy means fixation of

fixation

a displaced ovary. **-pexy** is a suffix that means _____. Fixation of a

orchi/o/pexy *or*
ōr′ kē ō peks′ ē
orchid/o/pexy
or′ kid ō peks′ ē

displaced testicle is _____/_____/_____.

6.69

An oophor/o/pexy is a surgical procedure. When an ovary is displaced, an

oophor/o/pexy
ō **of′** ə rō peks′ ē

_____/_____/_____ may be performed.

6.70

**TAKE A
CLOSER LOOK**

If you look up **oophor/o** in your medical dictionary, it will most likely show you
that the correct pronunciation of terms that begin with **oophor/o** is "o of′" or "o."
However, in practice it has become acceptable to use the usual English
pronunciation for oo as an "oo" sound. For example, the term oophorectomy may
be pronounced both as "o͞o fôr **ek′** tō mē" and "ō ôf′ ôr **ek′** tō mē."

6.71

The surgical procedure to fixate a prolapsed (dropped or sagged) ovary is called

oophoropexy

an _____.

6.72

In the male, fixation of a prolapsed or undescended testicle is called

-pexy

orchid/o/pexy (orchiopexy). The suffix that means fixation is _____.

6.73

salping/o, from the Greek word *salpinx*, meaning trumpet (describing the shape),
is used to build words about the fallopian tube(s). A salping/o/scope is an

fallopian tube(s)

instrument used to examine the * _____.

6.74

A new surgical opening made in a fallopian tube is called a

salping/o/stomy
sal pin **gos′** tō mē

_____/_____/_____.

6.75

Using what you need of **salping/o**, build words meaning inflammation of a
fallopian tube (or eustachian tubes)

salping/itis
sal pin **jī′** tis

_____/_____;

(continued)

ANSWER COLUMN

excision of a fallopian tube (uterine tube)

salping/ectomy
sal pin **jek′** tə mē

_____/_____.

NOTE: **salping/o** is also used to refer to the eustachian tubes in the ears. The context of the medical report should tell you if it refers to ears or uterine tubes.

6.76

When you are building compound medical words and use three like vowels between word roots or combining forms, separate them with a hyphen. For a model use salpingo-oophorectomy. Build a word that means inflammation of the fallopian tube and ovary.

salping/o-/oophor/itis
sal ping′ gō ō ə fôr ī′ tis

_____/_____-/_____/_____

6.77

SPELL
CHECK

Do not drop the _o_ in **salping/o** when joining it to **oophor/o** because the combining form **o/o** means egg. Remember to use a hyphen: salpingo-oophoritis.

6.78

A hernia that encloses the fallopian tube and ovary is

salping/o-/oophor/o/cele
sal ping′ gō ō **of′** ə rō sēl

a _____/_____-/_____/_____/_____.

6.79

colp/o is used in words about the vagina. Colp/itis means

inflammation of the vagina

* _____.

6.80

vaginal pain

Colp/o/dynia means * _____. Any disease of the vagina

colp/o/pathy
kol **pop′** ə thē

is called _____/_____/_____ or vaginopathy.

**External genitalia
of the female** _Delmar/
Cengage Learning_

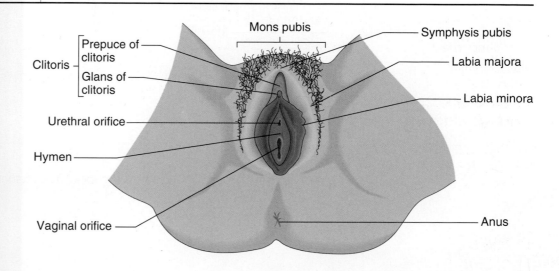

Mons pubis

Symphysis pubis

Prepuce of
clitoris

Clitoris

Glans of
clitoris

Labia majora

Labia minora

Urethral orifice

Hymen

Vaginal orifice

Anus

ANSWER COLUMN

6.81

vaginal spasm

colp/ectomy

kol **pek′** tə mē

Colp/o/spasm is a * _____ . Excision of a part of the vagina

is a _____/_____ or vaginectomy.

6.82

Build words meaning
fixation of the vagina

colp/o/pexy
kol′ pō peks ē

_____/_____/_____;

surgical repair of the vagina

colp/o/plasty
kol′ pō plast′ ē

_____/_____/_____ or vaginoplasty.

6.83

Build words meaning
instrument for examining the vagina

colp/o/scope
kol′ pō skōp

_____/_____/_____;

incision into the vaginal wall

colp/o/tomy
kol **po′** tōm ē

_____/_____/_____ .

6.84

Explanation for
next frame

In words built from **laryng/o**, **pharyng/o**, **salping/o**, and **mening/o**, the g is
pronounced as a hard "g" when followed by o, u, a, or a consonant. The g in good,
gut, gate, and glad is a hard "g."

NOTE: Listen to the Audio CD that accompanies *Medical Terminology:
A Programmed Systems Approach*, 10th edition, for assistance with these rules.

6.85

In laryng/oscope and salpingocele, the "g" of the word root is pronounced hard,
as in goat. In pharyngalgia and meningocele, the "g" is also given a

hard
(Pronounce them)
pharyng/algia
far in **gal′** jē ə
mening/o/cele
men **in** gō sēl

_____ pronunciation.

6.86

In laryngostomy, pharyngotomy, salpingopexy, and meningomalacia, the "g" is

hard

given a _____ sound.

ANSWER COLUMN

6.87

o
u
a
consonant

A hard "g" precedes the vowels _____, _____, and _____ or a _____.

6.88

Explanation for
next frame

In words built from **laryng/o**, **pharyng/o**, **salping/o**, and **mening/o**, the "g" is soft when followed by e, i, or y. The "g" in germ, giant, and gymnast is soft.

6.89

soft
mening/eal
men **in'** jē əl
pharyng/itis
far in **jī'** tis

In laryngectomy and salpingitis, the "g" is a soft "g," as in germ. In meningeal and pharyngitis, the "g" also is given a _____ pronunciation.

6.90

soft
(Pronounce them)

In meningitis, salpingectomy, laryngitis, and pharyngectomy, the "g" is given a _____ sound.

6.91

e
i
y

A soft "g" precedes the vowels _____, _____, and _____.

6.92

a
o
u

e
i
y

"g" is given a hard sound when followed by the vowels _____, _____, and _____.

"g" is given the soft "j" sound when followed by the vowels _____, _____, and _____.

6.93

three like vowels
join word roots or
combining forms

In compound words a hyphen (-) is used when

* _____

_____.

EXAMPLE: salpingo-oophoritis.

CASE STUDY INVESTIGATION (CSI)

Interval History and Physical Exam

Ms. S. Pingo, a 45-year-old female, was seen on 9/12/2009 after an eight-year absence from this **gynecology** office. She was referred from Dr. L's family practice following an abnormal **Pap smear** result on 9/4/2009 describing a squamous cell **carcinoma** in situ. An in-office **colposcopy** was performed on the same day with minimal abnormalities noted on visualization of the cervix. Biopsies were taken and the **pathologist** reported severe **dysplasia** and/or **carcinoma in situ** with glandular atypia. **D&C** with laser conization was recommended. Risks and benefits of the procedure were discussed with the patient and her family and informed consent was obtained. The surgery was scheduled for 9/27/2009.

CSI Vocabulary Challenge

Use your dictionary if necessary to look up the following terms presented in this case study and write their definition in the space provided. Analyze terms by dividing them into their word parts and drawing the slashes.

gynecology	_____
Pap smear	_____
carcinoma	_____
colposcopy	_____
pathologist	_____
dysplasia	_____
carcinoma in situ	_____
D&C	_____

ANSWER COLUMN

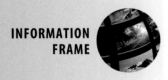

INFORMATION FRAME

6.94

The spermatozoon is the male germ cell; the ovum is the female egg cell. When they unite in the fallopian tube, fertilization occurs. The fertilized ovum moves to the uterus, implants itself into the endometrium, and grows until birth.

6.95

hyster/o is of Greek origin and is used to build words about the uterus as an

uterus
y$\overline{oo}$′ ter əs

organ. A hyster/ectomy is an excision of the _____.

6.96

uterus
uterus

A hyster/o/tomy is an incision into the _____, and a hysterospasm is a spasm of the _____.

ANSWER COLUMN

6.97

A hyster/o/gram is an x-ray (picture) of the uterus. A special x-ray (HSG) procedure is performed to determine patency (openness) of the fallopian tubes by injecting a contrast medium. This "picture," an x-ray of the uterus and fallopian tubes, is

hyster/o/salping/o/gram
his' tər ō sal **ping'** ō gram

called a _____/_____/_____/_____/_____ .

6.98

A general term for any disease of the uterus is

hyster/o/pathy
his' tər **op'** ə thē

_____/_____/_____ .

6.99

A hyster/o/salping/o-/oophor/ectomy is the excision of the uterus, fallopian tubes, and ovaries. Analyze this word:

hyster/o

_____/_____   combining form for uterus

salping/o

_____/_____   combining form for fallopian tubes

oophor

_____   word root for ovary

-ectomy

_____   suffix—excision

Look at the large words you now know. Good job!

6.100

WORD ORIGINS

Dimeter (of the womb) was the goddess of the harvest and the seasons. **metr/o** comes from the Greek word *metra*, meaning womb. The endometrium is the inner layer of tissues of the uterus. Mitra is also a woman's name.

6.101

hyster/o is used in words pertaining to the uterus as an organ. In order to view the uterus more closely, an instrument (**-scope**) with a light source is used to see into the uterus.

This instrument is called a

hyster/o/scope
his' ter ō skōp

_____/_____/_____ .

The procedure is called

hyster/o/scopy
his' ter **os'** kō pē

_____/_____/_____ .

6.102

Uterus (word root uter) comes from a Latin word meaning womb. The adjectival form is uterine. The tubes that attach to the uterus leading to the ovaries are

uter/ine
yōō' ter in

the _____/_____ (fallopian) tubes.

ANSWER COLUMN

(A) Hysterectomy
(B) Total hysterectomy—hysterosalpingo-oophorectomy *Delmar/ Cengage Learning*

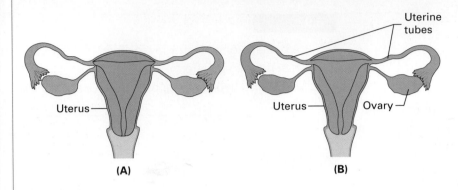

(A)   **(B)**

6.103

There are exceptions to the rule, but in general **hyster/o** means the uterus

as an _____. **metr/o** refers to the uterine _____.

organ
tissues

6.104

Metr/itis means an inflammation of the uterine musculature. Metr/o/paralysis

and metr/o/plegia mean paralysis of the * _____

_____.

uterus or uterine
   musculature

6.105

Using **metr/o** (mē' trō) and **-rrhea**, build a word meaning abnormal flow or
discharge from the uterine tissues:

_____/_____/_____.

NOTE: **-metry** and **-meter** are suffixes meaning measure and instrument used
to measure. They are pronounced me' trē and me' ter, as in audiometry
(aw dē **om'** et rē) and cytometer (sī **tom'** et er).

metr/o/rrhea
mē trō **rē'** ə *or*
met rō **rē'** ə

6.106

Build words meaning any uterine disease

_____/_____/_____

or _____/_____/_____;

herniation of the uterus

_____/_____/_____

or _____/_____/_____.

metr/o/pathy
mē **trop'** ə thē
hyster/o/pathy
his' ter **op'** ə thē

metr/o/cele
mēt' rō sēl
hyster/o/cele
his' ter ō sēl

6.107

The endo/metr/ium is the lining of the uterus.
Build words meaning inflammation of the uterine lining

_____/_____/_____;

endo/metr/itis
en dō mē **trī'** tis

(continued)

ANSWER COLUMN

metr/o/pathy
mē **trop'** ə thē

disease of the uterine tissue

_____/_____/_____ .

6.108

Endo/metr/iosis is a condition in which tissue that looks and acts like endometrial tissue is found in places other than the lining of the uterus. When endometrial-like tissue is found on the outside of the uterus, the ovaries, or bowel, this

condition is called _____/_____/_____ .

endo/metr/iosis
en' dō mē trē **ō'** sis

6.109

Build the word that means excision of the uterus, fallopian tubes, and ovaries:

_____/_____/_____/_____-/

_____/_____ .

Excellent!

hyster/o/salping/o-/
oophor/ectomy
his' te rō sal ping' gō-/ō' ə
fôr **ek'** tə mē

CASE STUDY INVESTIGATION (CSI)

Intestinal Endometriosis

A 45-year-old **perimenopausal** woman was admitted complaining of abdominal pain and vomiting for the past 15 days. Two years prior to admission she had a **hysterosalpingo-oophorectomy**. Abdominal **radiography** showed a **dilated** bowel with air and fluid indicating a bowel **obstruction**. An emergency **laparotomy** was performed revealing the ileum as rigid and shortened and perforated. Histological exam results showed **endometriosis** in the muscle and **mucosal** layers of the ileum. The patient had an uneventful postoperative recovery and was discharged with follow-up instructions.

CSI Vocabulary Challenge

Use your dictionary if necessary to look up the following terms presented in this case study and write the definition in the space provided. Analyze the terms by dividing them into their word parts and drawing the slashes.

perimenopausal   _____

hysterosalpingo-oophorectomy   _____

radiography   _____

dilated   _____

(continued)

obstruction   _____

laparotomy   _____

endometriosis   _____

mucosal   _____

ANSWER COLUMN

6.110

INFORMATION FRAME

-ptosis is a suffix meaning prolapse or downward displacement. Ptosis is also a word by itself meaning a condition of displacement. Ptotic is the adjectival form.

6.111

Hyster/o/ptosis means prolapse of the uterus. *Ptosis* is a Greek word that means

prolapse, falling, or to fall   * _____.

6.112

Hyster/o/ptosis is a compound word constructed from

hyster/o

ptosis   _____/_____ the combining form for uterus;

                                    _____ a word meaning prolapse.

6.113

When prolapse occurs, a fixation is usually done. A hyster/o/pexy would be done to correct or fixate

hyster/o/ptosis
his′ tər op **tō′** sis   _____/_____/_____.

6.114

Many organs can prolapse or sag. When the uterus prolapses, it is

hysteroptosis   called _____.

Hysteroptosis *Delmar/Cengage Learning*

Normal position

Prolapsed uterus

ANSWER COLUMN

6.115

Build a word meaning prolapse of the vagina:

colp/o/ptosis
kol′ pop **tō′** sis

_____/_____/_____ .

6.116

A word meaning surgical fixation of the uterus is

hyster/o/pexy
his′ tə rō pek sē

_____/_____/_____ .

A word meaning uterine hernia is

hyster/o/cele
his′ tə rō sēl

_____/_____/_____ .

6.117

Use **cervic/o** to refer to the cervix, which is the neck of the uterus. Cervic/o/plasty is a surgical procedure to repair the cervix.
Build a word that means
inflammation of the cervix

cervic/itis
ser vi **sī′** tis

_____/_____ ;

pertaining to the cervix

cervic/al
ser′ vi kal

_____/_____ .

6.118

SPELL
CHECK

Cervic/o is also used as a combining form referring to the neck (cervical) area of the spine. The first seven vertebral bones of the neck are the cervical vertebrae. Use the context of your subject and look up terms in the dictionary to know if you are using **cervic/o** correctly in a term when referring to either the neck of the uterus or the neck area of the spine.

6.119

TAKE A
CLOSER LOOK

One surgical procedure that may be performed on the cervix is a con/ization. A cone-shaped cut is made in the cervix to remove endo/cervical tissue. This may be done using electr/o/cautery (cautery conization) or a cold knife blade (cold conization).

6.120

con/ization
kō ni **zā′** shun
endo/cervical _or_
en′ dō **ser′** vi kal
cervic/al

Using what you have just learned, complete the following statement.
A _____/_____ may be performed to remove a
cone-shaped sample of _____/_____ tissue.

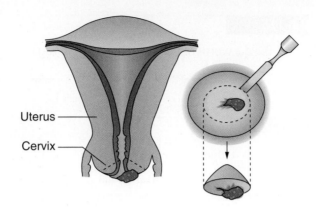

Uterus

Cervix

6.121

gynec/o and gyn/e come from the Greek word *gyne*, which means woman.

women

The field of medicine called gynec/o/logy deals with diseases of _____.

6.122

gynec/o/logist
gī nə **kol'** ə jist *or*
jin ə **kol'** ə jist
gynec/o/log/ic
gīn nə kō **lo'** jik *or*
jin ə kō **lo'** jik

Gynec/o/log/ic is the adjectival form of gynecology (GYN). The physician who

specializes in female disorders is called a _____/_____/_____.
This physician may perform a

_____/_____/_____/_____ exam.

6.123

gynec/oid
gī' nə koid *or* **jin'** ə koid
gynec/o/pathy
gī' nə **kop'** ə thē *or*
jin ə **kop'** ə thē
gyn/e/phobia
gī nə **fō'** bē ə *or*
jin ə **fō'** bē ə

Build words meaning
resembling woman

_____/_____;

any disease peculiar to women

_____/_____/_____;

abnormal fear of women

_____/_____/_____.

6.124

Vas is a Latin word meaning vessel, duct, or tube. vas/o is another combining
form for blood vessel. Vas/o/dilatat/ion means enlarging the diameter of a

vessel

_____.

NOTE: Dilatation and dilation are synonyms.

ANSWER COLUMN

6.125

Vas/o/constrict/ion is the opposite of vas/o/dilatat/ion.

decreasing the size of the
diameter of a vessel

Vas/o/constrict/ion means * _____

_____ .

6.126

Nitroglycerine is a vas/o/dilat/or. People with angina pectoris experience chest
pain due to vas/o/constrict/ion of the blood vessels to the heart. After taking a

vas/o/dilator
vas′ ō **dĭ′** lā tor

_____/_____/_____, the vessels allow more blood to

flow to the heart, and the pain stops.

6.127

**SPELL
CHECK**

Dilate, dilated, dilating, dilation, dilator, and dilatation are word forms that all
mean to increase in diameter. When a blood vessel enlarges the diameter of
the lumen vessel, it is dilated. When it becomes smaller in diameter, it constricts.
Here is a grammar test. Think of how you would use each of the following terms
in a sentence. State the part of speech (noun or verb) of each of the following.

dilate   _____

dilated   _____

dilating   _____

dilation   _____

dilator   _____

dilatation   _____

6.128

vessel

Vas/o/motor is an adjective that refers to nerves that control the tone of the

blood _____ walls.

6.129

Using **vas/o**, build words meaning
pertaining to a vessel

vas/al
vā′ səl or **vā′** zəl
vas/o/spasm
vas′ ō spaz əm or
vā′ zō spaz əm

vas/o/tripsy
vas′ ō trip sē or
vā′ zō trip sē

_____/_____;

spasm of a vessel

_____/_____/_____;

crushing of a vessel (with forceps to stop hemorrhage)

_____/_____/_____tripsy_____ .

INFORMATION FRAME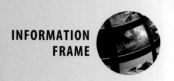

6.130

vas/o can be used to mean many types of vessels, ducts, or tubes. Look at the words used in your dictionary beginning with vas or **vas/o**. They could be confused with **angi/o**.
The four words in Frame 6.131 refer to the vas deferens only—no other vessel. The vas deferens is shown in the illustration of vasectomy.

6.131

vas/o/tomy
vas **ot'** ə mē

vas/o/rrhaphy
vas **or'** ə fē

vas/o/stomy
vas **os'** tə mē

vas/ectomy
vas **ek'** tə mē

Build words meaning
incision into the vas deferens

_____/_____/_____ ;

suture of the vas deferens

_____/_____/_____ ;

making a new opening into the vas deferens

_____/_____/_____ ;

removal of a segment of the vas deferens

_____/_____ .

NOTE: Tubal ligation is the excision of the fallopian tubes and is the sterilization surgery in women.

Vasectomy—excision of a section of the right and left vas deferens *Delmar/Cengage Learning*

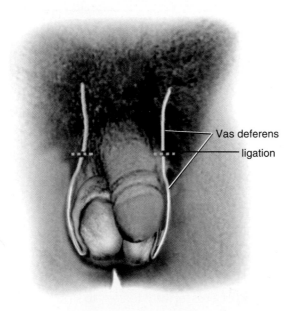

Vas deferens

ligation

ANSWER COLUMN

Abbreviation	Meaning
AID	artificial insemination (donor's sperm)
AIH	artificial insemination (husband's sperm)
BPH	benign prostatic hyperplasia (hypertrophy)
CIS	carcinoma in situ
cysto	cystoscopy
D&C	dilation and currettage
ESRD	end-stage renal disease
F, ♀	female
GYN	gynecology (ist)
HSG	hysterosalpingogram
IVP	intravenous pyelogram
KUB	kidney ureter bladder
M, ♂	male
MD	doctor of medicine
Pap	Papanicolaou test (smear)
PID	pelvic inflammatory disease
PSA	prostate specific antigen
RPG	retrograde pyelogram
sp gr, SpG	specific gravity
TAH	total abdominal hysterectomy
TSE	testicular self-exam
TUR (P)	transurethral resection (prostate)
UA	urinalysis
UTI	urinary tract infection

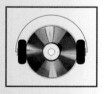

To complete your study of this unit, work the **Review Activities** on the following pages. Also, listen to the Audio CD that accompanies *Medical Terminology: A Programmed Systems Approach*, 10th edition, and practice your pronunciation.

STUDYWARE™ CONNECTION

To help you learn the content in this chapter, take a practice quiz or play an interactive game on your **StudyWARE™ CD-ROM**.

REVIEW ACTIVITIES

CIRCLE AND CORRECT

Circle the correct answer for each question. Then check your answers in Appendix E.

1. Sound made by g followed by e
   a. "k"
   b. "j"
   c. "s"
   d. "g" as in gut

2. Suffix for destruction
   a. -plasty
   b. -rrhexis
   c. -lysis
   d. -malacia

3. Plural form for sperm
   a. sperms
   b. spermat
   c. spermatozoon
   d. spermatozoa

4. Word root for penis
   a. penile
   b. pen
   c. balan
   d. orchid

5. Suffix for prolapse
   a. -ptosis
   b. -ectomy
   c. -cele
   d. -pexy

6. Suffix for surgical fixation
   a. -ptosis
   b. -ectomy
   c. -plasty
   d. -pexy

7. Suffix for suturing
   a. -rrhea
   b. -rrhaphy
   c. -rrhia
   d. -rrhagia

8. Word root for uterus (the organ)
   a. utero
   b. hyster
   c. metro
   d. meter

9. Adjective for testis
   a. testes
   b. orchidic
   c. testicular
   d. testicle

10. Suffix for instrument used to make a picture (x-ray)
    a. -graph
    b. -scope
    c. -meter
    d. -tome

11. Combining form for woman
    a. hystero
    b. andro
    c. gyneco
    d. femino

12. Adjective for ovary
    a. ovarian
    b. ova
    c. oophoral
    d. uterine

13. Combining form for kidney
    a. pyelo
    b. nephro
    c. oophoro
    d. renal

14. Suffix for abnormal bleeding
    a. -rrhea
    b. -rrhaphy
    c. -rrhagia
    d. -rrhia

15. Suffix for flow or discharge
    a. -clysis
    b. -trophy
    c. -rrhea
    d. -hydro

16. Adjective for kidney
    a. nephral
    b. nephroc
    c. cystic
    d. renal

17. Combining form for the tube that leads from the kidneys to the bladder
    a. cysto
    b. uretero
    c. urethro
    d. pyelo

18. Correct spelling for term meaning bleeding
    a. hemorage
    b. hematorrhagia
    c. hyperemia
    d. hemorrhage

SELECT AND CONSTRUCT

Select the correct word parts from the following list and construct medical terms that represent the given meaning.

algia	balano	centesis	cervic/o	colpo	crypt(o)
cyst(o)	dermato	dynia	ectomy	endo	genesis
gram	graph	gyneco	hystero	ic	ism
itis	logy(ist)	lysis	metro	nephr/o	oma
oo	oophoro	orchid(o)	osis	ostomy	pathy
pexy	plasty	prostato	ptosis	pyelo	reno(al)
rrhagia	rrhaphy	rrhea	salpingo	scope	scopy
spasm	testiculo	uretero	urethro	uro	

REVIEW ACTIVITIES

1. inflammation of the renal pelvis and the kidney _____

2. suture of the tube that goes from the kidney to the urinary bladder _____

3. process of examining the urinary bladder by looking through an instrument _____

4. prolapsed kidney _____

5. x-ray of the kidney _____

6. fixation of the urinary bladder _____

7. abnormal bleeding of the urethra _____

8. destruction of kidney tissue _____

9. make a new opening in the urinary bladder _____

10. inflammation of the inner lining of the uterus _____

11. prolapse of the uterus _____

12. undescended testicles _____

13. excision of the prostate gland _____

14. specialist in women's health _____

15. formation of ova _____

16. a discharge from the glans penis _____

17. vaginal pain _____

18. instrument used to look into the uterus _____

19. specialist in men's health _____

20. x-ray of uterus and fallopian tubes _____

21. fixation of a prolapsed testicle _____

22. process of viewing the inside of the vagina with a scope _____

23. inside the cervix _____

DEFINE AND DISSECT

Give a brief definition and dissect each term listed into its word parts in the space provided. Check your answers by referring to the frame listed in parentheses and your medical dictionary. Then listen to the Audio CD to practice pronunciation.

1. nephropexy (6.16)   _____/_____/_____

                                                       rt   v   suffix

   meaning _____

REVIEW ACTIVITIES

2. ureterocele (6.22)

_____/_____/_____
rt   v   suffix

_____

3. ureteropyelitis (6.23)

_____/_____/_____/_____
rt   v   rt   suffix

_____

4. cystorrhaphy (6.28)

_____/_____/_____
rt   v   suffix

_____

5. urethrotomy (6.31)

_____/_____/_____
rt   v   suffix

_____

6. nephroptosis (6.14)

_____/_____/_____
rt   v   suffix

_____

7. renopathy (6.10)

_____/_____/_____
rt   v   suffix

_____

8. nephrolith (6.17)

_____/_____/_____
rt   v   rt

_____

9. renal (6.10)

_____/_____
rt   suffix

_____

10. ureterocystostomy (6.24)

_____/_____/_____/_____/_____
rt   v   rt   v   suffix

_____

11. renogram (6.10)

_____/_____/_____
rt   v   suffix

_____

REVIEW ACTIVITIES

12. spermatozoa (6.36)

_____/_____/_____
rt   v   suffix

_____

13. orchidoplasty (6.45)

_____/_____/_____
rt   v   suffix

_____

14. testicular (6.42)

_____/_____
rt   suffix

_____

15. prostatorrhea (6.53)

_____/_____/_____
rt   v   suffix

_____

16. hysterosalpingogram (6.97)

_____/_____/_____/_____/_____
rt   v   rt   v   suffix

_____

17. salpingo-oophorocele (6.78)

_____/_____/_____/_____/_____
rt   v   rt   v   suffix

_____

18. colposcope (6.83)

_____/_____/_____
rt   v   suffix

_____

19. endometriosis (6.108)

_____/_____/_____
pre   rt   suffix

_____

20. hysteroptosis (6.113)

_____/_____/_____
rt   v   suffix

_____

21. seminal (6.50)

_____/_____
rt   suffix

_____

22. hysteroscopy (6.101)

_____/_____/_____
rt   v   suffix

_____

REVIEW ACTIVITIES

23. hysterosalpingo-oophorectomy (6.109)   _____/_____/_____/_____/_____/_____

rt   v   rt   v   rt   suffix

_____

24. orchidalgia (6.41)   _____/_____

rt   suffix

_____

25. spermicide (6.38)   _____/_____/_____

rt   v   suffix

_____

26. gynecologist (6.122)   _____/_____/_____

rt   v   suffix

_____

27. vasotripsy (6.128)   _____/_____/_____

rt   v   suffix

_____

28. vasectomy (6.130)   _____/_____

rt   suffix

_____

29. cervicoplasty (6.117)   _____/_____/_____

rt   v   suffix

_____

30. vasoconstriction (6.125)   _____/_____/_____/_____

rt   v   rt   suffix

_____

31. conization (6.119)   _____/_____

rt   suffix

_____

32. dysuria (6.5)   _____/_____/_____

pre   rt   suffix

_____

REVIEW ACTIVITIES

IMAGE LABELING

Match the combining forms with the numbered diagram. Write the structure name in the blank.

Combining Form   **Name of the Structure**

_____ rect/o   _____

_____ cyst/o   _____

_____ urethr/o   _____

_____ balan/o   _____

_____ prostat/o   _____

_____ vas/o   _____

_____ orchid/o   _____

_____ pen/o   _____

_____ ureter/o   _____

_____ scrot/o   _____

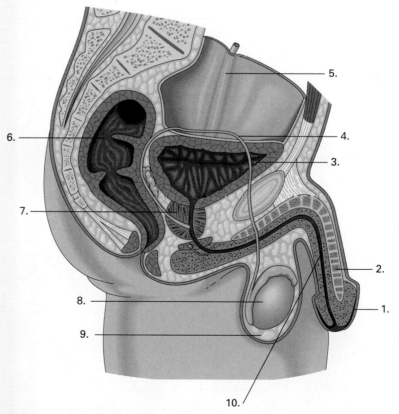

Male reproductive system *Delmar/Cengage Learning*

REVIEW ACTIVITIES

IMAGE LABELING

Label the structures of the female reproductive system by writing the number in front of the correct word part.
Write the body part indicated.

Combining Form	Body Part
_____ colp/o	_____
_____ hyster/o	_____
_____ oophor/o	_____
_____ metr/o	_____
_____ salping/o	_____
_____ cervic/o	_____
_____ rect/o	_____
_____ clitor/o	_____
_____ labi/o	_____
_____ urethr/o	_____
_____ an/o	_____
_____ ureter/o	_____
_____ cystovagin/o	_____
_____ cyst/o	_____

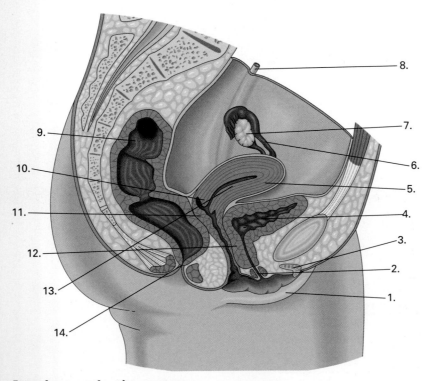

Female reproductive system *Delmar/Cengage Learning*

REVIEW ACTIVITIES

ABBREVIATION MATCHING

Match the following abbreviations with their definition.

_____ 1. HSG

_____ 2. cysto

_____ 3. BPH

_____ 4. F, ♀

_____ 5. TUR(P)

_____ 6. M, ♂

_____ 7. GYN

_____ 8. UTI

_____ 9. AID

_____ 10. TSE

_____ 11. RPG

_____ 12. IVP

_____ 13. UA

_____ 14. TAH

a. urinalysis (testing)

b. testicular self-exam

c. transluminal upper restoration

d. hysterectomy (total abdominal)

e. retrograde pyelogram

f. arteriosclerosis

g. benign prostatic hyperplasia (hypertrophy)

h. female

i. transurethral resection of the prostate

j. gynecophobia

k. artificial insemination using husband's sperm

l. intravenous pyelogram

m. male

n. artificial insemination by donor's sperm

o. gynecology (ist)

p. urinary tract infection

q. hysterosalpingogram

r. upper respiratory infection

s. cystoscopy

ABBREVIATION FILL-IN

Fill in the blanks with the correct abbreviation.

15. doctor of medicine   _____

16. prostate specific antigen _____

17. kidney, ureter, bladder   _____

18. artificial insemination using husband's sperm _____

19. end-stage renal disease   _____

20. Papanicolaou test   _____

REVIEW ACTIVITIES

CASE STUDY

Write the term next to its meaning given below. Then draw slashes to analyze the word parts. Note the use of medical abbreviations. Look these up in your dictionary or find them in Appendix B. If you have any questions about the answers, refer to your medical dictionary or check with your instructor for the answers in Appendix E.

CASE STUDY 6-1

Discharge Summary—Transurethral Resection of the Prostate

Pt: Male, age 72

Dx: Benign prostatic **hyperplasia** with retention and **hydronephrosis**

Mr. Travis Reese was brought to the hospital for a **TUR** for reasons itemized in the **H&P**. He underwent a **transurethral** resection of the trilobar gland on 9/21. On 9/22, **cystoclysis** was clear. He had one degree of temperature and went to straight drainage. On 9/23 his temperature was normal with slight **hematuria**. The **catheter** was removed. On 9/24 he was **afebrile**. Urine was light, diluted cherry Kool-Aid color. A **postoperative** instruction sheet was given to Mr. Reese. He read it and had no questions. He was given a prescription for Achromycin 250 **mg qid** and discharged.

Pathology report: 40 g of **benign** tissue with mild focal, acute and **chronic prostatitis**.

1. milligrams four times a day _____

2. noncancerous _____

3. study of disease _____

4. overdevelopment _____

5. inflammation of the prostate _____

6. long-term less severe _____

7. history and physical exam _____

8. urine (water) in the kidney _____

9. transurethral resection _____

10. blood in the urine _____

11. without a fever _____

12. irrigation of the bladder _____

13. tube inserted in the bladder _____

14. after surgery _____

15. across the urethra _____

REVIEW ACTIVITIES

CROSSWORD PUZZLE

Check your answers by going back through the frames or checking the solution in Appendix F.

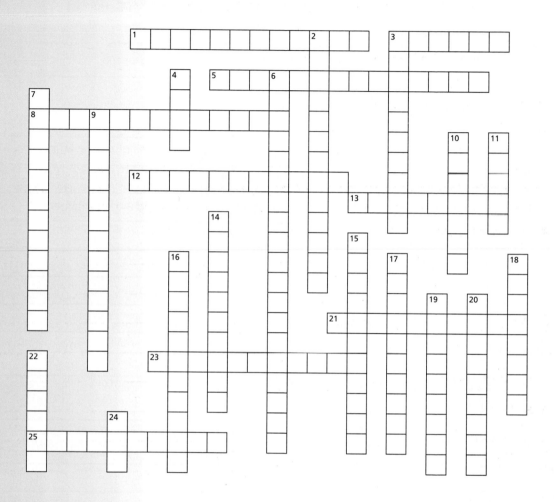

Across

1. suturing of the urinary bladder
3. pertaining to the penis
5. inflammation of the kidney and renal pelvis
8. condition of endometrial tissue on other organs
12. discharge from the glans penis
13. scant amount of urine
21. surgical fixation of orchidoptosis
23. stone in the tube from kidney to bladder
25. pertaining to the testes

Down

2. excision of the prostate gland
3. excessive hunger and eating
4. transurethral resection of the prostate
6. HSG
7. prolapsed kidney
9. surgical repair of testis
10. pertaining to the uterus
11. pertaining to the kidney
14. hysteropathy (synonym)
15. excessive bleeding with menses
16. metrocele (synonym)
17. inflamed ovaries
18. having more than two ears
19. colpodynia (synonym)
20. blood in the urine
22. combining form for hidden
24. pelvic inflammatory disease (abbr.)

REVIEW ACTIVITIES

GLOSSARY

antineoplastic	agent that works against tumor growth
anuria	unable to produce urine
balanoplasty	surgical repair of the glans penis
balanorrhea	discharge from the glans penis
cervical	pertaining to the neck and cervix
cervicitis	Inflammation of the cervix
cholelithiasis	Infestation with gallstones
colpalgia	vaginal pain
colpitis	inflammation of the vagina
colpopathy	any disease of the vagina (vaginopathy)
colpoptosis	prolapse of the vagina
colposcope	instrument used to examine the vagina and cervix
colposcopy	the process of using a colposcope to examine tissues of vagina and cervix
colpotomy	incision into the vaginal wall
conization	excision of a cone-shaped endocervical tissue
cryptorchidism	condition of an undescended testis
cystorrhagia	hemorrhage of the bladder
cystorrhaphy	suturing of the urinary bladder
dermatorrhaphy	suturing of the skin
dysplasia	abnormal development that may be cancerous
dysuria	difficult, painful urination
endocervical	inside the cervix
endometriosis	condition of endometrial tissue growing outside of the endometrium
endometritis	inflammation of the endometrium
glycosuria	glucose (sugar) in the urine

gynecoid	resembling a woman or female structures
gynecologist	physician specialist in health issues related to female reproductive organs and the breasts
gynecology	the science of studying diseases of the female reproductive organs and the breasts
gynecopathy	any disease peculiar to women
gyneophobia	abnormal fear of women
hematuria	blood in urine
hemorrhage	bleeding
hysterectomy	excision of the uterus
hysteropathy	any disease of the uterus
hysteropexy	fixation of a prolapsed uterus
hysterosalpingogram	x-ray of the uterus and fallopian tubes (uses contrast media)
hysterosalpingo-oophorectomy	total abdominal hysterectomy
hysteroscope	instrument used to examine the inside of the uterus closely
hysteroscopy	the process of using a hysteroscope
menorrhagia	abnormally excessive menstruation
metrocele	herniation of uterine tissues (hysterocele)
metropathy	any disease of the uterine tissues (hysteropathy)
metrorrhea	discharge from the uterine tissues
nephritis	inflammation of the kidney
nephrolith	kidney stone
nephromalacia	softening of kidney tissue
nephromegaly	enlargement of a kidney
nephropexy	surgical fixation of a prolapsed kidney
nephroptosis	prolapsed or displaced kidney

REVIEW ACTIVITIES

nephrorrhaphy	suturing of kidney tissue
neurorrhaphy	suturing of a nerve
nocturia	excessive urination at night
oliguria	abnormally low amount of urine
oogenesis	formation of ova
oophorectomy	excision of an ovary
oophoritis	inflammation of an ovary
oophoroma	tumor of an ovary
oophoropexy	surgical fixation of a prolapsed ovary
oophoroptosis	prolapsed ovary
orchidalgia	testicular pain (orchidodynia)
orchidectomy	excision of a testis (orchiectomy, orchectomy)
orchidocele	herniation of the testes
orchidoptosis	prolapsed condition of a testis
orchiopexy	fixation of an undescended testis (orchidopexy)
orchioplasty	surgical repair of the testes
orchiotomy	incision into a testis
penile	pertaining to the penis
penitis	inflammation of the penis
penoscrotal	pertaining to the penis and scrotum
polyarthritis	inflammation of many joints
polycystic	having many cysts
polyneuralgia	pain in many nerves
polyneuritis	inflammation of many nerves
polyotia	having more than two ears
polyphagia	excessive hunger and eating
polyphobia	having many fears
polyuria	abnormally excessive urination
prostatalgia	prostate pain
prostatectomy	excision of the prostate
prostatitis	inflammation of the prostate gland

prostatorrhea	discharge from the prostate
pyelitis	inflammation of the renal pelvis
pyelogram	x-ray of the renal pelvis
pyelonephritis	inflammation of the renal pelvis and the kidney
pyeloplasty	surgical repair of the renal pelvis
renal	pertaining to the kidney
renogastric	pertaining to the kidney and stomach
renogram	x-ray of the kidney (renograph)
renointestinal	pertaining to the kidney and intestine
renopathy	any disease of the kidney
salpingectomy	excision of a fallopian tube
salpingitis	inflammation of the fallopian tubes (or eustachian tubes)
salpingo-oophoritis	inflammation of the ovary and fallopian tube
salpingo-oophorocele	herniation of the ovary and fallopian tube
salpingostomy	forming a new opening in the fallopian tube
scrotum	saclike structure containing the testes
seminal	pertaining to semen
seminoma	tumor containing sperm
spermatoblast	immature sperm cell (spermoblast)
spermatocele	a herniated sac-like structure in the scrotum containing sperm
spermatocyst	saclike structure containing sperm
spermatoid	resembling sperm
spermatolysis	destruction of sperm (spermolysis)
spermatopathy	any disease of the sperm
spermicide	agent that kills sperm
testicular	pertaining to the testes
ureters	tubes from kidneys to bladder

REVIEW ACTIVITIES

ureterocele	herniation of the ureter
ureterocystostomy	procedure to form a new opening between the ureter and the urinary bladder
ureterolith	stone in the ureter
ureteropathy	any disease involving the ureter
ureteropyelitis	inflammation of the ureter and the renal pelvis
ureteropyosis	condition of pus in the ureter
ureterorrhagia	hemorrhage of the ureter
ureterorrhaphy	suturing of the ureter
urethra	tube from bladder to urinary meatus
urethrocystitis	inflammation of the urethra and urinary bladder
urethrorrhagia	hemorrhage of the urethra
urethrorrhaphy	suturing of the urethra
urethrospasm	spasm of the muscles of the urethra
urethrotomy	incision into the urethra

urogenital	pertaining to the urinary tract and genitals
urologist	physician specialist in disorders of the urinary and male reproductive systems
urology	the medical specialty that studies the urinary system
uropathy	any disease of the urinary system
uterine	pertaining to the uterus
vasectomy	excision of the vas deferens (for sterilization)
vasoconstriction	decrease in vessel diameter
vasodilation (vasodilatation)	increase in vessel diameter
vasorrhaphy	suturing of vessel or vas deferens
vasostomy	procedure to make a new opening in the vas deferens
vasotomy	incision into the vas deferens
vasotripsy	surgical crushing of a vessel

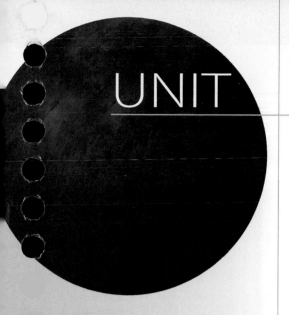

7

Gastroenterology

Read through the digestive system information in the following table. Locate the organs named by studying the illustration on page 250. Then work Frames 7.1–7.102.

Organ	Combining Form	Suffixes	Examples
mouth	stomat/o	-itis	stomat/itis
teeth	dent/o, odont/o	-ist	dent/ist
tongue	gloss/o, lingu/o	-plegia*	gloss/o/plegia
lips	cheil/o	-plasty	cheil/o/plasty
gums	gingiv/o	-ectomy	gingiv/ectomy
esophagus	esophag/o	-spasm	esophag/o/spasm
stomach	gastr/o	-ectasia*	gastr/ectasia
small intestine	enter/o	-logy	enter/o/logy
duodenum	duoden/o	-ostomy	duoden/ostomy
jejunum	jejun/o	-rrhaphy	jejun/o/rrhaphy
ileum	ile/o	-tomy	ile/o/tomy
large intestine	col/o	-clysis*	col/o/clysis
sigmoid colon	sigmoid/o	-scopy	sigmoid/o/scopy
rectum	rect/o	-cele	rect/o/cele
anus and rectum	proct/o	-scope	proct/o/scope
accessory organs			
liver	hepat/o	-megaly	hepat/o/megaly
gallbladder	cholecyst/o	-gram	cholecyst/o/gram
pancreas	pancreat/o	-lith	pancreat/o/lith

*New suffix.

7.1

Stoma is a Greek word meaning mouth. The combining form for mouth is

stomat/o

_____/_____ .

NOTE: The suffix **-ostomy** means forming a new opening like a mouth.

ANSWER COLUMN

7.2

inflammation of the mouth	Stomat/itis means * _____.
surgical repair of the mouth	Stomat/o/plasty means * _____.

7.3

Using the word root for mouth, form words meaning pain in the mouth

stomat/algia
stō mə **tal'** jē ə

_____/_____;

hemorrhage of the mouth

stomat/o/rrhagia
stō' mə tō **rā'** jē ə

_____/_____/_____.

7.4

Using the combining form **stomat/o** for mouth, build words meaning condition

stomat/o/myc/osis
stō' mə tō mī **kō'** sis
stomat/o/pathy
stō' mə **top'** ə thē

of mouth fungus (**myc/o**) _____/_____/_____/_____;

any disease of the mouth _____/_____/_____.

Digestive system
Delmar/Cengage Learning

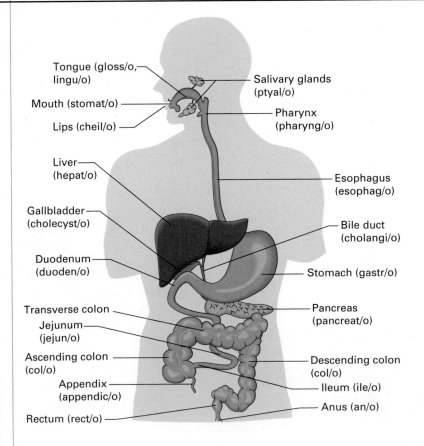

Tongue (gloss/o, lingu/o)
Salivary glands (ptyal/o)
Mouth (stomat/o)
Pharynx (pharyng/o)
Lips (cheil/o)
Liver (hepat/o)
Esophagus (esophag/o)
Gallbladder (cholecyst/o)
Bile duct (cholangi/o)
Duodenum (duoden/o)
Stomach (gastr/o)
Transverse colon
Pancreas (pancreat/o)
Jejunum (jejun/o)
Ascending colon (col/o)
Descending colon (col/o)
Appendix (appendic/o)
Ileum (ile/o)
Rectum (rect/o)
Anus (an/o)

ANSWER COLUMN

7.5

Recall that **-scope** is a suffix for an instrument used to examine. A micr/o/scope is an instrument for examining something small. An instrument for examining the

mouth is a _____/_____/_____ .

The process of examining with this instrument

is _____/_____/_____ .

stomat/o/scope
stō **mat'** ō skōp

stomat/o/scopy
stō mə **tos'** kə pē

7.6

SPELL CHECK

Be careful to use stomat/o for mouth, not stomach. Remember, **gastr/o** means stomach. A stoma is an opening or mouth.

7.7

The Greek combining form for tongue is **gloss/o** (think of a glossary of words).

inflammation of the tongue

Gloss/itis means * _____ .

excision of the tongue

Gloss/ectomy means * _____ .

7.8

Using the word root, build words meaning pain in the tongue

_____/_____ ;

gloss/algia
glos **al'** jē ə

pertaining to the tongue _____/_____ .

gloss/al
glos' əl

7.9

hypo- is a prefix meaning below or under. Cranial nerve XII is the hypo/gloss/al nerve. It supplies nerve impulses

* _____

_____ .

under the tongue or
to the tongue

A medication that is administered under the tongue is a

hypo/gloss/al *or*
hī pō **glos'** əl

_____/_____/_____ medication.

sub/lingu/al
sub **lin'** gwal

7.10

WORD ORIGINS

sub- and *lingual* are Latin word parts. **hypo-** and *glossal* are Greek word parts. Generally, original languages are not mixed when forming words. So, sublingual (Latin) and hypoglossal (Greek) are usually used. Think of linguistics and glossary. A person's native tongue is their native language.

ANSWER COLUMN

7.11

lingu/o is a Latin combining form for tongue (think of lingusitics or language). Lingu/al is the adjectival form. **sub-** is a prefix used with **lingu/o**. Build an adjective that means pertaining to under the tongue:

sub/lingu/al
sub **lin'** gwal

_____/_____/_____.

REMINDER: Do not use hypolingual; it is not a word.

7.12

Nitroglycerin tablets are administered sub/lingual/ly. This means they are placed

under the tongue

* _____.

7.13

Two words that you have learned that mean under the tongue

hypo/gloss/al

are _____/_____/_____ and

sub/lingu/al

_____/_____/_____.

7.14

Using **gloss/o** for tongue, build words meaning prolapse of the tongue

gloss/o/ptosis
glos op **tō'** sis

_____/_____/_____;
examination of the tongue

gloss/o/scopy
glos **os'** kə pē

_____/_____/_____.

7.15

-plegia is a suffix meaning paralysis. Build words meaning paralysis of the tongue

gloss/o/plegia
glos ō **plē'** jē ə

_____/_____/_____ (noun);
paralysis of the tongue

gloss/o/plegic
glos ō **plē'** jik

_____/_____/_____ (adjective).

7.16

cheil/o (note: e before i) is a combining form for lips. Cheil/itis means

inflammation of the lips

* _____.

plastic surgery of the lips

Cheil/o/plasty means * _____

_____.

7.17

cheil

The word root for lip is _____.

cheil/o
kī' lō

The combining form for lip is _____/_____.

NOTE: When pronouncing the diphthong "ei", the "e" is silent and the "i" is a long vowel sound.

ANSWER COLUMN

The oral cavity
Delmar/Cengage Learning

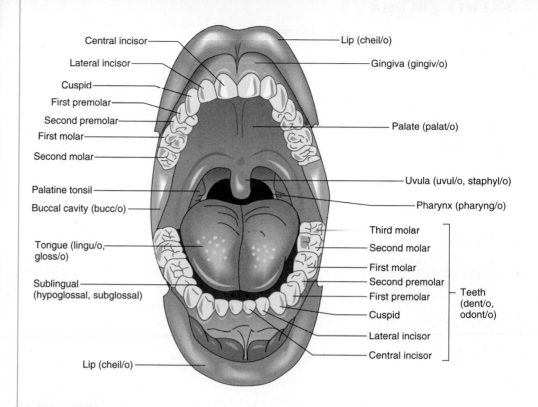

Central incisor

Lateral incisor

Cuspid

First premolar

Second premolar

First molar

Second molar

Palatine tonsil

Buccal cavity (bucc/o)

Tongue (lingu/o, gloss/o)

Sublingual (hypoglossal, subglossal)

Lip (cheil/o)

Lip (cheil/o)

Gingiva (gingiv/o)

Palate (palat/o)

Uvula (uvul/o, staphyl/o)

Pharynx (pharyng/o)

Third molar

Second molar

First molar

Second premolar

First premolar

Cuspid

Lateral incisor

Central incisor

Teeth (dent/o, odont/o)

7.18

cheil/o/tomy
kī **lot'** ə mē
cheil/osis
kī **lō'** sis

Build words meaning incision of the lips

_____/_____/_____;

condition or disorder of the lips _____/_____.

7.19

cheil/o/stomat/o/plasty
kī' lō stō **mat'** ō plas tē

A word meaning plastic surgery of the lips and mouth is

_____/_____/_____/_____/_____.

         lips   mouth   repair

7.20

pertaining to the gums

gingiv/o

gingiv/o is the combining form for gums. Gingiv/al means

* _____.

The combining form for gums is _____/_____.

7.21

gingiv/itis
jin ji **vī'** tis
gingiv/algia
jin ji **val'** jē ə

Build words meaning inflammation of the gums

_____/_____;

gum pain _____/_____.

ANSWER COLUMN

7.22

gingiv/ectomy
jin ji **vek'** tə mē

gingiv/o/gloss/itis
jin' ji vō glos **ī'** tis

lingu/o/gingiv/al
lin' gwō **jin'** ji vəl

Build words meaning excision of gum tissue

_____/_____;

inflammation of the gums and tongue

_____/_____/_____/_____;

tongue and gums (adjective)

_____/_____/_____/_____.

7.23

TAKE A CLOSER LOOK

Food is chewed (masticat/ion) by the teeth and mixed with saliva in the mouth. It is then pushed by the tongue into the pharynx and a series of smooth muscle contractions called peristalsis sends it down the esophagus to the stomach (ingest/ion). In the stomach, food is mixed with hydrochloric acid (HCl) and enzymes that begin chemical breakdown. Next, the mixture travels to the duodenum. Digestive enzymes are secreted from the duodenal wall and the pancreas, and bile is added from the gallbladder. The enzymes break up starches into glucose, proteins into amino acids, and the bile emulsifies fats (digest/ion). Nutrients including water are absorbed through the small and large intestinal walls into the blood and lymphatic system (absorp/tion). The undigested and unabsorbed food called feces (stool) travels through the large intestine to the rectum and is expelled through the anus (defecat/ion).

7.24

masticat/ion
ma sti **kā'** shun

ingest/ion
in **jest'** shun

digest/ion
dī **jest'** shun

absorp/tion
ab **sorp'** shun

defecat/ion
de fə **ka'** shun

From what you have just read, list the words that mean the following:
process of chewing

_____/_____;

process of swallowing

_____/_____;

chemical breakdown of food

_____/_____;

movement of nutrients from intestine to the blood

_____/_____;

expelling solid waste

_____/_____;

(continued)

STUDY WARE™ CONNECTION

View an animation on digestion on your **Study WARE™ CD-ROM.**

ANSWER COLUMN

feces
fē sēs

stool
sto͞ol

solid waste material

_____ or

_____ .

7.25

"Occult" is a word of Latin origin meaning to cover or hide. In English a "cult" is a hidden secret society with obscure rituals. Fecal occult blood is blood in the feces that is difficult to see. A guaiac test can be done to detect occult blood in a specimen of sputum, gastric secretion, or feces. A positive result of a fecal occult blood (FOB) test may indicate infection, ulcers, polyps, or tumors that are bleeding.

7.26

occult
ô **kult'**

fecal
fē' kəl

To detect gastr/o/intestinal bleeding a fecal _____ blood test may be performed.

A _____ specimen may be tested for the presence of blood by performing an FOB.

7.27

esophag/eal
ē so fə **jē'** əl

eso- means in or toward and **phag/o** means swallow. **esophag/o** is used in words about the esophagus. The adjective form of esophagus

_____ / _____ .

    word root   suffix

7.28

esophag/us
ē **so'** fə gus

sten/osis is a condition of narrowing that may occur in a tube or passageway. Mitral stenosis is a narrowing of the mitral valve opening in the heart.

Esophag/o/sten/osis is a narrowing of the _____ / _____ .

7.29

esophag/o/sten/osis
ē **so'** fə gō sten **ō'** sis

esophagus

A person experiencing dysphagia may have a narrowing of the esophagus or

_____ / _____ / _____ / _____ .

A para/esophag/eal hernia is a herniation around the

_____ .

7.30

esophag/o/gastr/ic

gastr/o/esophag/eal
(You pronounce)

Build an adjective meaning pertaining to the esophagus and stomach:

_____ / _____ / _____ / _____ or

_____ / _____ / _____ / _____ .

gastr/o/esophag/eal
gas′ trō ē sof ə **gē′** əl

7.31

Gastr/o/esophag/eal reflux disease (GERD) causes the gastric and duodenal juices to enter and irritate the esophagus. A person who has chronic heartburn and throat irritation may be suffering from

_____/_____/_____/_____ reflux disease.

CASE STUDY INVESTIGATION (CSI)

Paraesophageal Hernia with Perforated Duodenal Ulcer

An 84-year-old man presented in the emergency room in pre-shock after lunch with acute **epigastric** pain and **nausea** with belching. He has several medical conditions including: angina pectoris, COPD, type II diabetes, infected venous leg **ulcers** TURP, and percutaneous coronary artery intervention. Five years ago he was conservatively treated for a bleeding **gastric** ulcer. Upon examination his abdomen was soft and non-distended but severely tender to **palpation**. A CT scan of the thorax and abdomen showed a **paraesophageal** herniation into the right thorax containing a part of the **transverse** colon and a part of the distal stomach and proximal duodenum. A pronounced gastric **distension** was noted. No free fluid or gas was found in the abdominal cavity. Besides the herniation and an abundance of **fecal** content in the entire colon, the CT scan was normal. Fecal **occult** blood (FOB) test was positive and Hgb was 10gm. During surgery a **duodenal hernia** and perforated ulcer were discovered as the source of bleeding and were resected and repaired.

CSI Vocabulary Challenge

Analyze the terms by dividing them into their word parts and writing the definition. Use your dictionary if needed for assistance.

ulcers _____

gastric _____

epigastric _____

palpation _____

paraesophageal _____

transverse _____

distension _____

fecal _____

hernia _____

occult _____

duodenal _____

nausea _____

ANSWER COLUMN

7.32

Not eating just before going to bed, avoiding fatty foods, losing weight, and elevating the head of the bed are all recommendations for people who have GERD or * _____

gastroesophageal reflux
disease

_____ .

7.33

stomach hemorrhage

Gastr/o/rrhagia means * _____ .

inflammation of
the stomach

Gastr/itis means * _____ .

pertaining to the stomach

Gastr/ic means * _____

_____ .

7.34

**TAKE A
CLOSER LOOK**

An organism called *Helicobacter pylori* (H. pylori) has been found to be a common cause of gastritis in children and adults. It is transmitted through contamination with gastrointestinal substances such as vomit or feces. Symptoms of HP infection include epi/gastr/ic pain, nausea, vomiting, and dys/pepsia. This bacterial infection is treated with antibiotics and H2 antagonists (gastric secretion inhibitors).

7.35

-ectasia (or ectasis) is a suffix meaning stretching or dilatation.
Form words meaning
dilatation (stretching) of the stomach

gastr/ectasia
gas trek **tā'** shə

_____/_____;

prolapse of the stomach and small intestine

gastr/o/enter/o/ptosis
gas' trō en' ter op tō' sis

_____/_____/_____/_____/_____ .

7.36

enter/o is used in words about the small intestine or the intestine in general. Tablets that dissolve in the intestine may have an enter/ic coating. Inflammation

enter/itis
en ter **ī'** tis

of the intestine is _____/_____ .

7.37

The internal medicine specialty that studies diseases of the stomach and intestine

gastr/o/enter/o/logy
gas' trō en' ter **ol'** ō gē

is _____/_____/_____/_____/_____ .

7.38

Recall the prefix **dys-**, meaning difficulty or painful. Dys/entery is a disorder of the intestine characterized by inflammation, pain, and dia/rrhea. When caused by

dys/enter/y
dis' en tair ē

an amoeba-type parasite, it is called amoebic _____/_____/_____ .

ANSWER COLUMN

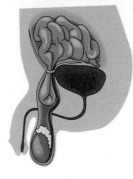
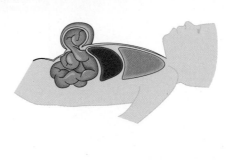

(A)   **(B)**   **(C)**

(A) Hiatal hernia (B) Inguinal hernia (C) Umbilical hernia *Delmar/Cengage Learning*

	7.39
dysentery	Drinking water contaminated with bacteria or parasites may cause _____.

	7.40
	Form words meaning
	pertaining to the stomach and small intestine
gastr/o/enter/ic	_____/_____/_____/_____;
gas′ trō en **tair′** ik	hemorrhage of the small intestine
enter/o/rrhagia	_____/_____/_____.
en tə rō **rā′** jē ə	

	7.41
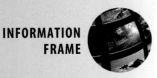 INFORMATION FRAME	The small intestine is divided into three sections: the duodenum (**duoden/o**), the jejunum (**jejun/o**), and the ileum (**ile/o**). The stomach empties the chyme (food mixed with gastric juices) into the duodenum. Bile formed in the liver and stored in the gallbladder, pancreatic enzymes, and duodenal wall enzymes enter the duodenum to break down the food into absorbable form. The lining and walls of the jejunum and ileum are rich in blood capillaries and lymphatic vessels into which the nutrients are absorbed. The three parts of the small intestine include the:
duodenum	_____;
dōō ō **dē′** nəm	
jejunum	_____; and the
je **jōō′** nəm	
ileum	_____.
il′ ē əm	

	7.42
	Recall the suffix **-cele** indicates a herniation. A hernia is a protrusion or rupture of an organ or tissues through an opening or weakened wall of a cavity. The illustration above shows types of digestive system hernias.

(continued)

ANSWER COLUMN

Build words meaning
intestinal hernia

enter/o/cele
en' ter ō sēl
_____ /_____ /_____ ;

washing or irrigation of the small intestine

enter/o/clysis
en ter **ok'** lə sis
_____ /_____ /_____ .

7.43

Build words meaning
paralysis of the small intestine

enter/o/plegia
en ter ō **plē'** jē ə
_____ /_____ /_____ ;

dilatation of the small intestine

enter/ectasia
en ter ek **tā'** shə
_____ /_____ .

7.44

prolapse of the
small intestine

Enter/o/ptosis means * _____

_____ .

surgical puncture of
the small intestine

Enter/o/centesis means * _____

_____ .

7.45

**INFORMATION
FRAME**

The large intestine (colon) includes the ascending colon, transverse colon, descending colon, and sigmoid colon leading to the rectum and anus. Digested and undigested food from the small intestine enters the ascending colon through the ile/o/cec/al valve. Water and water soluble nutrients like salts may still be absorbed through the colon wall. The solid waste or feces that remain is eliminated via the rectum and anus.

7.46

At the junction between the ileum and the cecum of the ascending colon is the

ile/o/cec/al
il ē ō **sē'** kəl
_____ /_____ /_____ /_____ valve.

Water and water-soluble nutrients are absorbed in the large intestine, also called

colon
kō' lən
the _____ .

rectum
rek' təm
Feces is eliminated through the _____

anus
a' nəs
and _____ .

7.47

Growing from the bottom of the cecum is a vermiform (worm-like) glandular structure called the appendix. **Append** is a word root and **appendic/o** is a combining form for appendix. Build words about the appendix from the phrases below:

(continued)

ANSWER COLUMN

inflammation of the appendix

appendic/itis
a pen di **si'** tis

_____/_____;

excision of the appendix

append/ectomy
a pen **dek'** tō mē

_____/_____;

plural of appendix

append/ices
a **pen'** di sēz

_____/_____.

7.48

col/o is the combining form for colon (large intestine).
Col/ic or colonic means

pertaining to the colon
or large intestine

* _____

_____.

surgical puncture
of the colon

Col/o/centesis means * _____

_____.

7.49

Build words meaning
surgical fixation of the colon

col/o/pexy
kō' lō pek sē or
kol' ō pek sē

_____/_____/_____;

making a new opening into the colon

_____/_____;

col/ostomy
ko **los'** tə mē

prolapse of the colon

col/o/ptosis
kōl' op **tō'** sis

_____/_____/_____.

7.50

**TAKE A
CLOSER LOOK**

Constipation, irritable bowel syndrome (IBS), and diverticular disease are all disorders associated with slow colonic motility (movement). Although each is treated with different medications, their treatments all include an increase in dietary fiber or a dietary fiber supplement. Chronic lack of moisture and bulk in the feces makes it more difficult for the intestinal muscles to push waste along. The intestine may develop weak walls, pouches, and/or infection.

7.51

Diverticula (singular, diverticulum) are outpouchings or pockets that develop in the colon wall. The presence of diverticula is a condition called diverticul/osis. Food may get trapped in these pockets, putrify, and irritate the tissues, causing infection and inflammation of the diverticula. Inflammation of the diverticula is

diverticul/itis
dī' ver tik yōō **li'** tis

called _____/_____.

ANSWER COLUMN

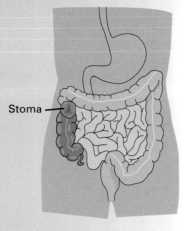
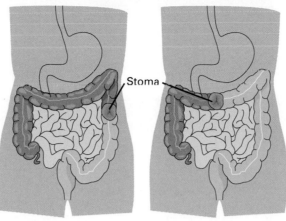
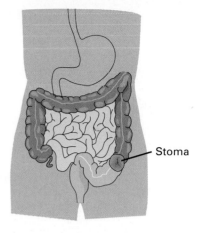

Ascending colostomy   Descending colostomy   Transverse colostomy   Sigmoid colostomy

Colostomy sites *Delmar/Cengage Learning*

7.52

Chronic abdominal pain, cramping, and changes in bowel habits may all be symptoms of either irritable bowel disease (condition) or

_____/_____ .

diverticul/osis
dī′ ver tik yōō lō′ sis

7.53

-clysis is a suffix meaning washing or irrigation. Build words meaning washing or irrigation of the colon

_____/_____/_____ ;

of the stomach

_____/_____/_____ .

col/o/clysis
kō **lok′** lə sis

gastr/o/clysis
gas **trok′** lə sis

Diverticulosis
Delmar/Cengage Learning

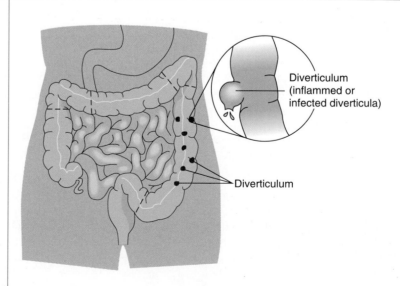

Diverticulum
(inflammed or
infected diverticula)

Diverticulum

ANSWER COLUMN

7.54

Irrigation of the small intestine using contrast media may be done to better view the small intestine on x-rays. This is called

enter/o/clysis
en' tr **ok**' lə sis

_____/_____/_____.

An instrument to examine the small intestine is the

enter/o/scope
en' tə rō skōp

_____/_____/_____.

7.55

sigmoid/o refers to the sigmoid colon. An instrument used to examine the

sigmoid/o/scope
sig **moid**' ō skōp

sigmoid colon is the _____/_____/_____.

sigmoid/o/scopy
sig moid **ōs**' kō pē

The procedure is called _____/_____/_____.

7.56

The combining form for rectum is **rect/o**. Rect/al means

pertaining to the rectum

* _____.

a rectal hernia or
    herniation of the rectum

A rect/o/cele is * _____

_____.

7.57

Build words meaning
washing or irrigation of the rectum

rect/o/clysis
rek **tok**' lə sis

_____/_____/_____;

instrument for examining the rectum

rect/o/scope
rek' tə skōp

_____/_____/_____;

pertaining to the colon and rectum

col/o/rect/al
kō lō **rek**' təl

_____/_____/_____/_____.

7.58

The process of examining the rectum with a rect/o/scope is called

rect/o/scopy
rek **tos**' kə pē

_____/_____/_____. In doing this, the physician has performed a

rect/o/scopic
rek tə **skop**' ik

_____/_____/_____ examination.
        (adjective)

NOTE: A more common procedure is a sigmoid/o/scopy. This is done using an endoscope introduced through the anus and rectum to the sigmoid colon.

ANSWER COLUMN

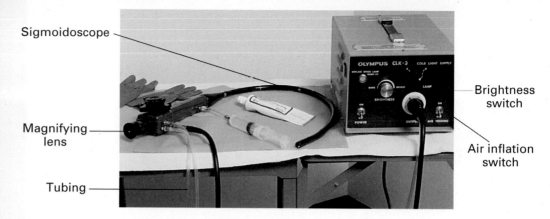

Sigmoidoscope

Magnifying lens

Tubing

Brightness switch

Air inflation switch

Parts of the sigmoidoscope *Delmar/Cengage Learning*

7.59

Build words meaning
plastic surgery of the rectum

rect/o/plasty
rek′ tə plas tē

_____/_____/_____;

suturing (stitching) of the rectum

rect/o/rrhaphy
rek **tôr′** ə fē

_____/_____/_____.

7.60

Build words meaning
pertaining to the rectum and urethra

rect/o/urethr/al
rek tō yoō **rē′** thrə l

_____/_____/_____/_____;

incision of the bladder through the rectum

rect/o/cyst/o/tomy
rek′ tō sis **tot′** ə mē

_____/_____/_____/_____/_____.

rectum   bladder   incision

7.61

proct/o is the combining form for anus and rectum.

specializes in diseases
of the anus and rectum

A proct/o/logist is one who * _____
_____.

the study of diseases of
the anus and rectum

Proct/o/logy is * _____
_____.

7.62

Build words meaning
washing or irrigation of anus and rectum

proct/o/clysis
prok **tok′** lə sis

_____/_____/_____;

paralysis of the anus and rectum

proct/o/plegia
prok tō **plē′** jē ə

_____/_____/_____.

(continued)

ANSWER COLUMN

proct/o/scope
prok′ tō skōp

proct/o/scopy
prok **tos′** kə pē

A proct/o/logist examines the rectum and anus with a

_____/_____/_____.

This examination is called

_____/_____/_____.

7.63

Build words meaning
suturing of the rectum and anus

proct/o/rrhaphy
prok **tôr′** ə fē

_____/_____/_____;

surgical fixation of the rectum and anus

proct/o/pexy
prok′ to peks ē

_____/_____/_____.

7.64

**WORD
ORIGINS**

Catharsis comes from the Greek word *katharsis* meaning purification. A catharsis may be an emotional release from anxiety caused by repressed events. In many ancient Greek plays, the purpose of the story was to produce catharsis for the audience members by acting out their anxieties and giving them an experience of relief. Today, psychoanalysis often works toward this goal by creating an experience of emotional release or catharsis.

7.65

Cathartics (laxatives) cause liquification of the stool or relaxation of the bowel to ease defecation, producing physical relief. Another name for laxative is

cathar/tic
ka **thar′** tik

_____/_____.

7.66

Eating a high-fiber diet and increasing water intake may also treat and prevent

constipation

infrequency of bowel movement (BM) or _____.

7.67

Infrequent or small amount of bowel movement is an indication of con/stip/ation. This term comes from Latin word parts meaning to withhold or press together. Slow bowel motility due to anesthesia use, aging, dehydration, or

con/stip/ation
kon sti **pā′** shun

low-fiber intake may be causes of _____.

7.68

The liver has many functions including the production of heparin, which affects the blood-clotting mechanism. It also produces bile. **hepat/o** is the combining form for liver. It comes from the Greek word *hepar*, meaning liver. Hepat/ic

pertaining to the liver

means * _____.

(continued)

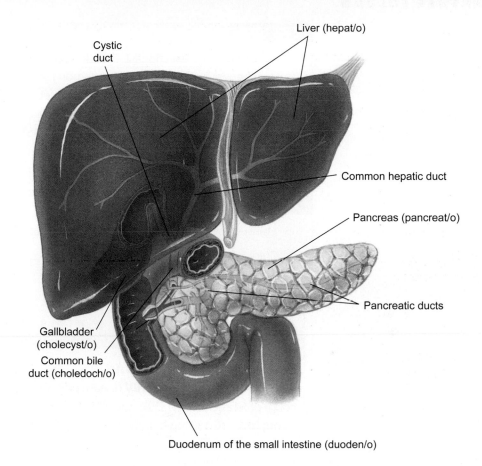

Cystic duct

Liver (hepat/o)

Common hepatic duct

Pancreas (pancreat/o)

Pancreatic ducts

Gallbladder (cholecyst/o)

Common bile duct (choledoch/o)

Duodenum of the small intestine (duoden/o)

---

enlargement of the liver

Hepat/o/megaly means * _____

_____ .

7.69

Build words meaning inspection (examination) of the liver

hepat/o/scopy
hep ə **tos'** kə pē

_____/_____/_____ ;

any disease of the liver

hepat/o/pathy
hep ə **top'** ə thē

_____/_____/_____ .

7.70

Build words meaning incision into the liver

hepat/o/tomy
hep ə **tot'** ə mē

_____/_____/_____ ;

excision of (part of) the liver

hepat/ēctomy
hep ə **tek'** tə mē

_____/_____ .

7.71

Hepat/itis is inflammation of the liver. Hepatitis B is a serious condition of the liver caused by a viral infection. Hepatitis B vaccine (HBV) may be administered as an

hepat/itis
hep ə **tīt'** is

immunization protection against _____/_____ .

TAKE A CLOSER LOOK

7.72

According to the National Center for Infectious Diseases, there are five types of viral hepatitis. The three most common forms are Hepatitis A, B, and C.
Hepatitis A (HAV infection) is an acute infection associated with food or water that is contaminated by human waste.
Hepatitis B (HBV infection) is classified as an STD and is transmitted by blood and body fluids.
Hepatitis C (HCV infection) is a chronic condition usually passed through the blood.

hepat/itis

7.73

Using standard precautions to avoid contact with the potentially infectious body fluids of others helps to prevent _____/_____ and other viral and bacterial infections.

CASE STUDY INVESTIGATION (CSI)

HIV with Hepatitis B and C

A 38-year-old male with B3 **HIV** disease presents on intake with a CD4 **lymphocyte** count of 542 cells/mm (31%), and HIV bDNA < 50 copies/ml. He is currently taking d4T 40 **mg bid**, 3TC 150 mg bid, and nelfinavir 1,250 mg bid with no **opportunistic** infections. Laboratory testing reveals mildly elevated liver enzymes (AST 76 and ALT 91) with normal LDH, bilirubin, albumin, prothrombin time, hematocrit, and platelet count. His current symptoms include: right flank pain, **lethargy**, depression, **insomnia**, and **anorexia**. Examination by systems is normal with tenderness on palpation of the liver. Enzyme immunoassay (EIA) shows positive results for **hepatitis** C virus (**HCV**) **antibody** and hepatitis B (**HBV**) core and surface antibody, but negative for hepatitis A (**HAV**).

CSI Vocabulary Challenge

Analyze the terms and abbreviations by writing the definition and dividing the terms into their word parts. Use your dictionary if needed for assistance.

HIV	_____
HBV	_____
HAV	_____
HCV	_____
mg bid	_____
lymphocyte	_____
opportunistic	_____
lethargy	_____
insomnia	_____
anorexia	_____
hepatitis	_____
antibody	_____

ANSWER COLUMN

7.74

The pancreas is both a digestive (producing amylase and lipase) and an endocrine (producing insulin) organ. **pancreat/o** is used in words about the pancreas.

Pancreat/ic means

pertaining to the pancreas

* _____.

Pancreat/o/lysis means

destruction of
   pancreatic tissue

* _____.

7.75

Build words meaning
a stone or calculus in the pancreas

pancreat/o/lith
pan krē **at′** ō lith

_____/_____/_____;

pancreat/o/pathy
pan′ krē ə **top′** ə thē

any pancreatic disease

_____/_____/_____.

7.76

Build words meaning
excision of part or all of the pancreas

pancreat/ectomy
pan′ krē ə **tek′** tə mē

_____/_____;

pancreat/o/tomy
pan′ krē ə **tot′** ə mē

incision into the pancreas

_____/_____/_____.

7.77

Recall that cholelithiasis is a condition in which gallstones have formed in the gallbladder. Choleliths can also lodge in the biliary duct blocking bile flow or in the pancreatic ducts causing pancreatitis. An x-ray of the gallbladder is called

chol/e/cyst/o/graph or
chol/e/cyst/o/gram

_____/_____/_____/_____/_____.

NOTE: -graph originally meant machine, but in practice it has come to mean the x-ray picture (film) itself.

7.78

Build words meaning inflammation of the pancreas

pancreat/itis
pan′ krē ə **tīt′** is

_____/_____;

chol/e/cyst/itis
kōl′ ē sis **tīt′** is

inflammation of the gallbladder

_____/_____/_____/_____.

ANSWER COLUMN

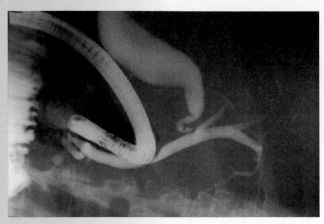

(A) Normal endoscopic retrograde cholangio-pancreatograph ERCP *Delmar/Cengage Learning*

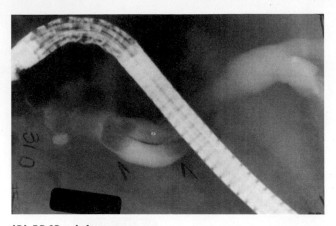

(B) ERCP with stones *Delmar/Cengage Learning*

7.79

TAKE A CLOSER LOOK

cholangi/o/pancreat/o/-graphy
kōl an′ jē ō pan′ krē ə **tog**′ ra fē

An end/o/scope can be used to insert a cannula (tube) into the common bile duct or the pancreatic duct. Contrast media is introduced and an x-ray taken. This procedure is known by its abbreviation ERCP, which stands for end/o/scop/ic retro/grade cholangi/o/pancreat/o/graphy. Look up ERCP in your dictionary or medical text reference and read about it. If a physician is trying to locate a stone that is difficult to see, a

_____/_____/_____/_____/_____.
may be ordered.

7.80

-ase is a suffix used to indicate an enzyme. Enzymes are specialized proteins that catalyze or speed up chemical reactions. In the digestive process enzymes assist in the breakdown of fats, proteins, and carbohydrates. Study the following table of enzyme terminology and their function.

Enzyme	Combining Form	Function
lip/ase **lī**′ pās	lip/o (fat)	breaks down fats into fatty acids
amyl/ase **am**′ ə lās	amyl/o (starch)	starch to glucose (simple sugar)
lact/ase **lak**′ tās	lact/o (milk sugar)	breaks down lactose into glucose (simple sugar)

7.81

lactase

A person who has difficulty digesting milk and milk products may be *lactose intolerant*. They may have a lack of the enzyme _____ that helps break down milk sugar.

ANSWER COLUMN

7.82

carb/o indicates the presence of a carbon (organic) compound. Carb/o/hydr/ates contain carbon (C), hydrogen (H), and oxygen (O). The most simple carbohydrate in your body is glucose ($C_6H_{12}O_6$). The metabolism of the

_____/_____/_____/_____

carb/o/hydr/ate
kär bō **hī′** drāt

glucose produces energy for the body.

7.83

Starch is a carbohydrate found in rice, potatoes, and flour. The enzyme

_____ breaks down starch into _____.

amylase
glucose

7.84

Malnutrition may be caused by over-nutrition or under-nutrition. Overeating and a sedentary lifestyle may lead to obesity. Obes/ity is the quality of being overweight for height and body frame size. An obese person is at risk for developing heart disease, hypertension, and arthritis. Overeating and lack of

exercise may lead to _____/_____.

obes/ity
ō **bē′** si tē

7.85

bar/o refers to weight. Bar/iatrics is the medical specialty that treats obesity. A bar/iatric medical center provides nutrition counseling, behavior therapy,

and if needed surgical interventions for the treatment of _____.
The specialty that treats obesity is _____/_____.

obesity
bar/iatrics
baer ē **a′** triks

7.86

Overeating disorder may increase the risk of heart disease _____
and _____.

hypertension
arthritis

7.87

Build words meaning
hemorrhage of the liver

_____/_____/_____;
suture of a wound of the liver
_____/_____/_____.

hepat/o/rrhagia
hep ə tō **rā′** jē ə
hepat/o/rrhaphy
hep ə **tôr′** ə fē

7.88

Build words meaning
hernia of the liver

_____/_____/_____;

hepat/o/cele
hep **at′** ō sēl

(continued)

ANSWER COLUMN

pain in the liver

hepat/o/dynia
hep at ō **din'** ē ə

_____ / _____ / _____ ;

stone in the liver

hepat/o/lith
hep **at'** ō lith

_____ / _____ / _____ .

7.89

A/tres/ia literally means not perforated or not open. Biliary atresia is a condition in which the bile ducts are not open. A congenital condition in which a part of the

a/tres/ia
a **trē'** zhē ə

intestine is closed is intestinal _____ / _____ / _____ .

7.90

Tresis is a Greek word for hole or opening. A/tres/ia is a condition in which an opening normally found in a structure fails to develop. For example, if the inside of the duodenum grew closed instead of open, this would be a condition called duodenal

a/tres/ia
a **trē'** zhē ə

_____ / _____ / _____ .

7.91

If a baby is born with esophageal atresia, the esophagus would be

closed

_____ .

In the heart, congenital closure of the mitral valve is mitral _____ .

atresia

7.92

Bile backs up into the liver if the ducts are closed or blocked. Biliary

atresia

_____ is a serious condition.

7.93

**TAKE A
CLOSER LOOK**

Another debilitating liver disease is cirrh/osis of the liver. In Greek, *kirrhos* means orange-yellow. This disease occurs as a result of malnutrition, alcoholism, poisoning, or a history of hepatitis. Treatment of cirrhosis depends on its cause and may include diet modifications, vitamin supplements, cessation of alcohol use with related support groups, energy conservation, and possibly surgery.

7.94

Chronic alcoholism or hepatitis may lead to a dysfunctional liver disease

cirrh/osis
si **rō'** sis

called _____ / _____ .

STUDYWARE™ CONNECTION

Remember, after completing this unit, you can play a championship or other interactive game on your **StudyWARE™ CD-ROM** that will help you learn the content in this chapter.

ANSWER COLUMN

7.95

splen/o is used in words about the spleen. Build words meaning
excision of the spleen

splen/ectomy
sple **nek'** tə mē
_____/_____;
enlargement of the spleen

splen/o/megaly
sple nō **meg'** ə lē
_____/_____/_____;
prolapse of the spleen

splen/o/ptosis
sple nop **tō'** sis
_____/_____/_____.

7.96

**SPELL
CHECK**

Watch your spelling in words about the spleen. The noun spleen has two *es*, but the combining form has one *e*, i.e., **splen/o**.

7.97

Build words meaning
surgical fixation of the spleen

splen/o/pexy
sple' nō peks ē
_____/_____/_____;
any disease of the spleen

splen/o/pathy
sple **nop'** ə thē
_____/_____/_____;
suture of the spleen

splen/o/rrhaphy
sple **nôr'** ə fē
_____/_____/_____;
hemorrhage from the spleen

splen/o/rrhagia
sple nō **rā'** jē ə
_____/_____/_____.

7.98

The spleen is one of the blood-forming organs.

pain in the spleen

Splen/algia means * _____.

7.99

pertaining to the spleen

Splen/ic means * _____.

ANSWER COLUMN

7.100

Recall the suffix **-ostomy**. Anastomosis is a surgical connection between tubular structures. The combining form for esophagus is **esophag/o**. When an entire gastrectomy is performed, a new connection is made between the esophagus and the duodenum. This particular anastomosis can also be called an

_____/_____/_____/_____.

esophag/o/duoden/-
    ostomy
i **sof'** ə gō dōō ə də **nos'**
    tə mē

7.101

All of the following operations are types of anastomoses. Using what you have learned about the digestive system, list the body parts indicated in these procedures.
gastr/o/enter/o/col/ostomy

*_____

stomach, small intestine,
    and large intestine

esophag/o/gastr/ostomy

esophagus, stomach

*_____

enter/o/cholecyst/ostomy

small intestine, gallbladder

*_____

7.102

Some medical words get pretty long. Insert the slashes and define the following terms.
jejunoileitis

jejun/o/ile/itis

inflammation of the
    jejunum and ileum

_____

*_____

chole/cyst/o/duoden/-
    ostomy

cholecystoduodenostomy

new opening between the
    duodenum and
    gallbladder

_____

esophag/o/gastr/o/-
    duoden/o/scopy

*_____

examination of the
    esophagus, stomach,
    and duodenum

esophagogastroduodenoscopy (EGD)

_____

chol/angi/o/pancreat/o/-
    graphy

*_____

x-ray of the biliary and
    pancreatic ducts

cholangiopancreatography

_____

*_____

Good!

ANSWER COLUMN

Abbreviation	Meaning
ALT	alanine aminotransferase (liver enzyme)
AST	aspartate aminotransferase (liver enzyme)
BE	barium enema
bid	twice a day (*bis in die*)
BM	bowel movement
Chol	cholesterol
EGD	esophagogastroduodenoscopy
ERCP	endoscopic retrograde cholangiopancreatography
FOB	fecal occult blood
GB	gallbladder
GERD	gastroesophageal reflux disease
GI	gastrointestinal
HAV	hepatitis A virus
HBV	hepatitis B virus
HCl	hydrochloric acid
HCV	hepatitis C virus
HDL	high density lipoproteins
Hep B	hepatitis B vaccine
H. pylori	*Helicobacter pylori*
IBS	irritable bowel syndrome
LDH	lactate dehydrogenase (cardiac enzyme)
LDL	low density lipoproteins
mg	milligram
NG	nasogastric
NPO, npo	nothing by mouth
PO	by mouth (Latin: *per os*), orally

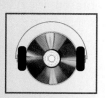

To complete your study of this unit, work the **Review Activities** on the following pages. Also, listen to the Audio CD that accompanies *Medical Terminology: A Programmed Systems Approach*, 10th edition, and practice your pronunciation.

STUDYWARE™ CONNECTION

To help you learn the content in this chapter, take a practice quiz or play an interactive game on your **StudyWARE™ CD-ROM**.

REVIEW ACTIVITIES

CIRCLE AND CORRECT

Circle the correct answer for each question. Then check your answers in Appendix E.

1. Suffix for dilatation or stretching
   - a. -dilatate
   - b. -clysis
   - c. -ectomy
   - d. -ectasia

2. Prefix for below
   - a. epi-
   - b. inter-
   - c. sub-
   - d. supra-

3. Combining form for small intestine or intestine
   - a. colpo
   - b. entero
   - c. duodeno
   - d. intestino

4. Combining form for liver
   - a. hepat
   - b. hepato
   - c. heparin
   - d. livo

5. Suffix for paralysis
   - a. -plasia
   - b. -phagia
   - c. -plegia
   - d. - phasia

6. Prefix for difficult or painful
   - a. sub-
   - b. dynia-
   - c. algia-
   - d. dys-

7. Combining form for spleen
   - a. spleno
   - b. spleeno
   - c. spleen
   - d. splenic

8. Suffix for making a new opening
   - a. -tomy
   - b. -ostomy
   - c. -tome
   - d. -scopy

9. Suffix for irrigation or washing
   - a. -colo
   - b. -ecstasia
   - c. -clysis
   - d. -enema

10. Word root for stomach
    - a. stomato
    - b. stomacho
    - c. cheilo
    - d. gastr

11. Stenosis means
    - a. dilation
    - b. discharge
    - c. tubelike
    - d. narrowing

12. The term for a congenital condition in which a tube is closed is:
    - a. stenosis
    - b. coloclysis
    - c. atresia
    - d. anastomosis

SELECT AND CONSTRUCT

Select the correct word parts from the following list and construct medical terms that represent the given meaning.

al	algia	cele	cheilo	chol(e)
cholangi/o	clysis	colo	duoden(o)	dys
ectasia	ectomy	entero(ic)	esophago(eal)	gastr(o)(ic)
gingiv(o)(a)	glosso(al)	graphy	hepato(i)c	hypo
ileo	itis	jejuno	linguo(al)	lith
megaly	myc(osis)	ostomy	pancreato	pathy
plasty	pleg(ic)(ia)	procto	ptosis	rect(o)(al)
rrhagia	rrhaphy	rrhea	scope(y)(ic)	sigmoid(o)
sis	spleno	stomato	sub	tomy

1. fungal infection of the mouth _____

2. below the tongue _____

3. surgical repair of the lips _____

REVIEW ACTIVITIES

4. inflammation of the gums _____

5. bleeding of the small intestine _____

6. process of examining the esophagus, stomach,
   and duodenum by looking with an instrument_____

7. prolapse of the small intestine _____

8. irrigation of the rectum _____

9. paralysis of the anus and rectum _____

10. stone in the pancreas _____

11. enlargement of the spleen _____

12. dilatation of the stomach _____

13. instrument for looking in the sigmoid colon _____

14. inflammation of the liver _____

15. herniation of the rectum _____

16. pertaining to stomach and esophagus _____

17. x-ray process of biliary and pancreatic ducts _____

18. pertaining to colon and rectum _____

DEFINE AND DISSECT

Give a brief definition and dissect each term listed into its word parts in the space provided. Check your answers by referring to the frame listed in parentheses and your medical dictionary. Then listen to the Audio CD to practice pronunciation.

1. cheilostomatoplasty (7.19)   _____ / _____ / _____ / _____ / _____

                                                  rt   v   rt   v   suffix

   meaning _____

2. gingivoglossitis (7.22)   _____ / _____ / _____ / _____

                                                  rt   v   rt   suffix

   _____

3. gastrorrhagia (7.33)   _____ / _____ / _____

                                                  rt   v   suffix

   _____

4. esophageal (7.27)   _____ / _____

                                                  rt   suffix

   _____

REVIEW ACTIVITIES

5. enterocentesis (7.44)

_____/_____/_____
rt   v   rt/suffix

_____

6. dysentery (7.38)

_____/_____/_____
pre   rt   suffix

_____

7. colopexy (7.49)

_____/_____/_____
rt   v   suffix

_____

8. rectocele (7.56)

_____/_____/_____
rt   v   suffix

_____

9. proctologist (7.61)

_____/_____/_____
rt   v   suffix

_____

10. hepatomegaly (7.68)

_____/_____/_____
rt   v   suffix

_____

11. pancreatolysis (7.74)

_____/_____/_____
rt   v   suffix

_____

12. splenorrhagia (7.97)

_____/_____/_____
rt   v   suffix

_____

13. esophagoduodenostomy (7.100)

_____/_____/_____/_____
rt   v   rt   v   suffix

_____

14. diverticulitis (7.51)

_____/_____
rt   suffix

_____

15. cathartic (7.65)

_____/_____
rt   suffix

_____

16. sigmoidoscopy (7.55)

_____/_____/_____
rt   v   suffix

_____

REVIEW ACTIVITIES

17. coloclysis (7.53)

_____/_____/_____
rt   v   suffix

_____

18. enterectasia (7.43)

_____/_____
rt   suffix

_____

19. glossoplegia (7.15)

_____/_____/_____
rt   v   suffix

_____

20. sublingual (7.11)

_____/_____/_____
pre   rt   suffix

_____

21. gastroenterology (7.37)

_____/_____/_____/_____/_____
rt   v   rt   v   suffix

_____

22. hepatitis (7.71)

_____/_____
rt   suffix

_____

23. esophagospasm (table page 249)

_____/_____/_____
rt   v   suffix

_____

24. gingivectomy (7.22)

_____/_____
rt   suffix

_____

25. stomatomycosis (7.4)

_____/_____/_____/_____
rt   v   rt   suffix

_____

26. esophagostenosis (7.29)

_____/_____/_____/_____
rt   v   rt   suffix

_____

27. cholangiopancreatography (7.79)

_____/_____/_____/_____/_____
rt   v   rt   v   suffix

_____

28. cirrhosis (7.94)

_____/_____
rt   suffix

_____

REVIEW ACTIVITIES

29. jejunoileitis (7.102)

_____/_____/_____/_____
     rt   v   rt   suffix

_____

30. appendectomy (7.47)

_____/_____
     rt   suffix

_____

31. carbohydrate (7.82)

_____/_____/_____/_____
     rt   v   rt   suffix

_____

IMAGE LABELING

Label the diagram of the digestive system by writing the number in the blank.

Write the correct word for the body part indicated.

_____ hepat/o	_____
_____ gastr/o	_____
_____ col/o	_____
_____ esophag/o	_____
_____ stomat/o	_____
_____ pancreat/o	_____
_____ sigmoid/o	_____
_____ pharyng/o	_____
_____ cholecyst/o	_____
_____ rect/o	_____
_____ duoden/o	_____
_____ appendic/o	_____

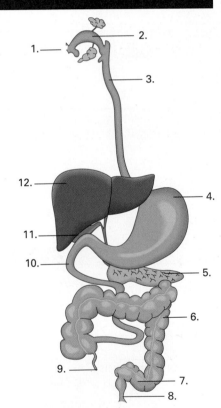

Digestive system *Delmar/Cengage Learning*

REVIEW ACTIVITIES

ABBREVIATION MATCHING

Match the following abbreviations with their definition.

_____ 1. GB

_____ 2. EGD

_____ 3. GI

_____ 4. po

_____ 5. npo

_____ 6. HBV

_____ 7. GERD

_____ 8. ERCP

_____ 9. NG

_____ 10. BM

_____ 11. HP

a. *Helicobacter pylori*

b. hepatomegaly

c. gums and incisors

d. sublingually

e. bowel movement

f. gallbladder

g. nothing by mouth

h. hepatitis B virus

i. gastrointestinal

j. orally (by month)

k. esophagogastroduodenostomy

l. esophagogastroduodenoscopy

m. AIDS virus

n. *Escherichia coli*

o. gastroesophageal reflux disorder

p. after meals

q. endoscopic retrograde cholangiopancreatography

r. nasogastric (tube)

SUFFIX MATCHING

Match the suffixes on the left with their meanings on the right.

_____ 1. -plegia

_____ 2. -clysis

_____ 3. -ectasia

_____ 4. -rrhagia

_____ 5. -megaly

_____ 6. -ostomy

a. stretching, dilation

b. uncontrolled twitching

c. new permanent opening

d. suturing

e. washing, irrigation

f. hemorrhage

g. herniation

h. enlarged

i. incision into

j. paralysis

REVIEW ACTIVITIES

CASE STUDY

Write the term next to its meaning given below. Then draw slashes to analyze the word parts. Note the use of medical abbreviations. Look these up in your dictionary or find them in Appendix B. If you have any questions about the answers, refer to your medical dictionary or check with your instructor for the answers in Appendix E.

CASE STUDY 7-1

Endoscopy Report

Pt: Female, age 89

Dx: **Gastrointestinal hemorrhage**, duodenal ulcer Tx: **EGD**

Ms. Dena Jitters was admitted through the emergency room because of **vomiting** coffee-grounds material, and passing **melenic** stools. The **nasogastric** tube was introduced and showed bright red blood. The patient became **hypotensive** and two units of packed red cells were given. Ms. Jitters became stable with a BP of 120/80. She was lavaged with iced **isotonic** saline and an endoscopy was performed.

REPORT: Premedication: Cetacaine locally. The **endoscope** was easily passed into the esophagus. Numerous amounts of **thrombi** were noted. The scope was introduced into the stomach, which showed increased amounts of bright red blood in the fundus. No **mucosal** lesions could be seen; however, half of the stomach was full of blood. The scope was then passed into the **duodenal** bulb, where clots were also noted. This patient could have a duodenal **ulcer** but because of the amount of blood, it is difficult to delineate an ulcer crater.

A great clot was located on the **anterior** wall. As the scope was withdrawn, the antrum of the stomach could be seen with no lesion noted. It was difficult to clean up all the blood clots and, because of the status of the patient, the procedure was discontinued. Ms. Jitters tolerated the procedure well and did not vomit or **aspirate**.

1. front _____

2. ejecting from the stomach
   through the mouth _____

3. bleed _____

4. pertaining to the nose and stomach _____

5. instrument used to look into _____

6. pertaining to mucosa _____

7. breathe in (suck in) _____

8. having the same concentration _____

9. sore _____

10. pertaining to the stomach and intestine _____

11. black, old blood (adjective) _____

12. low blood pressure (adjective) _____

13. first part of small intestine (adjective) _____

14. clots _____

15. esophagogastroduodenoscopy _____

REVIEW ACTIVITIES

CROSSWORD PUZZLE

Check your answers by going back through the frames or checking the solution in Appendix F.

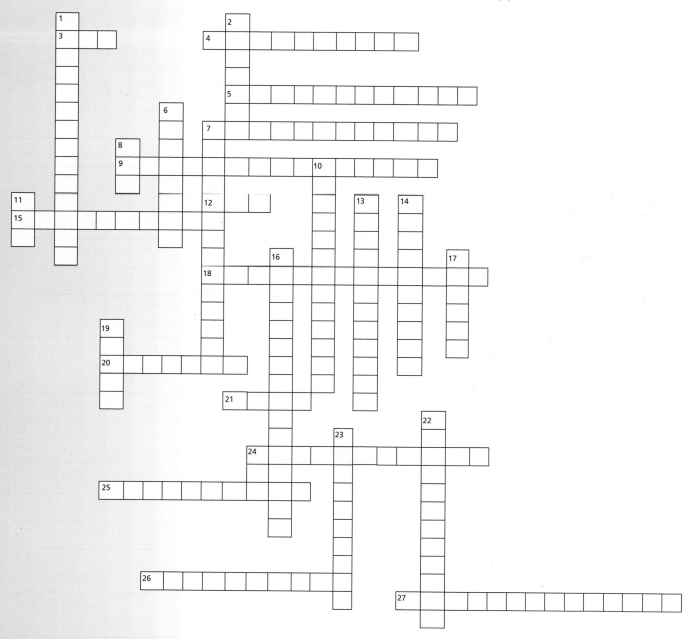

Down

1. x-ray of the gallbladder
2. condition of a closed tube or duct (may be congenital)
6. narrowing
7. around the esophagus (adj.)
8. nothing by mouth (abbr.)
10. surgical repair of the gums
11. hepatitis B virus (abbr.)
13. stretching of the stomach
14. upon the stomach
16. specialty in the study of stomach and the intestine
17. enzyme that breaks down fat
19. solid waste
22. irrigation of the anus and rectum
23. herniation of the small intestine

Across

3. high density lipoprotein (abbr.)
4. inflammation of the mouth
5. enlarged spleen
7. inflammation of the pancreas
9. choleangio_____, imaging bile ducts and pancreas
12. esophagogastroduodenoscopy (abbr.)
15. specialty that treats obesity
18. hemorrhage of the liver
20. stones
21. suffix for stone
24. process of examining the colon with a scope
25. condition of rupture of a structure through an opening
26. below the tongue
27. condition of diverticuli in the intestine

REVIEW ACTIVITIES

GLOSSARY

absorption	movement of nutrients from one layer to another	constipation	hard stool, infrequent bowel movements
anastomosis	connecting two tubular structures	diverticulitis	inflammation of diverticula of the intestine
amylase	enzyme that breaks down starch	digestion	breakdown of food
		defecation	expelling feces
appendicitis	inflammation of the appendix	diverticulosis	condition of having diverticula
atresia	closed ducts or tubes	dysentery	inflammation of the intestine, pain, diarrhea
bariatrics	specialty that treats obesity		
cathartic	agent that relieves constipation (synonym, laxative)	enterectasia	stretching of the intestine
		enteritis	inflammation of the intestine
cheiloplasty	surgical repair of the lips	enterocele	intestinal hernia
cheilosis	condition of the lips	enterocentesis	surgical puncture of the intestine to remove fluid
cheilostomatoplasty	repair of the lips and mouth		
cheilotomy	incision into the lip	enteroclysis	irrigation of the intestine
cholangiopancreatography	process of taking x-ray of the biliary and pancreatic ducts using contrast media	enteroplegia	paralysis of the intestine
		enteroptosis	prolapse of the intestine
		enterorrhagia	hemorrhage of the intestine
cholecystograph (cholecystogram)	x-ray picture of the gallbladder	enteroscope	instrument for examining the intestine
cirrhosis	chronic liver disease causing loss of liver function and resistance to blood flow through the liver. Etiology may include poor nutrition, alcoholism, previous hepatitis	epigastric	upon the stomach
		esophageal	pertaining to the esophagus
		esophagoduodenostomy	anastomosis between the esophagus and duodenum
colic	pertaining to the colon (synonym; colonic)	esophagogastric	pertaining to the esophagus and stomach
colocentesis	surgical puncture of the colon to remove fluid	esophagostenosis	narrowing of the esophagus
coloclysis	irrigation of the colon	feces	stool, solid waste adj. fecal
colopexy	surgical fixation of the colon	gastrectasia	dilatation of the stomach
coloptosis	prolapsed colon	gastric	pertaining to the stomach
colorectal	pertaining to the colon and rectum	gastritis	inflammation of the stomach
colostomy	making a new opening (stoma) in the colon	gastroclysis	irrigation of the stomach

REVIEW ACTIVITIES

gastroenteric	pertaining to the stomach and intestine
gastroenterology	the study of diseases of the stomach and intestine
gastroenteroptosis	prolapse of stomach and intestine
gastrorrhagia	hemorrhage of the stomach
gingival	pertaining to the gums
gingivalgia	gum pain
gingivectomy	excision of the gums
gingivoglossitis	inflammation of the gums and tongue
glossal	pertaining to the tongue
glossalgia	tongue pain
glossoplegia	tongue paralysis (adjective, glossoplegic)
glossoptosis	prolapse of the tongue
glossoscopy	examination of the tongue with a scope
hepatectomy	excision of the liver
hepatitis	inflammation of the liver
hepatocele	herniation of the liver
hepatodynia	liver pain (hepatalgia)
hepatolith	liver stone
hepatopathy	any disease of the liver
hepatorrhagia	hemorrhage of the liver
hepatorrhaphy	suture of the liver
hepatoscope	instrument for examining the liver
hepatoscopy	process of using a hepatoscope
hypoglossal	pertaining to below the tongue (synonym, sublingual)
ileocecal	between the ileum and the cecum
ingestion	swallowing, eating
linguogingival	pertaining to the gums and tongue

lactase	enzyme that breaks down lactose
lipase	enzyme that breaks down fat
mastication	chewing
nausea	feeling like one is going to vomit
obesity	quality of being overweight
occult	hidden
pancreatectomy	excision of the pancreas
pancreatic	pertaining to the pancreas
pancreatolith	stone in the pancreas
pancreatolysis	destruction of pancreatic tissue
pancreatopathy	any disease of the pancreas
paraesophageal	around the esophagus
proctoclysis	irrigation of the rectum and anus
proctologist	physician specialist in diseases of the anus and rectum
proctopexy	fixation of a prolapsed anus and rectum (synonyn, rectopexy)
proctoplegia	paralysis of the rectum and anus
proctorrhaphy	suture of the anus and rectum
proctoscope	instrument for examining the anus and rectum
proctoscopy	process of using a proctoscope
rectocele	herniation of the rectum
rectoclysis	irrigation of the rectum
rectocystotomy	incision into the urinary bladder through the rectum
rectoplasty	surgical repair of the rectum
rectorrhaphy	suturing of the rectum
rectoscope	instrument used to examine the rectum
rectoscopy	process of using a rectoscope (adjective, rectoscopic)
rectourethral	pertaining to the rectum and urethra

REVIEW ACTIVITIES

sigmoidoscope	instrument for examining the sigmoid and large colon
splenectomy	excision of the spleen
splenomegaly	enlarged spleen
splenopathy	any disease of the spleen
splenopexy	fixation of a prolapsed spleen
splenoptosis	prolapsed spleen
splenorrhagia	hemorrhage of the spleen
splenorrhaphy	suturing of the spleen
stomatalgia	mouth pain

stomatitis	inflammation of the mouth
stomatomycosis	fungal condition of the mouth
stomatopathy	any disease of the mouth
stomatoplasty	surgical repair of the mouth
stomatorrhagia	hemorrhage of the mouth
stomatoscope	instrument used to examine the mouth
stomatoscopy	process of using a stomatoscope
ulcer	craterlike sore

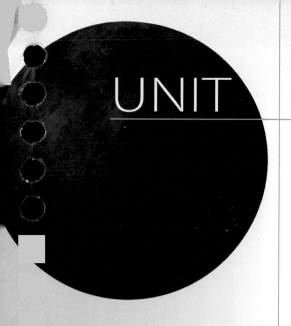

UNIT 8

Neurology, Psychology, Anesthesiology, and Vascular Terminology

Read through the list of word parts in the following table. Then work the frames in the first part of this unit. Refer back to this list when necessary.

Combining Form	Combining Form	Suffix
neur/o (nerve or neuron)	**blast/o** (germ or embryonic cell; gives rise to something else)	**-blast** (word itself)
angi/o (vessel)		**-spasm** (word itself)
		-osis (use with **scler/o**)
my/o (muscle)	**spasm/o** (involuntary contraction)	**-lysis** (use with all)
arteri/o (artery)	**scler/o** (hard)	**-oma** (use with **fibr/o**)
thromb/o (clot)	**lys/o** (breaking down, destruction)	**-pathy**, noun suffix (use with first column)
phleb/o (vein)		**-genesis**, noun suffix (use with **my/o**, **thromb/o**, **neur/o**)
hem/o, hemat/o (blood)	**fibr/o** (fibrous, fiber)	**-ectasia** (dilation, use with **angi/o, arteri/o, phleb/o**)
ather/o (fatty or porridgelike)		**-rrhexis** (rupture, use with **angi/o, arteri/o, phleb/o**)
ven/i (vein)		

ANSWER COLUMN

8.1

The nerv/ous system is made up of the brain, spinal cord, cranial nerves, and spinal nerves. It coordinates and regulates all types of body functions including movement, mental processes, and chemical balance. Neur/o/logy is the specialty that studies the anatomy, physiology, and pathology of the nervous system.

8.2

nerv/ous
ner′ vəs

neur/o/logy
nōō **ro′** lō jē

The adjective meaning pertaining to nerves is

_____/_____.

The study of the nervous system is

_____/_____/_____.

8.3

neur/o/surgeon
nōō rō **ser′** jən

A highly skilled physician specially trained to perform surgery on structures of the nervous system is a

_____/_____/_____.

Neurosurgeon performing repair of spondylolisthesis of the lumbar spine
Photo by Timothy J. Dennerll, RT(R), Ph.D., courtesy of Allegiance Health and Harrish Rawal, MD, Jackson, MI

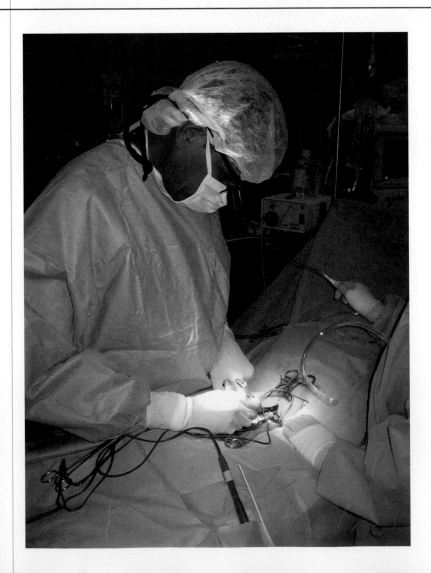

ANSWER COLUMN

8.4

An embryonic (germ or stem) cell from which a muscle cell develops is a my/o/blast. A germ cell from which a nerve cell develops is a

neur/o/blast
nōō rō blast

_____/_____/_____.

A germ cell from which vessels develop is an

angi/o/blast
an' jē o blast

_____/_____/_____.

8.5

A spasm is an involuntary twitching or contraction.
A spasm of a nerve is a neur/o/spasm.
A spasm of a muscle is a

my/o/spasm
mī' ō spaz əm

_____/_____/_____.

A spasm of a vessel is an

angi/o/spasm
an' jē ō spaz əm

_____/_____/_____.

Keep up the good work.

8.6

Build a term that means:
arterial spasm

arteri/o/spasm
är **tir'** ē ō spaz əm

_____/_____/_____;

gastric spasm

gastr/o/spasm
gas' trō spaz əm

_____/_____/_____;

softening of the stomach walls

gastr/o/malac/ia
gas' trō mə **lā'** shə

_____/_____/_____/_____.

8.7

My/o/pathy means a generalized disease condition of the muscles. Build words meaning
a generalized disease condition of the vessels

angi/o/pathy
an jē **op'** ath ē

_____/_____/_____;

a generalized disease condition of the nerves

neur/o/pathy
nōō **rop'** ath ē

_____/_____/_____.

REMINDER: The accent is on the **op'** in these terms.

8.8

A (condition of) hardening of nerve tissue is neur/o/scler/osis.
Hardening of a vessel is

angi/o/scler/osis
an' jē ō sklə **rō'** sis

_____/_____/_____/_____.

A hardening of muscle tissue is

my/o/scler/osis
mī' ō sklə **rō'** sis

_____/_____/_____/_____.

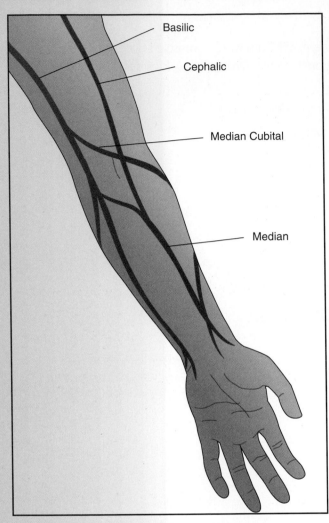

Superficial veins of the arm *Delmar/Cengage Learning*

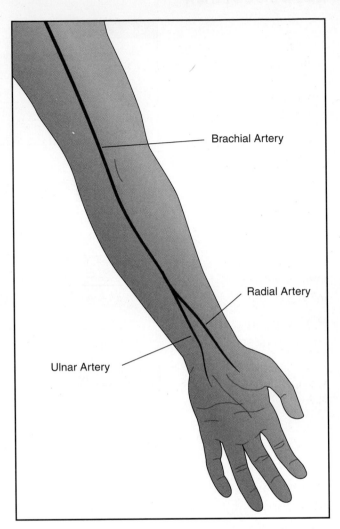

Arteries of the arm *Delmar/Cengage Learning*

8.9

Use **neur/o** plus suffixes you have learned in previous units to build words meaning a specialist who studies nervous system disorders

neur/o/logist
nōō **rol′** ō jist

_____/_____/_____;
the study of the nervous system

neur/o/logy
nōō **rol′** ō gē

_____/_____/_____;
inflammation of a nerve

neur/itis
nōō **rī′** tis

_____/_____.

8.10

A muscle tumor is a my/oma.
A nerve tumor is a

neur/oma
nōō **rō′** mə

_____/_____.

A vessel tumor is an

angi/oma
an jē **ō′** mə

_____/_____.

(continued)

ANSWER COLUMN

A fibrous tumor is a

fibr/oma
fī **brō′** mə

_____/_____.

8.11

The destruction of muscle tissue is my/o/lysis.
The destruction of nerve tissue is

neur/o/lysis
nōō **rol′** ə sis

_____/_____/_____.

The destruction or breaking down of vessels is

angi/ō/lysis
an′ jē **ol′** ə sis

_____/_____/_____.

8.12

nerve

Neur/algia means pain along the course of a _____.

nerves

Neuropathy refers to any disease of the _____.

8.13

nerves
joints

Neur/o/arthr/o/pathy is a disease of _____ and _____.

8.14

Build words meaning
inflammation of a nerve

neur/itis
nōō **ri′** tis

_____/_____;

(continued)

Afferent and efferent motor pathways of the CNS Delmar/Cengage Learning

ANSWER COLUMN

neur/o/lysis
no͞o **rol′** ə sis

neur/o/plasty
no͞o rō plas tē

neur/o/surgeon
no͞o′ rō **sur′** jən

destruction of nerve tissue

_____/_____/_____ ;

surgical repair of nerves

_____/_____/_____ ;

nervous system surgeon

_____/_____/_____ .

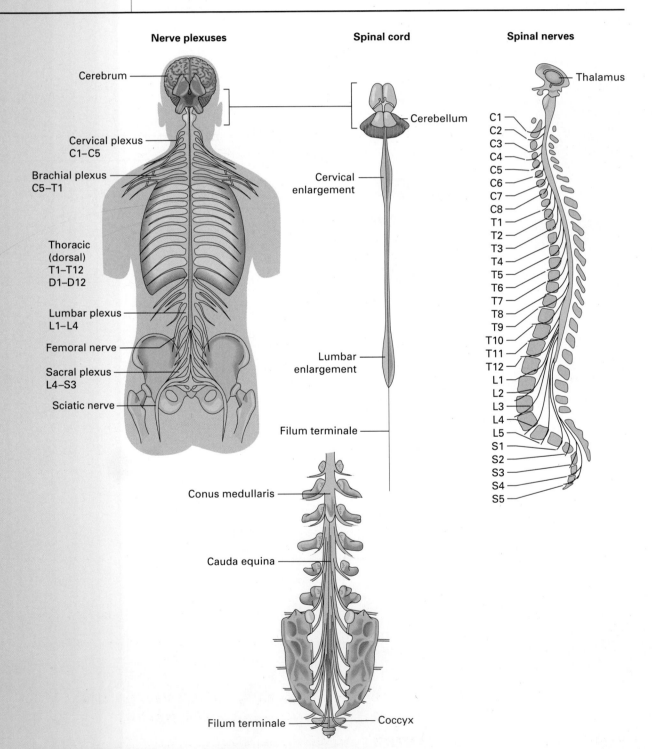

Nerve plexuses

Cerebrum

Cervical plexus
C1–C5

Brachial plexus
C5–T1

Thoracic
(dorsal)
T1–T12
D1–D12

Lumbar plexus
L1–L4

Femoral nerve

Sacral plexus
L4–S3

Sciatic nerve

Spinal cord

Cerebellum

Cervical
enlargement

Lumbar
enlargement

Filum terminale

Conus medullaris

Cauda equina

Filum terminale

Coccyx

Spinal nerves

Thalamus

C1
C2
C3
C4
C5
C6
C7
C8
T1
T2
T3
T4
T5
T6
T7
T8
T9
T10
T11
T12
L1
L2
L3
L4
L5
S1
S2
S3
S4
S5

Spinal cord (myel/o) and spinal nerves *Delmar/Cengage Learning*

ANSWER COLUMN

8.15

**TAKE A
CLOSER LOOK**

This table presents pairs of terms that are often confused in meaning because their spelling is so close. A simple difference between the term beginning with *e* or beginning with *a* makes a big difference in their correct use. Look them up in your dictionary for more information on word origins and use.

afferent	inflowing, *toward a center*, to bring to
efferent	outflowing, *away from a center*, to carry away
affect	to have *influence* upon, i.e. to change mood, thoughts, or actions
effect	the *result* or consequence of an action
accept	include, *bring toward*, embrace
except	exclude, *keep away*, reject
affusion	*pouring upon*, i.e. pouring of water *upon* the body for therapeutic purposes
effusion	the *escaping* of fluid or blood *from* its normal place, i.e. blood from vessels into the lungs or a joint cavity

8.16

State the term that begins with "a" that means:
include, bring toward

accept

_____ ;

inflowing, toward the center

afferent

_____ ;

have influence upon, to cause a change in mood or actions

affect

_____ .

8.17

State the term that begins with "e" that means:
exclude, keep away

except

_____ ;

outflowing, away from the center

efferent

_____ ;

the result of an action or consequence

effect

_____ .

8.18

Neur/o/trips/y means surgical crushing of a nerve. The word root for crushing

trips

(usually by rubbing or grinding) is _____ .

8.19

Tripsis, from which we get **-tripsy**, is a Greek word that means rubbing or massage. *Tripsis* can be carried to the point of crushing or grinding. Surgical

neur/o/tripsy
nōo′ rō trip sē

crushing of a nerve is _____/_____/_____ .

ANSWER COLUMN

8.20

In some cases of lith/iasis, it may be necessary to crush calculi so they may be passed. A word that means surgical crushing of stones, as in the bladder or

lith/o/tripsy
lith′ ō trip sē

ureters, is _____/_____/_____.

8.21

Therapeutic ultrasound (high-frequency sound waves) can be used to fragment

lithotripsy

stones in the kidney. This is ultrasonic _____/_____/_____.

8.22

**TAKE A
CLOSER LOOK**

Look up myel/itis in your dictionary. From the definition, you conclude that **myel** is the word root for spinal cord or bone marrow. Write two words for spinal cord and two words for bone marrow using **myel**.

_____

_____

_____

_____

8.23

Find the word myel/o/blast in your dictionary and write the meaning.

bone marrow germ cell

* _____.

myel/o

The combining form of myel is _____/_____.

8.24

Find words meaning
pertaining to myelocytes

myel/o/cyt/ic
mī′ el ō **sit′** ik

_____/_____/_____/_____;

herniation of the spinal cord

myel/o/cele
mī′ el ō sēl

_____/_____/_____.

8.25

-plasia means a condition of growth or development. It is used to indicate a change in the form of a structure or an abnormal number of cells. Write the meaning of the following terms.

poor or defective
development

dys/plasia * _____

overgrowth, too
much growth

hyper/plasia * _____

lack of development

a/plasia * _____

ANSWER COLUMN

8.26

Build a term that means defective (poor or bad) formation of the spinal cord:

myel/o/dys/plasia
mī el ō dis **plā'** zhə

_____/_____/_____/_____
(body part) + (disorder)

8.27

A/plasia means failure of an organ to develop properly. A word that means overgrowth or too many cells is

hyper/plasia
hī pər **plā'** zhə _or_
hī pər **plā'** zē ə

_____/_____ .

8.28

If growth of too many cells is hyper/plasia, underdevelopment or not enough

hypo/plasia
hī pō **plā'** zhə _or_
hī pō **plā'** zē ə

cells is expressed as _____/_____ .

NOTE: Review the text and illustrations in Unit 3 for information on hypertrophy and hypotrophy. The terms hyperplasia and hypoplasia mean something different.

8.29

Using myel/o/dys/plasia as a model, build words meaning defective formation of cartilage

chondr/o/dys/plasia
kon' drō dis **plā'** zhə

_____/_____/_____/_____ ;

oste/o/chondr/o/dys/plasia
os' tē ō kon' drō dis
   plā' zhə

defective formation of bone and cartilage

_____/_____/_____/_____/_____/_____ .

NOTE: **-plasia** may be pronounced either **plā'** zē ə or **plā'** zhə.

8.30

Form a word meaning inflammation of nerves and spinal cord

neur/o/myel/itis
nōō rō mī' ə **lī'** tis

_____/_____/_____/_____ .

8.31

SPELL CHECK

psych/o (sī' kō) refers to the mind. Look up **psych/o** in your dictionary and read the definition. See how many everyday terms begin with the word root psych. Be sure to watch your spelling on this one. The _p_ is silent and the _y_ sound is like an _i_.

8.32

The study of the mind, mental processes, and human behavior is

psych/o/logy
sī **kol'** ō jē

_____/_____/_____ .

ANSWER COLUMN

8.33

Using your dictionary, read and analyze the meanings of

psych/o/analysis
sī′ kō a **nal′** ə sis

psychoanalysis _____/_____/_____ ,

** _____ ;

psych/o/somatic
sī′ kō sō **mat′** ik

psychosomatic _____/_____/_____ ,

** _____ ;

psych/o/sexual
sī′ kō **sex′** ū əl

psychosexual _____/_____/_____ ,

** _____ .

8.34

Psychiatry is the field of medicine that studies and deals with mental and neurotic disorders. The physician who specializes in this field of medicine is called a

psych/iatrist
sī **kī′** ə trist

_____/_____ .

The treatment of mental disorders by a psychiatrist is called

psych/iatry
sī **kī′** ə trē

_____/_____ .

8.35

WORD
ORIGINS

In Greek mythology Psyche was Cupid's lover. She was the beautiful daughter of a king and the personification of fervent emotion. After many difficult trials, Psyche was made a goddess by Zeus and was united with Cupid on Mount Olympus. *Psyche* in Greek refers to the soul, spirit, or breath that creates life as distinguished from the physical aspects.

8.36

Psych/o/logy is the science that studies human behavior. The scientist or therapist

psych/o/logist
sī **kol′** ə jist

who works in this field is called a _____/_____/_____ .

8.37

Psych/o/therapy is a process of healing mental disorders using words, art, drama, or movement to express feelings. A clinical psych/o/logist helps clients with

psych/o/therapy
sī′ kō **thair′** ə pē

mental disorders by using _____/_____/_____ .

8.38

Psych/o/genesis means the formation of mental characteristics. A severe mental condition marked by loss of contact with reality and having delusions or

psych/osis
sī **ko′** sis

hallucinations is _____/_____ .

ANSWER COLUMN

8.39

psych/o/neur/osis
sī' kō nōō rō' sis
neur/osis
nōō rō' sis

Psych/o/neurosis (neur/o/sis), an emotional and behavioral disorder, is manifested by anxiety, phobias, and defense mechanisms. A psych/o/neur/o/tic behavior is exhibited in a person who suffers from a

_____ /_____ /_____ /_____ or

_____ /_____.

8.40

neurosis

The patient suffering from a neurosis knows the real from the unreal but will exaggerate reality. Individuals who will not touch others because they fear

contact with germs may suffer from _____ .

8.41

TAKE A CLOSER LOOK

neuro/sis

Obsessive-compulsive disorder (OCD) is a neurosis characterized by repeated distressing thoughts that produce anxiety (obsession) and uncontrollable repeated actions that must be done to relieve the anxiety (compulsion). A person may fear illness and think that they are being constantly exposed to germs. They may refuse to leave the house without wearing gloves and a mask, eat only boiled food, clean their house compulsively, and/or exclude social contact. OCD

is a type of _____ /_____ . Look up OCD and other neuroses in your dictionary.

8.42

INFORMATION FRAME

Psych/o/trop/ic (*trope*, Greek for turn) medications may be used to alter emotions or behavior.

8.43

psych/o/trop/ic
sī' kō trō' pik

A patient with a psychoneurosis may be given a

_____ /_____ /_____ /_____ medication to lower anxiety.

8.44

psych/o/trop/ic
sī' kō trō' pik

psych/osis
sī kō' sis

psych/o/motor
sī' kō mō' ter

psych/o/sexu/al
sī' kō seks' yōō al

Use **psych/o** to build words meaning
medication that alters mind and emotions

_____ /_____ /_____ /_____ ;

severe mental condition (delusional)

_____ /_____ ;

mental processes that cause movement

_____ /_____ /_____ ;

mental disorder related to sexual function

_____ /_____ /_____ /_____ .

Prescription psychotropic medication *Photo by Timothy J. Dennerll, RT(R), Ph.D.*

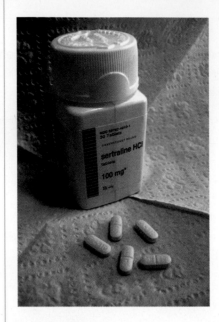

8.45

Psychoneuroses (neuroses, plural) take many forms. Obsessive-compulsive

reaction, conversion reaction, and phobias are forms of _____

_____ (plural form).

neuroses or
psychoneuroses

8.46

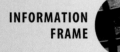

INFORMATION FRAME

In your dictionary read about the psychopath and the psychopathic personality. Also read the definition of psychopathy.

8.47

motor is a word root referring to movement. Mental processes that cause

movement are _____/_____/_____ functions.

psych/o/motor
sī' kō **mō'** ter

8.48

A neuron that innervates a muscle causes movement. It is called a

_____ neuron.

motor

8.49

TAKE A CLOSER LOOK

Let your eye wander down the columns of **psych** words in the dictionary. Read about those that interest you. Note the information following the words psychiatric and psychoanalysis. All **psych/o** words refer to

* _____

mental processes
(mental or soul)

ANSWER COLUMN

8.50

pharmac/o (as in pharmacy) means drugs or medicine. Neur/o/pharmacology is the study of drugs that affect the nervous system. The study of drugs that act on the mind and emotions is

psych/o/pharmac/o/logy
sī′ kō fär ma **kol′** ō jē

_____/_____/_____/_____/_____ .

8.51

**INFORMATION
FRAME**

Psych/o/pharmac/o/logy includes the study of using medications to treat mental illness. The following are examples of psychotropic medications: antidepressants (Prozac), tranquilizers (Thorazine), neuroleptics, sedatives, and anticonvulsants (Dilantin).

8.52

A pharmac/ist is licensed to dispense prescription and nonprescription medications from a pharmacy. To become a pharmacist, a person must study

pharmac/o/logy
fär′ ma **kol′** ō jē

_____/_____/_____ .

8.53

narc/o is the combining form for sleep. A narc/o/tic is a drug that produces sleep. Opium produces stuporous sleep. Opium is a

narc/o/tic
när **kot′** ik

_____/_____/_____ .

PROFESSIONAL PROFILE

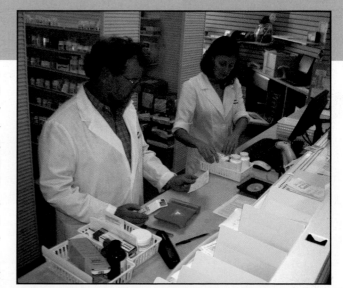

A **registered pharmacist (R.Ph)** is licensed by each state to prepare and dispense all types of medications as well as medical supplies related to medication administration. They may practice in hospitals and clinics or own and operate and/or be employed in private pharmacies. A license is required in all states, the District of Columbia, and all U.S. territories. In order to obtain a license, pharmacists must earn a Doctor of Pharmacy (Pharm.D.) degree from a college of pharmacy and pass several examinations.

Pharmacy technicians assist the pharmacist with preparation and administration of medications as well as with reception and billing duties. Professional certification of pharmacy technicians varies from state to state and is administered by state pharmacy associations.

Pharmacist and pharmacy technician preparing medication for dispensing _Photo by Timothy J. Dennerll, RT(R), Ph.D., courtesy of Brown's Advanced Care Pharmacy Services, Jackson, MI_

ANSWER COLUMN

8.54

A narcotic produces pain relief as well as numbness or stuporous sleep. A narcotic should be used only on the advice of a physician. Codeine produces pain relief

narcotic

and sleep. Codeine is a _____.

8.55

**WORD
ORIGINS**

Morpheus was the Greek god of dreams. Morphine is a narcotic derived from opium poppies and produces a dreamlike state as well as analgesia.

8.56

Morphine (MS-morphine sulfate) is used as a pain reliever (analgesic) and is also

narcotic

a _____.

8.57

Because narcotics can cause addiction, a physician must have a narcotic license

narcotics

to either dispense or write orders for _____ (plural).

8.58

narc/osis
när **kō′** sis

The condition induced by narcotics is called _____/_____.

8.59

**WORD
ORIGINS**

Epilepsia is a Greek word meaning to seize upon. In the past epilepsy has been classified by types of seizures described as petit mal (French: small bad) and grand mal (French: large bad). Today epilepsy is described by the area of the brain involved, and it is divided into two categories including partial and general. Medical and surgical therapies are used in treatment of seizure disorders

epilepsy
ep′ i lep sē

called _____.

8.60

-lepsy is used in words to mean seizure. Narc/o/lepsy means seizure or attacks of sleep. A person who is absolutely unable to stay awake suffers

narc/o/lepsy
när′ kō lep sē

from _____/_____/_____.

8.61

narcolepsy

Narcolepsy is a type of sleep disorder. A person may fall sound asleep standing at a bus stop. This is _____.

STUDYWARE™ CONNECTION

Remember, after completing this unit, you can complete a crossword puzzle or other interactive game on your **StudyWARE™ CD-ROM** that will help you learn the content in this chapter.

ANSWER COLUMN

	8.62
narcolepsy	Cerebroma, cerebral arteriosclerosis, and paresis (brain disease) are some causes of sleep seizures, which are called _____.
	8.63
sleep, stupor, or stuporous sleep	You may get "tired" of hearing this, but **narc/o** any place in a word should make you think of * _____ _____.
	8.64
lip/o/lysis li **pol'** ə sis cyt/o/lysis sī **tol'** ə sis	Build words meaning destruction (breakdown) of fat (lipids) _____/_____/_____; destruction (breakdown) of cells _____/_____/_____.
	8.65
arteri/o/scler/osis är tir' ē ō sklə **rō'** sis	**arteri/o** is used in words about the arteries. Arteries are blood vessels that carry blood away from the heart. A word meaning hardening of the arteries is _____/_____/_____/_____ (AS).
	8.66
arteri/o/fibr/osis är tir' ē ō fī **brō'** sis arteri/o/malacia är tir' ē ō mə **lā'** shə	Arteri/o/scler/osis means hardening of the arteries. Build words meaning a fibrous condition of the arteries _____/_____/_____/_____; a softening of the arteries _____/_____/_____.
	8.67
ather/o/scler/osis a' ther ō skler **ō'** sis	Refer to the diagram of atherosclerosis. Recall that **ather/o** means fatty or porridgelike. Hardening of the blood vessels (arteries) caused by a fatty substance (atheroma) is a condition called _____/_____/_____/_____.

ANSWER COLUMN

8.68

Atherosclerosis occurs primariy in medium to large blood vessels and can decrease vascular supply causing ischemia and necrosis. This leads to myocardial infarction (heart attack) or cerebral infarction (stroke). Fatty streaks inside the carotid arteries are an indication of

_____/_____/_____/_____.

NOTE: Look up ischemia and necrosis in your dictionary.

ather/o/scler/osis
a' ther ō skler ō' sis

8.69

If a large ather/oma develops from the fatty streak, an ather/ectomy may be performed. Excision of an ather/oma is called _____/_____

or _____/_____/_____. This procedure is most commonly performed on the carotid artery.

ather/ectomy
a' ther **ek'** tō mē
end/arter/ectomy
end är' ter **ek'** tō mē

Major arteries and vascular conditions associated with atherosclerosis
Delmar/Cengage Learning

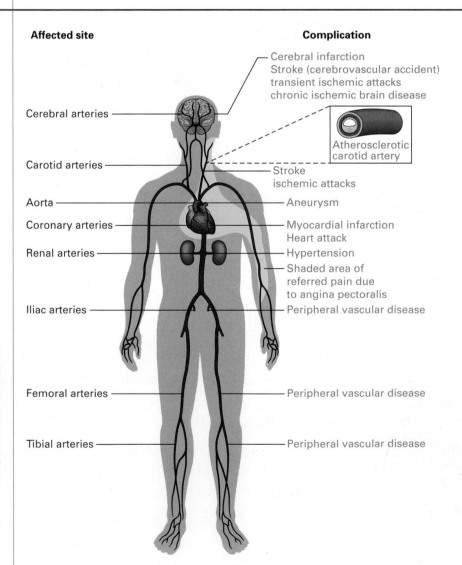

Affected site

- Cerebral arteries
- Carotid arteries
- Aorta
- Coronary arteries
- Renal arteries
- Iliac arteries
- Femoral arteries
- Tibial arteries

Complication

- Cerebral infarction
  Stroke (cerebrovascular accident)
  transient ischemic attacks
  chronic ischemic brain disease
- Atherosclerotic carotid artery
- Stroke
  ischemic attacks
- Aneurysm
- Myocardial infarction
  Heart attack
- Hypertension
- Shaded area of referred pain due to angina pectoralis
- Peripheral vascular disease
- Peripheral vascular disease
- Peripheral vascular disease

ANSWER COLUMN

8.70

Nonsurgical treatment of atherosclerosis includes bringing cholesterol to normal levels, increasing the high-density lipoproteins (HDL), decreasing the low-density lipoproteins (LDL), and stopping smoking. Diet, exercise, and lifestyle changes can

atherosclerosis

help reduce the risk of death from _____.

8.71

Ather/o/scler/o/tic coronary artery disease is the most common cause of angina pectoris. If the oxygen demand is higher than that supplied to the heart muscle,

angina pectoris
an **ji'** na pek **tor'** is   *or*
an' ji na pek **tor'** is

* _____ can occur.

NOTE: Look up angina pectoris in your dictionary.

8.72

hem/o refers to blood. A benign tumor of a blood vessel is a hem/angi/oma. (Note that the o is dropped.) An embryonic blood vessel cell is a

hem/angi/o/blast
hēm **an'** gē ō blast

_____/_____/_____/_____.

hem/arthr/osis
hēm är **thrō'** sis

A condition of blood in a joint is

_____/_____/_____.

8.73

hemat/o also refers to blood. Another word for destruction of blood cells

hemat/o/lysis
hēm ə **tol'** ə sis

is _____/_____/_____.
-phobia means fear. An abnormal fear of blood is

hemat/o/phobia
hēm' ə tō **fō'** bē ə

_____/_____/_____.

8.74

blood

Use **hemat/o** once more to mean _____.

hemat/o/logy
hēm ə **tol'** ə jē

The study of blood is _____/_____/_____.
One who specializes in the science of blood is a

hemat/o/log/ist
hēm ə **tol'** ə jist

_____/_____/_____/_____.

8.75

Hem/o/globin (hgb) blood lab test is measured to detect anemia. The red protein substance in erythrocytes that carries oxygen and carbon dioxide is hemoglobin. A range of 12–14 grams per decaliter of blood is a normal average amount

hem/o/globin
hēm' ō glō bin

of _____/_____/_____ for women.

ANSWER COLUMN

8.76

In addition to a hemoglobin measurement, a hemat/o/crit test may also be performed. The hematocrit (hct) measures the percent of formed elements (blood cells) compared to the total volume of blood. 36%–45% is a normal

hemat/o/crit
hem **at'** ō krit

average range for _____/_____/_____ levels.

8.77

The two combining forms used to refer to blood are

hem/o

_____/_____ and

hemat/o

_____/_____ .

8.78

thromb/o is the combining form that means blood clot.
Thromb/o/angi/itis means inflammation of a vessel with formation of a

blood clot

* _____ .

8.79

excision of a
    thrombus (clot)

Thromb/ectomy means * _____ .

8.80

The medical name for blood clot is thrombus.

thrombus
throm' bus

A synonym for clot is _____ .

thrombi
throm' bī

The plural form is _____ .

8.81

Recall **lymph/o** means lymphatic tissue. Thromb/o/lymph/ang/itis means

inflammation of a lymph
    vessel with formation
    of a thrombus (clot)

* _____
_____ .

8.82

phleb/o is a combining form for vein. Thromb/o/phleb/itis means

inflammation of a vein
    with thrombus formation

* _____
_____ .

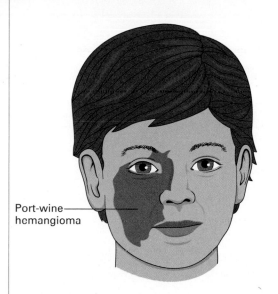

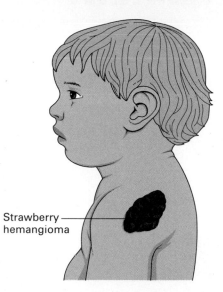

Port-wine hemangioma

Strawberry hemangioma

Delmar/Cengage Learning

8.83

See, you are great at figuring out meanings. Now, using **thromb/o**, build words meaning
a condition of forming a thrombus

thromb/osis
throm **bō′** sis

_____/_____;

a cell that aids clotting

thromb/o/cyte
throm′ bō sīt

_____/_____/_____;

resembling a thrombus

thromb/oid
throm′ boid

_____/_____.

8.84

Build words meaning
pertaining to the formation of a thrombus

thromb/o/gen/ic
throm′ bō **jen′** ik

_____/_____/_____/_____;

destruction of a thrombus

thromb/o/lysis
throm **bol′** ə sis

_____/_____/_____;

lack of cells that aid in clotting (platelets)

thromb/o/cyt/o/penia
throm′ bō sī′ tō **pē′** nē ə

_____/_____/_____/_____/_____.

Great! You are good at word building, too.

8.85

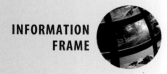

INFORMATION FRAME

A thrombus may block or "occlude" a vessel. This occlusion may cause isch/emia, stopping blood supply to the tissues and producing an infarct (necrosis of tissue). If this happens in the heart muscle, the condition is called myocardial infarction (MI).

8.86

Look up the following terms in your medical dictionary and write their definitions.

occlusion * _____

_____ ;

infarct * _____

_____ ;

myocardial * _____

_____ .

8.87

A thrombus or piece of a thrombus may move through blood vessels to another part of the body. This moving thrombus is called an embolus. An embolus may cause a block in a vessel called an _____/_____ .

occlus/ion
ō **klōō′** shun

8.88

If an artery of the heart muscle is occluded and an area of tissue has no blood supply, a * _____/_____/_____/_____ _____/_____/_____ (MI) may occur.

my/o/cardi/al in/farct/ion
mī ō **kär′** dē əl
in **fark′** shun

8.89

If an artery supplying the cerebrum (brain) is occluded, a * _____/_____ _____/_____/_____ (cerebrovascular accident [CVA] stroke) could occur.

cerebr/al in/farct/ion
se **rē′** bral in **fark′** shun

8.90

Recall that arteries (**arteri/o**) are vessels that carry blood away from the heart. Veins (**phleb/o**) are vessels that carry blood back to the _____ .

heart

8.91

One combining form for vein is **phleb/o**. Arteriosclerosis is hardening of the _____ . Hardening of veins is called _____/_____/_____/_____ .

arteries
phleb/o/scler/osis
fleb′ ō sklə **rō′** sis

8.92

Build words meaning
excision of a vein

_____/_____ ;
surgical fixation of a vein

_____/_____/_____ .

phleb/ectomy
fli **bek′** tə mē

phleb/o/pexy
fleb′ ō pek sē

CASE STUDY INVESTIGATION (CSI)

Endovenous Ablation (New Surgery for Varicose Veins)

Mr. J, an 80-year-old male, presented with **persistent** right leg pain, swelling, and a recurrent skin ulcer above the medial ankle. He had a history of **myocardial infarction (MI)** and deep vein **thrombosis (DVT). Angiogram** revealed a varicosed saphenous vein. **Phlebectomy** (vein stripping) was recommended. The **vascular** surgeon offered a new procedure, **endovenous ablation**, a venous closure radio-frequency system to heat and close the **varicosed** vein. Mr. J consented. Using guided real-time **ultrasound** visualization, the instrument **catheter** was inserted in the **proximal** end of the diseased vein and advanced through the length of the vein. The procedure was completed and Mr. J was discharged the same day wearing compression stockings. On follow-up Mr. J was pain-free and expected to resume activities of daily living as well as the gardening he enjoys.

CSI Vocabulary Challenge

Analyze the terms by dividing them into their word parts and writing the definition. Write the meaning of the abbreviations.

persistent	_____
myocardial infarction	_____
thrombosis	_____
angiogram	_____
phlebectomy	_____
endovenous	_____
ablation	_____
varicosed	_____
ultrasound	_____
catheter	_____
proximal	_____
MI	_____
DVT	_____

ANSWER COLUMN

8.93

Dilation and dilatation are synonyms for stretching or increase in diameter.
-ectasia is used as a suffix for dilatation.
Build words meaning
venous dilatation (stretching)

phleb/ectasia
fleb′ ek **tā′** zē ə

_____/_____;

(continued)

ANSWER COLUMN

arteri/ectasia
är tir' ē ek **tā'** zē ə

angi/ectasia
an' jē ek **tā'** zē ə

arterial dilatation

_____/_____ ;

vessel dilatation

_____/_____ .

NOTE: Remember the combining form rule from Unit 1. When the suffix begins with a vowel, use a word root. When the suffix begins with a consonant, use a combining form.

8.94

Phleb/o/plasty means

surgical repair of a vein

* _____ .

Phleb/o/tomy means

incision into a vein or
    venipuncture
vēn' i punk tyōōr

* _____ .

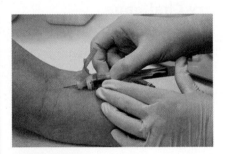

Phlebotomy *Delmar/Cengage Learning*

8.95

ven/i/puncture
vēn' i punk tyōōr

ven/o and **ven/i** are also combining forms for vein. To obtain a ven/ous blood

sample, a _____/_____/_____ is performed.

8.96

ven/ous
vēn' us
ven/ous

Venous blood is the dark blood in the veins. Blood flow through the veins back to

the heart is called _____/_____ return. Administering

medication within a vein is an intra/ _____/_____

injection.

STUDYWARE™ CONNECTION

After completing this unit, you can play a Spelling Bee game to help you learn the pronunciation of terms presented in the chapter or play other interactive games on your **StudyWARE™ CD-ROM** that will help you learn the content in this chapter.

ANSWER COLUMN

8.97

-**rrhexis** is a suffix meaning rupture. Hyster/o/rrhexis means

rupture of the uterus

* _____ .

8.98

With -**rrhexis** you learn the last of the Greek "rrh" forms. -**rrhea**, -**rrhagia**,

suffixes

-**rrhaphy**, and -**rrhexis** are _____ .

8.99

Cyst/o/rrhexis means

rupture of the bladder

* _____ .

Enter/o/rrhexis means

rupture of the small
   intestine

* _____ .

8.100

To summarize, the four "rrh" suffixes you have learned are

-rrhea, discharge or flow

_____ , meaning _____

-rrhagia, hemorrhage

_____ , meaning _____

-rrhaphy, suture

_____ , meaning _____

-rrhexis, rupture

_____ , meaning _____

8.101

Build words meaning
rupture of the heart

cardi/o/rrhexis
kär′ dē ō **rek**′ sis

_____/_____/_____ ;

rupture of a vessel

angi/o/rrhexis
an′ jē ō **rek**′ sis

_____/_____/_____ .

8.102

Build words meaning
rupture of an artery

arteri/o/rrhexis
är tir′ ē ō **rek**′ sis

_____/_____/_____ ;

rupture of a vein

phleb/o/rrhexis
fleb′ ō **rek**′ sis

_____/_____/_____ .

ANSWER COLUMN

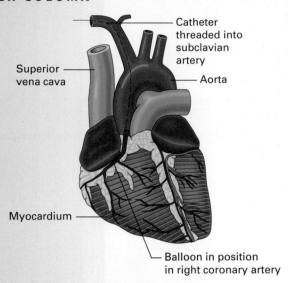

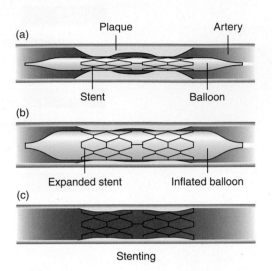

(A) Balloon angioplasty *Delmar/Cengage Learning*

(B) Stenting *Delmar/Cengage Learning*

8.103

Build terms that mean
repair of a vessel

angi/o/plasty
an' jē ō plas tē

_____/_____/_____;

process of obtaining an x-ray of a vessel

angi/o/graphy
an jē **og'** raf ē

_____/_____/_____;

process of using a looking device to examine a vessel

angi/o/scopy
an jē **os'** kō pē

_____/_____/_____;

image of a vessel

angi/o/gram
an' jē ō gram

_____/_____/_____.

8.104

Give the meaning of the following terms
phleb/o/plasty

repair of a vein

* _____;

phleb/o/graphy (ven/o/graphy)

process of obtaining
an x-ray of a vein

* _____
_____.

8.105

Rupture of the tissues of the uterus is called either

metr/o/rrhexis
mē trō **rek'** sis

_____/_____/_____

or

hyster/o/rrhexis
his' ter ō **rek'** sis

_____/_____/_____.

ANSWER COLUMN

8.106

Build words meaning
rupture of the liver

hepat/o/rrhexis
hep at ōr **eks'** is

_____/_____/_____ ;

hepat/o/rrhaphy
hep at **ōr'** a fē

suturing of the liver (wound)

_____/_____/_____ ;

hepat/o/rrhea
hep at ō **rē'** ə

excessive discharge of bile from the liver

_____/_____/_____ .

8.107

Build words meaning
rupture of the bladder

cyst/o/rrhexis
sis' tō **reks'** is

_____/_____/_____ ;

hemorrhage from the bladder

cyst/o/rrhagia
sis' tō **rā'** jē ə

_____/_____/_____ ;

discharge from the bladder

cyst/o/rrhea
sis tō **rē'** ə

_____/_____/_____ ;

suturing of the bladder

cyst/o/rrhaphy
sis **tōr'** a fē

_____/_____/_____ .

Good!

8.108

INFORMATION FRAME

Esthesia is a word meaning feeling or sensation. Think of the English word aesthetics, meaning that which we perceive or sense. **an-** is a form of the prefix **a-**. **an-** means without (e.g., anemia, lack of blood; anorexia, lack of appetite).

8.109

Recall that **a-** and **an-** are prefixes meaning without or lack of. Analyze the following words by dividing them into their word parts. Look up the meanings in your dictionary.
esthesiometer

esthesi/o/meter
es thēs' ē **om'** ə ter

_____/_____/_____

anesthesia

an/esthesi/a
an es **thēs'** ē ə

_____/_____/_____

anesthesiology

an/esthesi/o/logy
an es thēs' ē **ol'** o jē

_____/_____/_____/_____

anesthetist

an/esthet/ist
an **es'** the tist

_____/_____/_____

PROFESSIONAL PROFILE

Certified Registered Nurse Anesthetists (CRNAs) are advanced practice anesthesia nurses who safely administer *approximately 30 million anesthetics* to patients each year in the United States, according to the American Association of Nurse Anesthetists (AANA). They provide anesthesia in collaboration with surgeons, anesthesiologists (MD or DO specialists), dentists, podiatrists, and other qualified healthcare professionals. CRNAs earn a Bachelor of Science Degree in Nursing and a Master's Degree from an accredited CRNA educational program and maintain a license to practice.

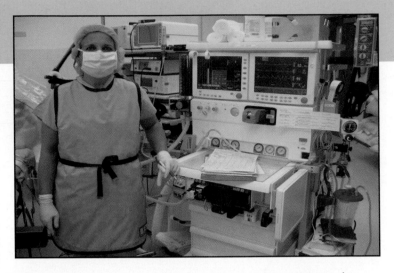

Certified Registered Nurse Anesthetist (CRNA) *Photo by Timothy J. Dennerll, RT(R), Ph.D.*

ANSWER COLUMN

	8.110
	Build words that mean without or lack of sensation
anesthesia	_____ ;
	a person who administers anesthetic agents
anesthetist	_____ ;
	a physician specialist in anesthesia
anesthesiologist	_____ .
	8.111
	Novocaine is used to remove sensation in a specific area. It is a local
an/esthet/ic an es **the'** tik	_____/_____/_____ .
	8.112
	Think of the meaning as you analyze the following words. dysesthesia
dys/esthesi/a dis es **thēs'** ē ə	_____/_____/_____
	hypoesthesia
hypo/esthesi/a hī' pō es **thēs'** ē ə	_____/_____/_____

ANSWER COLUMN

8.113

Alges/ia is a noun meaning oversensitivity to pain. Hyper/esthesi/a is a synonym for algesia. Algesia means

oversensitivity to pain or
hyperesthesia

* _____

_____ .

8.114

Use the word root alges to build words meaning
instrument used to measure pain

alges/i/meter
al jē **səm'** et er

_____/_____/_____ ;

pertaining to pain (adjective)

alges/ic
al **jēs'** ik

_____/_____ ;

condition without pain (noun)

an/alges/ia
an al **jēs'** ē ə

_____/_____/_____ .

8.115

**DICTIONARY
EXERCISE**

Look up the following words in your medical dictionary and write their meanings below.

analgesia

without pain

* _____

paralgesia

abnormal pain

* _____

paralgia

abnormal pain

* _____

paraplegia

paralysis of the lower body

* _____

8.116

para- is a Greek prefix that means beside, beyond, near, abnormal. Para/nephr/itis means

inflammation near
the kidney

* _____ .

Para/hepat/itis means

inflammation near
the liver

* _____ .

Para/medic means

works beside a physician
assisting in rescue
operation—EMT with
advanced training

* _____

_____ .

ANSWER COLUMN

8.117

Using the prefix **para-**, build terms that mean

inflammation near the kidney

para/nephr/itis
par' ə nef **rī'** tis

_____/_____/_____;

inflammation near the fallopian tubes

para/salping/itis
par' ə sal pin **jī'** tis

_____/_____/_____;

inflammation near the liver

para/hepat/itis
par' ə hep a **tī'** tis

_____/_____/_____;

disease near a bone and joint

para/oste/o/arthr/o/pathy
par' ə os' tē ō är **throp'**
ə thē

_____/_____/_____/_____/_____/_____.

8.118

Paralysis is a loss of muscle function and sensation. Para/plegia is

para/lysis
par **al'** ə sis

_____/_____ of the lower body.

8.119

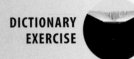

**DICTIONARY
EXERCISE**

Look up the following terms that begin with **par/a-** and write their meaning below.

partially paralyzed
(lower body)

delusions of persecution

part of the autonomic
nervous system

abnormal touch sensation

para/plegia _____

para/noid _____

para/sympathetic _____

par/esthesia _____

8.120

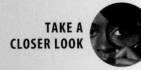

**TAKE A
CLOSER LOOK**

The autonomic nervous system (ANS) is the functional organization of the nervous system that responds during stress. The sym/path/etic nerves send signals to prepare the body for fight or flight when danger is either near or perceived. The para/sym/path/etic nerves return the body to its normal resting state.

8.121

Imagine that a person is driving and the car begins to slide out of control after hitting an ice patch. The person's eyes dilate, the heart and respiration rates increase, and epinephrine is released from the adrenal glands. This response to danger is brought on by the

sym/path/etic
sim pa **the'** tik

_____/_____/_____ nerves of the autonomic

nervous system.

(continued)

ANSWER COLUMN

After the danger has passed, the

para/sym/path/etic
par' ə sim pa **the'** tik

_____/_____/_____/_____

nerves return the body to a resting state.

8.122

INFORMATION FRAME

Paroxysmos is a Greek word meaning an irritation. A symptom that comes upon someone suddenly, for example difficulty breathing in the middle of the night, is called a paroxysm. Paroxysmal nocturnal dyspnea (PND) is the sudden onset of shortness of breath (SOB) at night.

8.123

paroxysm/al
par oks **iz'** mal

Waking in the middle of the night with difficulty breathing is called

_____/_____ nocturnal dyspnea.

Use the following combining forms and suffixes in Frames 8.124–8.134.

Combining Form	Meaning	Suffix
my/o	muscle	**-graph** (instrument for recording)
		-gram (record, picture)
		-algia (pain)
		-logy (study of)
kinesi/o	movement	**-oma** (tumor)
rhabd/o	rod shaped	**-pathy** (disease)
lip/o	fat	
fibr/o	fibrous	

8.124

muscles

Myon is a Greek word meaning muscle. Myocarditis means inflammation of the heart muscle. **my/o** is used in words referring to the _____.

8.125

INFORMATION FRAME

There are three main types of muscle found throughout the body. Study the table on page 317 to discover each type, its location, and main function.

8.126

myogram

myograph

myography

The words my/o/gram, my/o/graph, and my/o/graphy mean

_____ the tracing

_____ the instrument

_____ the process

8.127

muscles

My/asthenia gravis is a condition of the _____.

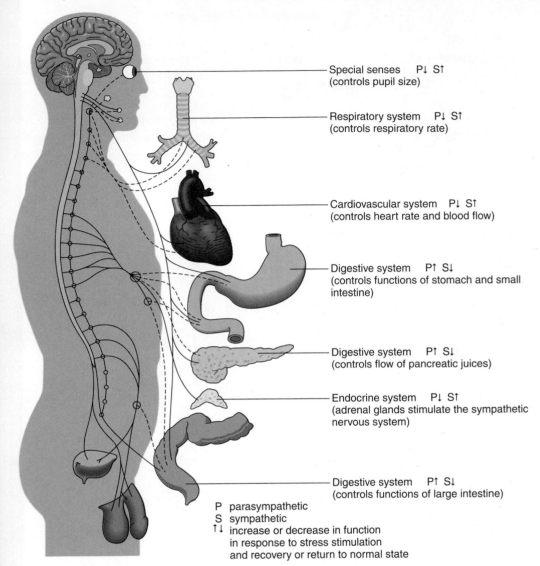

Special senses   P↓ S↑
(controls pupil size)

Respiratory system   P↓ S↑
(controls respiratory rate)

Cardiovascular system   P↓ S↑
(controls heart rate and blood flow)

Digestive system   P↑ S↓
(controls functions of stomach and small
intestine)

Digestive system   P↑ S↓
(controls flow of pancreatic juices)

Endocrine system   P↓ S↑
(adrenal glands stimulate the sympathetic
nervous system)

Digestive system   P↑ S↓
(controls functions of large intestine)

P parasympathetic
S sympathetic
↑↓ increase or decrease in function
in response to stress stimulation
and recovery or return to normal state

The autonomic nervous system controls the involuntary actions of the body
Delmar/Cengage Learning

8.128

my/o/fibr/oma
mī ō fib **rō′** mə
muscle

Using **my/o**, **fibr/o**, and **-oma**, build a term meaning a fibrous muscle tumor:

_____/_____/_____/_____. This is also

called a leiomy/oma uteri or fibroid tumor of the uterine _____
or my/o/metr/ium.

Muscle Type	Location	Function
striated (skeletal, voluntary) **rhabd/o/my/o**	covers skeleton Example: rhabdomyosarcoma	skeletal movement
smooth (visceral, involuntary) **leiomy/o**	organs, vessels Example: leiomyofibroma	movement of liquids, gases, and solids
cardiac **myocardi/o**	heart Example: myocardiopathy	maintain heartbeat

ANSWER COLUMN

8.129

Build words meaning
resembling muscle

my/oid
mī′ oid

_____/_____;

muscle tumor containing fatty elements

my/o/lip/oma
mī ō lip **ō′** mə

_____/_____/_____/_____;

muscle disease

my/o/pathy
mī **op′** ath ē

_____/_____/_____;

cardi/o/my/o/pathy   _or_
kär′ dē ō mi **op′** ə thē

heart muscle disease

my/o/cardi/o/pathy
mī′ ō kär dē **op′** ə thē

_____/_____/_____/_____/_____.

8.130

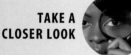

**TAKE A
CLOSER LOOK**

Look up words beginning with **my/o** in your dictionary. Count how many of the words you know. Write the number here:

more than 60

* _____

8.131

muscles

When you see **my/o**, you will think of _____.
When you see **leiomy/o**, you will think of

smooth muscle

* _____

When you see **myocardi/o**, you will think of

heart muscle

* _____

8.132

rhabd/o is a Greek combining form that means rod-shaped. It is used in names of rod-shaped parasites, such as the nematode worm _Rhabditoidea_. If you see the

rod-shaped

combining form **rhabd/o**, think of _____.

8.133

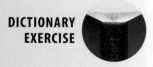

**DICTIONARY
EXERCISE**

A **blast** is an immature or stem cell. A my/o/blast is an immature muscle cell. A rhabd/o/my/o/blast is an abnormal rod-shaped muscle stem cell that may lead to the development of sarcoma. Use your dictionary to look up the following terms and write the definition below:
rhabdomyoma (rab′ do mi **o′** mə)

_____;

rhabdomyosarcoma (rab′ do mi′ o sar **ko′** mə)

_____

That's great. Your skills are building working with complex terms.

ANSWER COLUMN

SPELL CHECK

8.134

Notice the unusual spelling of the combining form **rhabd/o**. You may recall this "rh" blend is common in Greek origin words. The "h" is silent, but don't forget to put it in. Review the following terms with "rh" in their spelling:
rhabdomyoma
rhythm
rhino**rrh**ea
phlebo**rrh**agia
angio**rrh**exis
arterio**rrh**aphy

8.135

Electr/o/my/o/graphy (EMG) uses both surface and needle electrodes for recording muscle activity.
Electr/o/neur/o/my/o/graphy is a similar diagnostic tool that measures nerve function. Nerve and muscle function is assessed to confirm the need for carpal tunnel repair surgery.

electr/o/neur/o/my/o/
   graphy
ē lek′ trō no͞o rō mī **og′** ra fē

_____/_____/_____/_____/_____/_____/_____

is performed.

8.136

A test that creates an image of muscle function using electricity is

electr/o/my/o/graphy
ē lec′ trō mī **og′** ra fē

_____/_____/_____/_____/_____.

8.137

The main function of muscles is movement. **kinesi/o** is used in words to mean movement or motion. Brady/kinesi/a means

slowness of movement

* _____.

8.138

pain on movement or
   movement pain

Kinesi/algia means * _____.

8.139

Kinesi/algia occurs when you have to move any sore or injured part of the body.

kinesi/algia
ki nē′ sē **al′** jē ə

Moving a broken arm causes _____/_____.

8.140

After one's first ride on horseback, almost any movement causes

kinesialgia

_____.

Types of muscle tissue:
(A) skeletal muscle;
(B) smooth muscle;
(C) cardiac muscle
Delmar/Cengage Learning

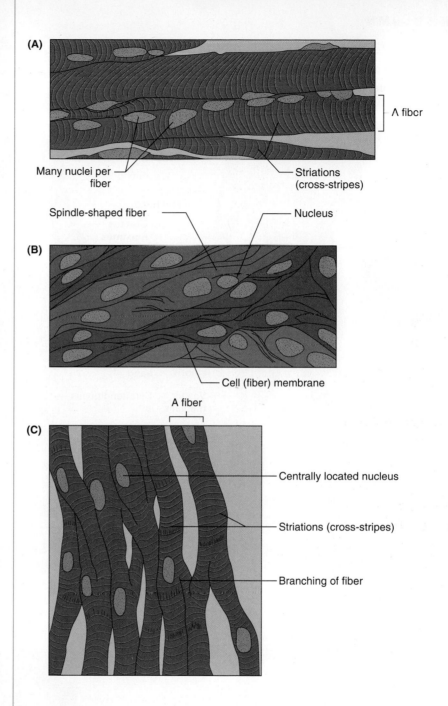

(A)

Many nuclei per fiber

A fiber

Striations (cross-stripes)

Spindle-shaped fiber

Nucleus

(B)

Cell (fiber) membrane

A fiber

(C)

Centrally located nucleus

Striations (cross-stripes)

Branching of fiber

8.141

kinesi/o/logy
ki nē′ sē **ol′** ə jē

-logy is used like a suffix to mean study of. (Remember **-logist**?) The study of muscular body movements is _____/_____/_____.

8.142

kinesiology

Kinesi/o/logy is the study of movement. The study of muscular movement during exercise would be done in the field of _____.

ANSWER COLUMN

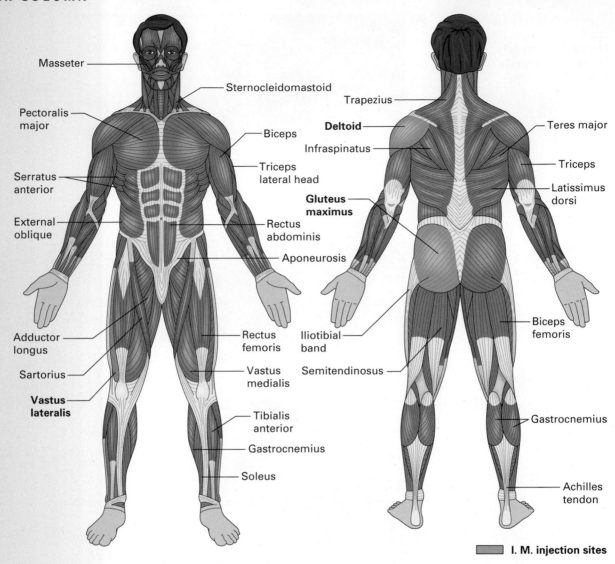

Anterior and posterior views of the muscles *Delmar/Cengage Learning*

Labels (anterior view):
- Masseter
- Pectoralis major
- Serratus anterior
- External oblique
- Adductor longus
- Sartorius
- **Vastus lateralis**
- Sternocleidomastoid
- Biceps
- Triceps lateral head
- Rectus abdominis
- Aponeurosis
- Rectus femoris
- Vastus medialis
- Tibialis anterior
- Gastrocnemius
- Soleus

Labels (posterior view):
- Trapezius
- **Deltoid**
- Infraspinatus
- **Gluteus maximus**
- Iliotibial band
- Semitendinosus
- Teres major
- Triceps
- Latissimus dorsi
- Biceps femoris
- Gastrocnemius
- Achilles tendon

I. M. injection sites

PROFESSIONAL PROFILE

Physical therapists (PTs) assess, prevent, and treat movement dysfunction and physical disabilities by using technological interventions as well as personal contact. In addition to patient care, the physical therapist may consult, supervise, administer, research, and provide community service through private practice or employment within an inpatient facility or clinic. **Physical therapy assistants** are supervised by the physical therapist and may administer physical therapy treatments as well as help with record keeping, billing, and reception. There are several professional organizations involved with education and credentialing of physical therapists. They include the American Association of Rehabilitation Therapy (AART), the American Physical Therapy Association (APTA), and the American Congress of Physical Medicine and Rehabilitation (ACPMR).

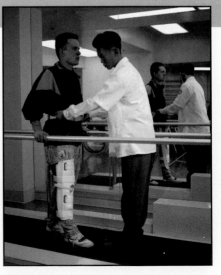

Physical therapist *Delmar/Cengage Learning*

ANSWER COLUMN

8.143

An exercise physiologist studies the science of how the body moves, called

kinesiology

_____ .

8.144

Recall **brady-** is the prefix for slow. Slowness of movement is

brady/kinesia

brād' i ki **nē'** sē ə   _or_

brād' ē ki **nē'** sē ə

called _____/_____ .

Abbreviation	Meaning
AANA	American Association of Nurse Anesthetists
AART	American Association of Rehabilitation Therapy
ACPMR	American Congress of Physical Medicine and Rehabilitation
ADL	activities of daily living
AOD	arterial occlusive disease
ANS	autonomic nervous system
APTA	American Physical Therapy Association
AS	arteriosclerosis
ASCVD	arteriosclerotic cardiovascular disease
ASHD	arteriosclerotic heart disease
C1–C8	cervical spinal nerve pairs
CABG	coronary artery bypass graft
CAD	coronary artery disease
CNS	central nervous system
CRNA	Certified Registered Nurse Anesthetist
C-section	cesarean section
EMG	electromyogram
HA	headache, hearing aid
Hct	hematocrit
HDL	high-density lipoproteins
Hgb	hemoglobin
IV	intravenous
L1–L5	lumbar spinal nerve pairs
MD	muscular dystrophy, medical doctor
MFT	muscle function test
MI	myocardial infarction
MS	multiple sclerosis, morphine sulfate
NVS	neurologic vital signs
OCD	obsessive-compulsive disorder
PND	paroxysmal nocturnal dyspnea, postnasal drip
PNS	peripheral nervous system
pro time, pt	prothrombin time
PT	physical therapy (therapist)
RPh	Registered Pharmacist

(continued)

ANSWER COLUMN

Abbreviation	Meaning
ROM	range of motion
S1–S5	sacral spinal nerve pairs
SOB	shortness (short) of breath
T1–T12 (D1–D12)	thoracic spinal nerve pairs (dyspnea), same as dorsal spinal nerve pairs
TENS	transcutaneous electric nerve stimulation

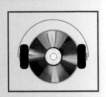

To complete your study of this unit, work the **Review Activities** on the following pages. Also, listen to the Audio CD that accompanies *Medical Terminology: A Programmed Systems Approach*, 10th Edition, and practice your pronunciation.

STUDYWARE™ CONNECTION

To help you learn the content in this chapter, take a practice quiz or play an interactive game on your **StudyWARE™ CD-ROM**.

REVIEW ACTIVITIES

CIRCLE AND CORRECT

Circle the correct answer for each question. Then, check your answers in Appendix E.

1. Suffix for surgical fixation
   a. -ptosis
   b. -plasty
   c. -pexy
   d. -ectasia

2. Combining form for vein
   a. phlebo
   b. ven
   c. venous
   d. thrombo

3. Suffix for rupture
   a. -ptosis
   b. -ectasis
   c. -rrhaphy
   d. -rrhexis

4. Suffix for most x-ray procedures
   a. -graphy
   b. -electric
   c. -Roentgen
   d. -graph

5. Prefix for without
   a. not-
   b. inter-
   c. an-
   d. dys-

6. Word root for oversensitivity to pain
   a. alges
   b. analgia
   c. esthesia
   d. algia

7. Prefix for abnormal, near, or beyond
   a. meta-
   b. para-
   c. ultra-
   d. ab-

8. Word root for movement
   a. my
   b. esthesi
   c. kinesi
   d. motor

9. Suffix for tumor
   a. -algia
   b. -itis
   c. -genic
   d. -oma

10. Combining form for hard
    a. cranio
    b. skullo
    c. osteo
    d. sclero

REVIEW ACTIVITIES

11. Word root for vessel
    - a. arterio
    - b. arter
    - c. angi
    - d. vesic

12. Suffix for destruction
    - a. -plasty
    - b. -rrhexis
    - c. -lysis
    - d. -malacia

13. Word root for blood clot
    - a. thromb
    - b. hem
    - c. hemat
    - d. embolism

14. Combining form for blood
    - a. hemato
    - b. penia
    - c. emia
    - d. thrombo

SELECT AND CONSTRUCT

Select the correct word parts from the following list and construct medical terms that represent the given meaning.

a	algeso(ic)	algia(esic)	an	analges/o
angio	arterio	ather/o	brady	cardio
dynia	dys	echo	ectasia	entero
esthesi/o(a)	fibr/o	gram	graph(y)	hepato
(c)ist	itis	kinesi/o(a)	logist	logy
meter	myo	neur/o	oma	osis
para	pathy	psych/o	pharm/o(a)	phlebo
plasty	plegia(ic)	rrhexis(ia)	sclero	scopy
spasm	tachy	thromb/o	tropic	veno

1. hardening of an artery _____

2. dilation of a vein _____

3. rupture of the intestine _____

4. x-ray of a vessel _____

5. instrument for measuring touch _____

6. physician specialist who prepares
   patients for painless surgery _____

7. pain-relieving medication (adjective) _____

8. inflammation near the liver _____

9. mental condition characterized by
   anxiety, phobias _____

10. instrument for measuring muscle function _____

11. difficult or painful movement _____

12. specialist in drug therapy _____

13. drugs that affect mental processes _____

14. paralysis of the lower body _____

15. fibrous and muscle tumor _____

16. large vessel hardening due to fatty streaks _____

REVIEW ACTIVITIES

17. repair of a vessel _____

18. condition of blood clots _____

19. abnormal muscle contraction _____

20. tumor of fiber and nerve _____

21. inflammation of vein caused by clots _____

22. specialist in nerve disorders _____

23. heart muscle disease _____

24. pertaining to heart muscle _____

DEFINE AND DISSECT

Give a brief definition and dissect each term listed into its word parts in the space provided. Check your answers by referring to the frame listed in parentheses and your medical dictionary. Then listen to the Audio CD to practice pronunciation.

1. neuroblast (8.4)

    _____ / _____ / _____
           rt   v   rt

   meaning _____

2. myelocele (8.24)

    _____ / _____ / _____
           rt   v   suffix

_____

3. arteriofibrosis (8.66)

    _____ / _____ / _____ / _____
       rt   v   rt   suffix

_____

4. hematolysis (8.73)

    _____ / _____ / _____
           rt   v   suffix

_____

5. thrombogenic (8.84)

    _____ / _____ / _____ / _____
       rt   v   rt   suffix

_____

6. occlusion (8.86)

    _____ / _____
           rt   suffix

_____

7. neurologist (8.9)

    _____ / _____ / _____
           rt   v   suffix

_____

REVIEW ACTIVITIES

8. myocardial (8.88)

_____/_____/_____/_____
rt   v   rt   suffix

9. hemangioma (8.72)

_____/_____/_____
rt   rt   suffix

10. phlebosclerosis (8.91)

_____/_____/_____/_____
rt   v   rt   suffix

11. arteriectasia (8.93)

_____/_____
rt   suffix

12. narcolepsy (8.60)

_____/_____/_____
rt   v   suffix

13. angioplasty (8.103)

_____/_____/_____
rt   v   suffix

14. phlebography (8.97)

_____/_____/_____
rt   v   suffix

15. anesthetist (8.109)

_____/_____/_____
pre   rt   suffix

16. dysesthesia (8.112)

_____/_____/_____
pre   rt   suffix

17. analgesia (8.114)

_____/_____/_____
pre   rt   suffix

18. paranephritis (8.116)

_____/_____/_____
pre   rt   suffix

REVIEW ACTIVITIES

19. paranoid (8.119)

                                                  _____ / _____
                                                        pre   suffix

_____

20. sympathetic (8.121)

_____ / _____ / _____
pre   rt   suffix

_____

21. cardiomyopathy (8.129)

_____ / _____ / _____ / _____ / _____
rt   v   rt   v   suffix

_____

22. myography (8.126)

_____ / _____ / _____
rt   v   suffix

_____

23. thrombophlebitis (8.82)

_____ / _____ / _____ / _____
rt   v   rt   suffix

_____

24. kinesiology (8.141)

_____ / _____ / _____
rt   v   suffix

_____

25. bradykinesia (8.137)

_____ / _____ / _____
pre   rt   suffix

_____

26. phlebotomy (8.94)

_____ / _____ / _____
rt   v   suffix

_____

27. anesthesiologist (8.110)

_____ / _____ / _____ / _____
pre   rt   v   suffix

_____

28. angioscopy (8.103)

_____ / _____ / _____
rt   v   suffix

_____

29. myofibroma (8.128)

_____ / _____ / _____ / _____
rt   v   rt   suffix

_____

30. paralysis (8.118)

_____ / _____
pre   suffix

_____

REVIEW ACTIVITIES

31. chondrodysplasia (8.29)

_____/_____/_____/_____
 rt   v   pre   suffix

_____

32. neurosurgeon (8.14)

_____/_____/_____/_____
 rt   v   rt   suffix

_____

33. paraplegia (8.119)

_____/_____
 pre   suffix

_____

34. endarterectomy (8.69)

_____/_____/_____
 pre   rt   suffix

_____

35. ischemia (8.85)

_____/_____
 rt   suffix

_____

36. infarction (8.88)

_____/_____/_____
 pre   rt   suffix

_____

37. paroxysmal (8.123)

_____/_____
 rt   suffix

_____

38. electroneuromyography (8.135)

_____/_____/_____/_____/_____/_____/_____
 rt   v   rt   v   rt   v   suffix

_____

39. psychoanalysis (8.33)

_____/_____/_____/_____
 rt   v   rt   suffix

_____

40. neurosis (8.45)

_____/_____
 rt   suffix

_____

41. rhabdomyoma (8.133)

_____/_____/_____/_____/_____
 rt   v   rt   v   suffix

_____

REVIEW ACTIVITIES

ABBREVIATION MATCHING

Match the following abbreviations with their definition.

_____ 1. CNS
_____ 2. MS
_____ 3. EMG
_____ 4. HA
_____ 5. AANA
_____ 6. ASHD
_____ 7. R.Ph
_____ 8. MFT
_____ 9. ROM
_____ 10. ADL

a. muscular dystrophy

b. milliamperes

c. arteriosclerotic heart disease

d. range of motion

e. arteriosclerotic cardiovascular disease

f. multiple fracture test

g. American Association of Nurse Anesthetists

h. electroencephalogram

i. American Association of Naturopaths

j. hearing aid

k. central nervous system

l. electromyogram

m. heartache

n. muscle function test

o. ad lib

p. Registered Pharmacist

q. above the elbow

r. activities of daily living

s. below the elbow, barium enema

t. multiple sclerosis

ABBREVIATION FILL-IN

Fill in the blanks with the correct abbreviations.

11. high-density lipoproteins _____

12. myocardial infarction _____

13. prothrombin time _____

14. coronary artery bypass graft _____

15. intravenous _____

16. hematocrit _____

17. muscular dystrophy _____

18. transcutaneous electrical nerve stimulation _____

19. paroxysmal nocturnal dyspnea _____

20. obsessive-compulsive disorder _____

REVIEW ACTIVITIES

CASE STUDY

Write the term next to its meaning given below. Then draw slashes to analyze the word parts. Note the use of medical abbreviations. Look these up in your dictionary or find them in Appendix B. If you have any questions about the answers, refer to your medical dictionary or check with your instructor for the answers in Appendix E.

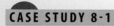
CASE STUDY 8-1

Summary

Pt: 83-year-old woman, Ht 5′2″, Wt 110, **BP** 104/60, **T** 98.9, **R** 20

Dx: 1. **Obsessive-compulsive disorder**

2. **Hypothyroidism**

3. **Incontinence**

This 83-year-old, single woman presented to the emergency room with complaints of anxiety, fear of impending death, panic, fatigue, and **diarrhea**. She has a history of hospitalization for obsessive-compulsive disorder between the ages of 35 and 55 when she was treated with **EST**, psychotropic medication, and psychotherapy. She was released to an adult foster care home where she lived for approximately 10 years, moving from home to home with difficulty conforming to house rules about bathroom privileges and having **paranoia**. She is currently living in an apartment. Although fully aware of her condition and advised of new treatments for **OCD**, she has refused medication and continues her daily routine of hand washing for as long as 30 minutes at a time several times a day. She explains that she is afraid people have entered her apartment and touched her bag of soaps and towels and that she had to throw it all away. She also states that the women in her building have tried to have her evicted because she looks so young for her age. She does not go out at night for fear of being raped. **Psychiatric** referral was ordered.

Physical examination reveals no significant abnormality, and she appears in remarkably good cardiovascular health. She states that she walks the equivalent of two miles a day from her apartment to the store or restaurant. The skin on her hands is thin, pink, and dry from hand washing. She does feel fatigued and has a history of hypothyroidism. She has taken no medication for several weeks since her prescription ran out. Rx 200 mcg Synthroid is recommended after lab results called. She has occasional accidents from incontinence and diarrhea. She was advised on the use of incontinence garments and will be assessed for **UTI**. Lab order: T3, T4, CBC, **Ua with C&S** if necessary, occult blood (OB) stool. Psychiatric consult ordered.

1. abnormally slow-acting thyroid

2. uncontrolled bowel movement or urination

3. pertaining to psychiatry

4. neurosis characterized by anxiety and ritual behavior

5. urinary tract infection

6. electroshock therapy

7. watery stool

8. blood pressure, temperature, respiration

9. urinalysis with culture and sensitivity

10. delusions of persecution and grandeur

REVIEW ACTIVITIES

CROSSWORD PUZZLE

Check your answers by going back through the frames or checking the solution in Appendix F.

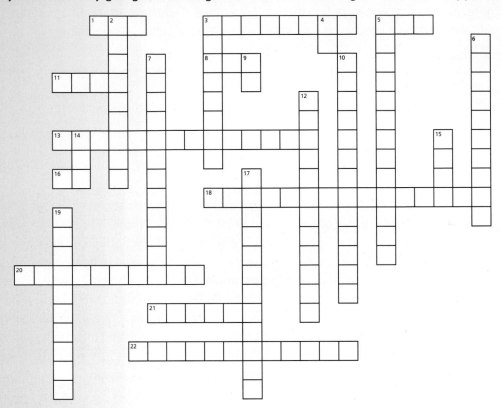

Across

1. obsessive-compulsive disorder (abbr.)
3. anxiety and phobia, nervous condition
5. high density lipoproteins (abbr.)
8. range of motion (abbr.)
11. combining form for vessel
13. study of producing loss of sensation for surgery
16. multiple sclerosis (abbr.)
18. condition; fatty deposits in large vessels, hardening
20. medication; produces loss of sensation
21. combining form for vein
22. pertaining to producing blood clots

Down

2. destruction of cells
3. medication; sleep-producing analgesic
4. intravenous (abbr.)
5. oversensitivity to touch
6. seizures of sleep
7. physician; treats mental disorders
9. myocardial infarction (abbr.)
10. dilation of an artery
12. medication; affects mental processes
14. neurologic vital signs (abbr.)
15. transcutaneous electric nerve stimulation (abbr.)
17. study of drugs
19. synonym for venipuncture

REVIEW ACTIVITIES

GLOSSARY

accept	include	atherectomy	excision of an atheroma or athermanous plaque from arteries
affect	influence or affect change	atheroma	fatty tissue tumor inside a large vessel
afferent	inflowing		
algesia	condition of pain sensitivity	atherosclerosis	fatty deposits on medium to large vessels, causing hardening
algesic	pertaining to algesia		
algesimeter	instrument for measuring level of pain	autonomic	self-controlling, stress response center of the nervous system
analgesia	condition without pain	cardiorrhexis	rupture of the heart
anesthesia	condition of no sensation	chondrodysplasia	defective development of cartilage
anesthesiology	science of studying the administration of anesthetics	cystorrhexis	rupture of the bladder
anesthetic	agent that produces loss of sensation	cytolysis	cell destruction
		dysesthesia	difficult or painful sensation
angiectasia	dilation of a vessel	effect	result
angioblast	immature vessel cell	efferent	outflowing
angiogram	x-ray of a vessel	electroneuromyography	process of making an image of nerve and muscle function using electricity
angiolysis	vessel destruction		
angioma	vessel tumor	enterorrhexis	rupture of the small intestine
angiopathy	vessel disease	esthesiometer	instrument used to measure the amount of sensation
angioplasty	surgical repair of a vessel		
angiorrhexis	rupture of a blood vessel	except	exclude
angiosclerosis	hardening of a vessel	fibroma	fibrous tumor
angioscopy	process of looking into a vessel using a scope	gastromalacia	softening of the stomach
		gastrospasm	stomach spasm
angiospasm	vessel spasm	hemangioblast	immature blood vessel cell
arteriectasia	dilation of an artery	hemarthrosis	blood in a joint
arteriofibrosis	condition of fibrous growth in the arteries	hematocrit	measurement of percent blood formed elements
arteriomalacia	softening of the arteries	hematologist	physician specialist in blood disorders
arteriorrhexis	rupture of an artery		
arteriosclerosis	hardening of the arteries	hematology	specialty of studying the blood
		hematolysis	destruction of blood (hemolysis)
arteriospasm	spasm of an artery	hematophobia	abnormal fear of blood

hepatorrhexis	rupture of the liver
hyperesthesia	oversensitivity to touch (may be painful)
hyperplasia	abnormal over growth of cells
hypoesthesia	below normal ability to feel (touch)
hysterorrhexis	rupture of the uterus
infarction	necrosis of tissue due to ischemia
ischemia	condition in which blood flow to tissues is temporarily slowed or stopped
lipolysis	lipid destruction
metrorrhexis	rupture of uterine tissues
myelocele	spinal cord herniation
myelocyte	bone marrow or spinal cord cell
myoblast	immature muscle cell
myocardial	pertaining to the heart muscle (myocardium)
myocarditis	inflammation of the myocardium
myofibroma	fibrous muscle tumor
myograph	instrument used to make a picture of muscle function
myography	the process of using a myograph to make a myogram
myolysis	muscle tissue destruction
myoma	muscle tumor
myopathy	muscle disease
myosclerosis	hardening of a muscle
myospasm	muscle spasm
narcolepsy	seizures of uncontrolled sleep
narcosis	condition of being affected by narcotics
narcotic	analgesic and sleep-producing drug
neuroblast	immature nerve cell

neurologist	physician specialist in nervous system disorders
neurolysis	nerve destruction
neuroma	nerve tumor
neuropathy	nerve disease
neurosis	nerve condition characterized by anxiety and phobias
neurospasm	nerve spasm
neurosurgeon	physician specialist who performs surgery on the brain and nerves
neurotripsy	surgical crushing of a nerve
parahepatitis	inflammation near the liver
paralgesia	pain in the lower body
paralgia	abnormal pain
paralysis	loss of muscle function and sensation
paramedic	emergency medical technician with advanced training
paranephritis	inflammation near the kidney
paraosteoarthropathy	disease near the bone and joint
paraplegia	paralysis in the lower body
parasympathetic	nerves that return the body to normal following stress
paroxysmal	pertaining to the sudden onset of an attack, symptoms, or emotion
pharmacist	specialist in drug therapy and dispensing drugs
pharmacology	study of drug therapy
phlebectasia	dilation of a vein
phlebectomy	excision of a vein
phlebography	process of taking an x-ray of a vein
phlebopexy	fixation of a prolapsed vein
phleboplasty	surgical repair of a vein
phleborrhexis	rupture of a vein

REVIEW ACTIVITIES

phlebosclerosis	hardening of a vein
phlebotomy	venipuncture
psychiatrist	physician specialist in treatment of mental disorders
psychoanalysis	analysis of mental and emotional state for treatment
psychology	study of the mind and mental processes
psychomotor	mental processes that control movement
psychosexual	mental processes related to sexuality
psychotherapy	therapy for mental disorders
psychotropic	agent that affects mental processes
thrombectomy	excision of a clot

thromboangiitis	blood clot in a vessel causing inflammation
thrombocyte	blood clotting cell (platelet)
thrombocytopenia	lack of platelets
thrombogenic	pertaining to producing clots
thromboid	resembling a clot
thrombolymphangitis	inflammation of a lymph vessel caused by a clot
thrombolysis	clot destruction
thrombophlebitis	inflammation of a vein caused by a clot (thrombus)
thrombosis	condition of forming clots
venipuncture	incision into a vein with a needle to remove a venous blood sample (synonym, phlebotomy)
venous	pertaining to veins

UNIT 9

Anatomic Terms

9.1

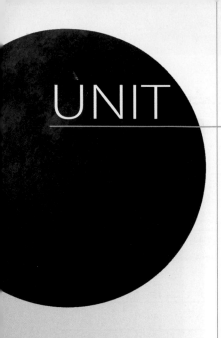

WORD ORIGINS

Ana/tomy comes from the Greek word *anatome* meaning cutting apart. Galen (A.D. 129–199), one of the earliest respected anatomists of the Western world, relied on animal experiments and dissecting corpses to identify and name body parts. As did many scholars of his day, he spoke and wrote in Greek and Latin. Those who followed him continued the creation of the anatomic and medical language that was later converted to English. You will notice that many anatomic terms have both Greek and Latin forms. The study of naming body structures is _____/_____ .

ana/tomy
a **na'** tō mē

9.2

Study the following table of new anatomic word parts. These will be used to build terms throughout this unit.

Directional Word	Combining Form	Meaning
dorsal	**dors/o**	near or on the back
ventral	**ventr/o**	near or on the belly side of the body
anterior (ant)	**anter/o**	toward the front or in front of
posterior (post)	**poster/o**	following or located behind
cephalic	**cephal/o**	upward, toward the head
caudal, caudad	**caud/o**	downward, toward the tail
medial	**medi/o**	toward the midline

(continued)

ANSWER COLUMN

Directional Word	Combining Form	Meaning
lateral	**later/o**	toward the side, away from the midline
superior	**super/o**	above
inferior	**infer/o**	below
proximal	**proxim/o**	near the point of origin
distal	**dist/o**	away from the point of origin
sagittal	**sagitt/o**	vertical, anteroposterior direction or plane dividing into left and right
coronal	**coron/o**	resembling a crown or encircling

Directions and planes of the body in anatomic position

Delmar/Cengage Learning

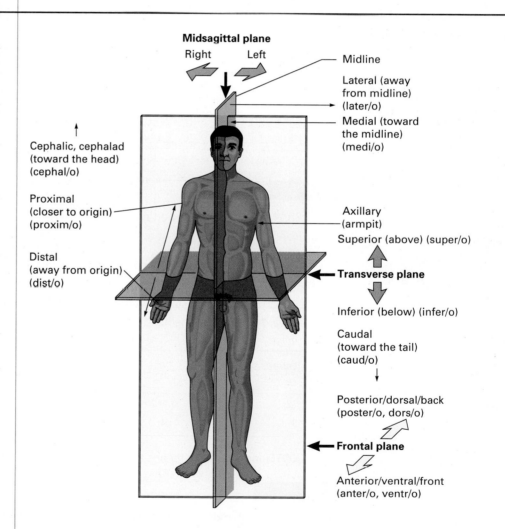

Midsagittal plane

Right   Left

Midline

Lateral (away from midline) (later/o)

Medial (toward the midline) (medi/o)

Cephalic, cephalad (toward the head) (cephal/o)

Proximal (closer to origin) (proxim/o)

Axillary (armpit)

Superior (above) (super/o)

Distal (away from origin) (dist/o)

Transverse plane

Inferior (below) (infer/o)

Caudal (toward the tail) (caud/o)

Posterior/dorsal/back (poster/o, dors/o)

Frontal plane

Anterior/ventral/front (anter/o, ventr/o)

9.3

The combining forms for anterior and posterior do not include the i. They are **anter/o** and **poster/o**. Using the information about directional terms in the table, build terms that mean pertaining to the

front and side

anter/o/later/al
an ter ō **lat′** er əl

_____/_____/_____/_____;

front and middle

anter/o/medi/al
an ter ō **mēd′** ē əl

_____/_____/_____/_____;

front and top

anter/o/super/ior
an ter ō sup **ēr′** ē or

_____/_____/_____/_____.

9.4

Build terms that mean pertaining to the

back and side

poster/o/later/al
pōst′ er ō **lat′** er əl

_____/_____/_____/_____;

back and outside of the body (external)

poster/o/extern/al
pōst′ er ō eks **ter′** nəl

_____/_____/_____/_____;

back and inside of the body (internal)

poster/o/intern/al
pōst er ō in **ter′** nəl

_____/_____/_____/_____.

9.5

Build terms that mean pertaining to the

front and back (from front to back)

anter/o/poster/ior
an′ ter ō pōst **ēr′** ē or

_____/_____/_____/_____ (AP)

or

ventr/o/dors/al
vent rō **dor′** səl

_____/_____/_____/_____;

toward the back of the head

dors/o/cephal/ad
dor sō **sef′** əl ad

_____/_____/_____/_____;

toward the front

ventr/ad (ventral)
vent′ rad (**ven′** trəl)

_____/_____

or

anter/ior
an **tēr′** ē or

_____/_____.

NOTE: **-ad** as a suffix means toward.

9.6

Proximal (**proxim/o**) means closer to a designated point (like the origin of a muscle or limb), and distal (**dist/o**) means further from a designated point. Because the elbow is closer to the shoulder than the hand is, the elbow is

proxim/al
proks′ i məl
dist/al
dis′ təl

_____/_____ to the head. Because the ankle is further from

the hip than the knee, the ankle is _____/_____ to the knee.

ANSWER COLUMN

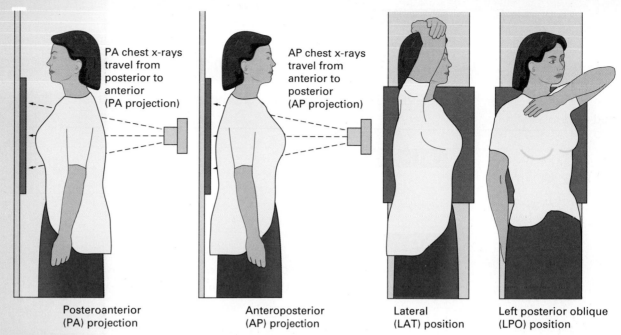

PA chest x-rays travel from posterior to anterior (PA projection)

AP chest x-rays travel from anterior to posterior (AP projection)

Posteroanterior (PA) projection

Anteroposterior (AP) projection

Lateral (LAT) position

Left posterior oblique (LPO) position

Radiographic projection positions *Delmar/Cengage Learning*

9.7

proximal

distal

A fracture in the upper part (closer to the hip) of the femur (thigh bone) is a fracture of the _____ end of the femur. A fracture in the lower part of the femur is a fracture of the _____ end.

9.8

distal

proximal

The bone in the tip of a finger (phalanx) is the _____ phalanx, because it is farther from the origin of the finger.

The phalanx close to the palm is the _____ phalanx.

9.9

middle and side

above and to the side

head to tail

After studying the table on pages 332 and 333 provide the meaning for the following terms

medi/o/later/al * _____ ;

super/o/later/al * _____ ;

cephal/o/caud/al * _____ .

STUDYWARE™ CONNECTION

View an animation on *Body Planes* on your **StudyWARE™ CD-ROM.**

ANSWER COLUMN

9.10

mid/sagitt/al
mid **saj**′ i təl

It is often necessary to look at anatomy by taking views of planes or slices of the body. This happens when using tomography and sonography. A sagittal cut is made in a vertical, anteroposterior direction. Such a cut made at the midline to divide the body into equal right and left halves is called the

_____/_____/_____ plane.

9.11

sagitt/al
saj′ i təl

Any vertical slice from front to back is a _____/_____ view.

9.12

axill/ary
ak′ si lair ē

The area under the fold of the arm, commonly known as the armpit, is the axilla or axill/ary region. A temperature taken under the arm is an

_____/_____ temperature and measures one degree Fahrenheit lower than an oral temperature.

9.13

mid/axill/ary
mid **ak**′ si lair ē

When performing an EKG one of the chest electrodes is placed in fifth intercostal space in line with the middle of the armpit, described as

_____/_____/_____.

9.14

WORD ORIGINS

In Latin *sagittalis* means arrowlike. The constellation and astrological sign Sagittarius is the shape of a mythological character, a Centaur, that is half man, half horse drawing a bow with a star for its arrow point. It is as if to say if struck with an arrow, a person would be cut into halves.

Electrocardiogram electrode placement
Delmar/Cengage Learning

Electro cardiogram electrode placement

Fourth intercostal space at right margin of sternum
Fourth intercostal space at left margin of sternum
Fifth intercostal space at junction of left midclavicular line
Midway between position 2 and position 4
At horizontal level of position 4 at left anterior axillary line
At horizontal level of position 4 at left midaxillary line

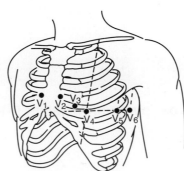

ANSWER COLUMN

9.15

The coron/al suture line of the skull sits at the crown of the skull. Coron/al comes from a Greek word root meaning crown or circle. The corona dentis is the

crown
circle (encircle)

_____ of a tooth. The coron/ary arteries _____ the heart to supply the muscle with blood.

9.16

coron/ary
kor' ən air ē
coron/ary

The arteries encircling the heart are the _____/_____ arteries.

The veins encircling the heart are the _____/_____ veins.

9.17

INFORMATION FRAME

To find a word root for navel, look up navel in the dictionary. A synonym for navel is the Latin word *umbilicus*. The Greek combining form **omphal/o** comes from *omphalos*.

9.18

omphal/itis
om fə lī' tis

Inflammation of the umbilicus is _____/_____.

9.19

In the dictionary, turn to words beginning with **omphal/o**. The combining form

omphal/o

for navel is _____/_____.

9.20

Using **omphal/o**, build words meaning
pertaining to the navel

omphal/ic
om **fal'** ik

_____/_____;
excision of the umbilicus

omphal/ectomy
om fə **lek'** tə mē

_____/_____;
herniation of the navel (umbilical hernia)

omphal/o/cele
om' fə lō sēl *or*
om **fal'** ō sēl

_____/_____/_____ or
_____/_____/_____

umbilic/o/cele
um bil' **i** kō sēl

9.21

Build words meaning
umbilical hemorrhage

omphal/o/rrhagia
om' fə lō **rāj'** ē ə

_____/_____/_____;

(continued)

ANSWER COLUMN

discharge flowing from the navel

omphal/o/rrhea
om′ fə lō **rē′** ə

_____/_____/_____ ;

rupture of the navel

omphal/o/rrhexis
om′ fə lō **reks′** is

_____/_____/_____ .

Good work!

9.22

navel

Words containing **omphal/o** refer to the _____, which is also called

umbilicus

the _____ .

9.23

ad- is used as a suffix meaning toward. Build words meaning
toward the head

cephal/ad
sef′ əl ad

_____/_____ and

toward the tail (lower spine)

caud/ad
kaw′ dad

_____/_____ .

9.24

Human development is usually in a head-to-body (tail) direction.
(The structures of the head develop first.) This is called

cephal/o/caud/al
sef′ əl ō **kaw′** dəl

_____/_____/_____/_____ development.

9.25

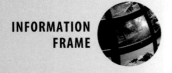

**INFORMATION
FRAME**

In your dictionary look at the words beginning with gnos. They come from the
Greek word meaning knowledge.

**Common terms for
body areas** *Delmar/Cengage
Learning*

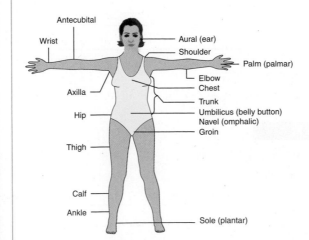

ANSWER COLUMN

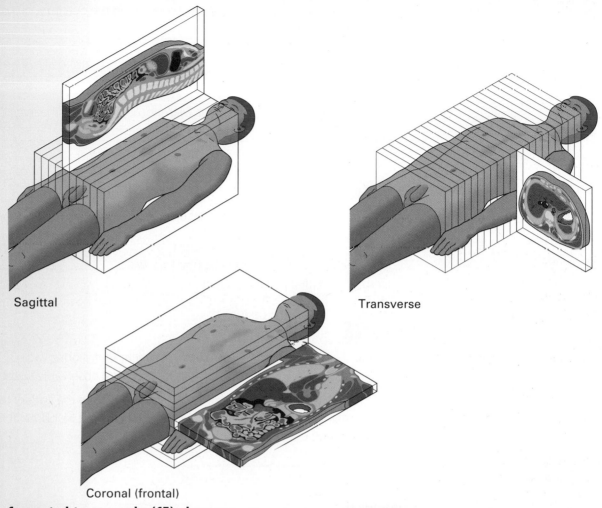

Sagittal

Transverse

Coronal (frontal)

Computed tomography (CT) planes *Delmar/Cengage Learning*

	9.26
knowledge	The words gnosia and gnosis are medical words built from the Greek word meaning _____.

	9.27
pro	**pro-** is a prefix meaning in front of; pro/gnos/is (P$_x$) means foreknowledge or predicting the outcome of a disease. The prefix that means before or in front of is _____.

	9.28
pro/gnos/is prog **nō'** sis	Leukemia is a serious disease associated with leukocytes. The _____/_____/_____ of acute leukemia is grave.

	9.29
pro/cephal/ic prō sə **fal'** ik	Procephalic means in the front of the head. Analyze procephalic _____/_____/_____.

(continued)

ANSWER COLUMN

pro/gnos/tic
prog **nos'** tik

Prognostic means giving an indication concerning the outcome of a disease.

Analyze prognostic: _____/_____/_____ .

9.30

knowing through or
know through

dia- means through or throughout. Dia/gnos/is (D$_x$) literally means

* _____

(identification of a disease through signs and symptoms).

9.31

dia/gnos/tic
dī ag **nos'** tik
dia/gnos/e
dī' ag nōs

Dia/gnos/tic is the adjectival form of diagnosis and dia/gnos/e is the verb.

When the results of the _____/_____/_____

(adjective) tests are complete, the physician will _____/_____/_____

(verb) the condition of the patient.

9.32

signs
sīnz'

sym/ptom/s
simp' təmz

A **sign** is objective information about the patient that is observable.
Skin color changes, lab tests, and measurements are observable so they

are _____. A **symptom** is subjective because the patient tells you
how he feels or what he has experienced, but it may not be observable. When a
patient complains of pain, nausea, or being tired, these are

_____/_____/_____ .

9.33

dia/gnos/is
dī əg **nō'** sis

A diagnosis (identification of a disease) is made by studying through its
symptoms. When a patient tells of having chills, hot spells, and a runny nose, the

physician may make the _____/_____/_____
of viral syndrome.

9.34

dia/gnos/is

dia/gnos/es
dī əg **nō'** sēs

Nurses observe patients for signs and symptoms of conditions that require
treatment. After careful observation, a nurse will summarize these findings by

writing a nursing _____/_____/_____ .

The International Classification of Diseases (ICD) lists and assigns code numbers

to thousands of _____ .

9.35

flowing through

The literal meaning of dia/rrhea (watery stool) is

* _____ .

ANSWER COLUMN

INFORMATION FRAME

9.36

Dia/lysis is the separation of substances in a solution.
Hem/o/dia/lysis removes waste from the blood by using an artificial kidney machine.

9.37

dia/lysis
dī **al′** i sis

Dialysis is a process of destroying waste products in the blood by diffusion through a membrane. People with kidney failure (ESRD, end-stage renal disease) may need _____/_____ to remove waste from their blood.

9.38

dialysis

Peritoneal dialysis and hemodialysis are two types of _____.

9.39

dia

A dia/scope is placed on the skin, and the skin is looked at *through* the instrument to see superficial surface lesions and other things. The word part for through is _____.

9.40

air

aer/o is used in words to mean air. You undoubtedly know the words aer/ial and aer/ialist. **aer/o** always makes you think of _____.

9.41

aer/o/phobia
air′ ō **fō′** bē ə

aer/o/therapy
air′ ō **thair′** ə pē

aer/o/cele
air′ ō sēl

Using what you need of **aer/o**, build words meaning
abnormal fear of air

_____/_____/_____;

treatment with air

_____/_____/_____;

herniation containing air

_____/_____/_____.

9.42

bi/o/logy
bī **o′** lə jē

Bios is the Greek word for life. Bi/o/chemistry is the study of chemical changes in living things. The science (study of) living things is _____/_____/_____.

9.43

living things or life

A bi/o/logist is one who studies

*_____.

living things

Bi/o/genesis is the formation of

*_____.

Peritoneal dialysis
Delmar/Cengage Learning

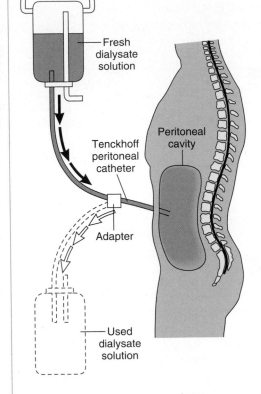

Fresh
dialysate
solution

Tenckhoff
peritoneal
catheter

Peritoneal
cavity

Adapter

Used
dialysate
solution

Hemodialysis
Delmar/Cengage Learning

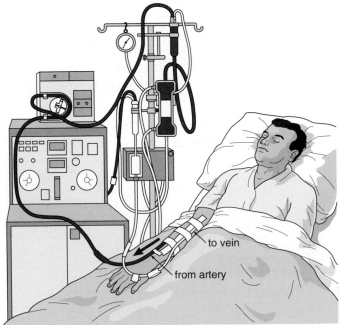

to vein

from artery

9.44

An an/aer/o/bic plant or animal cannot live in the presence of air (**an-**––without).
Analyze anaerobic:

an

prefix (without) _____ ;

aer/o

combining form (air) _____ / _____ ;

bic

suffix (life) _____ .

ANSWER COLUMN

Water aerobics is a type of exercise that is an excellent way to maintain cardiopulmonary fitness. It requires increased oxygen consumption, raises heart rate, improves lung capacity, and conditions muscles.
Photo by Timothy J. Dennerll, RT(R), Ph.D.

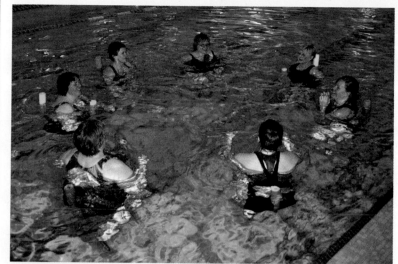

9.45

If anaerobic means existing without air (oxygen), build a word that means needing air (oxygen) to live (adjective);

aer/o/bic
air ō' bik

_____/_____/_____ .

9.46

Use aerobic or anaerobic in Frames 9.46–9.48.
The bacterium that causes pneumonia requires air to live. These bacteria are

aerobic

considered _____ bacteria.

9.47

The tetanus bacillus causes lockjaw. Lockjaw can develop only in closed wounds where air does not penetrate (e.g., stepping on an old nail). The tetanus bacillus

an/aer/o/bic
an air o' bik

is an _____/_____/_____/_____ bacterium.
Read about tetanus in your medical dictionary.

9.48

Botulism is a serious type of food poisoning. It occurs from eating improperly canned meats and vegetables. Cans do not admit air. The bacillus that causes

anaerobic

botulism is _____ .

9.49

A bi/o/psy is an excision of tissue for examination of

living or live

* _____ tissue.

9.50

A combining form that means color is **chrom/o**. The Greek word for a color is *chroma*. There are English words chroma and chrome. **chrom/o** makes you think

color

of _____ .

*Neisseria gonorrhoeae
in symovial fluid
(gram-negative
intracellular diplococci)*
Delmar/Cengage Learning

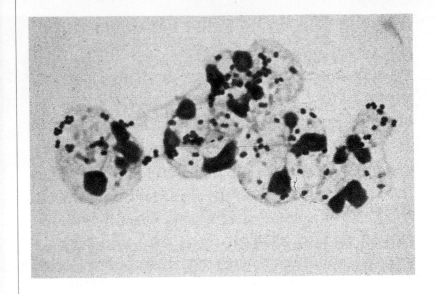

9.51

A chrom/o/cyte is any colored cell. An embryonic color (pigment) cell is called a

_____/_____/_____.

chrom/o/blast
krō′ mō blast

9.52

Build words meaning
destruction of color (in a cell)

_____/_____/_____;

formation of pigment (color)

_____/_____/_____/_____;

instrument for measuring amount of color in a substance

_____/_____/_____.

(chromat/o/graph)

chrom/o/lysis
krō **mol′** ə sis

chrom/o/gen/esis
krō′ mō **jen′** ə sis

chrom/o/meter
krō **mom′** ə ter

9.53

phil is a word root meaning attracted to or loves. A chrom/o/philic cell is one
that takes a stain easily (attracts stain). Some leukocytes stain deeper than others.

They are more _____/_____/_____ than the less easily
stained leukocytes.

chrom/o/philic
krō′ mō **fil′** ik

9.54

Some cells are chrom/o/phobic and will not stain at all. They are not

_____.

EXAMPLE: Gram-negative bacteria will not attract color from the Gram stain.

chromophilic

ANSWER COLUMN

9.55

staining easily

Chromophilic means * _____ .

The word that means something does not (without) stain easily is

a/chrom/o/philic
ā' krō mō **fil**' ik

_____/_____/_____/_____ .

9.56

abnormal, bad, painful, or
difficult

well or easy

dys- means * _____ .

The opposite of **dys-** is **eu-**, which means

* _____ .

9.57

Form the word that means the opposite of
dys/pepsia

eu/pepsia
yōō **pep**' sē ə

_____/_____ ;

dys/peptic

eu/peptic
yōō **pep**' tik

_____/_____ ;

dys/pnea

eu/pnea
yōōp **nē**' ə or
yōōp' nē ə

_____/_____ .

9.58

Form the opposite of
dys/kinesi/a

eu/kinesi/a
yōō ki **nē**' zhə

_____/_____/_____ ;

dys/esthesi/a

eu/esthesi/a
yōō es **thē**' zhə

_____/_____/_____ ;

dys/phor/ia

eu/phor/ia
yōō **fôr**' ē ə

_____/_____/_____ .

9.59

easy or normal labor
and childbirth

-tocia is a suffix meaning labor. Dys/tocia (dis tō' shə) means difficult labor.
Eu/tocia (ū tō' shə) means

* _____ .

STUDYWARE™ CONNECTION

After completing this unit, you can play a hangman or other interactive game on your
StudyWARE™ CD-ROM that will help you learn the content in this chapter.

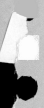

ANSWER COLUMN

9.60

If you work a frame and have forgotten what the word root means, look it up in your medical dictionary. Use this frame to take a breath and *say* the word, *listen* to it, *look* at it, *write* it, and *think* about it.

9.61

Thanatos is a Greek word meaning death. The word root for death is than. When someone has an easy or peaceful death, it is called

eu/than/asia
yōō tha **nā'** zhə

_____ / _____ / _____ .

euthanasia

Many ethical medical questions surround the subject of _____ .
If this interests you, you may want to learn about active and passive euthanasia.

9.62

Another area of ethics is the study of eu/gen/ics (good development). Researchers are working on ways to improve humans through genetic engineering. Look up eugenic in your dictionary and analyze the word parts

good

eu- _____ ;

form or produce

gen * _____ ;

adjective ending

-ic * _____ .

9.63

Eugenic sterilization is selective sterilization of individuals that society says have undesirable traits or would be unable to be good parents. One controversial topic of bi/o/ethics is whether severely mentally impaired adult patients may be

eu/gen/ic
yōō **jen'** ik

selected for _____ / _____ / _____ sterilization.

9.64

INFORMATION FRAME

Bi/o/ethics and medical ethics are topics that deal with decisions about life and medical treatments that concern right and wrong as seen by both society and individuals.

9.65

Euthanasia and eugenics are both controversial topics concerning

bi/o/ethics
bī ō **eth'** iks

_____ / _____ / _____ .

9.66

Recall that **enter/o** is the combining form for intestine. Infections of the intestine can be viral, bacterial, or parasitic and cause pain and diarrhea. This painful or difficult condition of the small intestine is

dys/enter/y
dis' en tair ē

called _____ / _____ / _____ .

(continued)

NOTE: **enter/o** is used more with words about the small intestine, and **col/o** is used for the large intestine.

	9.67
dysentery	Travelers are cautioned not to drink water in countries with poor sanitation systems to avoid contracting amebic _____.

	9.68
men/ses *or* **men'** sis men/struation men strōō ā' shun	**men/o** is used in words referring to the menses. In Latin *mensis* means month. Men/ses is another way of saying men/struation, which occurs in monthly cycles. **men/o** in any word should make you think of _____/_____.

	9.69
SPELL CHECK	Watch the spelling and pronunciation of menstruation. There is a "u" after the "str," and it is pronounced with a long "u" sound; men stru **a'** tion.

	9.70
men/o/rrhea men ō **rē'** ə dys/men/o/rrhea dis' men ō **rē'** ə	Men/arche (men ar' kē) comes from the Greek words *men* for month and *arche* for beginning. Menarche refers to a female's first menstrual period. Build words meaning flow of menses _____/_____/_____; painful (bad or difficult) menstrual flow _____/_____/_____/_____.

	9.71
menstruation or menses excessive menstruation or menstrual hemorrhage	Men/o/pause (men' ō paws) means permanent cessation of * _____. Men/o/rrhagia (men ō rā' jē ə) means * _____ _____.

	9.72
a/men/o/rrhea ā men ō **rē'** ə men/o/stasis mə **nos'** te sis	Build words meaning absence (without) menstrual flow _____/_____/_____/_____; stopping menstrual flow _____/_____/stasis_____.

ANSWER COLUMN

9.73

-**stasis** means the act or condition of stopping or controlling.

act of controlling
blood flow

Hem/o/stasis means * _____ .
A word meaning control of blood flow in veins is

phleb/o/stasis *or*
fli **bos'** tə sis
ven/o/stasis
vē **nos'** tə sis
arteri/o/stasis
är tir' ē **os'** tə sis
lymph/o/stasis
lim **fos'** tə sis

_____/_____/_____ .

Build words meaning
control of flow in arteries

_____/_____/_____ ;

control of lymph flow

_____/_____/_____ .

9.74

hem/o/stat
hēm' ō stat

A hem/o/stat is a instrument used in surgery to control blood flow by
clamping off an artery or vein. Hemostasis may be achieved by using

a _____/_____/_____ .

9.75

**SPELL
CHECK**

Take caution when using the terms hemostasis and homeostasis. There are just a
few letters difference but they are completely different words. Hem/o/stasis is
control of blood flow. Home/o/stasis is derived from the combining form home/o
from the Greek *homoios* meaning same and refers to the state of the internal
environment of the body staying in balance. If it helps, think of the thermostat
keeping your "home" at a set temperature. Write the correctly spelled term below
that means control of blood flow

hem/o/stasis

_____/_____/_____ ;

balance of body functions (staying the same)

home/o/stasis

_____/_____/_____ .

Hemostats *Courtesy of Miltex, Inc.*

Mosquito hemostatic forceps
(long)

Mosquito forceps tips

ANSWER COLUMN

INFORMATION FRAME

9.76

Medical terms ending in **-stasis** are formally pronounced as indicated in Frame 9.73. In practice and transcription you will probably hear the following instead

phlebostasis—flē bō **stā'** sis

venostasis—vē nō **stā'** sis

arteriostasis—är tir ē ō **stā'** sis

hemostasis—hē mō **stā'** sis

9.77

Syphilis is a sexually transmitted disease (STD). Read about the disease in your dictionary. Note the origin of the word. Look at the words beginning with syphil. The combining form used in words referring to this disease is

syphil/o   _____/_____ .

9.78

Using syphil, build terms that mean

mental condition caused by syphilis

syphil/o/psych/osis
sif' il ō sī **kō'** sis   _____/_____/_____/_____ ;

syphil/o/phobia   fear of contracting syphilis
sif' il ō **fōb'** ē ə
                                 _____/_____/_____ ;

syphil/o/therapy   therapy for syphilis
sif' il ō **ther'** a pē
                                 _____/_____/_____ .

9.79

Build words meaning

a syphilitic tumor

syphil/oma   _____/_____ ;
sif il ō' mə

                                 any syphilitic disease

syphil/o/pathy
sif il **op'** ə thē   _____/_____/_____ .

Syphilitic chancre
Delmar/Cengage Learning

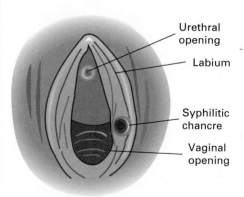

Urethral opening

Labium

Syphilitic chancre

Vaginal opening

ANSWER COLUMN

9.80

-cyesis comes from the Greek word *kyesis* meaning pregnancy. **pseudo-** means false. A pseud/o/cyesis (sōō dō sī ē' sis) or pseud/o/pregnancy is a false pregnancy. A pseud/o/science is a

false science

* _____ .

9.81

Pseud/o/mania is a psychosis in which patients have a false or pretended mental disorder. Pseud/o/paralysis means

false paralysis
(paralysis not due
   to nerve damage)

* _____ .

9.82

Build words meaning
a false cyst

pseud/o/cyst
sōō' dō sist

_____/_____/_____ ;

false edema

pseud/o/edema
sōō' ə dē' mə

_____/_____/_____ ;

false or imaginary sensation

pseud/o/esthesi/a
sōō' dō es thē' zhə

_____/_____/_____/_____ .

Look up and learn the meaning of edema.

9.83

Build words meaning
false hypertrophy

pseud/o/hyper/trophy

_____/_____/_____/_____ ;

false tuberculosis (TB)

pseud/o/tubercul/osis

_____/_____/_____/_____ ;

false nerve tumor

pseud/o/neur/oma
(You pronounce)

_____/_____/_____/_____ .

9.84

**SPELL
CHECK**

Words built with **pseud/o** often give students spelling and pronunciation problems. Remember, the *p* is silent and the *eu* has a long *u* sound.

9.85

The viscera (singular viscus) are the internal organs of the body. Viscer/ad means toward the viscera. Viscer/o/genic means development of organs. The combining

viscer/o

form for viscera is _____/_____ .

NOTE: Viscus is the singular for viscera. Viscous means having high viscosity or stickiness. They are both pronounced vis' kus.

ANSWER COLUMN

9.86

organs (internal)

In the words viscer/o/motor, viscer/o/pariet/al, and viscer/o/pleur/al, **viscer/o** refers to _____ .

9.87

periton/eum
per i tō **nē'** um

Locate the peritoneum on page 352. The membrane that lines the abdominal cavity is the _____/_____ .

9.88

pleur/al
plōōr' əl

Locate the pleura on page 352. The membrane that covers the lungs is the viscer/o _____/_____ membrane.

9.89

INFORMATION FRAME

pariet/o is the combining form for wall. Uses of visceral (vis' er **əl**) and parietal (pa **rī'** ətəl) include

visceral pleura	(membrane on the surface of the lung)
parietal pleura	(membrane on chest cavity wall)
visceral peritoneum	(membrane on the surface of the organs of the abdominal cavity)
parietal peritoneum	(membrane on the abdominal cavity wall)

9.90

viscer/al
vis' er əl

pariet/al
pa **rī'** ə təl

Name the membrane that covers the surface of the lungs

_____/_____ pleura;

is on the thoracic cavity wall

_____/_____ pleura.

9.91

viscer/o/ptosis
vis' ər op **tō'** sis

viscer/algia
vis' ər al' jē ə

viscer/al
vis' ər əl

Build words meaning
prolapse of organs

_____/_____/_____ ;

pain in organs

_____/_____ ;

pertaining to organs

_____/_____ .

Ventral cavity membrances *Delmar/Cengage Learning*

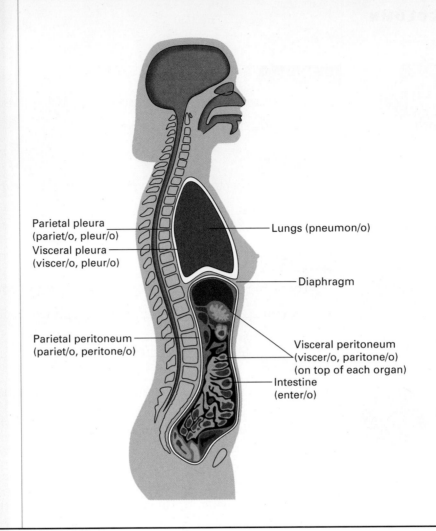

Parietal pleura
(pariet/o, pleur/o)

Visceral pleura
(viscer/o, pleur/o)

Lungs (pneumon/o)

Diaphragm

Parietal peritoneum
(pariet/o, peritone/o)

Visceral peritoneum
(viscer/o, paritone/o)
(on top of each organ)

Intestine
(enter/o)

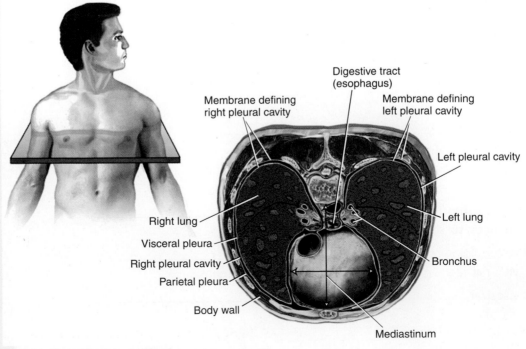

Membrane defining
right pleural cavity

Digestive tract
(esophagus)

Membrane defining
left pleural cavity

Left pleural cavity

Right lung

Left lung

Visceral pleura

Bronchus

Right pleural cavity

Parietal pleura

Body wall

Mediastinum

Thorax (transverse section) *Delmar/Cengage Learning*

ANSWER COLUMN

viscer/o/sensor/y vis′ er ō **sens′** ôr ē	
viscer/o/skelet/al vis′ er ō **skel′** e tal	
viscer/o/gen/ic vis′ er ō **jen′** ik	

9.92

Build words beginning with **viscer/o** that mean
sensory function of organs

_____/_____/_____/_____;

pertaining to organs and the skeleton

_____/_____/_____/_____;

pertaining to the development of organs

_____/_____/_____/_____.

The following table is for use in building words for Frames 9.93–9.125.

Prefix of Location	Meaning
ecto-	outer-outside
endo-	inner-inside
meso-	middle
retro-	backward-behind
para-	near

9.93

| endo/derm
en′ dō dûrm | The blast/o/derm is an embryonic disk of cells that gives rise to the three main layers of tissue in humans. The outer germ layer is called the ecto/derm. The inner germ layer is called the _____/_____. |

9.94

| meso/derm
mez′ ō dûrm | Between the ectoderm and endoderm is a middle germ layer called the _____/_____. |

9.95

| ecto/derm
ek′ tō dûrm | The ectoderm forms the skin. The nervous system arises from the same layer as the skin. This layer is the _____/_____. |

9.96

| ectoderm | Sense organs and some glands are also formed from the _____. |

9.97

| endoderm | The endo/derm forms organs inside the body. The stomach and small intestine arise from the _____. |

ANSWER COLUMN

9.98

The mesoderm forms the organs that arise between the ectoderm and

mesoderm

endoderm. Muscles are formed by the _____.

9.99

The blastoderm gives rise to the three germ layers. They are

ectoderm

outer _____;

mesoderm

middle _____;

endoderm

inner _____.

9.100

ecto- is a Latin prefix for outside. **exo-** is a Greek prefix for outside. Something

produced within an organism is said to be endo/gen/ous. Something produced

ecto/gen/ous

outside an organism is _____/_____/_____

ek **toj'** ə nəs

or

exo/gen/ous

_____/_____/_____ .

eks **oj'** ə nəs

9.101

Type 1 diabetics produce very little endogenous insulin. Therefore, they must take

ectogenous or exogenous

_____ (from an outside source) insulin.

9.102

People with type 1 diabetes have hyperglycemia and no insulin to carry the

glucose into the cells. Therefore they exhibit the three *P*s as classic symptoms.

Recall the prefix **poly-** and build words that represent these symptoms:

poly/ur/ia

excessive urination _____/_____/_____;

poly/dips/ia

excessive thirst _____/_____/_____;

poly/phag/ia

excessive hunger _____/_____/_____ .

9.103

Ecto/cyt/ic is an adjective meaning outside a cell. An adjective meaning inside a

endo/cyst/ic

bladder is _____/_____/_____ .

en' dō **sis'** tik

STUDY **WARE**™ C O N N E C T I O N

After completing this unit, you can play a Spelling Bee game to help you learn the pronunciation
of terms presented in the chapter or play other interactive games on your **StudyWARE**™ **CD-ROM**
that will help you learn the content in this chapter.

ANSWER COLUMN

9.104

-**plasm** is used as a suffix in words about the substance of cells (cyt/o/plasm). **proto-** means first. Think of prot/o/type. Prot/o/plasm is the substance of life. The protoplasm that forms the outer membrane of the cell is called

ecto/plasm
endo/plasm   *or*
cyt/o/plasm
(You pronounce)

_____/_____ . The protoplasm within the cell is called

_____/_____/_____ .

9.105

Endo/crani/al is an adjective meaning within the cranium. An adjective meaning

endo/chondr/al
en' dō **kon'** drəl

within cartilage is _____/_____/_____ .

9.106

Endo/enter/itis means inflammation of the lining of the small intestine.
Build words meaning
pertaining to the lining of the heart (adjective)

endo/cardi/al   *or*
endo/cardi/ac

_____/_____/_____;
inflammation of the lining of the colon

endo/col/itis
(You pronounce)

_____/_____/_____.

9.107

An endo/scope is an instrument used to look into a hollow organ or cavity of the body, as in viewing the stomach. The process of viewing the stomach through an

endo/scopy
en' **dos'** kō pē

instrument is called _____/_____
or

gastr/o/scopy
gas **tros'** kō pē

_____/_____/_____ .

9.108

endoscopy

Esophag/o/gastr/o/duoden/o/scopy (EGD) is one type of _____.

WORD BUILDING
■ ■ ■ ■ ■

ESOPHAG/O
combining form

+

GASTR/O
combining form

+

DUODEN/O
combining form

+

SCOPY
suffix

9.109

Using what you know about **endo-**, **arter**, and **-ectomy**, complete the definition of this term
end/arter/ectomy—removal of a substance (usually an atheroma) from the

inside

_____ of an artery.

ANSWER COLUMN

INFORMATION FRAME

9.110

Note the involved development of the word ectopic (out of place)
ect/o—outside
top/o—place (combining form)
-ic—adjectival suffix

9.111

An ectopic pregnancy occurs outside of the uterus (usually in a fallopian tube).
A salpingectomy may be required after the rupture of an

_____/_____/_____ pregnancy.

ec/top/ic
ek **top'** ik

9.112

If endometrial tissue occurs in the fallopian tubes, a fertilized egg can lodge in it,

thus causing pregnancy. This is an _____ pregnancy.

ectopic

9.113

An embryo's development in the abdominal cavity is another example of an

_____ pregnancy.

ectopic

9.114

meso- is a prefix for middle. Build words meaning peritoneum attaching intestine
to the abdominal wall (literally: middle intestine)

_____/_____/_____;
peritoneum attaching large intestine to the abdominal wall (mesentery of the colon)
_____/_____;
pertaining to middle-sized teeth
_____/_____/_____.

mes/enter/y
mez' en tair ē

meso/colon
mez' ō **kol'** in

meso/dont/ic
mez' ō **don'** tik

Ectopic (tubal) pregnancy _Delmar/Cengage Learning_

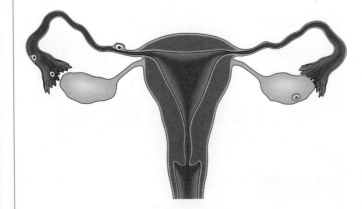

ANSWER COLUMN

9.115

retro- is a prefix meaning behind. Build adjectives meaning
behind the colon

retro/colic
ret′ rō **kol′** ik

_____/_____;
behind the breast (mammary glands)

retro/mammary
ret′ rō **mam′** ə rē

_____/_____;
behind the stern/um

retro/stern/al
ret′ rō **stûr′** nəl

_____/_____/_____.

9.116

Ante/version means turning forward. The word for turning backward is

retro/vers/ion
ret′ rō vûr zhən

_____/_____/_____.

9.117

behind

The retro/periton/eum is the space _____ the peritoneum.
An inflammation of this space is called

retro/periton/itis
ret′ rō per′ i tə **nī′** tis

_____/_____/_____.

9.118

Recall that ERCP is an x-ray procedure in which an endo/scope is used to inject
a contrast medium into the ducts of the pancreas and gallbladder so that any
obstructions can be viewed. Using what you know about the word parts you
have already learned, draw the slashes for the ERCP terms:

endo/scop/ic

endoscopic _____;

retro/grade

retrograde _____;
cholangiopancreatography

cholangi/o/pancreat/o/-
graphy

_____.

Refer to the illustration on page 268.

9.119

Flex/ion is bending or shortening of a body part (usually at a joint). **ante-** is the
prefix for front or forward. Therefore, the word ante/flexion means

bending forward

* _____.

9.120

retro- means behind (or backward). Build a term meaning bending backward:

retro/flex/ion
re′ trō flek shən

_____/_____/_____.

Uterine positions
Delmar/Cengage Learning

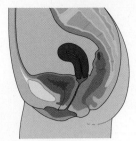
Anteversion

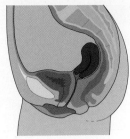
Marked retroversion

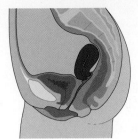
Retroflexion

	9.121
	Retro/flex/ion of the uterus means that the uterus is
bending backward	* _____.

	9.122
	para- as a prefix means near, beside, or around.
near the center or around the center	Para/centr/al means * _____ _____.
inflammation around the appendix	Para-/appendic/itis means * _____ _____.

	9.123
	Build words meaning inflammation around (near) the bladder
para/cyst/itis par' ə sis **tī'** tis	_____/_____/_____; inflammation of tissues around (near) the vagina
para/colp/itis par' ə kol **pī'** tis	_____/_____/_____.

	9.124
	Build words meaning inflammation of tissues near the liver
para/hepat/itis	_____/_____/_____; near the kidney
para/nephr/itis (You pronounce)	_____/_____/_____.

	9.125		
outer	**ecto-**	means	_____.
inner	**endo-**	means	_____.
middle	**meso-**	means	_____.
around (near)	**para-**	means	_____.
behind	**retro-**	means	_____.

ANSWER COLUMN

Abbreviation	Meaning
ā	before (ante)
AD*	right ear (auris dextra)
AP	anterior to posterior, anteroposterior
AS*	left ear (auris sinstra)
AU*	both ears (auris uterque)
AX	axillary
Bx	biopsy
CT	computed tomography
DRG	diagnostic-related group
Dx	diagnosis, diagnoses
ESRD	end-stage renal disease
ERCP	endoscopic retrograde cholangiopancreatography
Hx	history
LAT	lateral
LMP	last menstrual period
LOA	left occiput anterior
LPO	left posterior oblique
OD*	right eye (ocula dextra)
OS*	left eye (ocula sinistra)
OT	occupational therapy
OU*	both eyes (ocula uterque), each eye
PA	posterior to anterior, posteroanterior
p̄	after (post)
Px	prognosis, prognoses
ROP	right occiput posterior
RPO	right posterior oblique
RPR, VDRL	syphilis test (blood test)
STD, STI	sexually transmitted disease (infection)
TB	tuberculosis
VD	venereal disease (old use STD)

*Abbreviation use warning. These abbreviations have been judged to be dangerous and should not be used.

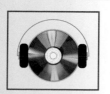

To complete your study of this unit, work the **Review Activities** on the following pages. Also, listen to the Audio CD that accompanies *Medical Terminology: A Programmed Systems Approach*, 10th edition, and practice your pronunciation.

STUDYWARE™ CONNECTION

To help you learn the content in this chapter, take a practice quiz or play an interactive game on your **StudyWARE™ CD-ROM**.

REVIEW ACTIVITIES

CIRCLE AND CORRECT

Circle the correct answer for each question. Then check your answers in Appendix E.

1. Prefix for in front of
   a. sub-   b. pro-
   c. post-   d. an-

2. Prefix for through
   a. gnosis-   b. pre-
   c. pro-   d. dia-

3. Suffix for substance that affects
   a. -pathic   b. -tropic
   c. -trophic   d. -phobic

4. Word root for front
   a. frontal   b. post
   c. ante   d. anter

5. Combining form for back
   a. posto   b. posterio
   c. ventr   d. postero

6. Adjectival form for side
   a. anterial   b. dorsal
   c. lateral   d. laterial

7. Combining form for umbilicus
   a. omphalo   b. onycho
   c. umbilical   d. omphalic

8. Combining form for without air
   a. pneumo   b. apnea
   c. anaero   d. aerobic

9. Suffix for attraction to
   a. -philic   b. -phobic
   c. -phagic   d. -appeal

10. Prefix for false
    a. fraud-   b. psycho-
    c. pseudo-   d. mal-

11. Prefix for easy or good
    a. a-   b. eu-
    c. dys-   d. eas-

12. Prefix or suffix for toward
    a. rrhexis   b. al
    c. ad   d. to

13. Word root for color
    a. chrom   b. chlor
    c. xanth   d. philic

14. Combining form for menstruation
    a. metro   b. metrio
    c. orrhea   d. meno

15. Suffix for controlling or stopping
    a. -rrhagia   b. -centesis
    c. -stasis   d. -dilation

16. Combining form for wall
    a. peritoneo b. parieto
    c. viscero   d. septum

SELECT AND CONSTRUCT

Select the correct word parts from the following list and construct medical terms that represent the given meaning.

a/an	aero	anter/o/ior	bio/bic	caud/al
cephal/o/ic	chrom/o	cyesis	derm	dia
dist/o	dys	ecto (ec)	edema	endo
eu	gastr/o	gen/ous	gnosis	hemo
hyper	itis	later/o/al	log/y/ist	lysis
medi/o	men/o	meso	omphal/o	omphal/o/ic
osis	pariet/o/al	pepsia	peritone/o/um/al	philia/ic
phobia	phoria	pleur/o/al	poster/o/ior	pro
proxim/o/al	pseud/o	retro	rrhea	scopy
stasis	syphil/o/is	thanat/o	topic	tropic
ventr/o/al	viscer/o/al	thanas/ia		

1. looking into the stomach with a scope _____

2. behind the peritoneum (adjective) _____

3. filtering blood through a membrane (artificial kidney) _____

REVIEW ACTIVITIES

4. inner germ layer that gives rise to organs _____

5. outside of the normal location (i.e., pregnancy) _____

6. pertaining to direction from back to front _____

7. pertaining to in front of the head _____

8. identification of a disease through signs and symptoms _____

9. inflammation of the umbilicus (navel) _____

10. pertaining to the side and front _____

11. pertaining to a direction from head to tail _____

12. lack of digestion _____

13. false pregnancy _____

14. feeling of well-being (good) _____

15. easy (peaceful) death _____

16. difficult (painful) menstruation _____

17. membrane attached to the lung _____

18. control of blood flow _____

19. uses air to live (metabolism with oxygen) _____

20. absorbs stain easily _____

21. membrane that lines the abdominal wall _____

22. discharge from the navel _____

23. fear of contracting syphilis _____

24. pertaining to the middle and the side _____

25. formed outside of the body (from another source) _____

DEFINE AND DISSECT

Give a brief definition and dissect each term listed into its word parts in the space provided. Check your answers by referring to the frame listed in parentheses and your medical dictionary. Then listen to the Audio CD to practice pronunciation.

1. diagnostic (9.31)   _____/_____/_____
                                                    pre   rt   suffix

   meaning _____

2. dialysis (9.37)   _____/_____
                                                    pre   suffix

   _____

REVIEW ACTIVITIES

3. ectoderm (9.95)

_____/_____
pre   rt

_____

4. exogenous (9.100)

_____/_____/_____
pre   rt   suffix

_____

5. polyphagia (9.102)

_____/_____/_____
pre   rt   suffix

_____

6. endoscopy (9.107)

_____/_____
pre   suffix

_____

7. mesentery (9.114)

_____/_____/_____
pre   rt   suffix

_____

8. retroversion (9.116)

_____/_____/_____
pre   rt   suffix

_____

9. prognosis (9.28)

_____/_____/_____
pre   rt   suffix

_____

10. hemodialysis (9.36)

_____/_____/_____/_____
rt   v   pre   suffix

_____

11. cholangiopancreatography (9.118)

_____/_____/_____/_____/_____/_____
rt   rt   v   rt   v   suffix

_____

12. para-appendicitis (9.122)

_____-/_____/_____
pre   rt   suffix

_____

13. paranephritis (9.124)

_____/_____/_____
pre   rt   suffix

_____

REVIEW ACTIVITIES

14. proximal (9.6)

_____/_____
rt   suffix

_____

15. dorsocephalad (9.5)

_____/_____/_____/_____
rt   v   rt   suffix

_____

16. posterolateral (9.4)

_____/_____/_____/_____
rt   v   rt   suffix

_____

17. omphalocele (9.20)

_____/_____/_____
rt   v   suffix

_____

18. dysentery (9.66)

_____/_____/_____
pre   rt   suffix

_____

19. anaerobic (9.47)

_____/_____/_____/_____
pre   rt   v   suffix

_____

20. biopsy (9.49)

_____/_____/_____
rt   v   suffix

_____

21. chromolysis (9.52)

_____/_____/_____
rt   v   suffix

_____

22. eukinesia (9.58)

_____/_____/_____
pre   rt   suffix

_____

23. euthanasia (9.61)

_____/_____/_____
pre   rt   suffix

_____

24. menorrhea (9.70)

_____/_____/_____
rt   v   suffix

_____

25. syphilopsychosis (9.78)

_____/_____/_____/_____
rt   v   rt   suffix

_____

REVIEW ACTIVITIES

26. pseudoesthesia (9.82)

       _____/_____/_____/_____
           rt   v   rt   suffix

27. pseudoneuroma (9.83)

       _____/_____/_____/_____
           rt   v   rt   suffix

28. visceroptosis (9.91)

       _____/_____/_____
           rt   v   suffix

29. visceropleural (9.88)

       _____/_____/_____/_____
           rt   v   rt   suffix

30. distal (9.6)

       _____/_____
           rt   suffix

31. mediolateral (9.9)

       _____/_____/_____/_____
           rt   v   rt   suffix

32. omphalorrhagia (9.21)

       _____/_____/_____
           rt   v   suffix

33. dyspnea (9.57)

       _____/_____
           pre   suffix

34. cephalocaudal (9.24)

       _____/_____/_____/_____
           rt   v   rt   suffix

35. achromophilic (9.55)

       _____/_____/_____/_____
           pre   rt   v   suffix

36. phlebostasis (9.73)

       _____/_____/_____
           rt   v   suffix

37. visceromotor (9.86)

       _____/_____/_____
           rt   v   rt/suffix

REVIEW ACTIVITIES

38. chromoblast (9.51)

_____/_____/_____
      rt   v   suffix

_____

39. midaxillary (9.13)

_____/_____/_____
     pre   rt   suffix

_____

40. symptoms (9.32)

_____/_____/_____
     pre   rt   suffix

_____

DIAGRAM LABELING

From what you have learned about directional terms, complete the diagram below by labeling the blanks with the proper direction term or word part.

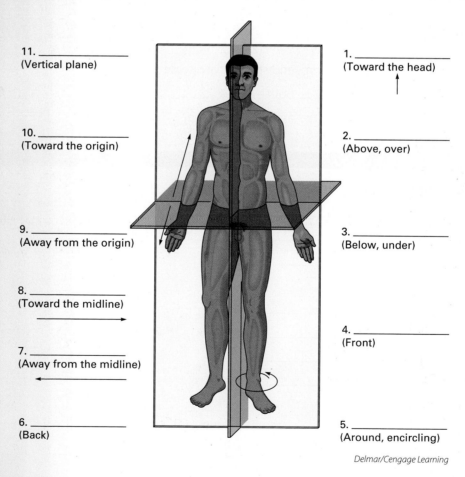

11. _____
(Vertical plane)

10. _____
(Toward the origin)

9. _____
(Away from the origin)

8. _____
(Toward the midline)

7. _____
(Away from the midline)

6. _____
(Back)

1. _____
(Toward the head)

2. _____
(Above, over)

3. _____
(Below, under)

4. _____
(Front)

5. _____
(Around, encircling)

Delmar/Cengage Learning

REVIEW ACTIVITIES

ABBREVIATION MATCHING

Match the following abbreviations with their definition.

_____ 1. Dx

_____ 2. Bx

_____ 3. Hx

_____ 4. OD

_____ 5. Px

_____ 6. ESRD

_____ 7. AP

_____ 8. LMP

_____ 9. DRG

_____ 10. ANT

a. treatment

b. prescribe

c. diagnosis-related group

d. anterior

e. prognosis

f. last menstrual period

g. certified pharmacy technician

h. diagnosis

i. esophagogastric disease

j. physician's assistant

k. history

l. biopsy

m. right eye

n. end-stage renal disease

o. both eyes

p. anterior to posterior

ABBREVIATION FILL-INS

Fill in the blanks with the correct abbreviations.

11. left occiput anterior _____

12. sexually transmitted disease _____

13. syphilis test _____

14. lateral _____

15. last menstrual period _____

16. posterior to anterior _____

17. occupational therapy _____

18. tuberculosis _____

REVIEW ACTIVITIES

CASE STUDY

Write the term next to its meaning. Then draw slashes to analyze the word parts. Note the use of medical abbreviations. Look these up in your dictionary or find them in Appendix B. If you have any questions about the answers, refer to your medical dictionary or check with your instructor for the answers in Appendix E.

CASE STUDY 9-1

Pt: Female, age 34

Dx: 1. Obesity **hypoventilation syndrome**

2. **Diabetes mellitus type 1**

Ms. Betty Sweet presented with a history of morbid obesity and a previous admission for respiratory insufficiency. She entered the emergency room complaining of progressive fatigue, sleepiness, **cephalalgia, narcolepsy**, general weakness, and **dyspnea**. She admits to a dry nonproductive cough without congestion, **URI symptoms**, recent fevers, sweats, and chills. For her headache she had been taking an occasional nonprescription **analgesic** amounting to 2 aspirins/week and she denied any other drug use. Ms. Sweet has a history of type 1 diabetes and had been maintained on 25 **U** of insulin until August 11 when she was increased to 40 U. A urinary tract infection was an incidental finding. She has done no blood sugar checks at home. No **hypoglycemic** reactions have been recorded. Ms. Sweet has progressive, increasing lethargy and feels unrested. Past history is also significant for a hospitalization in 1988 for which she required **ventilatory** support for obstructive **apnea**. She was discharged home on nasal **CPAP** and was able to lose 20–30 pounds with marked improvement in her symptoms. She has gained the weight back over the last 6 months and is dieting again. Of note at that time was Swan-Ganz **catheterization**, which revealed elevated pulmonary artery pressures.

1. introduction of a tube to evacuate or irrigate a body cavity   _____

2. cessation of breathing   _____

3. DM Type 1   _____

4. upper respiratory infection   _____

5. sleep seizures   _____

6. continuous positive air pressure   _____

7. reduced depth of breaths   _____

8. symptoms that run together   _____

9. how the patient feels   _____

10. units   _____

11. low blood sugar (adjective)   _____

12. pain reliever   _____

13. headache   _____

14. difficulty breathing   _____

15. getting air in lungs (adjective)   _____

REVIEW ACTIVITIES

CROSSWORD PUZZLE

Check your answers by going back through the frames or checking the solution in Appendix F.

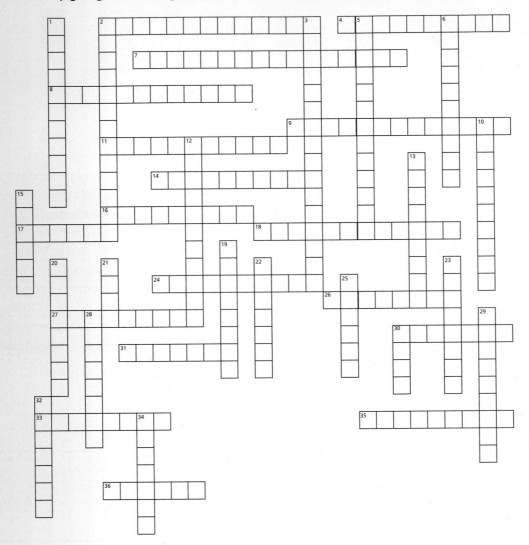

Across

2. does not absorb stain
4. partial paralysis (lower body)
7. inflammation behind the peritoneum
8. twisting backward
9. pertaining to the back and head
11. bending forward
14. formed outside the body (adj.)
16. grows without air
17. synonym for posterior
18. inflammation near the bladder
24. below normal amount of growth
26. filtration of blood with artificial kidney
27. examination by looking into the body
30. pregnancy outside of the uterus
31. difficulty breathing
33. choosing good genetic traits only
35. cessation of reproductive cycle
36. synonym for menorrhea

Down

1. hemorrhage during menstruation
2. pertaining to the front and side
3. defective cartilage development
5. control of blood flow in the arteries
6. easy death
10. absence of menstruation
12. crushing of a stone
13. opinions of good and bad choices for living things
15. middle (adj.)
19. toward the head
20. below or bottom
21. outer (prefix)
22. side
23. difficult labor
25. away from the point of origin
28. flowing of watery stool
29. identifying a disease
30. inner (prefix)
32. synonym for anterior
34. pertaining to the crown

REVIEW ACTIVITIES

GLOSSARY

achromophilic	resisting color (stain)		diagnosis	identifying a disease
aerobic	requiring air to live		dialysis	separating of substances in a solution (filtration)
aerocele	herniation containing air		diarrhea	abnormally loose watery bowel movement
aerophobia	abnormal fear of air			
aerotherapy	treatment using air (respiratory therapy)		distal	away from a point of origin or designated point
amenorrhea	cessation of menstruation		dorsal	back (posterior)
anaerobic	able to live without air		dorsocephalad	toward the back of the head
anterolateral	front and side		dysentery	inflammation of the intestine
anteromedial	front and middle		dysmenorrhea	difficult or painful menstruation
anteroposterior	from front to back		dyspepsia	poor digestion
anterosuperior	front and top		dyspnea	difficulty breathing
arteriostasis	control of flow through arteries		dystocia	difficulty in labor
axillary	underarm, armpit		ectocytic	outside the cell (extracellular, adjective)
bioethics	study of what is good and bad for living things		ectoderm	outer embryonic (germ) layer
biology	science studying living things		ectogenous	formed outside the body (from another source, adjective)
blastoderm	embryonic disk that gives rise to the endoderm, mesoderm, ectoderm		ectopic	outside of the normal location (adjective)
caudad	toward the tail (sacrum)		ectoplasm	outer membrane of the cell
cephalad	toward the head		endocardium	inner membrane layer of the heart
cephalocaudal	from head to tail		endochondral	within the cartilage (adjective)
chondrodysplasia	defective development of cartilage		endocolitis	inflammation of the lining of the colon
chromogenesis	formation of color		endocystic	inside the urinary bladder or inside a cyst (adjective)
chromolysis	destruction of color			
chromometer	measuring color		endoderm	inner embryonic (germ) layer
chromophilic	attracting color (stain)		endoenteritis	inflammation of the lining of the small intestine
coronal	pertaining to the crown or encircling		endogenous	made by one's own body (adjective)
coronary	pertaining to the crown or encircling (reference to around the heart)		endoscopy	process of using a scope to look into the body

REVIEW ACTIVITIES

eugenics	choosing good genetic traits to propagate	para-appendicitis	inflammation of near the appendix
eupepsia	good digestion	paracentral	pertaining to near the center (adjective)
eupnea	easy breathing	paracolpitis	inflammation near the vagina
euthanasia	easy death	paracystitis	inflammation near the urinary bladder
eutocia	easy labor	parahepatitis	inflammation near the liver
hemostasis	control blood flow	paranephritis	inflammation near the kidney
hyperplasia	overdevelopment (too many cells)	parietal	pertaining to the wall
hypoplasia	underdevelopment (too few cells)	peritoneum	membrane of the abdomen
inferior	below	phlebostasis	control of flow through a vein (venostasis)
lateral	side	pleura	membrane of the lungs
lithotripsy	surgical crushing of a stone	posteroanterior	from back to front
lymphostasis	control or stoppage of lymph flow	posteroexternal	back and outside
medial	middle	posterointernal	back and inside
menopause	cessation of menstruation, ovulation, and atrophy of female reproductive system	posterolateral	back and side
		procephalic	in front of the head
menorrhagia	hemorrhage during menstruation	prognosis	predicting the outcome of a disease
menses	menstruation (menorrhea), menses: plural and singular		
mesoderm	middle germ layer	prognostic	pertaining to a prognosis
midaxillary	middle of the armpit	proximal	near the point of origin or a designated point
midsagittal	the plane dividing the body into equal right and left halves	pseudocyesis	false pregnancy (pseudopregnancy)
neurotripsy	surgical crushing of a nerve	pseudocyst	false cyst
omphalectomy	excision of the umbilicus	pseudoedema	false swelling
omphalic	pertaining to the umbilicus	pseudoesthesia	false sensation (i.e., phantom limb)
omphalitis	inflammation of the umbilicus	retrocolic	behind the colon (adjective)
omphalocele	umbilical hernia (umbilicocele)	retroflexion	bending (flexing) backward
omphalorrhagia	hemorrhage of the umbilicus	retroperitoneum	behind the peritoneum
omphalorrhea	discharge from the umbilicus	retroperitonitis	inflammation of the area behind the peritoneum
omphalorrhexis	rupture of the umbilicus		
osteochondrodysplasia	defective development of bone and cartilage	retrosternal	behind the sternum (adjective)
		retroversion	twisting (turning) backward

REVIEW ACTIVITIES

sagittal	vertical plane or slice, divides into left and right
signs	objective observable Information
superior	above
symptoms	subjective self-reported information
syphilophobia	abnormal fear of syphilis

syphilopsychosis	severe mental condition caused by untreated syphilis
syphilotherapy	treatment for syphilis
ventral	front (anterior)
viscera	organs
visceropleura	membrane surrounding and attached to the lung

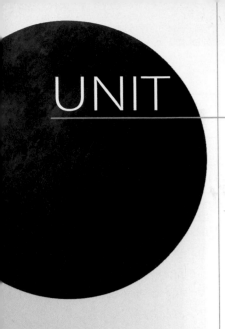

10

Surgery, Diabetes, Immunology, Lesions, and Prefixes of Numbers and Direction

10.1

lapar/o means abdominal wall. A laparectomy is an excision of part of the

abdominal wall

* _____ .

10.2

The process of examining the abdominal cavity with an end/o/scope is called

lapar/o/scopy
lap ər **os'** kō pē

_____ / _____ / _____ .

10.3

INFORMATION
FRAME

A lapar/o/scope is a special instrument that allows a physician to view the inside of the abdominal cavity and its organs. Surgery can also be performed while using a laparoscope (usually attached to a video screen). See the illustration on page 374.

10.4

Lapar/o/scop/ically assisted vaginal hyster/ectomy (LAVH) is actually the removal of the uterus through the vagina assisted by looking through

lapar/o/scope
lap' är ō skōp

the _____ / _____ / _____ from within the abdominal cavity.

10.5

lapar/o/scop/ic
lap' är ō **skō'** pik

Chole/cyst/ectomy can also be performed with the assistance of the laparoscope.

This would be called _____ / _____ / _____ / _____ cholecystectomy.

CASE STUDY INVESTIGATION (CSI)

Laparoscopic Procedure Description

The most common **laparoscopic** procedure is laparoscopic **cholecystectomy** performed with 5–10 mm diameter instruments **introduced** into the abdomen through **trocars** (hollow tubes with a seal). Rather than a 20 cm **incision** in the traditional gallbladder removal, four incisions of 0.5–1.0 cm are used. The gallbladder is small flexible sack that may be removed from the abdomen by first suctioning out the bile and then removing the empty gallbladder through the 1 cm **omphalotomy**. The advantage of laparoscopic procedures is that the **postoperative** stay is minimal often with a same-day discharge. Other laparoscopically assisted surgeries include: **colectomy**, nephrectomy, hysterectomy, appendectomy, ovarian cyst **I&D**, and tubal **ligations**.

CSI Vocabulary Challenge

Use a medical dictionary to analyze the term or abbreviation listed from the case study. Divide the term into word parts by drawing in the slashes and write the definition in the space provided.

laparoscopic   _____

cholecystectomy   _____

introduced   _____

trocars   _____

incision   _____

omphalotomy   _____

postoperative   _____

colectomy   _____

I&D   _____

ligations   _____

ANSWER COLUMN

10.6

lapar/o/tomy
lap′ ərot′ əmē

lapar/o/rrhaphy
lap′ ərôr′ əfē

An incision into the abdominal wall is a _____/_____/_____.

Suturing of the abdominal wall is _____/_____/_____.

10.7

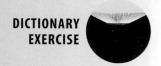

DICTIONARY EXERCISE

Use your dictionary to give the meaning for the following words about the abdomen.

laparohepatotomy (lap′ ə rō hep′ **tot′** ō mē)

* _____ ;

(continued)

laparocolostomy (lap′ ə rō kō **los′** tō mē)

* _____;

laparogastrotomy (lap′ ə rō gas **trot′** ō mē)

* _____

Great job!

10.8

There may be longer words than this, but not many. Analyze it for fun. Think of the word parts.

Laparohysterosalpingo-oophorectomy *_____

_____

abdomen, uterus, fallopian tubes, ovaries, excision

lap′ ə rō **his′** ter ō sal **ping′** ō-ōō for **ek′** tō mē

10.9

pyr/o is used in words to mean heat, fever, or fire. The early Greeks and Romans burned their dead on funeral pyres. A pyr/o/maniac is one who has a madness (excessive preoccupation) for starting or seeing _____.

fires

10.10

Pyr/exia (pi **reks′** ē ə) means fever. A condition of heat (heartburn) is

pyr/osis
pī **rō′** sis

_____/_____.

hyper/pyrexia
hī′ per pī **reks′** ē ə

A condition of high fever (over 102°F) is _____/_____.

Laparoscopy performed with hysteroscopy
Delmar/Cengage Learning

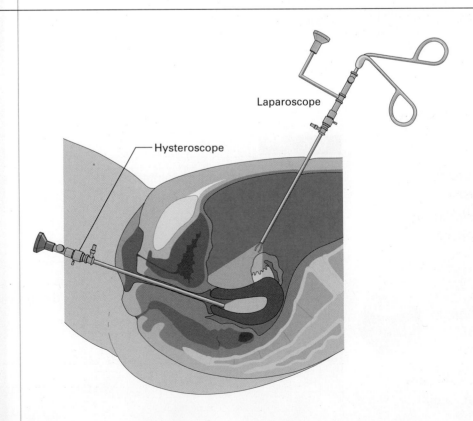

Laparoscope

Hysteroscope

PROFESSIONAL PROFILE

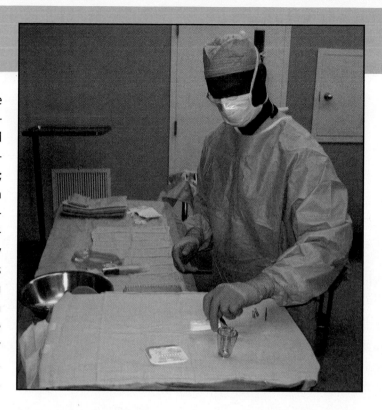

Certified surgical technologists (CSTs) are an integral part of a surgical team. They prepare the operating room by selecting and opening sterile supplies; assembling, adjusting, and checking nonsterile equipment; and operating sterilizers, lights, suction machines, electrosurgical units, and diagnostic equipment. The CST most often functions as a member of the surgical team by passing instruments, sutures, and sponges during surgery, holding retractors, receiving specimens, as well as assisting other team members in gowning and gloving. They give preoperative care to surgical patients by providing physical and emotional support, checking charts, and observing vital signs. The Accreditation Review Committee on Education in Surgical Technology (ARC-ST) recommends educational standards and accredits programs. Voluntary professional certification is obtained from the Association of Surgical Technologists (AST) upon passing a CST national certification examination.

Surgical technician using aseptic techniques to prepare a sterile field with supplies *Photo by Timothy J. Dennerll, RT(R), Ph.D., courtesy of Allegiance Health, Jackson, MI*

ANSWER COLUMN

10.11

Build words meaning
instrument for measuring heat (thermometer)

pyr/o/meter
pī **rô'** mə ter

_____/_____/_____;

destruction by fever

pyr/o/lysis
pī **rô'** lə sis

_____/_____/_____;

abnormal fear of fire

pyr/o/phobia
pī rō **fō'** bē ə

_____/_____/_____;

madness (obsession) for setting fires

pyr/o/mania
pī rō **mā'** nē ə

_____/_____/_____.

10.12

A pyr/o/toxin is a toxin (poison) produced by

fever or high body
temperature

* _____.

ANSWER COLUMN

10.13

hydro- (a combining form and prefix) means water or fluid. **hidro-**
(from the Greek *hidros*) means sweat. A hidro/cyst/aden/oma is a cystic tumor

sweat

of a _____ gland.

10.14

inflammation of
  sweat glands

Hidr/aden/itis means *_____

_____ .

10.15

The three words below mean sweating; define and divide them into their word
parts.

hidr/osis
hī **drō'** sis
condition of sweating

hidrosis _____/_____ ,

*_____ ;

hyper/hidr/osis
hī per hī **drō** sis
profuse sweating

hyperhidrosis _____/_____/_____ ,

*_____ ;

hidr/o/rrhea
hī drō **rē'** ə
flow of sweat

hidrorrhea _____/_____/_____ ,

*_____ .

10.16

The word an/hidr/osis (an hī **drō'** sis) means

absence of sweat

*_____ .

10.17

Both **hydro-** and **hidro-** are pronounced alike.

water or fluid

Hydro, with a *y*, means *_____ .

sweat

Hidro, with an *i*, means _____ .

10.18

**DICTIONARY
EXERCISE**

glyc/o (glycos) and **gluc/o** (glucos) are different translations of Greek word parts
meaning sweet or sugar. Here are some examples of sweet words:

glycogenesis/glucogenesis: formation of sugar
glycoprotein/glucoprotein: substance made of sugar and protein
glycosuria/glucosuria: (glycos/glucos) sugar in the urine
glycohemoglobin: sugar and hemoglobin

Look up terms beginning with **gluco** and **glyco** in your dictionary. They are
interchangeable in some words, but notice many in which they have a unique use.

ANSWER COLUMN

10.19

glyc/o/gen
glī′ kō jen

Glycogen is "animal starch" formed from simple sugars and stored as reserve fuel. The cells of the body use a simple sugar, glucose, to release energy. To use its reserve fuel supply of animal starch, the body must convert

_____/_____/_____ to glucose.

10.20

gluc/o/gen/esis
glōō kō **jen′** ə sis

glyc/o/gen/esis
glī′ kō **jen′** ə sis

gluc/o is a combining form for glucose. The formation of glucose from glycogen stores is called _____/_____/_____/_____.
The formation of glycogen from carbothydrates is

_____/_____/_____/_____.

10.21

glycogen

Glucose is used by the muscles to release energy. Glycogen is the reserve food supply of glucose. Glucose is the usable form of stored _____.

10.22

glyc/o/hem/o/globin
glī kō **hē′** mə glō bin

Glyc/o/hem/o/globin is a combination of sugar (glucose) and hemoglobin in the blood. This substance, also called glyc/ated hem/o/globin (GHB) remains permanently in the red blood cells which live up to 90 days. If a person has experienced chronic high blood sugar levels, an increase in the level of

_____/_____/_____/_____/_____ may be expected.

NOTE: The hemoglobin A1c (Hb A1c or Hgb A1c) test measures the glycohemoglobin levels which indicate the average blood glucose levels during the 60 to 90 days prior to the test.

10.23

TAKE A CLOSER LOOK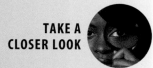

Diabetes mellitus has many forms, all of which are characterized by hypoglycemia and other metabolic disturbances. Listed on the next page are three types of diabetes mellitus and their characteristics.

(continued)

Glucose tolerance test (GTT) graph *Delmar/Cengage Learning*

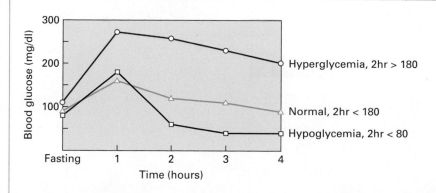

Type 1 (insulin-dependent diabetes mellitus, IDDM) is characterized by onset in youth, exogenous insulin dependency, tendency to ketoacidosis, viral etiology, autoimmune basis, and genetic predisposition.

Type 2 (noninsulin-dependent diabetes mellitus, NIDDM) is characterized by onset in adults over 40, some endogenous insulin production, obesity or normal weight, and can be treated with diet modification and oral hypoglycemic agents.

Gestational diabetes mellitus (GDM) occurs in individuals not previously diabetic who develop hyperglycemia during pregnancy. These women may progress to another diabetes mellitus or return to normal glucose levels postpartum.

10.24

Recall that **-emia** means condition in the blood. Glyc/emia means sugar in the blood. A symptom of diabetes is hyper/glyc/emia. This means

*_____

_____.

too much sugar in the
blood (high blood
sugar)

10.25

Hyper/glyc/emia means high blood sugar. The word that means low blood sugar

is _____/_____/_____.

hypo/glyc/emia
hī′ pō glī **sē′** mē ə

10.26

When a person produces too much of the hormone insulin, the blood glucose level may decrease to below normal. This is called _____.

hypoglycemia

10.27

If glucogenesis is the formation of glucose, then the formation of glycogen from food is _____/_____/_____/_____.

glyc/o/gen/esis
glī′ kō **jen′** ə sis

10.28

The breakdown of glycogen to glucose is _____/_____/_____.
The discharge (flow) of sugar from the body is

_____/_____/_____.

glyc/o/lysis
glī **kol′** ə sis

glyc/o/rrhea
glī′ kō **rē′** ə

10.29

Glyc/o/lipid should make you think of two foods: _____ and

_____.

sugar

fat

STUDYWARE™ CONNECTION

Remember, after completing this unit, you can play a concentration or other interactive game on your **StudyWARE™ CD-ROM** that will help you learn the content in this chapter.

ANSWER COLUMN

10.30

immun/o/logy
im' yoo **nol'** ō jē

immun/o is the combining form for immune. Immun/ity is one of the body's defenses against disease. The study of the function of the immune system is called _____/_____/_____.

10.31

immun/o/therapy
im' yoo nō **thair'** a pē

immun/i/zations
im' yoo nə **zā'** shunz

Immun/ization (vaccination) injections are given to stimulate an immune response to infections. The process is known as immun/o/therapy. DPT (diphtheria, pertussis, tetanus) and IPV (inactivated polio vaccine) are two types of _____/_____/_____
or
_____/_____/_____.

10.32

immun/o/deficiency
im' yoo nō de **fish'** en cē

Immun/o/logists are studying HIV (human immun/o/deficiency virus), which causes AIDS (acquired immunodeficiency syndrome). Because it is characterized by inability to fight off disease, AIDS is a type of _____/_____/_____ disease.

10.33

INFORMATION FRAME

When an antigen (such as a foreign protein from a virus) invades the body, special leukocytes (lymphocytes) produce antibodies to disable the invader. This antigen-antibody reaction is called the immune response.

10.34

TAKE A CLOSER LOOK

Natural immunity is part of human physiology. The immunity passed from a mother to the fetus during pregnancy or when breastfeeding is called natural *passive* immunity. If a child is infected with chickenpox by being exposed to another child with chickenpox and then develops antibodies against Varicella, this is *naturally acquired active immunity*.

ANSWER COLUMN

10.35

Artificial immunity has been scientifically designed. An individual who has a failing natural immune system may be given immun/o/globulin (IG) injections to boost their immune response. This type of immunity is *artificial passive immunity*. Vaccines are designed to contain pathogen-specific antigens that stimulate the lymphatic system to produce specific matching antibodies. Vaccination against infectious diseases like measles, mumps, rubella (MMR) is *artificially acquired active immunity*.

10.36

Chickenpox is caused by the virus *Varicella zoster*. When first infected, the person becomes ill. If infected again, the person will most likely not become ill due to

immun/ity
im **yoo'** ni tē

acquired active _____/_____.

10.37

A breastfed infant receives antibodies from its mother's body through the breast

immunity

milk. This type of immunity is called passive _____.

10.38

WORD
ORIGINS

The word "vaccine" comes from *vacca,* the Latin word for cow. Edward Jenner first innoculated a young boy with a substance from the sore of a milkmaid infected with cowpox. At a later time, he exposed the boy to smallpox and the boy resisted the disease. This was the first vaccination (immunization).

vaccin/a/tion
vak sin **ā'** shun

10.39

vaccin/e
vak **sēn'**

The inactivated polio _____ (IPV) stimulates resistance to poliomyelitis.

10.40

TAKE A
CLOSER LOOK

Eleven immunizations are recommended before age seven for the general population. To learn about these recommendations, study the immunization schedule on page 381.

10.41

self

aut/o is a combining form that means self. You already recognize **aut/o** in such ordinary English words as aut/o/mobile (a self-propelled vehicle) and aut/o/bi/o/graphy. **aut/o** means _____.

ANSWER COLUMN

Vaccine ▼ Age ▶	Birth	1 month	2 months	4 months	6 months	12 months	15 months	18 months	19–23 months	2–3 years	4–6 years
Hepatitis B	HepB	HepB			HepB						
Rotavirus			RV	RV	RV						
Diphtheria, Tetanus, Pertussis			DTaP	DTaP	DTaP		DTaP				DTaP
Haemophilus influenzae type b			Hib	Hib	Hib	Hib					
Pneumococcal			PCV	PCV	PCV	PCV					PPSV
Inactivated Poliovirus			IPV	IPV		IPV					IPV
Influenza						Influenza (Yearly)					
Measles, Mumps, Rubella						MMR					MMR
Varicella						Varicella					Varicella
Hepatitis A						HepA (2 doses)				HepA Series	
Meningococcal										MCV	

■ Range of recommended ages

■ Certain high-risk groups

This schedule indicates the recommended ages for routine administration of currently licensed vaccines, as of December 1, 2008, for children aged 0 through 6 years. Any dose not administered at the recommended age should be administered at a subsequent visit, when indicated and feasible. Licensed combination vaccines may be used whenever any component of the combination is indicated and other components are not contraindicated and if approved by the Food and Drug Administration for that dose of the series. Providers should consult the relevant Advisory Committee on Immunization Practices statement for detailed recommendations, including high-risk conditions: http://www.cdc.gov/vaccines/pubs/acip-list.htm. Clinically significant adverse events that follow immunization should be reported to the Vaccine Adverse Event Reporting System (VAERS). Guidance about how to obtain and complete a VAERS form is available at http://www.vaers.hhs.gov or by telephone, 800-822-7967.

Recommended immunization schedule for persons aged 0 through 6 years—United States · 2009 *Approved by the Advisory Committee on Immunization Practices (www.cdc.gov./vaccines/recs/acip), the American Academy of Pediatrics (http://www.aap.org), and the American Academy of Family Physicians (http://www.aalp.org)*

10.42

Aut/o/dia/gnos/is means diagnosing one's own diseases. Aut/o/derm/ic pertains to dermat/o/plasty with

one's own skin

* _____.

10.43

Aut/o/nom/ic means self-controlling, as in the autonomic nervous system. Aut/o/lysis (aw **tol'** ə sis) means

self-destruction or
self-destroying

aut/o/nom/ic
aw' tō **nom'** ik

* _____.

The self-controlling part of the nervous system is the

_____/_____/_____/_____ nervous system (ANS).

10.44

aut/o/immun/ity
aw' tō im **yōō'** ni tē

If one's own body produces antibodies to one's own tissues (like being allergic to oneself), _____/_____/_____/_____ has occurred.

EXAMPLE: Rheumatoid arthritis and lupus erythematosus are often seen in the same patient and are autoimmune disorders.

ANSWER COLUMN

10.45

Aut/o/phagia means biting one's self. A word that means abnormal fear of being

aut/o/phobia
aw tō **fō'** bē ə

alone is _____/_____/_____.

aut/o/immun/ity

_____/_____/_____/_____ is being
allergic to one's own tissues.

10.46

Build terms that mean therapy with one's own blood (transfusion)

aut/o/hem/o/therapy
aw' tō hēm' ō **thair'** a pē

_____/_____/_____/_____/_____;

aut/o/plasty
aw' tō plas tē

surgery using grafts from one's own body _____/_____/_____.

10.47

Aut/o/logous is an adjective meaning originating in itself or coming from one's
own body. Persons anticipating surgery can have blood drawn and saved for

aut/o/logous
aw **tol'** ō gus

their own use if needed. This would be an _____/_____/_____
blood transfusion.

10.48

Keeping the previous frame in mind, think of what an aut/o/graft might be.
A burn victim needing a skin graft may use his or her own healthy skin as

aut/o/graft
aw' tō graft

an _____/_____/_____.

10.49

The term aut/o/genous has a similar meaning to aut/o/logous. If a vaccine
is made from a culture of a patient's own bacteria, this is called an

aut/o/gen/ous
aw **to'** jen us

_____/_____/_____/_____ vaccine.

10.50

Great! When you analyze a word, think of its meaning. If you have forgotten a part
of the word, look it up. Analyze the following

aut/o/phobia

autophobia _____/_____/_____,

abnormal fear of one's
self or being alone

_____;
meaning

aut/o/phagia

autophagia _____/_____/_____.

biting one's self

_____.
meaning

ANSWER COLUMN

Study this table. Notice the specific use of each prefix.

Numeric Prefixes				
Greek	**Latin**	**Meaning**	**Symbol**	**Examples**
hemi-	semi-	half	0.5, ss	hemiplegia, semiconscious
mono-	uni-	one	1, i	monocyte, uniparous
prot-	prim-	first		protozoan, primigravida
di(plo)-	bi-	two	2, ii	diplococci, bifurcation
tri-	tri-	three	3, iii	triglyceride, triceps
tetra-	quadr-	four	4, iv	tetramastia, quadriplegia
penta-	quint-	five	5, v	pentadactyl, quintuplets
hexa-	sex/ta-	six	6, vi	hexapodia, sexagenarian
hepta-	sept/a-	seven	7, vii	heptachromic, septuplet
octa-	oct-	eight	8, viii	octodont, octogenarian
enne(a)-	non(i)-	nine	9, ix	ennead, nonipara
deca- (10)	dec(i)- (0.1)	ten, tenth	10, x	decaliter, deciliter
hecto- (100)	cent(i)- (0.01)	one hundred, one hundredth		hectogram, centigram
kilo- (1,000)	mill(i)- (0.001)	one thousand, one thousandth		kilometer, millimeter

Then use this knowledge to work the rest of the frames in this unit.

10.51

one

mono- means one or single. You know it in the ordinary English words monorail, monopoly, and monogamy. When you see **mono-**, think of _____.

10.52

one

A mono/graph deals with a single subject. A mono/nucle/ar cell has

_____ nucleus.

10.53

Mono/mania is an abnormal preoccupation with one subject only. Build words meaning

mono/cyte
mon' ō sīt

one cell _____/_____ (a type of leukocyte);

mono/oma
mon ō' mə

one tumor _____/_____ .

10.54

Build words that begin with **mono-**.
paralysis of one muscle

mono/my/o/plegia
mon' ō mī ō **plē'** jē ə

_____/_____/_____/_____;

(continued)

ANSWER COLUMN

pertaining to one nerve

mono/neur/al
mon ō **nōōr'** əl   _____/_____/_____ ;

mono/cyt/osis   condition of increase in monocytes

mon' ō sī **tō'** sis   _____/_____/_____ .

10.55

Mono/nucle/osis (mono) is a condition caused by a viral infection that can damage the liver. One sign is an abnormally high monocyte count. Mono/cyt/osis

mono/nucle/osis
mon' ō nōō klē **ō'** sis   may be an indication of _____/_____/_____ .

10.56

multi- means the opposite of **mono-**. **multi-** (as in multiply) means

many or more than one   *_____ .

10.57

In ordinary English, you are acquainted with **multi-** in the words multiply and

many   multitude. Something composed of multiple parts has _____ parts.

10.58

many capsules   Something that is multi/capsular has *_____ .

10.59

Multi/glandular is an adjective meaning

many glands   *_____ .

                                      Multi/cellular is an adjective meaning

many cells   *_____ .

                                      Multi/nuclear is an adjective meaning

many nuclei   *_____ .

10.60

INFORMATION FRAME

Para is a whole word, a suffix (**-para**) and a prefix (**para-**). **Para** and **-para** refer to a woman who has given birth one or more times. Par/ity is the quality of having given birth. **Para** followed by a number indicates the number of times she has given birth. Examples: para ll, para 2, para IV, para 4.

10.61

A multi/para is a woman who has brought forth (borne) more than one child. par is one word root meaning to bear. Multi/par/ous is the adjectival form

multi/para
mul **tip'** ə rə   of _____/_____ .

Gravida II, para I. Pregnant mother with her son. *Photo by Timothy J. Dennerll, RT(R), Ph.D.*

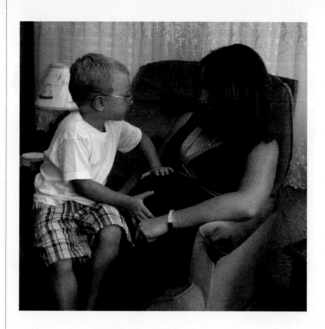

10.62

Multi/para always refers to the mother. Multi/par/ous may refer to a mother who has had many children or may mean multiple birth (twins or triplets). When desiring to indicate that a woman has borne more than one child, use the

multipara | noun _____ .

10.63

multi/para
multi/par/ous
mul **tip′** ər əs

Multi/par/ous is the adjectival form of _____/_____ .
To indicate that twins are born, say _____/_____/_____
birth.

10.64

multiparous
multiparous

To indicate that triplets are born, say _____ birth. If ten
children were born, you would still use the adjective _____.

10.65

nulli- means *none.* To nullify something is to bring it to nothing. There
are not many medical words using **nulli-**; but when you do see it, it

none | means _____ .

10.66

a woman who has
never borne a child

A nulli/para is *_____.

primi/para
prī **mip′** ər ə

primi- means first. A woman who is having her first child is a
_____/_____ (noun).

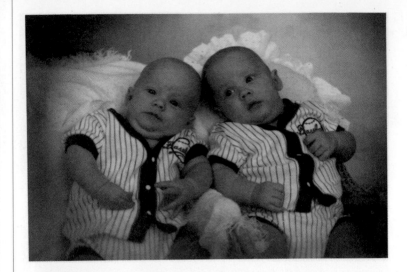

10.67

Gravida is a Latin word meaning heavy or weighted down. In medical terms it is used to mean pregnant. A woman experiencing her first pregnancy is called a

primi/gravida
prim′ i **grav**′ i da

_____/_____.

10.68

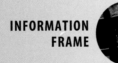

**INFORMATION
FRAME**

Gravida refers to pregnancies, whereas **para** refers to live births. A woman who has been pregnant four times and had two spontaneous abortions (miscarriages) and two live births would be described on the chart as grav 4, ab 2, para 2 (G4, AB2, P2).

10.69

Analyze the following and define:

nulli/para
nu **lip**′ ar ə
no live births

nullipara _____/_____ (noun),

*_____;

nulli/par/ous
nu **lip**′ ar us
pertaining to no live
  births

nulliparous _____/_____/_____ (adjective),

*_____;

primi/para
prī **mip**′ ar ə
first live birth

primipara _____/_____ (noun),

*_____.

10.70

Give the prefix for

nulli-

none _____;

mono-

one (single) _____;   *(continued)*

ANSWER COLUMN

multi-

para-

primi-

many _____ ;	
bear _____ ;	
first _____ .	

10.71

deca- and **deci-** both mean ten but are used differently. **deca-** is used in words meaning the whole number ten. **deci-** is used in words meaning the fraction one

ten

tenth

tenth. A decaliter (dal) is _____ liters.

A deciliter (dL) is one _____ of a liter.

10.72

kilo- and **milli-** both refer to thousand but are used differently. **kilo-** is used in words to mean one thousand. **milli-** is used in words to mean one thousandth.

thousand

thousandth

A kilometer (km) is one _____ meters.

A millimeter (mm) is one _____ of a meter.

10.73

Build words that mean
one thousand grams

kilo/gram
ki′ lo gram

_____/_____ (kg);
one thousandth of a gram

milli/gram
mi′ li gram

_____/_____ (mg);
one thousand meters

kilo/meter
kil **om′** ə ter

_____/_____ (km);
one thousandth of a meter

millī/meter
mil′ ə mē ter

_____/_____ (mm).

10.74

Build words that mean:
one thousandth of a second

milli/second
mil′ ē se kund

_____/_____ (ms);
one thousandth of a mole

milli/mole
mil′ ē mōl

_____/_____ (mmol).
Now you've got it!

10.75

A volume measurement that is frequently used when giving injections is the cubic centimeter (cc). It is the amount of fluid in one centimeter cubed. If the physician writes an order to give 0.5 cc of tetanus toxoid, the medical assistant

cubic centimeter

will inject one half of a *_____ .

ANSWER COLUMN

10.76

Do the work on this frame using the table on page 383.
Build words that mean
one hundred meters

hecto/meter
hek **tom'** ə ter

_____/_____ (hm);
one hundredth of a meter

centi/meter
sen' ti mē ter

_____/_____ (cm);
one hundred grams

hecto/gram
hek' to gram

_____/_____ (hg);
one hundredth of a gram

centi/gram
sen' ti gram

_____/_____ (cg);
one thousandth of a liter

milli/liter
mil' ə lē ter

_____/_____;
Good work!

Prefixes representing place often cause difficulty in word building because of their similarity. Use this information carefully while working through Frames 10.77–10.109.

Prefix	Meaning	Sense of Meaning
ab-	from	away from
de-	from	down from or from—resulting in less than
ex-	from	out from

10.77

away from

Recall ab/duction and ad/duction. You have already learned **ab-** is the opposite of **ad-**. ad- means toward; **ab-** means _____.

10.78

away from

away from

Ab/duct/ion (ab **duk'** shun) means moving away from the midline.
Ab/norm/al means going *_____ normal.
Ab/or/al means away from the mouth. Ab/errant (ab **er'** ənt) means wandering
*_____ the normal course.

10.79

ab/duct/ion
ab **duk'** shun

ab/norm/al
ab **nor'** məl

ab/errant
ab **air'** ant
ab' er ant

Swinging the arm away from the side of the body is

_____/_____/_____.
A sign or symptom that is unusual is

_____/_____/_____.
A blood vessel that is not located where it should be is an

_____/_____ vessel.

ANSWER COLUMN

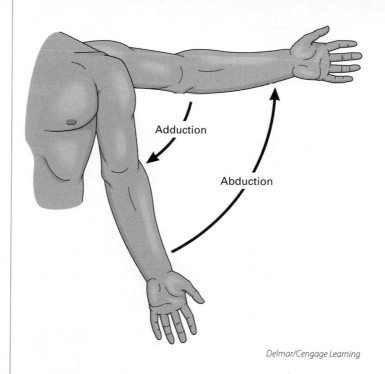

Adduction

Abduction

Delmar/Cengage Learning

10.80

away from

away from

An ab/irritant is something that takes irritation *_____
the patient. Ab/lact/ation means takes the baby *_____
the breastfeeding or the cessation of milk secretion.

10.81

ab/ort/ion

a **bôr'** shən

ab/ort/ed

Ab/ort was, literally, built by joining **ab-** to a word part meaning to be born (Latin: *oriri,* to be born). A naturally occurring termination of pregnancy (miscarriage) is

called a spontaneous _____/_____/_____.
In an induced abortion, the products of conception are taken away from the

uterus or _____/_____/_____.

10.82

**DICTIONARY
EXERCISE**

Look up the following terms that begin with **ab-** in your medical dictionary and
write their definitions below.

ab/duction   _____

ab/lation   _____

ab/rasion   _____

ab/sorption   _____
ab/oral   _____

ab/scess   _____

ab/sence   _____

ab/stinence   _____

ANSWER COLUMN

INFORMATION FRAME

10.83

Three types of wounds are lacerations (cuts), contusions (bruises), and abrasions (scrapes).

10.84

away from

ab/rasion

a **brā′** shən

To ab/rade (a **brād′**) the skin is to scrape some of the skin

*_____ the surface of the body. A scrape type

of injury is called an _____/_____.

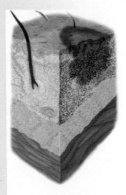

A. Bruise, also known as a contusion, results from damage to the soft tissues and blood vessels, which causes bleeding beneath the skin surface. A bruise in a light-skinned individual will change from red to purple to greenish yellow before fading. In a dark-skinned person, the bruise will first look dark red, then darker red, brown, or purple, and slowly fade.

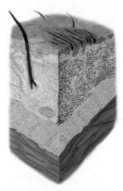

B. Abrasion, also known as a scrape or rug burn, results when the outer layer of skin is scraped or rubbed away. Exposure of nerve endings makes this type of wound painful, and the presence of debris from the scraped surface (rug fibers, gravel, sand) makes abrasions highly susceptible to infection.

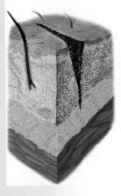

C. Laceration, cut, or incision, are caused by sharp objects such as knives or glass, or from trauma due to a strike from a blunt object that opens the skin, such as a baseball bat. If the wound is deep, the cut may bleed profusely; if nerve endings are exposed, it could also be painful.

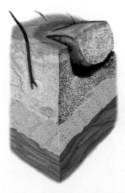

D. Avulsion results when the skin or tissue is torn away from the body, either partially or completely. The bleeding and pain depends on the depth of tissue affected.

Skin Injuries *Delmar/Cengage Learning*

STUDYWARE™ CONNECTION

View an animation on *Tissue Repair* on your **StudyWARE™ CD-ROM**.

ANSWER COLUMN

	10.85
ab/lation ab **lā'** shun	End/o/metr/ial ab/lation is a surgical procedure that destroys (takes away) the uterine lining. A special cutting instrument may be used with a hyster/o/scope to perform endometrial _____ / _____ .
	10.86
take away, destroy	Endo/venous ab/lation is used to *_____ the varicosed vein by collapsing the vessel wall. **NOTE:** Refer back to Unit 8 Case Study on page 305.
	10.87
ab	These gynecologic procedures get pretty technical for the nonsurgeon, but remember, the part of the term ablation that means something is taken away is _____ .
	10.88
from	**de-** is another prefix that means _____ .
	10.89
down from	One who de/scends the stairs comes down from a higher level. A de/scend/ing nerve tract comes *_____ the brain.
	10.90
de/cid/uous dē **sij'** o͞o əs	De/ciduous leaves fall from a tree. "Baby teeth" that fall from a child's mouth to make room for permanent teeth are called _____ / _____ / _____ teeth.
	10.91
deciduous	There are thirty-two secondary (permanent) and twenty primary (_____) teeth.
	10.92
from	When water is taken from a moist substance, the substance has less water. De/hydr/ation takes water _____ a wet substance.

**Primary teeth
(deciduous, baby
teeth)** *Delmar/Cengage Learning*

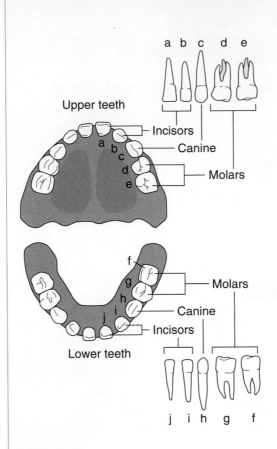

Upper teeth

a b c d e

Incisors
Canine
Molars

a b c d e

Lower teeth

f g h i j

Molars
Canine
Incisors

j i h g f

10.93

de/hydr/ation
dē hī **drā**′ shən

When water is taken from plums to make prunes, de/hydr/ation occurs. When
water is taken from a cell, _____ / _____ / _____
also occurs.

10.94

de/hydr/ated
dē hī **drā**′ tid

When something is dehydrated, it has less water than it did before. When
water is lost from the body due to excessive vomiting or diarrhea, the patient
is _____ / _____ / _____ .

10.95

dehydration

Vomiting can cause dehydration. A high fever can also cause

_____ .

10.96

de/calci/fication
dē kal′ si fi **kā**′ shən

When calcium is removed from the bones, there is less calcium than before. This
process is called _____ / _____ / _____ .

10.97

decalcification

De/calci/fication can occur from many causes. When a pregnant woman does
not eat enough calcium for the growing baby, her own bones will be robbed of
calcium, and _____ will occur.

ANSWER COLUMN

10.98

decalcification

Because vitamin D helps control calcium metabolism, inadequate vitamin D in the diet can account for some _____.

10.99

decalcification

Oste/o/por/osis may occur in postmenopausal women due to _____ of the bones.

10.100

out from

ex- also means from, but in the sense of *_____.

10.101

out

ex/cis/ed

ek **sīz'** d

To ex/cise is to cut _____ and remove a part. A diseased gallbladder may be _____/_____/_____.

10.102

from

To ex/hale (ex/pire) is to breathe out waste matter _____ the body.

10.103

ex/cretion

eks **krē'** shən

Ex/cretion is the process of ex/pelling (or getting out from the body) a substance. Expelling urine is urinary _____/_____.

10.104

excretion

excretion

Expelling carbon dioxide is respiratory _____.

Expelling sweat is dermal _____.

10.105

excretion

excretion

Expelling menses is menstrual _____. Expelling fecal matter is gastrointestinal (GI) _____.

10.106

SPELL
CHECK

Excretions are usually waste substances. Secretions, such as hormones, are useful substances, so do not use them as synonyms. You may think "exit—out," "keep the secret—in."

10.107

ex/tract/ion

eks **trak'** shən

An ex/traction is a procedure in which something is pulled out. When all of a patient's teeth have to be pulled out, it is called a full-mouth _____/_____/_____(FME).

ANSWER COLUMN

10.108

Recall the word flexion, meaning to bend or shorten. The opposite of flexion is ex/tension, meaning to straighten or lengthen. Bending flexes the arm.

ex/tends
eks **tendz'**

Straightening _____/_____ the arm.

10.109

Contracting the biceps muscle of the upper arm causes flex/ion of the arm.

ex/tens/ion
eks **ten'** shun

Relaxing this muscle causes _____/_____/_____.

10.110

Try to work this summary frame without referring to page 388.
Give the prefix meaning from in the following sense:

ab-

away from _____;

ex-

out from _____;

de-

down from or from, resulting in less than _____.

10.111

iso- is used in words to mean equal or the same. Something that is iso/metr/ic

equal

is of _____ dimensions.

10.112

equal

Something that is iso/cellular is composed of cells of _____ size.

10.113

An isotonic solution has the same osmotic pressure as red blood cells. Normal

iso/ton/ic
ī sō **ton'** ik

saline is an _____/_____/_____ solution.

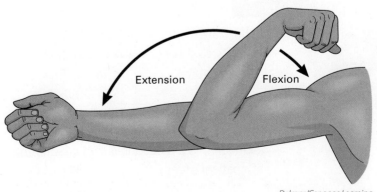

Extension   Flexion

Delmar/Cengage Learning

ANSWER COLUMN

10.114

isotonic

Intra/ven/ous glucose is another _____ solution.

10.115

isotonic

Any solution that will not destroy red blood cells because it is of equal osmotic pressure is an _____ solution.

10.116

higher

lower

same or equal

Hyper/tonic solutions have a _____ osmotic pressure than blood cells, hypo/tonic solutions have a _____ osmotic pressure than blood cells, and iso/tonic solutions have the _____ osmotic pressure as blood cells.
Good try!

10.117

DICTIONARY EXERCISE

Use your dictionary to look up the following terms about types of movement of solids, liquids, and gases.

diffusion _____

osmosis _____

filtration _____

10.118

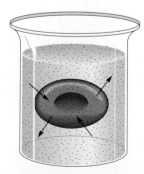

TAKE A CLOSER LOOK

Many physiologic processes rely on the movement of fluids and substances in and out of the cells and bloodstream. You may think it would be nice if you could learn through osmosis just by holding this book.

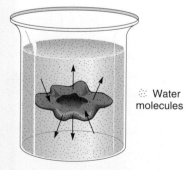

✦ Water molecules

Hypertonic solution (sea-water) a red blood cell will shrink and wrinkle up because water molecules are moving out of the cell.

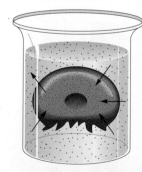

Hypotonic solution (fresh-water) a red blood cell will swell and burst because water molecules are moving into the cell.

Isotonic solution (human blood serum) a red blood cell remains unchanged, because the movement of water molecules into and out of the cell are the same.

Movement of water molecules through membranes in solutions of different osmolalities *Delmar/Cengage Learning*

ANSWER COLUMN

10.119

Build words meaning

fingers or toes of equal length

iso/dactyl/ism
ī sō **dak'** til izm

_____/_____/ism;

pertaining to equal temperature

iso/therm/al (ic)
ī sō **thûr'** məl (ik)

_____/_____/_____.

10.120

iso- is a prefix for equal. **an-** is a prefix meaning without or lack of. Something that is without equality is unequal. The combining form for unequal is

aniso

_____.

10.121

unequal

Aniso/mastia means that a woman's breasts are of _____ size.

10.122

Mastos (or *mazos*) is the Greek word for breast. Inflammation of the breast is mast/itis. Surgical excision of part or all of the breast is a

mast/ectomy
mast **ek'** tōm ē

_____/_____.

10.123

mastectomy

Radical and simple are the two main types of surgery for excising diseased breast

tissue or _____.

10.124

Build a term that means a cancerous tumor of the breast

mast/o/carcin/oma
mast' ō kär si **nō'** mə

_____/_____/_____/_____. See the case study on mastectomy at the end of this unit.

10.125

WORD ORIGINS

A legendary tribe of female warriors in Asia Minor were known to have removed one breast so that they could more powerfully draw their bows. They were named the Amazons, meaning without a breast (a, *without;* mazos, *breast*). In the 1500s, a Spanish explorer named a river the Amazon after doing battle with a South American tribe that included its women in the fight.

10.126

Aniso/cyt/osis means that cells are of unequal sizes. This word is commonly limited to red blood cells in medical usage. A word indicating a condition of

aniso/cyt/osis
an ī' sō sī **tō'** sis

inequality in cell size is _____/_____/_____.

ANSWER COLUMN

10.127

anisocytosis

Normal red blood cells are the same size (7.2 μm). An abnormal condition resulting in unequal size of red blood cells is _____.

10.128

anisocytosis

Red blood cells are formed in the bone marrow. An unhealthy bone marrow can result in unequal red blood cells, or _____.

Use the following information to work Frames 10.129–10.155. This is another group of prefixes of place.

Prefix	Meaning	Differentiation
dia-	through, complete	used with the combining forms for medical terminology
per-	through	prefix from Latin used more often in ordinary English
peri-	around	prefix from Greek used with the combining forms for medical terminology
circum-	around	Latin prefix used more often in ordinary English

10.129

around the tonsil

Peri/articular means around articulations or joints. Peri/tonsill/ar means

*_____.

10.130

around the colon or
    pertaining to around
    the colon

Peri/col/ic means *_____

_____.

10.131

peri/chondr/al
per i **kon'** drəl

peri/odont/al
per i ō **don'** təl

Peri/odont/al means pertaining to diseases of the support structures around (**peri-**) the teeth (**odont/o**). A word that means around a cartilage is

_____/_____/_____. Gum disease may require

_____/_____/_____ surgery.

ANSWER COLUMN

10.132

Build words meaning
inflammation around a gland

peri/aden/itis
per′ i ad en ī′ tis

_____/_____/_____;

inflammation around the vagina

peri/colp/itis
per′ i kol **pī**′ tis

_____/_____/_____;

inflammation around the liver

peri/hepat/itis
per′ i hep ə **tī**′ tis

_____/_____/_____;

excision of tissue (pericardium) around the heart

peri/cardi/ectomy
per′ i kär′ dē **ek**′ tō mē

_____/_____/_____.

10.133

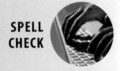

SPELL CHECK

para- and **peri-** are similar prefixes. They are often confused as homonyms (sound alike) and as synonyms (mean the same). They are seldom interchangeable and you should look up terms that begin with **para-** and **peri-** in your medical dictionary before you use them, just to make sure. Here are some patterns that may help.
para- is used more often for conditions with **-ia**, **-osis**, **-itis**, and **-oma** suffixes, as in paranoia and para-appendicitis.
para- is also used as a chemical name prefix in para-aminobenzoic acid.
peri- is a common anatomic term prefix as in peri/cardium, peri/toneum, and peri/osteum.

10.134

Another prefix that means around is **circum-**.
Moving toward is ad/duction. Moving away is ab/duction.
Moving around (circular motion) is

circum/duct/ion
sûr kəm **duk**′ shən

_____/_____/_____.

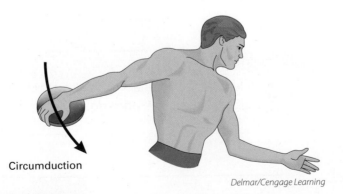

Circumduction

Delmar/Cengage Learning

10.135

around

Circum/ocul/ar means _____ the eyes.

ANSWER COLUMN

around	**10.136** Circum/oral means _____ the mouth.
circum/scrib/ed **sûr′ kəm skrīb′d**	**10.137** Circumscribed means limited in space (as though a line were drawn around it). A hive is limited in space—does not spread. A hive may be called a _____/_____/_____ wheal.
circumscribed	**10.138** A boil is also limited in the space it covers. A boil is a _____ lesion.
circumscribed	**10.139** Round-shaped pimples and pustules are also _____ lesions.

SURFACE LESIONS

A.

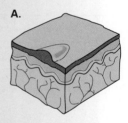

Papule
Solid, elevated lesion less than 0.5 cm in diameter
Example
Warts, elevated nevi, papilloma

B.

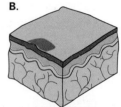

Macule
Localized changes in skin color of less than 1 cm in diameter
Example
Freckle, age spot

C.

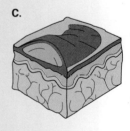

Wheal
Localized edema in the epidermis causing irregular elevation that may be red or pale
Example
Insect bite or a hive

D.

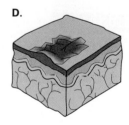

Crust
Dried serum, blood, or pus on the surface of the skin
Example
Impetigo, scab

FLUID FILLED

E.

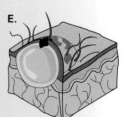

Boil (Furuncle)
Skin infection originating in gland or hair follicle
Example
Furunculosis, folliculitis

F.

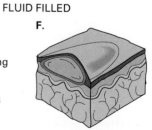

Vesicle
Blister
Bullae
Same as a vesicle only greater than 0.5 cm
Example
Contact dermatitis, large second-degree burns, bulbous impetigo, pemphigus

G.

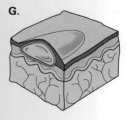

Pustule
Vesicles or bullae that become filled with pus, usually described as less than 0.5 cm in diameter
Example
Acne, impetigo, furuncles, carbuncles

H.

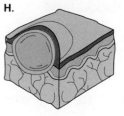

Cyst
Encapsulated fluid-filled or a semi-solid mass in the subcutaneous tissue or dermis
Example
Sebaceous cyst, epidermoid cyst

Lesions *Delmar/Cengage Learning*

STUDY WARE™ CONNECTION

After completing this unit, you can play a Spelling Bee game to help you learn the pronunciation of terms presented in the chapter or play other interactive games on your **StudyWARE™ CD-ROM** that will help you learn the content in this chapter.

ANSWER COLUMN

	10.140
to cut around (actually a surgical procedure for removing the foreskin of the penis)	From the word parts you have already learned, think of the meaning for the following term and write it below. circum/cision *_____ _____ _____
	10.141
circum/cis/ion **sûr′** kum si shun	The pediatrician performed a _____/_____/_____ on the new baby boy soon after birth.
	10.142
dia	There are two prefixes that mean through. The one that you would expect to use more often in medical terminology is _____.
	10.143
through through dia/rrhea dia/therm/y **dī′** əthûr mē	You have already learned dia/gnosis, which means knowing _____, and dia/thermy, which means heating _____. Build a term that means flow through _____/_____; heat through _____/_____/_____.
	10.144
	-esis is a suffix meaning action or process. Dia/phor/esis is an action of profuse sweating. Diaphoretic is the adjectival form. Can you think of the reason for using **dia-** as the prefix in these terms?
	10.145
di/ur/esis **dī** yōō rē′ sis	Arthr/o/desis is the action of immobilizing (binding) a joint. Hemat/o/poi/esis is the process of forming blood. The process of causing urine to flow through more rapidly is _____/_____/_____. **NOTE:** In the term diuretic the **dia-** is shortened to **di-** and still means through.

ANSWER COLUMN

10.146

A substance that causes increase in urine output (water excretion) is called a

di/ur/etic
di yōō re′ tik

_____/_____/_____.

10.147

From what you have just learned in the past few frames, decipher and recall the meaning of this condition.

noct/urnal en/ur/esis

nighttime bedwetting

* _____

10.148

Per- is a prefix meaning through. Per/for/ation (noun) means a puncture or hole.

through

Per/for/ate (verb) means the act of making a hole _____ something.

10.149

The past tense verb of per/for/ate is per/for/ated.
An ulcer that has eaten a hole through the stomach wall is

per/for/ated
per′ fôr ā t′d

a _____/_____/_____ ulcer.

per/for/ate
per′ fôr āt

An ulcer may also _____/_____/_____
(present tense verb) the stomach wall.

10.150

per/for/ation
per fôr ā′ shən

When ulcers make a hole in an organ, a _____/_____/_____ (noun) is formed.

10.151

Per/cuss/ion (noun) means a striking through. Read the section on percussion in a dictionary. Analyze the word here.

per/cuss/ion
per **kush′** ən

_____/_____/_____

NOTE: A drum is a percussion instrument that is struck to make sounds.

10.152

Supplying tissues with oxygen and nutrients through the blood supply or other tissue fluids is called per/fus/ion. The passage of blood through the arteries of the

per/fus/ion
per **fyōō′** shun

heart is called coronary _____/_____/_____.

10.153

per/fuse
per **fyōōz′**

A per/fus/ate is a fluid used to _____/_____ (verb form) tissues.

1. stethoscope
2. penlight
3. guaiac/occult blood test developer
4. guaiac/occult blood test
5. flexible tape measure
6. urine specimen container
7. metal nasal speculum
8. tuning fork
9. percussion hammer
10. tongue depressor
11. ophthalmoscope head
12. okastic ear/nose speculum
13. otoscope head attached to base handle
14. sphygmomanometer
15. latex gloves

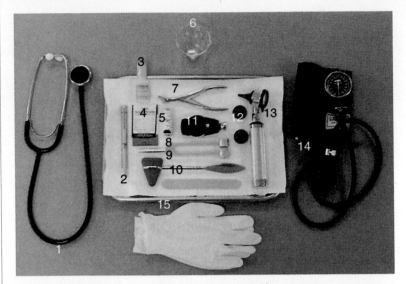

Instruments and supplies used in the physical examination for auscultation, percussion, inspection, and palpation
Delmar/Cengage Learning

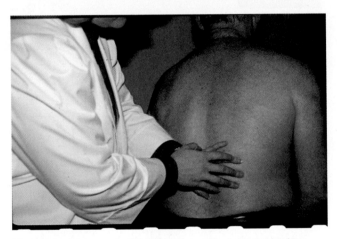

The examiner uses blunt percussion to examine the kidney *Delmar/Cengage Learning*

10.154

per, dia

circum, peri

Summarize. Two prefixes meaning through are _____ and _____.

Two prefixes meaning around are _____ and _____.

10.155

Look up the following terms in your dictionary. Notice that medical specialists use the word-building system to name new procedures. Write the meaning of each term.

through the skin

across the lumen

heart

vessel repair

per/cutane/ous *_____;

trans/lumin/al *_____;

coron/ary *_____;

angi/o/plasty *_____;
(abbreviation: PTCA).

ANSWER COLUMN

10.156

Necros is a Greek word meaning corpse. **necr/o** is used in words pertaining to

death. Necr/o/cyt/osis is cellular _____.

death

A necr/o/parasite is one that lives on _____ organic matter.

dead

10.157

Necr/osis refers to a condition in which dead tissue is surrounded with healthy

necr/osis
ne **krō′** sis

tissue. Infections can cause _____/_____ of the bones.

When blood supply is cut off from a toe, gangrene sets in. This results in

necrosis

_____ (death) of the toe's tissue.

10.158

Build words meaning
excision of dead tissue

necr/ectomy
ne **krek′** tō mē

_____/_____;
incision into (dissection of) a dead body

necr/o/tomy
ne **krot′** ō mē

_____/_____/_____;
abnormal fear of death

necr/o/phobia
ne krō **fōb′** ē ə

_____/_____/_____.

10.159

There are three ways of saying post/mort/em (after death) examination. One

necr/o
nek′ rop sē

is aut/o/psy. Another is _____/_____/psy and the third is
necr/o/scopy.

10.160

aut/o/psy *or*
aw′ top sē

If the cause of death is unknown, a(n) _____/_____/_____

necr/o/scopy *or*
ne **kros′** kō pē

may be required to examine the body.

necropsy *or*
postmortem exam

10.161

Cyan/o/tic is the adjectival form of cyanosis. Build the adjectival form of necrosis:

necr/o/tic
ne **krō′** tik

_____/_____/_____.

10.162

De/bride/ment (dā brēd **mən′**) of dead tissue is often done for patients with severe

necr/o/tic
ne **krō′** tik

burns. The _____/_____/_____ (dead) tissue is removed.

CASE STUDY INVESTIGATION (CSI)

Autopsy (Postmortem Exam)

External Examination: The body is that of a normally developed, well-nourished 65-year-old male who appears appropriate for his reported age. The body length is 70 inches and weight 176.6 lbs and is well preserved in the absence of embalming. **Lividity** is posterior and fixed. **Rigidity** is complete. The head is **normocephalic** and balding of the vertex and frontal scalp is noted with straight gray hair up to 2 inches long. No **petechiae** are seen on the conjunctivae or sclerae. The **periorbital** regions are not remarkable. The nose is intact to palpation. The teeth are natural. No oral or buccal mucosal lesions are seen. The neck, chest, and abdomen have normal contour without deformity. All four extremities are present and normally developed. The penis is **circumcised** and both testicles **descended**.

CSI Vocabulary Challenge

Use a medical dictionary to analyze the term listed from the case study. Divide the term into word parts by drawing in the slashes and write the definition in the space provided.

autopsy   _____

postmortem   _____

lividity   _____

rigidity   _____

normocephalic _____

petechiae   _____

periorbital   _____

circumcised   _____

descended   _____

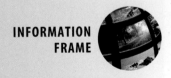

INFORMATION FRAME

10.163

-**philia** is the opposite of -**phobia**. -**phobia** is abnormal fear of; -**philia** is abnormal or unusual attraction to.

10.164

Words that can end in -**phobia**, can also end in -**philia**.
Necr/o/phobia is an abnormal fear of dead bodies. Necr/o/philia is

abnormal attraction to dead bodies

*_____.

(continued)

ANSWER COLUMN

hydro/phobia
(You pronounce)

hydro/philia
hī drō **fil'** ē ə

Morbid fear of water is

_____ / _____.

Strong attraction to water is

_____ / _____.

| 10.165 |

Think of the meaning while building words opposite of

hemat/o/philia

pyr/o/philia

aer/o/philia

aut/o/philia
(You pronounce)

hemat/o/phobia _____ / _____ / _____ ;

pyr/o/phobia _____ / _____ / _____ ;

aer/o/phobia _____ / _____ / _____ ;

aut/o/phobia _____ / _____ / _____ .

| 10.166 |

attraction to, liking,
    loving

phil/o is the combining form that means

* _____.

| 10.167 |

philosopher, philosophy,
    Philadelphia, etc.

Can you think of a nonmedical word that involves **phil/o**? If so, write it here:

_____.

Abbreviation	Meaning
†	death
μm*, mcm	micrometer
2 h pc, 2 hr pc, 2° pc	two hours postcibum (after meal)
2 h pg, 2 hr pg, 2° pg	two hours postglucose (after drinking glucose)
2 h pp, 2 hr pp, 2° pp	two hours postprandial (after meal)
Ab 1,2,3, AB	abortion (number of)
AIDS	acquired immunodeficiency syndrome
bid	*bis in die*, twice a day
Ca	calcium
cc*	cubic centimeter(s)
cm	centimeter
CST	certified surgical technologist
D/W	dextrose in water
DPT, DTP, DTaP	diphtheria, pertussis, tetanus (vaccine)
exc	excision
FBS	fasting blood sugar
FME	full mouth extraction
grav 1,2,3	pregnancy (number of)

(continued)

ANSWER COLUMN

Abbreviation	Meaning
GHB	glycosylated hemoglobin
GTT	glucose tolerance test (3 hr–5hr)
Hb A1c, Hgb A1c	Hemoglobin A1c (test)
HepB	hepatitis B vaccine
Hib	*Haemophilus influenzae* vaccine
HIV	human immunodeficiency virus
HPV	human papilloma virus
hs*	hour of sleep, bed time
I&D	incision and drainage
IDDM	insulin dependent diabetes mellitus
IPV	inactivated poliovirus vaccine (injectable)
kg	kilogram
LAVH	laparoscopically assisted vaginal hysterectomy
mcg, μg*	microgram
mg	milligram
mgdl or mg/dL	milligram/deciliter(s)
ml or mL	milliliter
mm	millimeter
MMR	measles, mumps, rubella (vaccine)
mono	mononucleosis
NIDDM	noninsulin dependent diabetes mellitus
NS	normal saline (isotonic saline)
para 1,2,3	live births past 20 weeks gestation (numbers of)
PCV	pneumococcal vaccine
PTCA	percutaneous transluminal coronary angioplasty
q 2 h, q 2 hr, q 2°*	*quaque 2 hora*, every 2 hours
qid	*quarter in die*, four times a day
SA, S&A	sugar and acetone
Td	Tetanus toxoid (vaccine)
tid	*ter in die*, three times a day
Var	chickenpox vaccine (*Varicella zoster*)

Also, study the weights and measures abbeviations in Appendix B.

*Abbreviation use warning. These abbreviations have been judged to be dangerous and should not be used.

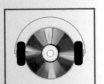

To complete your study of this unit, work the **Review Activities** on the following pages. Also, listen to the Audio CD that accompanies *Medical Terminology: A Programmed Systems Approach,* 10th edition, and practice your pronunciation.

STUDYWARE™ CONNECTION

To help you learn the content in this chapter, take a practice quiz or play an interactive game on your **StudyWARE™ CD-ROM**.

REVIEW ACTIVITIES

PREFIX AND WORD

Write the prefix that represents the direction, then build a word using that prefix.

Prefix   Word

_____ 1. away from   move away from
                                    the body   _____

_____ 2. down from   part of the aorta that moves
                                    down from the heart   _____

_____ 3. out of   to cut out   _____

_____ 4. equal/same   equal osmotic
                                    pressure (solution)   _____

_____ 5. unequal   condition of unequal sized cells _____

_____ 6. through   treatment by heating
                                    through tissues   _____

_____ 7. through   to strike through
                                    (part of physical examination) _____

_____ 8. around   membrane around the heart _____

_____ 9. around   circular motion   _____

_____ 10. under   below the tongue   _____

CIRCLE AND CORRECT

Circle the correct answer for each question. Then, check your answers in Appendix E.

1. Word root for abdominal wall
   a. abdomeno   b. lapar
   c. hepar   d. hyster

2. Suffix for destruction
   a. -tripsy   b. -stasis
   c. -pexy   d. -lysis

3. Combining form for sweat
   a. hidro   b. hydro
   c. sudoriferous   d. hyper

4. Suffix meaning in the urine
   a. -urea   b. -uria
   c. -uric   d. -uro

5. Term indicating high blood sugar
   a. glycogen   b. hypoglycemia
   c. hypertension   d. hyperglycemia

6. Suffix meaning producing or generating
   a. -lysis   b. -trophy
   c. -genesis   d. -stasis

7. Physician specialist in immunity
   a. immunology   b. immunologist
   c. immunization   d. immunotherapist

8. An autologous donor gives blood
   a. to a family member b. to self
   c. to a friend   d. frequently

9. The opposite of -philia
   a. hemato   b. genesis
   c. phobia   d. phagia

10. Word part indicating pregnancy
    a. para   b. genesis
    c. partum   d. gravida

REVIEW ACTIVITIES

COUNT WITH PREFIXES

Count and write the prefix. Then build a word using that prefix.

Prefix   Word

_____ 1. none   no pregnancies   _____

_____ 2. first   first live birth   _____

_____ 3. one   one cell   _____

_____ 4. two   two branches
                                 (use your dictionary)   _____

_____ 5. three   three sided   _____

_____ 6. four   paralysis, four limbs   _____

_____ 7. five   five infants born at the same
                                 time (use your dictionary)   _____

_____ 8. six   sixth pregnancy   _____

_____ 9. seven   seventh live birth   _____

_____ 10. eight   person 80 years old
                                 (use your dictionary)   _____

_____ 11. nine   ninth pregnancy   _____

_____ 12. ten   ten liters   _____

_____ 13. one hundred(th) 1/100th of a meter   _____

_____ 14. one thousand(th) 1,000 calories   _____

_____ 15. many   many glands   _____

SELECT AND CONSTRUCT PART I

Select the correct word parts from the following list and construct medical terms that represent the given meaning.

cyst/o/ic	deca	deci	emia	enter(o)(y)	gluco
glyco	gram	hecto	hidro	hyper	hypo
itis	kilo	laparo	lipid	lysis	mammary
meter	milli	(o)sis	ous	peri	plasm
pyro	retro	rrhea	scope (ic)		

1. instrument for looking into the abdomen _____

2. condition of heat (fever) _____

3. excessive sweating _____

REVIEW ACTIVITIES

4. breakdown of sugar _____

5. inflammation around the bladder _____

6. low blood sugar _____

7. containing sugar and fat _____

8. ten grams _____

9. one thousandth of a meter _____

10. behind the breast _____

SELECT AND CONSTRUCT PART II

Select the correct word parts from the following list and construct medical terms that represent the given meaning.

a(b)	aden	a(n)	aniso	a/t/ion	blat	bort
brade	bras	calcific	carcin	cardium	circum	cision
coction	cre(t)	cussion	cyt	de	dia	duct
ecto	ex	fusion	hale	hepat	hydr	irritant
iso	itis	lact/ation	lation	lepsy	mast/o	narco
oma	osis	per	peri	rade	tic	tion
tonic						

1. removal of waste from the body _____

2. to take away the products of conception _____

3. sleep attacks (seizures) _____

4. cancer of the breast _____

5. take away skin by scraping (verb) _____

6. inflammation around the liver _____

7. drug that produces sleep _____

8. process of taking calcium from bone _____

9. IV solutions are _____ compared to blood cells _____

10. process of cutting around (usually the foreskin for removal) _____

11. take away tissue (i.e., endometrial _____) _____

12. striking through (i.e., hammer) _____

13. condition of cells of unequal size _____

14. taking the baby away from the breast (weaning) _____

15. condition of water taken away from the body _____

16. process of supplying blood through tissue _____

REVIEW ACTIVITIES

17. circular motion _____

18. breathe out _____

19. destroying and scraping away _____

20. membrane around the heart _____

MATCHING

Match the following skin lesions with a synonym or example.

_____ 1. pustule   a. scab

_____ 2. papule   b. sore

_____ 3. macule   c. pimple

_____ 4. vesicle   d. blister

_____ 5. crust   e. boil

_____ 6. ulcer   f. hive

_____ 7. wheal   g. freckle

_____ 8. furuncle   h. papilloma

DEFINE AND DISSECT

Give a brief definition, and dissect each term listed into its word parts in the space provided. Check your answers by referring to the frame listed in parentheses and your medical dictionary. Then listen to the Audio CD to practice pronunciation.

1. laparotomy (10.6)

         _____ / _____ / _____
                 rt   v   suffix

    meaning _____

2. laparohepatotomy (10.7)

     _____ / _____ / _____ / _____ / _____
        rt   v   rt   v   suffix

    _____

3. pyrolysis (10.11)

         _____ / _____ / _____
                 rt   v   suffix

    _____

4. pyrexia (10.10)

                 _____ / _____
                      rt   suffix

    _____

5. glucogenesis (10.20)

       _____ / _____ / _____ / _____
         rt   v   rt   suffix

    _____

REVIEW ACTIVITIES

6. glycogenesis (10.20)

_____ / _____ / _____ / _____
rt   v   rt   suffix

7. hypoglycemia (10.25)

_____ / _____ / _____
pre   rt   suffix

8. glucosuria (10.18)

_____ / _____
rt   suffix

9. laparoscopic (10.5)

_____ / _____ / _____ / _____
rt   v   rt   suffix

10. glycoprotein (10.18)

_____ / _____ / _____
rt   v   rt

11. glycolipid (10.29)

_____ / _____ / _____
rt   v   rt

12. immunology (10.30)

_____ / _____ / _____
rt   v   suffix

13. immunodeficiency (10.32)

_____ / _____ / _____
rt   v   rt/suffix

14. autoimmunity (10.44)

_____ / _____ / _____ / _____
pre   v   rt   suffix

15. autophagia (10.45)

_____ / _____ / _____
pre   v   rt/suffix

16. mononucleosis (10.53)

_____ / _____ / _____
pre   rt   suffix

17. multiparous (10.60)

_____ / _____ / _____
pre   rt   suffix

REVIEW ACTIVITIES

18. primigravida (10.64)

_____/_____
pre   rt/suffix

_____

19. kilometer (10.69)

_____/_____
pre   suffix

_____

20. centigram (10.72)

_____/_____
pre   rt

_____

21. quadriplegia (table)

_____/_____
pre   suffix

_____

22. sexagenarian (table)

_____/_____/_____
pre   rt/suffix

_____

23. septuplets (table)

_____/_____
pre   rt/suffix

_____

24. immunization (10.31)

_____/_____/_____
rt   v   suffix

_____

25. autohemotherapy (10.46)

_____/_____/_____/_____/_____
pre   v   rt   v   suffix

_____

26. monocytosis (10.54)

_____/_____/_____
pre   rt   suffix

_____

27. hemiplegia (table)

_____/_____
pre   suffix

_____

28. deciliter (table)

_____/_____
pre   rt

_____

29. nullipara (10.69)

_____/_____
pre   rt/suffix

_____

REVIEW ACTIVITIES

30. bifurcation (table)

_____/_____/_____
pre   rt   suffix

31. aberrant (10.79)

_____/_____
pre   rt/suffix

32. abrasion (10.84)

_____/_____
pre   rt/suffix

33. deciduous (10.90)

_____/_____/_____
pre   rt   suffix

34. dehydrated (10.94)

_____/_____/_____
pre   rt   suffix

35. decalcification (10.96)

_____/_____/_____
pre   rt   suffix

36. excised (10.101)

_____/_____/_____
pre   rt   suffix

37. isotonic (10.113)

_____/_____/_____
pre   rt   suffix

38. anisocytosis (10.126)

_____/_____/_____
pre   rt   suffix

39. mastectomy (10.122)

_____/_____
rt   suffix

40. circumscribed (10.137)

_____/_____
pre   rt/suffix

41. perforated (10.149)

_____/_____/_____
pre   rt   suffix

REVIEW ACTIVITIES

42. diaphoresis (10.144)

_____/_____/_____
pre   rt   suffix

_____

43. percutaneous (10.155)

_____/_____/_____
pre   rt   suffix

_____

44. necrotic (10.161)

_____/_____/_____
rt   v   suffix

_____

45. necrophobia (10.158)

_____/_____/_____
rt   v   suffix

_____

46. circumcision (10.141)

_____/_____
pre   rt/suffix

_____

47. extension (10.109)

_____/_____
pre   rt/suffix

_____

48. flexion (10.109)

_____/_____
rt   suffix

_____

49. diuresis (10.145)

_____/_____/_____
pre   rt   suffix

_____

50. percussion (10.151)

_____/_____
pre   rt/suffix

_____

51. pericardiectomy (10.132)

_____/_____/_____
pre   rt   suffix

_____

52. ablation (10.85)

_____/_____
pre   rt/suffix

_____

53. perfusion (10.152)

_____/_____
pre   rt/suffix

_____

REVIEW ACTIVITIES

ABBREVIATION MATCHING PART I

Match the following abbreviations with their definition.

_____ 1. 2 h pc   a. sugar and acetone

_____ 2. GTT   b. noninsulin dependent diabetes (NIDDM)

_____ 3. FBS   c. quad

_____ 4. Type II diabetes   d. two hours after meal

_____ 5. S&A   e. acid-fast bacillus

_____ 6. Type I diabetes   f. fasting blood sugar

_____ 7. AB 2   g. glucose tolerance test

_____ 8. IPV   h. insulin dependent diabetes (IDDM)

_____ 9. mono   i. human immunodeficiency virus

_____ 10. HepB   j. diphtheria, pertussis, tetanus

_____ 11. AIDS   k. one

_____ 12. para 2   l. oral poliovirus vaccine

_____ 13. DPT   m. acute autoimmune disease

       n. herpes influenza virus

       o. two abortions

       p. acquired immunodeficiency syndrome

       q. mononucleosis

       r. hepatitis B vaccine

       s. two live births (viable)

       t. inactivated poliovirus vaccine

ABBREVIATIONS—WEIGHTS AND MEASURES

State the correct abbreviation for the following weights and measures.

_____ 1. kilogram

_____ 2. milligram

_____ 3. cubic centimeter

_____ 4. deciliter

_____ 5. millimeter

_____ 6. microgram

REVIEW ACTIVITIES

ABBREVIATION MATCHING PART II

Match the following abbreviations with their definition.

_____ 1. bid   .

_____ 2. q2h

_____ 3. PTCA

_____ 4. exc

_____ 5. hs

_____ 6. Ca++

_____ 7. tid

_____ 8. μm, mcm

a. every night

b. micrometer

c. three times a day

d. normal saline

e. parent-teacher agency

f. at bedtime

g. twice a day

h. every two hours

i. excision

j. calcium

k. full-mouth extraction

l. dextrose in water

m. percutaneous transluminal coronary angioplasty

n. millimeter(s)

ABBREVIATION FILL-INS

Fill in the blank with the correct abbreviation.

9. every four hours   _____

10. dextrose in water   _____

11. normal saline   _____

12. four times a day   _____

13. death (symbol)   _____

CASE STUDY

Write the term next to its meaning. Then draw slashes to analyze the word parts. Note the use of medical abbreviations. Look these up in your dictionary or find them in Appendix B. If you have any questions about the answers, refer to your medical dictionary or check with your instructor for the answers in Appendix E.

CASE STUDY 10-1

Mastectomy

Pt: 50-year-old female

Surgeon: Sharon Rooney-Gandy, D.O.

REVIEW ACTIVITIES

Preoperative Dx: **Multifocal** ductal **carcinoma in situ**, left breast

Postoperative Dx: Multifocal ductal carcinoma in situ, left breast, pathology pending

Operation performed: Left simple **mastectomy**

Preop History: The patient was noted to have calcifications on routine **mammogram**. She does not practice breast self-exam and felt no lumps herself. Upon needle localization left breast **biopsy**, she was found to have multifocal ductal carcinoma in situ, noncomedo type with tumor extending to margin of excision and **microcalcifications**. *Hx:* Grav 0, Para, AB 0, and is in menopause with history of ependymoma and radiation of her spine, paternal grandmother with bilateral breast cancer, paternal aunt with bilateral breast cancer. Physical examination of the right breast was essentially unremarkable. The left breast revealed a well-healed upper medial quadrant curvilinear incision from previous biopsy. There was no **retraction**, discharge, masses, or axillary nodes. After biopsy she was evaluated by an oncologist for treatment of carcinoma in situ. Dr. Peter, radiation oncologist, evaluated her for radiation therapy. It was felt best that the patient undergo simple mastectomy, not so much because of previous radiation therapy, but because of the residual multicalcifications remaining in her left breast. The patient did understand this. Because of her small breasts, we thought she would be best treated cosmetically with a left simple mastectomy. The patient tolerated the procedure well and was taken to the recovery room in satisfactory condition.

Procedure: The patient was taken to the operating room, given general **anesthesia**, prepped and draped in a **sterile** manner. Elliptical incisions were made in a horizontal fashion incorporating the previous biopsy site. The skin was incised with minor bleeding controlled using Bovie cautery. The breast tissue was **dissected** down to the pectoral fascia and up to the clavicle, elevating the superior skin flap. The lower skin flap was developed using Bovie cautery down to the pectoral fascia. The breast was excised using Bovie cautery, **hemostasis** secured with Bovie cautery. The incision was irrigated with saline. No other masses or **axillary** nodes could be palpated. The skin was closed with interrupted 4-0 Vicryl followed by a continuous **subcuticular** 4-0 Prolene. Prior to closing the skin a JP drain was placed through a separate stab incision. Steri-strips were applied and the drain was sutured in place. A sterile pressure dressing was applied. Postoperative condition was stable. The case was clean and elective.

1. pertaining to below the epidermis   _____

2. condition creating no sensation   _____

3. having more than one focus (location)   _____

4. type of cancer in one location   _____

5. was cut apart   _____

6. area under the arm   _____

7. control of blood flow   _____

8. excision of the breast   _____

9. breast x-ray   _____

10. absence of organisms   _____

11. pulling and holding back   _____

12. small calcium deposits   _____

13. examination of living tissue   _____

REVIEW ACTIVITIES

CROSSWORD PUZZLE

Check your answers by going back through the frames or checking the solution in Appendix F.

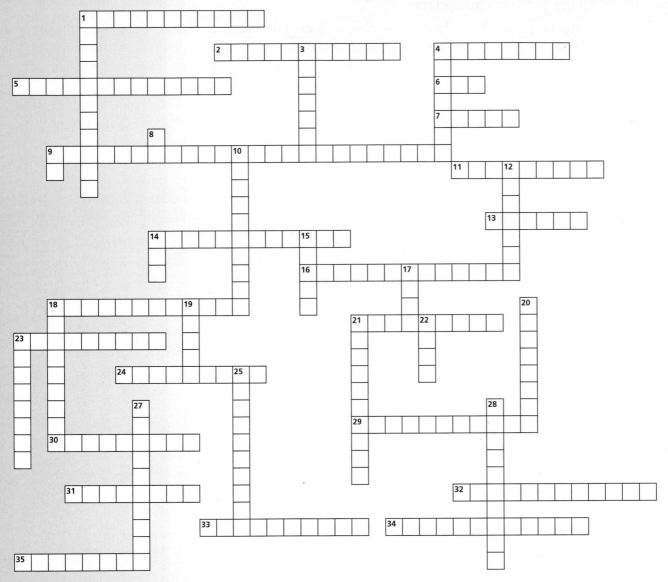

Across

1. condition of increase in monocyes
2. fear of water (rabies)
4. surgical destruction by scraping layers of tissue
5. pertaining to many capsules
6. three time a day
7. prefix for first
9. x-ray process, biliary and pancreatic vessels
11. make a hole (verb)
13. breathe out
14. across the lumen (blood vessel)
16. movement in a circle
18. immune response to one's self
21. teeth that fall out (primary)
23. movement toward the midline
24. 0.01 gram
29. loss of water
30. night (adjective)
31. removal
32. attraction to blood
33. excision of a breast
34. same length fingers or toes
35. scraping wound

Down

1. pertaining to many live births
3. fever
4. exam of a dead body
8. kilogram
9. symbol for calcium
10. seizures of sleep
12. bending
14. prefix for three
15. combining form for dead
17. prefix for one tenth
18. movement away from the body
19. prefix for none
20. termination of pregnancy
21. The _____ colon moves down.
22. prefix for ten
23. wandering from the norm
25. pertaining to self generating
27. striking or tapping
28. 0.001 meter

REVIEW ACTIVITIES

CROSSWORD PUZZLE

Check your answers by going back through the frames or checking the solution in Appendix F.

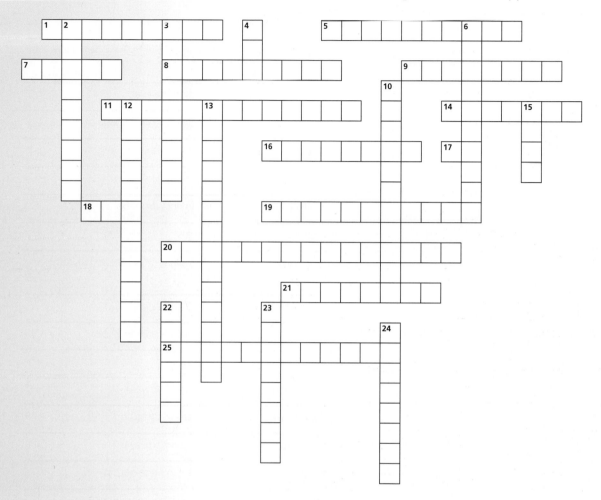

Across

1. make a hole in (verb)
5. seizures of sleep
7. combining form for dead
8. teeth that fall out (primary)
9. agent that causes diuresis
11. encircled
14. synonym for necropsy
16. seizure disorder
17. hour of sleep, at bedtime (abbr.)
18. excision (abbr.)
19. water loss (noun)
20. excision of the pericardium
21. wandering from the norm
25. loves blood

Down

2. waste removal
3. movement away from the midline
4. twice a day (abbr.)
6. striking to examine
10. different size breasts
12. same size digits
13. breast cancer
15. percutaneous transluminal coronary angioplasty (abbr.)
22. breathe out
23. termination of pregnancy
24. sleeping drug

REVIEW ACTIVITIES

GLOSSARY

abduction	movement away from the midline
aberrant	wandering away from the norm
ablactation	weaning a baby from the breast
ablation	takes away a layer or destroys a tissue layer
abnormal	unusual (not normal)
aboral	away from the mouth
abortion	termination of pregnancy
abrasion	scraping
adduction	movement toward the midline
aerophilia	attraction to air
anhidrosis	absence of sweating
anisocytosis	cells of unequal sizes
anisomastia	breasts of unequal size
autodermic	plastic surgery and grafting using one's own skin (dermatoplasty)
autodiagnosis	diagnosing one's self
autogenous	made by or from one's own tissues (adjective)
autograft	graft of tissue from one's own body
autohemotherapy	transfusion with one's own blood (autologous donor)
autoimmunity	reaction of immune response to one's own tissues
autologous	originating from one's self
autonomic	self-controlling part of the nervous system (adjective)
autophagia	biting one's self
autophilia	attraction to one's self
autophobia	abnormal fear of one's self, being alone
autopsy	necropsy, postmortem examination, exam to confirm cause of death
centigram	one hundredth of a gram (0.01 g)
centimeter	one hundredth of a meter (0.01m)

cholangio-pancreatography	X-ray of bile ducts and pancreatic ducts using contrast medium
circumduction	moving as to describe a circle with a body part
circumocular	encircling the eye
circumscribed	encircling or in the shape of a circle
cytoplasm	substance within the cell
decagram	ten grams
decalcification	calcium loss (from bone)
decaliter	ten liters
deciduous	falls down (primary teeth that come out)
decigram	one tenth of a gram (0.1 g)
deciliter	one tenth of a liter (0.1 L)
dehydration	water loss
descending	moving downward
diaphoresis	profuse sweating
diathermy	heat through tissues
diuresis	increase in urine output
diuretic	agent that causes diuresis
epilepsy	disorder characterized by seizures
excision	removing a body part
excretion	removal of waste (urination, defecation)
exhale	breathe out (expire)
extension	to straighten or lengthen a body part
extraction	removal or pulling out of a body part
flexion	to shorten or bend a body part
glycogenesis	formation of glycogen or sugar
glycohemoglobin	hemoglobin with attached glucose
hematophilia	attraction to blood
hidrosis	condition of sweating
hydrophilia	attraction to water

REVIEW ACTIVITIES

hydrophobia	fear of water (symptom of rabies)	necroparasite	organism that lives off dead tissue
hyperpyrexia	high fever	necrophobia	abnormal fear of dead bodies
hyperglycemia	high blood glucose level	necrotic	pertaining to necrosis (condition of dead tissue)
hypoglycemia	low blood glucose level	necrotomy	incision into dead tissue
immuno-deficiency	deficient (poor) immune system	nocturnal enuresis	bedwetting
immunotherapy	vaccination, immunization	nullipara	having no pregnancies carried to the third trimester
isocellular	equal size cells	omphalotomy	incision into the navel
isodactylism	digits the same length	percussion	striking or tapping
isometric	measures the same on all sides	percutaneous	through the skin
isotonic	osmotic pressure equal to the inside of a cell	perforation	puncturing
laparoscopy	examination of the abdomen with a scope	perfusion	supplying blood to tissues
laparotomy	incision into the abdomen	periarticular	area surrounding a joint
mastectomy	excision of breast tissue	pericardiectomy	excision of the membrane around the heart
mastocarcinoma	breast cancer	pericolic	area surrounding the colon
milligram (mg)	one thousandth of a gram (0.001 g)	perihepatitis	inflammation around the liver
millimeter (mm)	one thousandth of a meter (0.001 m)	peritonsillar	area surrounding the tonsils
monocyte	one cell (type of leukocyte)	postmortem	after death
monocytosis	increase in the number of monocytes	primigravida	first pregnancy
monoma	a single tumor	primipara	first live birth
monomyoplegia	paralysis of one muscle	pyrexia	fever (hyperthermia)
mononeural	involving one nerve	pyrolysis	destruction of tissue caused by fever
mononuclear	having one nucleus	pyromania	compulsion (madness) for setting fires
mononucleosis	viral infection causing monocytosis	pyrometer	thermometer
multicapsular	having more than one capsule (adjective)	pyrophilia	attraction to fire
multicellular	having or involving many cells (adjective)	pyrophobia	abnormal fear of fire
multiglandular	having or involving many glands (adjective)	pyrosis	heartburn
multinuclear	a cell having more than one nucleus (adjective)	pyrotoxin	poisonous by-product of metabolism created during fever
multipara	having many live births (born in third trimester)	transluminal	across the lumen
necrectomy	excision of dead tissue	vaccination	immunization
necrocytosis	condition of cell death or decomposition	vaccine	substance used to stimulate an immune response for immunization

UNIT

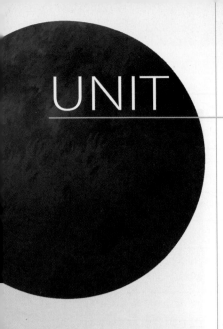

11

Descriptive Prefixes, Asepsis, and Pharmacology

INFORMATION FRAME

11.1

In medicine it is important to be clear and precise in describing qualities, quantities, locations, the nature of conditions observed, and symptoms presented by patients. It can be harmful to the patient if the wrong location of an injury is named or the opposite condition is described because someone did not use the proper term.

11.2

Prefixes are placed in front of a word root or whole word to change its meaning and make the term a clear descriptor. Many of the descriptive medical terms that begin with a prefix are used in their adjectival form. The word part placed in front

prefix

of a word root to change the use of its meaning is a _____.

adjectives

Often terms that begin with prefixes are descriptors or _____.

Study the table of descriptive prefixes below as an introduction. You will use them as you work the frames in Unit 11.

Prefix	Meaning	Example
homo-	same	homolateral (same side)
hetero-	different	heteropsia (different vision in each eye)
syn-	joined	syndactylism (joined fingers or toes)
sym-	joined	symbiosis (organisms living together)
super-	excess, above	superficial (above or on the surface)
supra-	above, more than	supralumbar (above the lumbar spine)
anti-	against	antiseptic (against infective organisms)
contra-	against	contraceptive (against conception)
trans-	across	transverse (travel across or sideways)
a-	absence of, lack of	agenesis (absence of development)
an-	absence of, lack of	anemia (lack of blood)

ANSWER COLUMN

	11.3
	homo- means same. Homo/genized milk has the same amount of cream throughout. Homo/gland/ular means pertaining to the
same gland	* _____ .
	11.4
same	Homo/therm/al means having the _____ body temperature all the time (i.e., 98.6°F [37°C]).
	11.5
same	Homo/later/al means pertaining to the _____ side.
	11.6
	Homo/sex/ual means being attracted to the same sex. When men are sexually attracted to men, they are said to be
homo/sex/ual	_____ / _____ / _____ .
hŏ′ mō **sek**′ shōō əl	
	11.7
	When women are attracted to women rather than to men, they too are called
homosexual	_____ .
	11.8
	hetero- is the opposite of **homo-**. **hetero-** means
different	_____ .
	Heter/opsia (het ûr **op**′ sē ə) means
different	_____ vision in each eye.
	11.9
different	Hetero/sex/ual means being attracted to a _____ sex.

Sexuality and Identity Terms Table	
hetero/sexual	Person whose predominant sexual attraction is to the opposite sex, also known as "straight."
homo/sexual	Person whose predominant sexual attraction is to the same sex, also known as gay (men or women, mostly men) or lesbian (homosexual women).
bi/sexual	Person with sexual attraction to both males and females.
crossdresser	Person who dresses in clothing generally identified with the opposite gender/sex. Syn: trans/vestite

(continued)

Sexuality and Identity Terms Table	
trans/sexual	Person who physically alters his or her body to be more like the opposite of his or her birth sex using hormones, implants, or surgery.
trans/gender	Umbrella term for all gender-variant people who by nature do not conform to gender-based expectations.
gender cues	Observable characteristics that may demonstrate the gender of another person. Examples include hairstyle, gait, vocal inflection, body shape, facial hair, etc. Cues vary by culture.
gender identity	A person's sense of being masculine, feminine, or other gendered.
inter/sexed person	Someone who is born with characteristics difficult to categorize as either male or female. A person whose combination of chromosomes, internal and external genitalia, and hormones differ from patterns of being completely male or female.
sex identity	How a person identifies as physically female, male, in between, beyond, or neither.
sexual orientation	The desire for intimate emotional and/or sexual relationships with people of the same gender/sex, another gender/sex, or multiple genders/sexes.

11.10

Look up the meanings of homogeneous and heterogeneous. Draw the slashes and write the definitions below

homo/gen/eous
hō′ mō **jē′** nē us
pertaining to the same
   throughout
hetero/gen/eous
het′ ûr ō **jē′** nē us
pertaining to different
   throughout

_____,
* _____;
_____,
* _____.

11.11

Open your dictionary and look up these terms. While you think of their meanings, form *opposites* of the following.
homo/gen/esis

hetero/gen/esis
het′ ûr ō **jen′** ə sis

_____/_____/_____

hetero/sex/ual
het′ ûr ō **seks′** ū əl

homo/sex/ual

_____/_____/_____

ANSWER COLUMN

11.12

Think of their meanings while you recall these or other opposites

anterior

posterior _____;

iso

aniso- (prefix) _____;

hyper

hypo- (prefix) _____;

adduction

abduction _____.

11.13

Good. Now you'll study **syn-** and **sym-**. They are different forms of the same prefix. **syn-** and **sym-** mean

together or joined

* _____.

11.14

Review: You have already learned **syn-** in the words syndactylism, synergetic, synarthrosis, and syndrome.

11.15

syn- is the form of the prefix that is used to mean fixed or joined, except when it is

sym-

followed by the sound of "b," "m," "f," "ph," or "p." Then, _____ is used.

EXAMPLE: symbol, symphony, sympathy

11.16

Sym/pathy is an ordinary word that has a special medical meaning. From either a medical or regular English dictionary, find what it takes to fill this blank:

suffering (medical) or
feeling (standard)

sym- + path/os, the Greek word for _____.

11.17

blephar/o means eyelid. A sym/physis is a growing together of parts.

eyelids have grown
together, or adhesions
of the eyelids

Sym/blepharon means * _____

_____.

11.18

pod/o is one combining form for foot. Build words meaning lower extremities are grown together (united)

sym/podia
sim **pō′** dē ə

_____/_____/_____;

excision of a sympathetic nerve

sym/path/ectomy
sim pa **thek′** tō mē

_____/_____/_____;

tumor of a sympathetic nerve

sym/path/oma
sim pa **thō′** mə

_____/_____/_____.

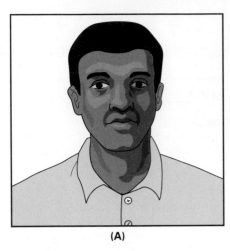

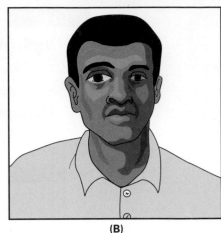

(A)   (B)

11.19

Find a fairly common word in your medical dictionary in which **sym-** is followed by *m*. (There are only two or three choices.)

One is _____/_____/_____.

sym/metr/y, sym/metr/ic,
or sym/metric/al

11.20

Find a common word in your medical dictionary that is used in ordinary English in which **sym-** is followed by "b"

symbol or symbolism

* _____.

11.21

syn- and **sym-** both mean together. **sym-** is used when followed by the sound

b
m
p
f
ph

of the letters _____, _____, _____, _____, and _____. **syn-** is used in other medical words.

11.22

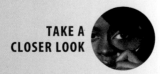

**TAKE A
CLOSER LOOK**

super- and **supra-** are both Latin origin prefixes that mean above, beyond, or excessive. **super-** is used in descriptive common English terms and a few medical terms. **supra-** is used more in terms that are describing anatomical locations. Look up **super-** and **supra-** in your dictionary and read and study the terms that begin with these prefixes.

ANSWER COLUMN

11.23

Finish writing the definitions of the following terms beginning with the prefix **super-**.

surface

super/ficial—above or on the _____ ;

eyebrow

super/ciliary—above the _____ ;
super/infection—an infection on top of another

infection

_____ ;

above or better than

super/iority—quality of being * _____ ;

deadly

super/lethal—pertaining to excessively _____ ;

number

super/numerary—too many to _____ .

11.24

Build adjective using the prefix **supra-** that means above the:

supra/lumb/ar
sōō' pra **ləm'** bar

lumbar spine _____/_____/_____ ;

supra/pub/ic
sōō' pra **pyoo'** bik

pubis _____/_____/_____ ;

supra/mamm/ary
sōō' pra **ma'** mair ē

breasts _____/_____/_____ ;

supra/ren/al
sōō' pra **re'** nəl

kidneys _____/_____/_____ ;

supra/inguin/al
sōō' pra **ing'** win əl

inguinal region (groin) _____/_____/_____ .

11.25

Draw a conclusion about **super-** and **supra-** from your answers in the last two frames.

used more frequently in
modern English

super- is * _____
_____ .

used more frequently in
medical words

supra- is * _____
_____ .

11.26

**DICTIONARY
EXERCISE**

a- and **an-** are prefixes that mean without or lack of.
Examine the following words that begin with **a-** or **an-**.
First try to think of the meanings from what you have previously learned.
Then, look up the terms in your dictionary and write the definition in the blank.
See how many you get right!

ANSWER COLUMN

a-	Definition	an-	Definition
a/bort	_____	an/algesia	_____
a/cephal/y	_____	an/aphylaxis	_____
a/chrom/ia	_____	an/emia	_____
a/chol/ia	_____	an/encephaly	_____
a/dactyl/y	_____	an/esthesia	_____
a/febr/ile	_____	an/iso/cytosis	_____
a/galact/o/rrhea	_____	an/hidr/osis	_____
a/kinesia	_____	an/hydr/ous	_____
a/men/o/rrhea	_____	an/onych/osis	_____
a/phas/ia	_____	an/orch/ism	_____
a/plas/ia	_____	an/orex/ia	_____
a/pne/a	_____	an/ovul/ation	_____
a/rhin/ia	_____	an/ops/ia	_____
a/rrhythm/ia	_____	an/ox/ia	_____
a/sep/sis	_____	an/odont/ia	_____
a/symmetr/y	_____	an/ur/ia	_____
a/troph/y	_____	an/ur/esis	_____

11.27

Draw a conclusion.

consonant

Use **a-** if it is followed by a (choose one) _____
(vowel/consonant).

vowel

Use **an-** if it is followed by a (choose one) _____
(vowel/consonant).

More prefixes! Use this table to work Frames 11.28–11.66.

Prefix	Meaning	Special Comment
epi-	over, upon	epicenter of an earthquake
extra-	outside of, beyond, in addition to	extracurricular activities
infra-	below, under	almost always below a part of the body; almost always adjectival in form; there are fewer words beginning with **infra-** than with **sub-**
sub-	under, below	many words of all kinds begin with **sub-**
meta-	beyond, after, occurring later in a series	also used with chemical names

---

11.28

epi- means upon or over. The epi/gastr/ic region is the region

over the stomach

* _____ .

ANSWER COLUMN

	11.29
over the spleen	Epi/splen/itis means inflammation of the tissue * _____ .
	11.30
	Build words meaning inflammation of the area over the bladder
epi/cyst/itis ep' i sis **tī'** tis	_____/_____/_____ ; inflammation (of the tissue) upon the kidney
epi/nephr/itis ep' i ne **frī'** tis	_____/_____/_____ .
	11.31
	Build words meaning excision of the tissue upon the kidney
epi/nephr/ectomy ep' i ne **frek'** tə mē	_____/_____/_____ ; suture of the region over the stomach
epi/gastr/o/rrhaphy ep' i gas **trôr'** ə fē	_____/_____/_____/_____ .
	11.32
	Build words meaning pertaining to (the tissue) upon the skin (outermost layer)
epi/derm/al	_____/_____/_____ ; (the tissue) covering the cranium
epi/crani/al	_____/_____/_____ ; the area above the sternum
epi/stern/al	_____/_____/_____ ; the tissues upon the heart
epi/cardi/um (You pronounce)	_____/_____/_____ .

Direction prefixes *Delmar/ Cengage Learning*

Directional prefixes

INFORMATION FRAME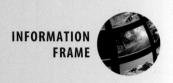

11.33

Didymos is another Greek word for testis. The epi/didymis is a small oblong body resting upon the testicle, containing convoluted tubules. The epididymis is involved in sperm production and transportation.

11.34

epi/didym/itis
ep' i did i **mī'** tis

epi/didym/ectomy
ep' i did i **mek'** tō mē

Build words that mean
inflammation of the epididymis

_____/_____/_____;

excision of the epididymis

_____/_____/_____.

The meninges *Delmar/Cengage Learning*

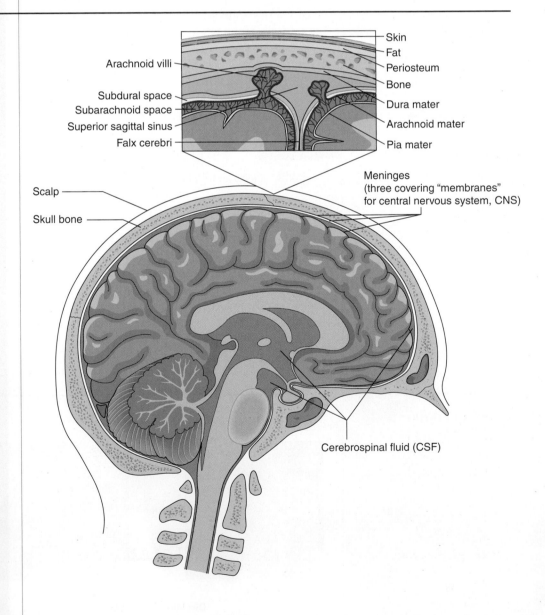

- Skin
- Fat
- Periosteum
- Bone
- Dura mater
- Arachnoid mater
- Pia mater

Arachnoid villi
Subdural space
Subarachnoid space
Superior sagittal sinus
Falx cerebri

Meninges
(three covering "membranes"
for central nervous system, CNS)

Scalp
Skull bone

Cerebrospinal fluid (CSF)

STUDYWARE™ CONNECTION

Remember, after completing this unit, you can play a championship or other interactive game on your **StudyWARE™ CD-ROM** that will help you learn the content in this chapter.

ANSWER COLUMN

	11.35
	Recall your previous study of the meninges, the membranes that surround the brain and spinal cord. The dura (dur) mater is a layer of the meninges.
upon	The epi/dur/al layer is located _____ the dura.

	11.36
	Anesthetic can be administered in the layer or space upon the dura. This is
epi/dur/al ep′ i **dur′** əl	_____/_____/_____ anesthesia.

	11.37
	Using dur/al, build words meaning below the dura mater
sub/dur/al sub **dur′** əl	_____/_____/_____;
	upon the dura mater
epi/dur/al ep′ i **dur′** əl	_____/_____/_____.

	11.38
SPELL CHECK	derm/al and dur/al look and sound similar but have completely different meanings. The **derm/is** is the middle layer of the skin, and the **dura mater** is the outer layer of the meninges. Look up the following terms in your dictionary, and be watchful of their use and spelling.
	epi/derm/al _____
	epi/dur/al _____

	11.39
	extra- means outside or beyond. Think of extraterrestrial. Extra/nuclear
outside of or beyond	(eks tra **nōō′** klē är) means * _____ the nucleus of a cell.

	11.40
outside of or beyond	Extra/uterine is an adjective meaning * _____ the uterus.

ANSWER COLUMN

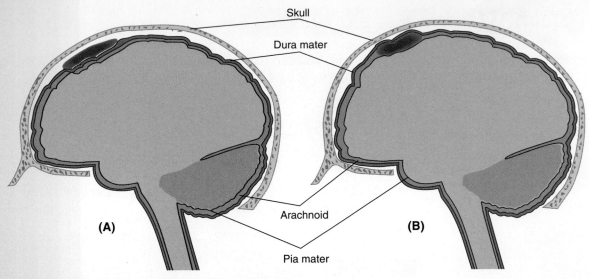

Cranial hematomas: (A) epidural, (B) subdural *Delmar/Cengage Learning*

	11.41
	Build words meaning
	outside of the joint
extra-/articul/ar	_____/_____/_____ ;
eks' trə är **tik'** yə lər	urinary bladder
extra/cyst/ic	_____/_____/_____ ;
eks' trə **sis'** tik	dura mater (meninges)
extra/dur/al	_____/_____/_____ ;
eks' trə **dōōr'** əl	genitals
extra/genit/al	_____/_____/_____ ;
eks' trə **jen'** i təl	liver
extra/hepat/ic	_____/_____/_____ ;
eks' trə hep **at'** ik	cerebrum
extra/cerebr/al	_____/_____/_____ .
eks' trə ser **ē'** brəl	

	11.42
	Look at the words in the last frame. Draw a conclusion. **extra-** is used as a prefix in
adjectives	words that are usually (choose one) _____ (nouns/adjectives).

	11.43
	Recall that **mamm/o** is one combining form for breast. An x-ray picture of the
	breast is a mammogram. The process of taking this x-ray is called
mamm/o/graphy	_____/_____/_____ .
mam **og'** raf ē	

During a mammography, the breast is gently flattened and then radiographed *Delmar/Cengage Learning*

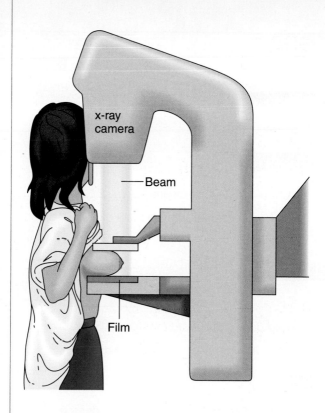

x-ray
camera

— Beam

Film

11.44

Build a term that means:
incision into breast tissue

mamm/o/tomy
ma **mot'** ō mē

_____/_____/_____;

surgical repair of the breast

mamm/o/plasty
ma' mō pla stē

_____/_____/_____;

above the breast

supra/mamm/ary
sōō' pra **ma'** mair ē

_____/_____/_____ .

11.45

bi- means both or two. When a procedure is performed on both sides, it is said

both sides

to be bilateral. A bilateral hernia repair is on * _____ .

both breasts

A bilateral mammogram is a radiograph of * _____ .

11.46

In humans, because most body parts are in pairs, the opposite of unilateral is

bi/later/al
bī **lat'** er əl

_____/_____/_____ .

11.47

infra- means below or under. Infra/mammary means

below or under

* _____ the mammary gland.

ANSWER COLUMN

11.48

below or under

Infra/patell/ar means * _____ the patella (kneecap).

11.49

sub

Below the tongue is _____/lingual.

11.50

under or below

under

sub- is a prefix that means * _____.

A sub/dural hematoma is a mass of clotted blood _____ the dura mater.

11.51

under

below

below

Sub/abdominal means _____ the abdomen. aur from the Latin word *auris* is one word root for ear. Sub/aur/al means _____ the ear.

Sub/cutaneous (subcu, subq, s.c) means _____ the skin.

11.52

Build words that mean below or under the
 dura mater

sub/dur/al

sub **dûr′** əl

_____/_____/_____;

ear

sub/aur/al

sub **aw′** rəl

_____/_____/_____;

skin

sub/cutane/ous

sub′ kyo͞o **tān′** ē əs

_____/_____/_____.

11.53

The prefixes **infra-** and **sub-** are sometimes confusing in word building. For that reason, you will build words that can take either prefix. When you see **sub-** or

under

below

infra-, you will think of _____ or _____.

11.54

Using **stern/o**, build two words meaning below the sternum

infra/stern/al

in′ fra **stûr′** nəl

_____/_____/_____

and

sub/stern/al

sub′ **stûr′** nəl

_____/_____/_____.

A word meaning above the sternum is

supra/stern/al

so͞o′ pra **stûr′** nəl

supra/_____/_____.

ANSWER COLUMN

11.55

Using **cost/o**, build two words meaning under the ribs

infra/cost/al
_____/_____/_____;

sub/cost/al
_____/_____/_____.

supra/cost/al
A word meaning above the ribs is _____/_____/_____.

inter/cost/al
(You pronounce)
The _____/_____/_____ muscles are between the ribs.

11.56

Using **pub/o**, build two words meaning under the pubis:

infra/pub/ic
_____/_____/_____ and

sub/pub/ic
_____/_____/_____.

supra/pub/ic
(You pronounce)
A word meaning above the pubis is _____/_____/_____.

INFORMATION FRAME

11.57

meta- is a prefix used in many ways. Look at the table on page 428 to discover its meanings.

11.58

Analyze the term metaphysics. It is the study of things

beyond the physical or of the spirit
* _____.

11.59

The bones of the hand that are beyond the carpals (wrist) are the

meta/carpals
me′ tə **kar′** palz
_____/_____.

11.60

The bones of the foot that are beyond the tarsals (ankle) are the

meta/tarsals
me′ tə **tar′** salz
_____/_____.

STUDYWARE™ CONNECTION

After completing this unit, complete an exercise *Labeling the Bones of the Wrist and Hand* on your **StudyWARE™ CD-ROM** that will help you learn the content in this chapter.

ANSWER COLUMN

Bones of the wrist and hand *Delmar/Cengage Learning*

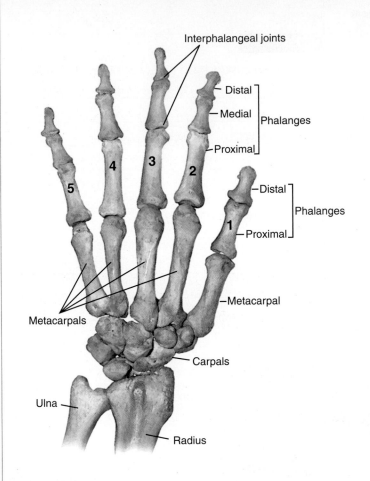

Interphalangeal joints

Distal
Medial Phalanges
Proximal

4 3 2

5

Distal
Phalanges
1
Proximal

Metacarpal

Metacarpals

Carpals

Ulna

Radius

11.61

A meta/stasis occurs when a disease spreads beyond its point of origin.
A meta/static (adjective) tumor is a secondary growth from a malignant tumor.

This secondary growth is a _____/_____ (singular noun).
The plural form of this word is

_____/_____.

meta/stasis
me **tas'** tə sis

meta/stases
me **tas'** tə sēz

11.62

The area of the origin of cancer or the first discovered site in a patient is said to be

the primary site. If a secondary site is found, it is a _____.

metastasis

11.63

ultra- is a prefix meaning beyond or in excess. Light waves that are beyond the

violet frequency are _____/_____ (UV).

ultra/violet
ul' tra **vī** ō let

11.64

Sound waves that are beyond the audible frequency are ultra/son/ic. The process
of making an image using ultrasound (US) is called

_____/_____/_____/_____ or sonography.

ultra/son/o/graphy
ul' tra son **og'** raf ē

ANSWER COLUMN

	11.65
ultrasonography ultrasonography	Ultra/sound may be used for therapy or for diagnostic testing. To detect gallstones in a diseased gallbladder, the sonographer uses diagnostic _____. To treat a patient with kidney stones, the sonographer uses therapeutic _____.
	11.66
Do it!	You have now learned many prefixes of location. Review them by making a list with their meaning plus anything special about them.
	11.67
a/seps/is ə **sep'** sis, ā **sep'** sis	Recall that path/o/genic refers to disease production. Sepsis is a noun meaning a poisoned state or infection caused by absorption of pathogenic bacteria and their products into the bloodstream. A noun meaning a state without (or lack of) sepsis _____/_____/_____.
	11.68
a/sept/ic ə **sep'** tik, ā **sep'** tik	Sept/ic is the adjectival form of sepsis. The adjectival form for the word meaning free from infection is _____/_____/_____.

Urinary catheterization requires strict asepsis
Delmar/Cengage Learning

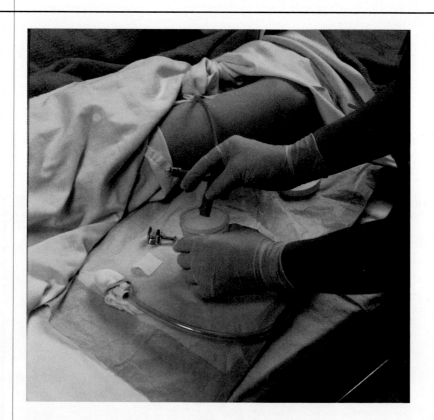

PROFESSIONAL PROFILE

Registered diagnostic medical sonographers (RDMSs) are highly skilled allied health professionals who use ultrasound (high-frequency sound) to create images of organs and tissues that are displayed on a computerized monitor in real time and on still films (sonograms). Knowledge of sectional anatomy, pathology, computer technology, and medical ethics is essential. The American Registry of Diagnostic Medical Sonographers (ARDMS) determines educational requirements and criteria for registration of diagnostic medical sonographers.

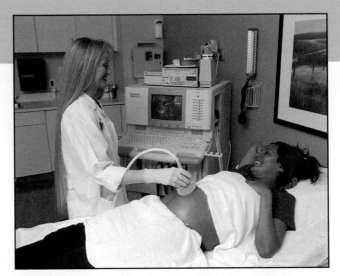

Sonographer performing fetal ultrasound *Delmar/ Cengage Learning*

ANSWER COLUMN

	11.69
infection with pus in the bloodstream	Septic/emia is an infection (poisoned state) in the bloodstream. Septic/o/py/emia means * _____ _____ . NOTE: **sept/i, sept/o, septic/o,** and **seps/o** are combining forms for infection.
	11.70
sept/i (used most often) or septic/o	Study the last two frames. A combining form for infection is _____ / _____ .

Fetal ultrasound *Prepared by Lynne Schreiber, MA, RDMS, RT(R)*

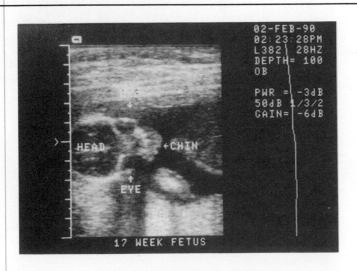

ANSWER COLUMN

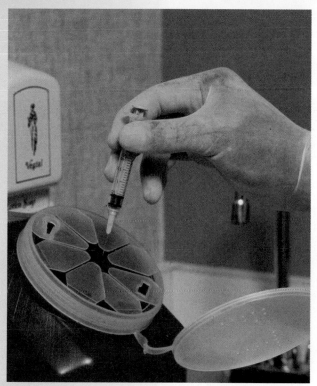

Proper disposal of contaminated needles and syringes (sharps) into biohazard containers prevents accidental exposure to potentially infectious body fluids *Delmar/Cengage Learning*

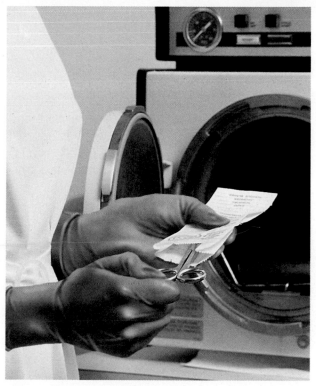

This medical assistant places an instrument into an envelope package for sterilization using an autoclave *Delmar/Cengage Learning*

11.71

Review the material from Frames 11.67–11.70. Give words that mean

seps/is

sept/ic

a/seps/is
ā **sep'** sis

a/sept/ic
ā **sep'** tik

noun for infection _____/_____;

adjective for infected _____/_____;

noun for state free from infection _____/_____/_____;

adjective for free from infection _____/_____/_____ .

11.72

against

against

toxin

anti- is a prefix meaning against. An anti/pyretic is an agent that

works _____ a fever. An anti/toxin is an agent that

works _____ a toxin. A pyr/o/toxin

is a _____ produced by fever (heat).

NOTE: A toxin is a poisonous substance produced by an organism.

The following table lists categories of drugs that work against something.

Drug Category	Works Against
ant/acid	acid
anti/anemic	anemia
anti/arrhythmic	irregular heartbeats
anti/arthritic	arthritis
anti/biotic	bacteria
anti/cholinergic	parasympathetic impulses
anti/coagulant	clotting
anti/convulsant	seizures
anti/depressant	depression
anti/diarrheal	diarrhea
anti/emetic	vomiting
anti/fungal	fungi
anti/histamine	histamine (allergic reactions)
anti/hypertensive	high blood pressure
anti-/inflammatory	inflammation
anti/manic	manic-depression
anti/narcotic	narcotics
anti/neoplastic, anti/tumor	tumors
anti/pruritic	dry skin (itching)
anti/psychotic	psychosis
anti/pyretic	fever
anti/spasmodic	muscle spasms
anti/toxin	poisons (toxins)
anti/tussive	coughs

11.73

against

An anti/narcotic is an agent that works _____ narcotics.

11.74

against

An anti/biotic is an agent that works _____ living bacterial infections.

11.75

anti/bio/tic
an' ti bī **ot'** ik

Erythromycin is prescribed to fight bacteria and is one type of

_____/_____/_____.

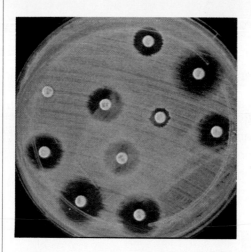

The following table differentiates between various methods of providing medications.

Method	Description
Administration	General term for giving medications by any form or method
Dispensing	Preparing and giving medications (or other treatment items) to those who will use them
Prescription	Written orders for medication or treatment
Injection	Parenteral administration of medication through a needle and syringe (IM, IV, subcu, ID)
Topical	Applying agents directly to the treatment area (lotions, sprays, creams, ointments, drops)
Transdermal	Medication is absorbed through the skin via patch, cream, or lotion
Oral	Medication is swallowed (tablets, liquids)
Inhalation	Medications are breathed in through inhalers or respiratory treatments

Confused about agents that fight pathogenic organisms? Study the following table.

AGENTS THAT FIGHT AGAINST PATHOGENIC ORGANISMS

Antiseptics are agents that prevent sepsis by inhibiting growth of causative organisms. They may be inorganic, such as mercury and iodine preparations, or organic, such as carbolic acid (phenol) and alcohol.

Antibiotics are mostly prescription drugs that inhibit growth or destroy microorganisms, especially bacteria. Antibiotics can be used topically or taken internally for a systemic effect. Examples: penicillin, Keflex, erythromycin. Antibiotics can be bacteriocidal (kill bacteria) or bacteriostatic (inhibit growth, keep the numbers down).

Disinfectants are chemical or physical agents that prevent infection by killing microorganisms. They are used to clean equipment or surfaces rather than in or upon the body (e.g., Virex, bleach).

(continued)

ANSWER COLUMN

AGENTS THAT FIGHT AGAINST PATHOGENIC ORGANISMS

Sanitization is the process of cleaning instruments, surfaces, and other items in the environment that are in contact with patients and workers. This step is taken before disinfection or sterilization.

Sterilization is a process that kills organisms of all sorts. An autoclave uses pressure and steam and is the most effective form of sterilization. Chemical sterilization using disinfectants such as bleach kills most organisms but not the ones that form spores.

11.76

Now, build words describing the agents that work against

rheumatic disease

anti/rheumat/ic
an' ti rōō **ma'** tik

_____/_____;

spastic muscle

anti/spasmod/ic
an' ti spaz **mod'** ik

_____/_____;

toxins

anti/tox/in
an' ti **toks'** in

_____/_____.

11.77

Build adjectives describing the agents that work against

convulsive states

anti/convuls/ive
an' ti kon **vul'** siv

_____/_____;

arthritic diseases

anti/arthr/itic
an' ti ar **thri'** tik

_____/_____;

toxic states

anti/tox/ic
an' ti **toks'** ik

_____/_____;

sepsis

anti/sept/ic
an' ti **sep'** tik

_____/_____.

11.78

contra- is a prefix that means against. contra- is usually used with modern

against

English words. To contra/dict someone is to speak _____ what the person is saying.

STUDY WARE™ CONNECTION

After completing this unit, you can play a Spelling Bee game to help you learn the pronunciation of terms presented in the chapter or play other interactive games on your **StudyWARE™ CD-ROM** that will help you learn the content in this chapter.

ANSWER COLUMN

11.79

against

against

Contra/ry things are _____ each other. A contra/ry person is one who is _____ your wishes.

11.80

Analyze these three words
contraindication

contra/indica/tion
kon' tra in di **kā'** shun

_____/_____/_____;

contraceptive

contra/cept/ive
kon' tra **sep'** tiv

_____/_____;

contralateral

contra/later/al
kon' tra **lat'** ur əl

_____/_____/_____.

11.81

Using the words in Frame 11.80, fill the following blanks with a word whose literal meaning is

contraindication

against indication _____;

contraceptive

against conception _____;

contralateral

opposite (against) side _____.

11.82

Using the noun contra/indication, build other parts of the same word

contra/indicate

_____/_____ (present tense verb);

contra/indicated
(You pronounce)

_____/_____ (past tense verb).

11.83

Before beginning a drug therapy of any kind on a pregnant patient, a physician will consult a drug reference guide to see if the medication is safe for use during pregnancy. If it is not, the guide will say the medication is contra/indicat/ed during pregnancy. Narcotic medications are not advisable during pregnancy; therefore, they are _____/_____/_____.

contra/indicated
kon' tra **in'** di kā ted

CASE STUDY INVESTIGATION (CSI)

Unintentional Drug Overdose Death

The Centers for Disease Control and Prevention (CDC) has reported that since 1999 there has been an increase in unintentional drug **overdose** deaths attributed to three categories of drugs: **narcotic** medications, other and unspecified drugs,

(continued)

and **psychotherapeutics**. Narcotic overdose is the most common. **Prescription analgesics** such as OxyContin, Vicodin (**opioid** painkillers) as well as cocaine, heroine, and methadone are in this group. The second most common group includes a wide variety of drug substances that are "other and unspecified." Psychotherapeutic or **psychotropic** drugs are the third group comprised of sedatives like Valium and **antidepressants**. Misuse and abuse of prescription medications in these three categories of drugs coupled with alcohol abuse constitute a serious health threat from unintentional drug overdose.

CSI Vocabulary Challenge

Use a medical dictionary to analyze the terms below from the case study. Divide each term into word parts by drawing in the slashes and write the definition in the space provided.

overdose   _____

narcotic   _____

analgesics   _____

opioid   _____

prescription   _____

psychotherapeutics   _____

psychotropic   _____

antidepressants   _____

ANSWER COLUMN

Study the following list of drug categories that **do not** begin with **anti-**. Can you analyze their meaning from word parts you have already learned? If not, look them up in your dictionary for more information.

Drug	Action
bronch/o/dilat/or	dilates or enlarges bronchi
de/congest/ant	reduces respiratory congestion
di/ur/etic	increases urine flow
ex/pector/ant	assists in removing respiratory secretions
hem/o/stat/ic	controls bleeding
hormon/es	endocrine secretions that affect control mechanisms
hypn/o/tic	sleep agent, produces state of hypnosis
hypo/glyc/em/ic	agent that lowers blood sugar (glucose)
lax/a/tive	loosens or liquifies stool for relief of constipation
muscle re/lax/ant	relieves tension in skeletal muscle
sed/a/tive	calms nervous excitement
tran/quiliz/er	lowers anxiety and mental tension
vas/o/dilat/or	dilates blood vessels
vas/o/press/or	constricts blood vessels, increases blood pressure

ANSWER COLUMN

11.84

across or over

trans- is a Latin prefix meaning across or over. To trans/port a cargo is to carry it
* _____ the ocean or land.

11.85

across or over

Trans/position means literally position * _____.

11.86

trans/position
trans' pə **zish'** ən

When an organ is placed across to the other side of the body from where it is
normally found (e.g., liver on the left side), _____/_____
occurs.

11.87

transposition

Cardi/ac transposition means that the heart is on the right side of the body. If the
stomach is on the right side of the body, the condition is gastr/ic
_____.

11.88

across or over

When a trans/fusion is given, blood is passed
* _____ from one person to another.

11.89

trans-

Recall that the procedure performed across the lumen of an artery of the heart is
percutaneous _____/luminal angioplasty (PTA).

**Transurethral resection
of the prostate (TURP)**
Delmar/Cengage Learning

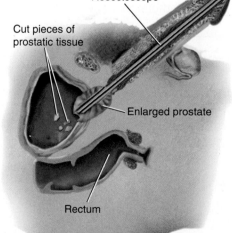

Resectoscope

Cut pieces of
prostatic tissue

Enlarged prostate

Rectum

ANSWER COLUMN

11.90

Analyze the following by drawing the slashes and writing the meaning

trans/sex/ual

transsexual   _____ ,   _____

                                                 meaning

trans/illumin/ation

transillumination _____ ,   _____

                                                   meaning

trans/vagin/al

transvaginal   _____ ,   _____

                                                   meaning

trans/thorac/ic

transthoracic   _____ ,   _____

                                                   meaning

trans/urethr/al

transurethral   _____ ,   _____

                                                   meaning

trans/fusion

transfusion   _____ ,   _____

                                                   meaning

(You pronounce)

INFORMATION FRAME

11.91

A catheter (**kath'** e ter) is a flexible tube. When a sterile urine specimen is needed, the urologist may introduce a catheter through the urethra into the bladder to obtain the specimen.

INFORMATION FRAME

11.92

A procedure for enlarging heart vessels is called trans/catheter therapy or angioplasty. It is possible to introduce an intravascular occlusion balloon "through" a catheter. Look up these terms in your dictionary and note the use of the prefix **trans-**.

11.93

Inserting a catheter for urine collection is called

catheter/ization

_____/_____.

11.94

Cardiac catheterization allows the physician to view the inside of the vessels

heart

of the _____.

Abbreviation	Meaning
A, B, O, AB	blood types
AAMA	American Association of Medical Assistants
ARDMS	American Registry of Diagnostic Medical Sonographers
c̄	with
cath	catheter

(continued)

ANSWER COLUMN

Abbreviation	Meaning
cm	centimeter (centimeters)
CMA	certified medical assistant
C&S*, C and S	culture and sensitivity (antibiotic)
ftm	female to male
inf	infusion
met., metas., mets.	metastasis/metastases
mtf	male to female
RDMS	registered diagnostic medical sonographer
s̄	without (sans)
subcu, subq, sc*	subcutaneously
trans	transverse
TURP	transurethral resection of the prostate
US	ultrasound
UV	ultraviolet
XM	cross match (as in blood type and cross match)

*Abbreviation use warning. These abbreviations have been judged dangerous and should not be used.

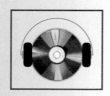

To complete your study of this unit, work the **Review Activities** on the following pages. Also, listen to the Audio CD that accompanies *Medical Terminology: A Programmed Systems Approach*, 10th edition, and practice your pronunciation.

STUDY WARE™ CONNECTION

To help you learn the content in this chapter, take a practice quiz or play an interactive game on your **StudyWARE™ CD-ROM**.

REVIEW ACTIVITIES

CIRCLE AND CORRECT

Circle the correct answer for each question. Then check your answers in Appendix E.

1. Heteropsia indicates _____ visual acuity in each eye.
   - a. the same
   - b. blurred
   - c. different
   - d. changed

2. If a substance is blended or the same throughout, it is _____
   - a. homozygous
   - b. hypertrophic
   - c. isocellular
   - d. homogenous

3. If the next letter is b, m, f, or ph, use _____ as the prefix for joined.
   - a. sym-
   - b. syn-
   - c. iso-
   - d. inter-

4. In anatomic terms indicating a location above, use _____ as a prefix.
   - a. hydro-
   - b. antero-
   - c. superio-
   - d. supra-

REVIEW ACTIVITIES

5. The fluid outside of the cell is _____
   cellular fluid.
   a. extra-
   b. intra-
   c. sub-
   d. exo-

6. If the next letter is a vowel, use _____
   as the prefix meaning not or lack of
   a. a
   b. an
   c. either a or an

7. Epicystitis is inflammation _____
   the urinary bladder.
   a. in
   b. outside of
   c. upon
   d. under

8. Which of the following is spelled correctly?
   a. extra-articular
   b. extra-genital
   c. extra-cerebral
   d. extra-hepatic

9. Which of the following refers to a layer of the meninges?
   a. dermal
   b. pneumonic
   c. myelo
   d. dural

10. If a procedure is performed on both sides it is
    a. diplocellular
    b. bilateral
    c. laterodiploid
    d. bifurcated

SELECT AND CONSTRUCT

Select the correct word parts from the following list and construct medical terms that represent the given meaning.

a(an)	algesia	aniso	anti	bi
ceptive	contra	cyst/o(ic)	cyt(o)(ic)	derm/o(al)
didym/o(is)	dur/a(al)	ectomy	epi	extra
gastr/o	graph/o(y)(er)	hetero	homo	infra
iso	itis	later/o(al)	lumb/ar	mamm/o
meta	oma	osis	otic	path(o)(y)
pod/o(ia)	ren/o(al)	rrhaphy	sept/o(ic)	sex(ual)
son/o	stasis	stern/o(al)	sub	sym
syn	tox/o(in)(ic)	tri	ultra	

1. agent that works against bacterial infection _____

2. agent that works against fertilization of an ovum _____

3. attracted to the same sex _____

4. cells of different sizes _____

5. feet joined (grown) together _____

6. below the sternum _____

7. breast x-ray procedure _____

8. one who uses reflected sound to make images _____

9. upon the dura mater _____

10. outside of the urinary bladder _____

11. three sides _____

12. disease that goes beyond its original growth _____

REVIEW ACTIVITIES

PREFIX AND WORD

Write the prefix that represents the direction. Then build a word using that prefix.

Prefix   Word

_____ 1. same   attracted to the same sex   _____ _____

_____ 2. different   made of different   _____
                                  substances

_____ 3. join   feet grown together   _____
                                  (followed by b, m, f, ph, p)

_____ 4. above   above the surface   _____

_____ 5. above   above the kidneys   _____

_____ 6. without   absence of menstruation   _____

_____ 7. without   without feeling or sensation   _____

_____ 8. upon/over   upon the stomach (adjective)   _____

_____ 9. outside of   outside of the cell (adjective) _____

_____ 10. below/under   below the sternum (adjective)   _____

_____ 11. beyond   bones beyond the carpals   _____

_____ 12. beyond   beyond audible sound waves   _____

_____ 13. both   including both sides (adjective) _____

_____ 14. against   against arthritis (adjective)   _____

_____ 15. against   against indications (not indicated) _____

_____ 16. across   across the urethra (adjective)   _____

DEFINE AND DISSECT

Give a brief definition and dissect each term listed into its word parts in the space provided. Check your answers by referring to the frame listed in parentheses and your medical dictionary. Then listen to the Audio CD to practice pronunciation.

1. homolateral (11.5)   _____/_____/_____
                                                   pre   rt   suffix

   meaning _____

2. heterosexual (11.11)   _____/_____/_____
                                                   pre   rt   suffix

   _____

3. sympathectomy (11.18)   _____/_____/_____
                                                   pre   rt   suffix

   _____

REVIEW ACTIVITIES

4. symmetrical (11.19)

_____/_____/_____
pre   rt   suffix

_____

5. superinfection (11.23)

_____/_____/_____
pre   rt   suffix

_____

6. suprarenal (11.24)

_____/_____/_____
pre   rt   suffix

_____

7. analgesia (table p. 428)

_____/_____/_____
pre   rt   suffix

_____

8. asepsis (11.71)

_____/_____
pre   rt/suffix

_____

9. episplenitis (11.29)

_____/_____/_____
pre   rt   suffix

_____

10. extra-articular (11.41)

_____/_____/_____
pre   rt   suffix

_____

11. extracerebral (11.41)

_____/_____/_____
pre   rt   suffix

_____

12. inframammary (11.47)

_____/_____
pre   rt/suffix

_____

13. mammography (11.43)

_____/_____/_____
rt   v   suffix

_____

14. metastasis (11.61)

_____/_____
pre   rt/suffix

_____

REVIEW ACTIVITIES

15. ultrasonography (11.64)

_____/_____/_____/_____
pre   rt   v   suffix

16. anti-inflammatory (table p. 440)

_____/_____/_____/_____
pre   pre   rt   suffix

17. contraceptive (11.80)

_____/_____
pre   rt/suffix

18. transcatheter (11.92)

_____/_____
pre   rt/suffix

19. homogeneous (11.10)

_____/_____/_____
pre   rt   suffix

20. antiseptic (11.77)

_____/_____/_____
pre   rt   suffix

21. antibiotic (11.75)

_____/_____/_____
pre   rt   suffix

22. bacteriostatic (table p. 441)

_____/_____/_____/_____
rt   v   rt   suffix

23. epididymitis (11.34)

_____/_____/_____
pre   rt   suffix

24. epidural (11.36)

_____/_____/_____
pre   rt   suffix

25. contraindication (11.80)

_____/_____/_____
pre   rt   suffix

26. heteropsia (11.8)

_____/_____/_____
pre   rt   suffix

REVIEW ACTIVITIES

27. transposition (11.86)

_____/_____/_____

pre   rt   suffix

_____

28. catheterization (11.93)

_____/_____

rt   suffix

_____

ABBREVIATION MATCHING

Match the following abbreviations with their definition.

_____ 1. c̄   a. ultraviolet

_____ 2. trans   b. transurethral

_____ 3. C&S   c. blood group types

_____ 4. CMA   d. catheter

_____ 5. UV   e. fractured metatarsals

_____ 6. mets.   f. across, through

_____ 7. RDMS   g. with

_____ 8. A, B, O, AB   h. certified medical assistant

                              i. culture and sensitivity

                              j. metastases

                              k. registered dietitian

                              l. registered diagnostic medical sonographer

                              m. without

                              n. infrared

                              o. certified physicians' assistant

ABBREVIATION FILL-IN

Fill in the blank with the correct abbreviation.

9. American Association of Medical Assistants _____

10. without _____

11. infusion _____

12. crossmatch _____

13. subcutaneously _____

14. female to male _____

15. transurethral resection of the prostate _____

REVIEW ACTIVITIES

CASE STUDY

Write the term next to its meaning given below. Then draw slashes to analyze the word parts. Note the use of medical abbreviations. Look these up in your dictionary or find them in Appendix B. If you have any questions about the answers, refer to your medical dictionary or check with your instructor for the answers in Appendix E.

CASE STUDY 11-1

Neurology Operative Report

Pt: Male, age 46

Preoperative diagnosis: Left **hemiparesis** with right **subdural** hygroma

Diagnosis (Dx): Left hemparesis with right subdural hygroma

Procedure: Bur hole with evacuation of subdural fluid

Anesthesia: 1% Xylocaine with standby **anesthesiologist**

Having shaved his head and properly positioned him, the patient was turned slightly to the left. IV Valium was given by the anesthetist who was monitoring his vital signs, including oxygenation.

The right **temporoparietal** region was prepared and draped in the usual fashion. Xylocaine 1% was administered locally and thereafter a scalp **incision** was carried out, which was deepened down through the **subcutaneous** tissue. The galea was incised. **Hemostasis** was achieved. The muscle fascia and muscle fibers were incised; thereafter, the wound was **retracted**, and the **pericranium** was thus opened and incised. Using McKenzie's **perforator**, a bur hole was made, which was widened and thereafter the **dura mater** was thus exposed. Cauterization was carried out. Bone wax was applied to the scalp margin, and thereafter a cruciate incision was carried out. Clean fluid with pressure was obtained; however, there was no evidence of any blood. The fluid was allowed to seep out, was suctioned out, and a small amount of dura was removed, using Kerrison rongeur. I felt no drain would be necessary in the absence of blood. The wound was closed in layers, closing the temporalis muscle fascia, the galea, and skin. Steri-strips were applied and the patient was **transferred** to his room in stable condition.

1. below the dura mater _____

2. physician specializing in painless surgery _____

3. making a cut into (noun) _____

4. controlling blood flow _____

5. below the skin _____

6. membrane surrounding the skull _____

7. pulled back _____

8. instrument used to make a hole _____

9. outermost layer of the meninges _____

10. placed in another location _____

11. half (partially) paralyzed _____

12. pertaining to the temporal and parietal region _____

REVIEW ACTIVITIES

CROSSWORD PUZZLE

Check your answers by going back through the frames or checking the solutions in Appendix F.

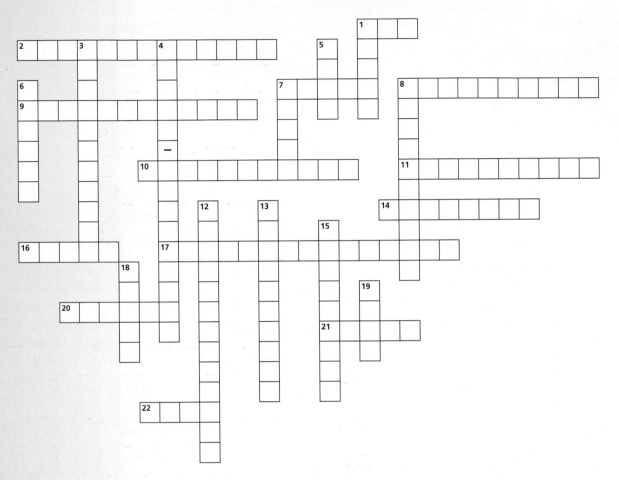

Across

1. synonym for syn-
2. prevents pregnancy
7. prefix meaning between
8. infection in the blood
9. inflammation upon the kidney
10. x-ray of the breast (process)
11. drug that fights bacteria
14. below the dura mater
16. prefix meaning across
17. process of inserting a catheter
20. prefix meaning against
21. prefix meaning outside
22. prefix meaning same

Down

1. prefix meaning above
3. Donors give blood for a _____.
4. outside of a joint
5. prefix meaning against
6. prefix meaning different
7. prefix meaning within
8. above the pubic bone
12. made of different substances or tissues
13. cleans the skin before surgery
15. both sides
18. prefix meaning beyond
19. prefix meaning beyond

GLOSSARY

analgesics	pain relievers	antidepressants	agent that works against depression
antiarthritic	agent that works against arthritis	antinarcotic	agent that works against the effects of narcotics
antibiotic	agent that works against organisms, especially bacteria	antipyretic	agent that works against fever
anticonvulsant	agent that prevents seizures	antirheumatic	agent that works against rheumatic disease

REVIEW ACTIVITIES

antiseptic	agent that protects against infection (external cleaner)
antispasmodic	agent that prevents muscle spasms
antitoxin	agent that works to destroy toxins
asepsis	without poisons or infection
bilateral	including both sides (adjective)
catheterization	using a tube (catheter) inserted into the bladder or vessels to obtain specimens, to look, or to keep the vessel open
contraceptive	agent that prevents conception
contraindicated	not recommended under these circumstances
contravolitional	against one's will
disinfectants	chemical or physical agents that kill organisms; not used on the human body
epicystitis	inflammation upon the urinary bladder
epidermal	pertaining to the epidermis
epidural	pertaining to the layer upon the dura mater (adjective)
epigastric	upon the stomach
epigastrorrhaphy	suturing of tissue in the region upon the stomach
epinephrectomy	excision of tissue upon the kidney
epinephritis	inflammation upon the kidney
episplenitis	inflammation upon the spleen
extra-articular	outside of a joint (adjective)
extracerebral	outside of the cerebrum (adjective)
extracystic	outside of the bladder (adjective)
extradural	outside of the dura mater (adjective)
extragenital	outside of the genital area (adjective)
extranuclear	outside of the nucleus (adjective)
heterogeneous	different throughout (adjective)
heteropsia	different vision in each eye
heterosexual	attracted to the opposite sex (adjective)

homogeneous	the same throughout (adjective)
homoglandular	same gland (adjective)
homosexual	attracted to the same sex (adjective)
infracostal	below the ribs (adjective)
inframammary	below the breast (adjective)
infrapatellar	below the patella (adjective)
infrapubic	below the pubic bone (adjective)
injection	give agent through needle and syringe
mammogram	breast x-ray film or x-ray picture
mammography	process of taking a breast x-ray
mammoplasty	surgical repair of the breast
metacarpals	bones of the hand beyond the wrist bones (carpals)
metastasis (pl. metastases)	disease that spreads beyond its origin
metacarpals	bones of the hand beyond the carpals
metatarsals	bones of the foot beyond the ankle (tarsals)
oral	by mouth
prescription	written order for treatment
psychotherapeutics	medications and treatments that treat psychological disorders
pyrotoxin	toxin produced by fever or heat
sanitization	cleaning items or surfaces
septicemia	infection in the blood
septicopyemia	infection and pus in the blood
sterilization	process that kills all organisms
subaural	below the ear
subcutaneous	below the skin, fat layer
subdural	below the dura mater (adjective)
superciliary	pertaining to the eyebrow
superficial	on the surface (adjective)
superinfection	an infection on top of another infection

REVIEW ACTIVITIES

supracostal	above the ribs (adjective)
suprainguinal	above the groin
supralumbar	above the lumbar spine (adjective)
suprapubic	above the pubic bone (adjective)
suprarenal	above the kidney
suprarenopathy	disease of the suprarenal glands (adrenals)
symmetry	the same size and shape all around or on both sides
sympathetic	suffering along with, functional part of the autonomic nervous system
sympathoma	tumor of a sympathetic nerve
sympodia	feet that have grown united
transcatheter	performed through the lumen of a catheter
transdermal	through the skin

transfusion	transferring blood from one person to another
transillumination	the passage of strong light through a body structure, to permit inspection by an observer on the opposite side
transluminal	across the lumen of a vessel
transposition	placement of an organ on the opposite side
transsexual	a person who has changed sexes
transurethral	performed through the urethra
transvaginal	performed through the vagina
ultrasonography	process of making a computer image using reflected high frequency sound waves
ultrasound	high-frequency sound waves (inaudible)
ultraviolet	high-frequency light waves beyond the violet frequency

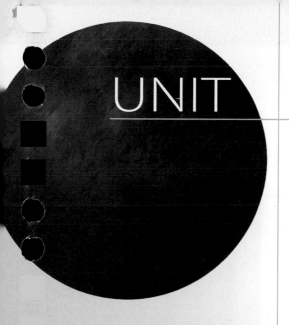

UNIT 12

Prefixes of Location and Medication Administration

12.1

Spirare is a Latin word meaning to breathe. Breathing is respiration. Breathing consists of the following two processes: expiration and inspiration. Think of the meaning as you analyze:

ex/pir/ation
eks spə **rā'** shun
in/spir/ation
in spə rā' shun

expiration _____/_____/_____ (noun);

inspiration _____/_____/_____ (noun);

12.2

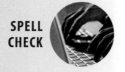

SPELL CHECK

Notice that the "s" is dropped from **spire** when preceded by **ex**.

EXAMPLES: inspire, expire, inspiration, expiration.

12.3

inspiration
expiration

inspire
expire

The noun that means breathing in is _____ and breathing out is _____ .

The verb that means breath in is _____ and breath out is _____ .

12.4

not

in- is a prefix that means in, into, within or **not**. In/compatible drugs are drugs that do _____ mix well with each other.

ANSWER COLUMN

12.5

not able

In/compet/ence occurs in an organ when it is * _____ to perform its function.

Incompetence is a noun. When the ile/o/cec/al valve cannot perform its function,

in/compet/ence
in **kom′** pə təns

the result is ileocecal valve _____/_____/_____.

12.6

in/compet/ent
in **kom′** pə tent

In/compet/ent is an adjective. An _____ cervix cannot help to hold a pregnancy.

12.7

incompetence

When blood seeps back through the aortic valves, aortic _____ or insufficiency occurs.

12.8

incompetence
incompetent

When a person is not able to think rationally enough to care for himself or herself, it may be called ment/al _____ (noun). You may even say the person is mentally _____ (adjective).

12.9

in/continence
in **kon′** ti nəns
in/continent
in **kon′** ti nent

Continence is the ability to control defecation and urination. Lack of bowel control is called _____/_____ (noun). The person who loses bladder control is _____/_____ (adjective).

12.10

in/sane
in **sān′**
in/somnia
in **som′** nē ə
in/coherent
in **kō hēr′** ənt

Build words meanings

not sane _____/_____ ;

unable to sleep _____/_____ ;

not coherent _____/_____ .

12.11

in/cis/ion
in **sizh′** ən
in/cis/ed
in **sīz′** ′d

in- also means into. To in/cise (verb) is to cut into. The noun form of in/cise is _____/_____/_____. The past tense verb form of incise is _____/_____/_____.

ANSWER COLUMN

12.12

ex/cise
ek′ sīz′
ex/cis/ion
ek si′ zhun

To cut into is to incise (verb). To cut out (remove) is to _____/_____
(verb). An _____/_____/_____ (noun)
removes an organ or tissue.

12.13

In/flamma/tion (noun) comes from a Latin term meaning "to set on fire." Our
bodies are not literally set on fire, but, redness, swelling, pain, and heat occurs in
irritated or infected tissues. The in/flamma/tory (adjective) response is part of our
defense system. Tissues that are invaded by pathogens or receive physical injury
become in/flamed (verb).
Complete the following statements:

in/flam/ed
in **flām′** ′d
in/flamma/tion
in flə **mā′** shun

The infected wound looked _____/_____/_____ (verb).

_____/_____/_____ was one sign of an
allergic reaction to the bee sting.

NOTE: Recall the suffix **–itis** means inflammation.

12.14

In/ject means to introduce a substance into the body (usually through a needle).
Define the following

verb form of inject
one who (thing which)
   injects

procedure of injecting

inject, injected * _____;
injector * _____
_____;
injection * _____.

**Intravenus infusion
using an IV infusion
pump** *Photo by Timothy J. Dennerll,
RT(R), Ph.D.*

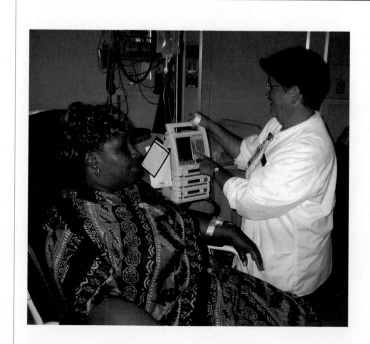

ANSWER COLUMN

---

in/fus/ion
in **fyoo'** shən
infusion

12.15

Fluids such as normal (isotonic) saline with 5% dextrose may be introduced into a vein. This is an IV _____/_____/_____.

The pump used to regulate the speed of flow of an IV is called an _____ pump.

---

in/filtr/ation
in fil **tra'** shun

12.16

In/filtr/ation is the permeation or penetration of a dissolved substance into a tissue. Local anesthetic may be in/filtr/ated by injection into tissues around a lesion that is going to be removed. The process of injecting an anesthetic solution such as lidocaine to numb an area before surgery is

_____/_____/_____.

---

in/filtr/ated
in **fil'** tra ted

12.17

If an intra/ven/ous needle slips out of position in the vein and the IV solution seeps into the surrounding tissues it has _____/_____/_____.
(past tense verb)

---

in/still/ation
in stil **ā'** shən
in/still
in **stil'**

12.18

In Latin *stillare* means to drip. In/stillation is putting medicated drops into an eye or body cavity. Medication (otic solution) dropped into an ear is

an _____/_____/_____. To put in medication in droplet form is to _____/_____ (verb) a medication.

Instillation—eye drops
Delmar/Cengage Learning

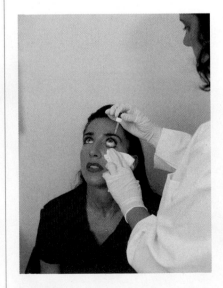

ANSWER COLUMN

12.19

Recall that semen is a fluid substance that contains sperm. *Semin/o* is the combining form. Artificial in/semin/ation is a process of placing semen into the opening of the cervix using either husband (AIH) or donor (AID) sperm. Couples having difficulty with conception may be successful using artificial

in/semin/ation
in sem i **nā'** shun

_____ / _____ / _____ .

12.20

Use of a husband's sperm to fertilize an egg is called artificial

insemination

_____ by husband (AIH).

12.21

Now, see how many new vocabulary words you have just learned.
Build words that mean

ex/pire or ex/hale

to breath out (verb) _____ / _____ or _____ / _____ ;

ex/cis/ion

cutting out (noun) _____ / _____ / _____ ;

in/spir/ation

breathing in (noun) _____ / _____ / _____ ;

in/cise

to cut into (verb) _____ / _____ .

12.22

Build words that mean

in/compentence

not competent (noun) _____ / _____ ;

in/compatible

not compatible _____ / _____ ;

in/coherent

not able to be understood _____ / _____ ;

in/fus/ion

solution introduced Into a vein _____ / _____ / _____ ;

in/still/ation

medication administration by drops _____ / _____ / _____ ;

in/flam/ed

red, swollen, painful, warm _____ / _____ / _____ (verb).

12.23

**TAKE A
CLOSER LOOK**

Use your dictionary
if you need help.

Analyze the following **in-** words by writing their meaning and indicating the part of speech

	meaning	*part of speech*
injected	_____	(_____)
incision	_____	(_____)
inflamed	_____	(_____)
infusion	_____	(_____)
infested	_____	(_____)

ANSWER COLUMN

bad

12.24

Mal is a French word that means bad. **mal-** is also a prefix that means bad or poor.

Mal/odor/ous means having a _____ odor.

---

poorly formed or
poor formation

12.25

Mal/aise (ma lāz') means a general feeling of illness or feeling poorly.

Mal/formation means * _____

_____ .

---

poor nutrition

poor absorption
(as of nutrients)

12.26

Good nutrition is essential for good health. Mal/nutrition means

* _____ .

Mal/absorption means

* _____ .

---

mal/aise
ma **lāz'**

mal/nutrition
mal noo **trī'** shun

mal/absorbtion
mal ab **sorb'** shun

mal/formation
mal fôr **mā'** shun

12.27

Build a "bad" word that means
feeling bad

_____/_____ ;

bad (poor) nutrition

_____/_____ ;

bad (poor) absorption

_____/_____ ;

bad (poor) formation

_____/_____ .

Good!

**DICTIONARY
EXERCISE**

12.28

Mal/nutrition may take the form of overnutrition or undernutrition.
Malnutrition may be caused by lack of nutrients, starvation, overeating,
socioeconomic conditions, or emotional eating disorders. Hyper/phagia
(overeating), anorexia nervosa (not eating), and bulimia (binging and purging)
are all eating disorders. Look up the following terms in your dictionary and write
more information about their meanings here.

hyperphagia _____

anorexia _____

anorexia nervosa _____

bulimia _____

compulsive overeating _____

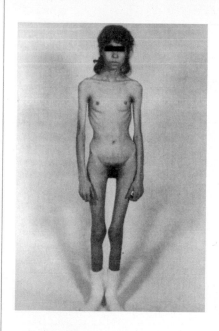

12.29

-**orexia** is a Greek word part meaning appetite.

A person who is obsessed about being thin, and severely limits his or her food

intake may have * _____.

an/orexia nervosa
an ôr **eks'** ē ə ner **vō'** sa

12.30

Diseases which cause anorexia (loss of appetite) such as ulcers and cancer make it difficult for a person to maintain normal weight. They begin wasting away. Cach/exia is a word built from the Greek *kakos*, meaning bad, and *hexia*, for condition. A person who has unhealthy loss of weight because of chronic illness

has _____/_____.

cach/exia
ka **keks'** ē ə

12.31

Cachexia means

** _____.

wasting away due to
illness and anorexia

12.32

A person who may overeat and then take laxatives or force himself or herself to vomit to purge the stomach of the food may be suffering from

_____/_____.

bul/imia
boo **lē'** mē ə

ANSWER COLUMN

---

malari/o

12.33

Look at the words in the next two frames. Now find the combining form for the disease malaria: _____/_____ .

12.34

malari/a
mə **lair'** ē ə

Before people knew that mosquitoes carry the malaria parasite (*Plasmodium vivax*), they thought this disease was caused by "bad" night air. Analyze malaria (means bad air): _____/_____ .

CASE STUDY INVESTIGATION (CSI)

Malaria
Malaria, a disease producing 500 million cases a year, results from **infection** following the bite of an *Anopheles* mosquito **infested** with Plasmodium. The severity and course **malaria** takes depends on the malarial species, patient age, genetic constitution, immune status, general health, and nutritional status of the patient. The parasites first multiply in **hepatocytes** of the liver before invading the blood. Malaria is an **erythrocytic** parasite that causes fever, **diaphoresis**, rigor, headache, **malaise**, anemia, and complications that may lead to death. The **incubation** period is **asymptomatic** and parasites may be undetectable for up to 16 days. The **diagnosis** of malaria must be based on laboratory findings and **intravenous** drug therapy is the most effective treatment.

CSI Vocabulary Challenge
Use a medical dictionary to analyze the term listed from the case study. Divide the terms into word parts and write the definition in the space provided.

infection _____

infested _____

malaria _____

hepatocytes _____

erythrocytic _____

diaphoresis _____

malaise _____

incubation _____

asymptomatic _____

diagnosis _____

intravenous _____

ANSWER COLUMN

12.35

Analyze these words involving the disease malaria by drawing the diagonals and giving the part of speech:

part of speech

malari/al (adjective)

malari/ous (adjective)

malari/o/logy (noun)

malari/o/therapy (noun)
(You pronounce)

malarial _____ (_____)

malarious _____ (_____)

malariology _____ (_____)

malariotherapy _____ (_____)

12.36

three

three

three

uni- means one. **bi-** means two. **tri-** means three. The tri/ceps muscle has

_____ heads. A tri/cuspid valve has _____ cusps.

The tri/gemin/al nerve has _____ branches.

Look back to the numeric prefix table on page 383 to review Latin and Greek word parts.

12.37

tri/ceps

trī′ seps

The three-headed muscle in the posterior upper arm is the

_____/_____.

NOTE: triceps is both a singular and plural form.

12.38

tri/plets

trip′ letz

Quintuplets are five infants born at the same time. Giving birth to three infants during the same pregnancy is having _____/_____.

12.39

tri/gemin/al

trī **jem′** i nəl

The three-branched cranial nerve is the _____/_____/_____ nerve.

Antagonistic muscle pair: (A) extension— biceps relaxed, triceps contracted; (B) flexion—biceps contracted, triceps relaxed *Delmar/Cengage Learning*

Triceps contracted

Biceps relaxed

Triceps relaxed

Biceps contracted

Biceps relaxed

(A)

(B)

ANSWER COLUMN

Blood vessels of the head and neck
Delmar/Cengage Learning

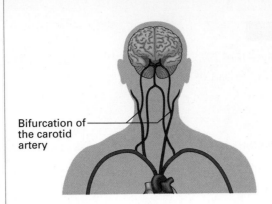

Bifurcation of the carotid artery

12.40

bi- means two. **furco-** means branching or dividing. To bi/furc/ate is to divide into two branches. When an artery divides into two, it

bi/furc/ates
bī′ fər kāts

_____/_____/_____ (verb) (e.g., cartoid artery; see the illustration).

NOTE: The word root **furc** should make you think of "fork."

12.41

bi/furc/ation
bī fer **kā′** shən

Bi/furc/ate is a verb. The noun is bi/furc/ation. When a nerve divides into

two branches, a _____/_____/_____ (noun) is formed.

12.42

bifurcations

Lymphatic vessels or ducts also form _____ (plural).

12.43

two

two

two

two

The bi/ceps brachii is a muscle with _____ heads or muscle bundles.

A bi/cusp/id is a tooth with _____ cusps.

Bi/foc/al glasses have _____ foci in one lens.

A bi/furc/ation has _____ branches.

12.44

bi/cuspid
bī **kus′** pid

bi/focals
bī′ fō kəlz

bi/sexual
bī **sex′** yōō əl

Build words that mean
a tooth with two cusps

_____/_____/_____;

lenses with two areas of focus

_____/_____/_____;

one who is sexually attracted to both males and females

_____/_____/_____;

(continued)

ANSWER COLUMN

bi/furcation
bī fer **kā'** shun

bi/ceps
bī' seps

the part of a structure that divides into two branches

_____/_____/_____;

a muscle with two heads

_____/_____ brachii.

12.45

SPELL
CHECK

Biceps is used both as a singular and as a plural form. The biceps brachii is the name of the muscle.

12.46

one

one

one

uni- means one. A uni/corn has _____ horn. Uni/ovul/ar pertains to twins who develop from _____ ovum. Uni/vers/al means combined into _____ whole.

12.47

uni/later/al
yōō ni **lat'** er əl

bi/later/al
bī' lat er əl

tri/later/al
trī' lat er əl

Later/al means pertaining to the side. Build words meaning pertaining to one side

_____/_____/_____;

two sides

_____/_____/_____;

three sides

_____/_____/_____.

12.48

bi/cell/ular
bī **sel'** yōō lar

uni/cell/ular or
yōō' nē **sel'** yōō lar
mono/cell/ular
mon ō **sel'** yōō lar

multi- means many. Multi/cell/ular means made of many cells. Build words meaning
made of two cells

_____/_____/_____;

made of one cell only

_____/_____/_____.

STUDYWARE™ CONNECTION

Remember, after completing this unit you can play a championship or other interactive game on your **StudyWARE™ CD-ROM** that will help you learn the content in this chapter.

ANSWER COLUMN

12.49

Some cells are multi/nucle/ar in nature. Build words meaning
having one nucle/us (adjective)

uni/nucle/ar *or*
yōō ni **nōō'** klē är
mono/nucle/ar
mon ō **nōō'** klē är

bi/nucle/ar
bī **nōō'** klē ar

_____/_____/_____ ;

having two nucle/i

_____/_____/_____ .

NOTE: Nucleus is singular, nuclei is plural, and nuclear is the adjectival form.

12.50

A person with physical characteristics of both males and females is a
hermaphrodite.
A person with both male and female genitals may be said to be a

herm/aphrodite
herm **af'** rō dīt

_____/_____ .

NOTE: Refer back to Unit 11 Information Table of Sexuality Terms.

12.51

WORD ORIGINS

Hermaphrodites was the child of the god Hermes and the goddess Aphrodite.
S/he exhibited characteristics of both the father and mother, male and female
genders. Today the term hermaphrodite (Hermes and Aphrodite) or intersexual
means having both male and female characteristics.

12.52

Affective disorders are disturbances in emotional mood or mental state. Some
people experience severe mood swings from a manic (excited) to a depressive state.

bi/polar
bī **pōl'** ar

This experience of two polar extremes is called _____/_____
affective disorder.

12.53

Build words that mean
sexually attracted to both sexes

bi/sex/ual

_____/_____/_____ ;
having two poles (as in manic/depressive)

bi/polar

_____/_____ .

12.54

Review

one
two
three
many

uni- means _____ ;

bi- means _____ ;

tri- means _____ ;

multi- means _____ .

ANSWER COLUMN

12.55

Give the meaning of the following terms
bifurcation

dividing into two
branches

* _____ ;

bisexual

attracted to both males
and females

* _____ ;

pertaining to both sides

bilateral

* _____ ;

uninuclear

pertaining to having one
nucleus

* _____ ;

hermaphrodite

individual possessing both
male and female genitals

* _____ .

Prefix	Meaning	Explanation
semi-	half	used with modern English words or words closer to modern English
hemi-	half	used more with medical terms

12.56

semi-

hemi-

There are two prefixes that mean half. They are _____ and
_____ .

12.57

Form words that mean

half circle _____ / _____ ;

semi/circle

semi/conscious

semi/private

half conscious _____ / _____ ;

half private (hospital room) _____ / _____ .

12.58

Build words meaning
presence of only half a heart (noun)

hemi/cardi/a
hem ē **kär'** dē ə

_____ / _____ / _____ ;

removal of half the stomach

hemi/gastr/ectomy
hem ē gast **rek'** tom ē

_____ / _____ / _____ ;

paralysis of half the body (on one side)

hemi/plegia *or*
hem ē **plē'** jē ə
hemi/paralysis
hem ē par **al'** ə sis

_____ / _____ .

ANSWER COLUMN

12.59

TAKE A CLOSER LOOK

Note the difference between these two words: hemi/plegia (paralysis of one side of the body) and paraplegia (paralysis of the lower half of the body). Look up para/plegia, hemi/plegia, and quadri/plegia in your dictionary and read about these conditions.

12.60

Build words meaning

semi/circul/ar

half circular _____/_____/_____;

semi/norm/al

half normal _____/_____/_____;

semi/coma/tose
(You pronounce)

half comatose _____/_____/_____.

12.61

Build words with the literal meaning of paralysis of half (one side) of the body

hemi/plegia
hem′ ē **plē′** jē ə

_____/_____;

half of a sphere (e.g., cerebral)

hemi/sphere
hem′ i sfēr

_____/_____;

anesthesia of half the body

hemi/an/esthesi/a
hem′ ē an es **thēs′** ē ə

_____/_____/_____/_____.

12.62

INFORMATION FRAME

genit/o comes from the Greek word *genesis,* meaning the beginning or formation. The reproductive system structures are called genit/als.

12.63

genit/al
jen′ i təl

A herpes simplex virus (HSV) infection in the area around the external genitalia is called _____/_____ herpes.

12.64

with

con- is a prefix that means with. Con/genit/al means born _____.

12.65

born with

A child with con/genit/al cataracts is * _____ cataracts.

12.66

con/genit/al
kon **jen′** i təl

There are many con/genit/al deformities. A child born with a lateral curvature of the spine has _____/_____/_____ scoliosis.

ANSWER COLUMN

12.67

congenital

Another way of saying a deformity with which one is born, is to say congenital anomaly. A child born with kyphosis (posterior curvature of the spine) has a

_____ anomaly (abnormality).

12.68

congenital

A child born with hydr/ophthalm/os has _____ glaucoma (increased fluid pressure condition of the eye).

12.69

congenital

A child born with syphilis has _____ syphilis.

Child with Down syndrome, a congenital anomaly, with his sister *Photo by Timothy J. Dennerll, RT(R), Ph.D.*

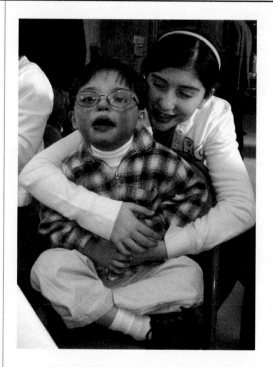

Abnormal curvatures of the spine: (A) kyphosis; (B) lordosis; (C) scoliosis *Delmar/Cengage Learning*

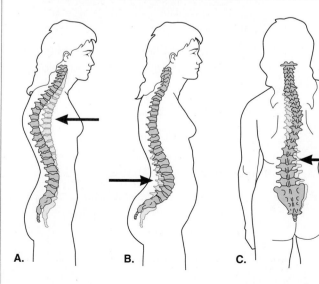

A.   B.   C.

ANSWER COLUMN

12.70

con- prefix—with
sanguin/o combining form—blood
-ity noun suffix—quality
Using what you need of the above word parts, build a word meaning literally with blood or, in usage, blood relationship:

con/sanguin/ity
kon' sang **gwin'** i tē

_____/_____/_____ .

12.71

Con/sanguin/ity is a relationship by descent from a common ancestor. The noun

consanguinity

that expresses the relationship of cousins is _____ .

12.72

sanguin/o means bloody. Build a word meaning having bloody drainage on a

sanguin/eous _or_
sang **gwin'** ē us
sanguin/ous
sang' gwin us

dressing: _____/_____ .
NOTE: The suffix -ous means having, possessing, or full of.

12.73

Build words meaning

con/sanguin/ity

having blood relationship _____/_____/_____;

san/guin/ous _or_
    san/guin/eous

bloody _____/_____/_____;

con/genit/al

born with _____/_____/_____ .

12.74

dis- is a prefix that means to free of, to separate, or to undo. Dis/ease means,

free of ease

literally, * _____ .

12.75

To dis/sect is to cut a tissue or to undo it (into parts) for purposes of study. Write the following forms of the word dissect below
verb

dis/sect
dis **sekt'**

_____/_____;

noun

dis/sect/ion
dis **sek'** shən

_____/_____/_____;

past tense verb

dis/sect/ed
dis **sek'** ted

_____/_____/_____ .

ANSWER COLUMN

12.76

To dis/infect is to free of infective agents. Analyze the following terms and check definitions

dis/infect

disinfect _____/_____;

dis/infect/ant

disinfectant _____/_____/_____;

dis/infect/ion

disinfection _____/_____/_____;

dis/infect/ed

disinfected _____/_____/_____.

12.77

People with multiple personality disorder (MPD) dis/associate and experience various personas. Analyze and check definitions

dis/associate

disassociate _____/_____;

dis/sociate

dissociate _____/_____;

dis/sociated

dissociated _____/_____;

dis/sociation

dissociation _____/_____.

12.78

Recall that **dys-** means difficult or painful.

to free of, to undo

dis- is a prefix that means * _____ .

with

con- is a prefix that means _____ .

Use the following table to work Frames 12.79–12.89.

Prefix	Meaning	Look Up Meanings
post-	behind	postnasal
	after	postmastectomy
ante-	before	antecubital
	forward	anteverted
pre-	before	premolar
	in front of	pretibial

12.79

post- means after.

after

Post/prandial (pp) means _____ meals.

after

Post/cibal (pc) means _____ food.

after

Post/glucose (pg) means _____ ingesting glucose.

behind

Post/esophageal means _____ the esophagus.

after

Post/menopausal means _____ menopause.

ANSWER COLUMN

12.80

pre- means before or in front of.

before

in front of

Pre/an/esthetic means _____ anesthesia.

Pre/hyoid means * _____ the hyoid bone.

12.81

ante- means before or forward.

before

forward

Ante/pyr/etic means _____ the fever.

Ante/flex/ion means _____ bending.

12.82

Peri/nat/al concerns events that are around birth. Nat/al means birth.
Think of the meaning while you analyze
postnatal

post/nat/al

pōst **nā'** təl

_____/_____/_____ ;

pre/nat/al

prē **nā'** təl

prenatal

_____/_____/_____ ;

ante/nat/al

an tē **nā'** təl

antenatal

_____/_____/_____ .

12.83

Febris in Latin means fever. Febr/ile means pertaining to fever.
Build words meaning
pertaining to after a fever

post/febr/ile

pōst' **fē'** brəl

_____/_____/_____ ;

ante/febr/ile

an' tē **fē'** brəl

pertaining to before a fever

_____/_____/_____ .

NOTE: Natal refers to birth and terms related to the newborn baby.
Partum refers to delivery and terms related to the mother.

12.84

Build words meaning pertaining to
after an operation

post/operat/ive

pōst **op'** er a tiv

_____/_____/_____ (PO);

post/coit/al

pōst **kō'** it əl

after coitus (intercourse)

_____/_____/_____ ;

post/part/um

pōst **par'** tum

after delivery (refers to the mother)

_____/_____/_____ ;

post/nat/al

pōst **nāt'** al

after delivery or birth (refers to the baby)

_____/_____/_____ .

ANSWER COLUMN

12.85

pre/operative

pre/mature

pre/scribe

pre/cancer/ous
(You pronounce)

pre- means before. Build a word that means

before an operation _____/_____;

before maturity (readiness) _____/_____;

write before you can take (Rx) _____/_____;

before cancer develops _____/_____/_____.

12.86

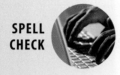

SPELL CHECK

A prescription is written before a medication may be dispensed. It is prescribed (Rx). "Perscription" is <u>not</u> a word.

Medical Specialists PC

500 W. Care Street • Health City PA • (800) 999-1000

Name <u>Jean Green</u>	**Date** <u>12/9/2009</u>
Address <u>3500 W Nile</u>	**DOB** 12/12/1950
	Wt: 160

Rx   Zoloft 50 mg
Disp #30
Sig: Take 1 tab qd

Generic permissible   <u>Holly Helpful DO</u>
Lic# A55555
DEA#AH 5555555

Refills   <u>3</u>

Delmar/Cengage Learning

12.87

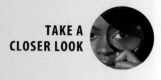

TAKE A CLOSER LOOK

Medications may be prescribed, dispensed, and administered. These three processes are often confused. "Prescribing" is writing an order for a drug. The pharmacy, office, or clinic that fills a prescription by handing the medication to the patient to give to themselves is "dispensing" the medication. If the healthcare worker injects a medication or applies a topical medicated ointment that is ordered, they are "administering" the medication.

ANSWER COLUMN

12.88

Build terms that begin with **ante-**
turning forward

ante/vers/ion
an' tē ver shən

_____/_____/_____ ;

before delivery

ante/part/um
an tē **par'** tum

_____/_____/_____ ;

position in front

ante/posit/ion
an tē po **si'** shən

_____/_____/_____ .

12.89

Mortem means death (think of mortal). What do these terms mean?

after death

postmortem * _____ ;

before death

antemortem * _____ .

NOTE: A.M. means **ante-** meridiem—before noon.
      P.M. means **post-** meridiem—after noon.

12.90

In medicine mort/ality refers to the death rate and morbid/ity refers to the rate of occurrence of disease. Statistics giving the ratio of deaths in a given population

mort/ality
mor **tal'** it ē
morbid/ity
mor **bid'** it ē

is the _____/_____ rate. The ratio of disease in a given

population is the _____/_____ rate.

12.91

Recall that **inter-** means between. **intra-** means within. Intra-abdominal means

within the abdomen

* _____ .

12.92

within a cell

Intra/cellular means * _____ .

within the uterus

Intra/uterine means * _____ .

12.93

Using **intra-** and the adjectives ven/ous, spin/al, and lumb/ar,
build words meaning
within a vein

intra/ven/ous
in' tra **vēn'** us

_____/_____/_____ ;

within the spine

intra/spin/al
in' tra **spīn'** əl

_____/_____/_____ ;

within the lumbar region

intra/lumb/ar
in' tra **lum'** bar

_____/_____/_____ .

PROFESSIONAL PROFILE

A **nurse** is a health care professional who provides a wide variety of services including the most simple patient care tasks, sophisticated lifesaving procedures, management of health care teams, education, and research. The level of responsibility of each nurse is related to education, licensure, and experience. The following are descriptions of various levels and credentials.

Licensed practical nurse (LPN) is a graduate of a practical nursing program who has passed a state practical nursing licensing exam; most programs grant a certificate of completion.

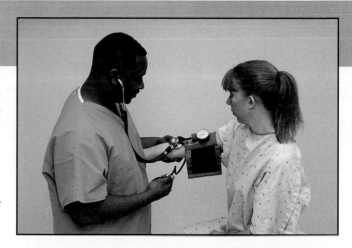

This nurse is assessing a young adult's blood pressure as part of a health program to enhance patient wellness *Delmar/Cengage Learning*

Registered nurse (RN) is a graduate of a state board-approved school of nursing who has passed a state registered nurse exam; he or she may earn an associate degree, diploma, or bachelor's degree.

Nurse practitioner (NP) is an RN with advanced preparation for practice including clinical experience in diagnosis and treatment of illnesses. NPs may be allowed to practice independently depending upon state laws; this is a master's degree level.

Certified registered nurse anesthetist (CRNA) is an RN who administers anesthesia under the supervision of an anesthesiologist and receives specialized training and certification recognized by the American Association of Nurse Anesthetists.

Clinical nurse specialist is an RN with a master's degree with a special competence in an area such as obstetrics, cardiology, or intensive care nursing.

Masters of Science in Nursing (MSN) is completion of a board-approved MSN program including clinical practicum and research. MSNs may work directly with patients, manage teams, or serve as administrators and educators in nursing programs.

RNs with Doctorate Degrees in Nursing (PhDs) work as educators and researchers in colleges and universities, or they may serve as hospital administrators.

ANSWER COLUMN

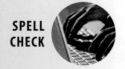

SPELL CHECK

12.94

Intravenous ends in -ous, not -eous. Also watch the pronunciation: in' tra **vēn'** us.

ANSWER COLUMN

Angle of injection for parenteral administration of medications *Delmar/Cengage Learning*

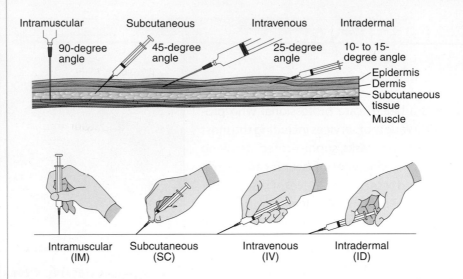

12.95

Using **intra-**, build adjectives meaning
within an artery

intra-/arteri/al
in' tra är **tēr'** ē əl

_____/-_____/_____;

within the cranium

intra/crani/al
in' tra **krā'** nē əl

_____/_____/_____;

within the bladder

intra/cyst/ic
in' tra **sis'** tik

_____/_____/_____;

within the aorta

intra-/aort/ic
in' tra ā **ôr'** tik

_____/-_____/_____.

NOTE: Take notice of the hyphen in intra-arterial and intra-aortic.

12.96

Build adjectives meaning

intra/derm/al

within the skin _____/_____/_____;

intra/duoden/al

within the duodenum _____/_____/_____;

intra/thorac/ic
(You pronounce)

within the thoracic cavity _____/_____/_____.

Abbreviation	Meaning
ac	before meals (ante cibal)
ad lib	as desired (ad libetum)
AID	artificial insemination by donor's sperm
AIH	artificial insemination by husband's sperm
am, A.M.	morning, before noon (ante meridiem)
bid	twice a day (bis in die)
caps	capsules

(continued)

ANSWER COLUMN

Abbreviation	Meaning
CRNA	certified registered nurse anesthetist
DAW	dispense as written
exc	excision
gt/gtt, gtts	drop/drops
I&O*	intake and output
IABP	intra-aortic balloon pump
ID	intradermal, identification
IM	intramuscular
inf	infusion
instill	instillation
IU*	international unit
IUD	Intrauterine device
IV	intravenous
LPN	licensed practical nurse
MSN	Masters of Science in Nursing
NP	nurse practitioner
pc	after meals (post cibal)
pm, P.M.	after noon (post meridiem)
postop	postoperative
PO	by mouth (per os)
prn	as needed or required (pro renata)
RN	registered nurse
sc, subcu, sq, subq*	subcutaneous
tab	tablet(s)
tid	three times a day (ter in die)
ī, īi, īii, īv, v̄	one, two, three, four, five (apothecary numbers)
†	death

*Abbreviation use warning. These abbreviations have been judged dangerous and should not be used.

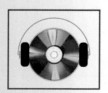

To complete your study of this unit, work the **Review Activities** on the following pages. Also, listen to the Audio CD that accompanies *Medical Terminology: A Programmed Systems Approach*, 10th edition, and practice your pronunciation.

STUDYWARE™ CONNECTION

To help you learn the content in this chapter, take a practice quiz or play an interactive game on your **StudyWARE™ CD-ROM**.

REVIEW ACTIVITIES

CIRCLE AND CORRECT

Circle the correct answer for each question. Then check your answers in Appendix E.

1. Which of the following means breathing out?
   a. excise
   b. incising
   c. exhale
   d. inspiration

2. If an organ does not function properly it may be said to be
   a. incontinent
   b. inflamed
   c. instilled
   d. incompetent

3. Which of the following is a noun form?
   a. inject
   b. injection
   c. injectable
   d. injecting

4. Which of the following prefixes does not mean bad or poor?
   a. mal-
   b. dys-
   c. mis-
   d. eu-

5. Anorexia literally means
   a. underweight
   b. starvation
   c. lack of appetite
   d. malnutrition

6. The three-headed muscle of the back upper arm is the
   a. triangle
   b. deltoid
   c. tricuspid
   d. triceps

7. A person who switches from mania to depression and experiences mood swings may have

   _____ disorder.
   a. multiple personality disorder
   b. hyperglycemia
   c. bipolar
   d. schizophrenia

8. Which of the following prefixes means with?
   a. con-
   b. contra-
   c. in-
   d. intra-

PREFIX AND WORD

Write the prefix that represents the direction. Then build a word using that prefix.

Prefix			Word
_____	1. out	breathe out (verb)	_____
_____	2. in	cut into (verb)	_____
_____	3. not	not competent	_____
_____	4. bad/poor	poor nutrition	_____
_____	5. three	three-branched nerve	_____
_____	6. two	two foci in one lens	_____
_____	7. one	one sided	_____
_____	8. half	half conscious	_____
_____	9. half	paralysis of half the body (one side)	_____
_____	10. with	born with	_____
_____	11. to free of	substance used to free of infective agents	_____
_____	12. after	after mastectomy	_____
_____	13. before	before surgery	_____
_____	14. in front of	in front of the frontal lobe	_____
_____	15. behind	behind the esophagus	_____
_____	16. before	before a fever	_____
_____	17. within	within the dermis	_____
_____	18. between	between the cells (review)	_____
_____	19. below	below the cutaneous (dermis) layer (review)	_____

REVIEW ACTIVITIES

SELECT AND CONSTRUCT

Select the correct word parts from the following list and construct medical terms that represent the given meaning.

ante	aria(l)	bi	cancer/o	card/ia(o)	cell/ular
cibal	coit(us)(al)	comatose	con	continence(y)	febrile
fest(ed)(ing)	formation	fus(ed)(ion)	glucose	hemi	in
intra	ject(ion)(ed)	mal	natal	nuclear(us)	partum
plegia	post	pre	sane	semi	tri
uni					ous

1. before birth _____

2. after delivery _____

3. half of a heart _____

4. partially (half) in a coma _____

5. pertaining to one cell _____

6. having one nucleus _____

7. before the development of cancer _____

8. put in using a needle (verb) _____

9. not able to control urination _____

10. not sane _____

11. poor growth _____

12. parasitic disease caused

    by *Plasmodium vivax* _____

13. after intercourse _____

14. before a fever _____

15. after a meal _____

DEFINE AND DISSECT

Give a brief definition and dissect each term listed into its word parts in the space provided. Check your answers by referring to the frame listed in parentheses and your medical dictionary. Then listen to the Audio CD to practice pronunciation.

1. expiration (12.1) _____/_____/_____

                                                                        pre   rt   suffix

    meaning _____

2. incompetence (12.5) _____/_____/_____

                                                                        pre   rt   suffix

_____

REVIEW ACTIVITIES

3. inflammation (12.13)

_____/_____/_____
      pre   rt   suffix

_____

4. malaise (12.25)

_____/_____/_____
      pre   rt   suffix

_____

5. infusion (12.15)

_____/_____
      pre   rt/suffix

_____

6. malariology (12.35)

_____/_____/_____
      rt   v   suffix

_____

7. bicuspid (12.44)

_____/_____
      pre   rt/suffix

_____

8. uniovular (12.46)

_____/_____
      pre   rt/suffix

_____

9. bifurcation (12.41)

_____/_____/_____
      pre   rt   suffix

_____

10. semicomatose (12.60)

_____/_____/_____
      pre   rt   suffix

_____

11. hemigastrectomy (12.58)

_____/_____/_____
      pre   rt   suffix

_____

12. consanguinity (12.70)

_____/_____/_____
      pre   rt   suffix

_____

13. dissection (12.75)

_____/_____/_____
      pre   rt   suffix

_____

14. postfebrile (12.83)

_____/_____/_____
      pre   rt   suffix

REVIEW ACTIVITIES

15. precancerous (12.85)

_____/_____/_____
pre   rt   suffix

_____

16. anteversion (12.88)

_____/_____/_____
pre   rt   suffix

_____

17. intravenous (12.93)

_____/_____/_____
pre   rt   suffix

_____

18. incontinence (12.9)

_____/_____
pre   rt/suffix

_____

19. insemination (12.18)

_____/_____/_____
pre   rt   suffix

_____

20. bisexual (12.53)

_____/_____/_____
pre   rt/suffix

_____

21. triplets (12.38)

_____/_____
pre   rt/suffix

_____

22. hemiplegia (12.58)

_____/_____
pre   suffix

_____

23. disassociate (12.77)

_____/_____
pre   rt/suffix

_____

24. perinatal (12.82)

_____/_____/_____
pre   rt   suffix

_____

25. intradermal (12.96)

_____/_____/_____
pre   rt   suffix

_____

26. excision (12.12)

_____/_____/_____
pre   rt   suffix

_____

REVIEW ACTIVITIES

27. anorexia (12.29)

_____/_____/_____
pre   rt   suffix

_____

28. cachexia (12.30)

_____/_____
rt   suffix

_____

29. infiltration (12.16)

_____/_____/_____
pre   rt   suffix

_____

ABBREVIATION MATCHING

Match the following abbreviations with their definition.

_____ 1. IUD
_____ 2. IM
_____ 3. PO
_____ 4. IV
_____ 5. ac
_____ 6. bid
_____ 7. pc
_____ 8. IU

a. drops
b. international units
c. intravenous
d. subcutaneous
e. intake and output
f. intramuscular
g. intrauterine device
h. before meals
i. postoperative
j. intradermal
k. twice a day
l. after meals
m. infusion
n. input and outtake
o. postprandial

ABBREVIATION FILL-IN

Fill in the blanks with the correct abbreviation.

9. excision _____
10. artificial insemination (husband) _____
11. intradermal _____
12. apothecary number three _____
13. before noon _____
14. infusion _____
15. as needed _____

REVIEW ACTIVITIES

CASE STUDY

Write the term next to its meaning. Then draw slashes to analyze the word parts. Note the use of medical abbreviations. Look these up in your dictionary or find them in Appendix B. If you have any questions about the answers, refer to your medical dictionary or check with your instructor for the answers in Appendix E.

CASE STUDY 12-1

Operative Report

Preoperative diagnosis: **Bilateral** adnexal masses, probable pelvic endometriosis, and **endometriomata**

Postoperative diagnosis: Bilateral adnexal masses, probable pelvic endometriosis, and endometriomata

Procedure: Total abdominal hysterectomy, bilateral **salpingo-oophorectomy**, lysis of **adhesions**, incidental **appendectomy**

Technique and findings: Under adequate general anesthesia the patient was prepped and draped in the usual sterile fashion and placed in the supine position with an **intracystic** Foley catheter. A lower abdominal midline incision was made and the abdominal wall opened in the usual fashion. Upon entering the abdominal cavity, no unusual peritoneal fluid was noted. The upper abdomen was explored and found to be within normal limits. There were noted bilateral large ovarian endometriomata. The anterior cul-de-sac was free of adhesions, but the lower part of the sigmoid colon was adhered to the **posterior** wall of the cul-de-sac. The sigmoid adhesion was taken off the posterior wall of the uterus by sharp and blunt **dissection**, down past the uterosacral ligaments, freeing the cul-de-sac area. The bilateral endometriomata were ruptured, freeing the ovaries from the lateral pelvic walls. The round ligaments were bilaterally clamped, cut, and ligated with #1 chromic sutures. The **visceroperitoneum** between the round ligaments was **transversely incised** and the bladder bluntly **dissected** off the lower uterine segment of the cervix.

1. both sides _____

2. tumors of the endometrium _____

3. cut into (verb) _____

4. across (adverb) _____

5. the membrane on the abdominal organs _____

6. before surgery _____

7. cut apart (verb) _____

8. back _____

9. within the urinary bladder _____

10. excision of the appendix _____

11. excision of the ovaries and uterine tubes _____

12. tissues grown together _____

13. after surgery _____

14. cutting apart (noun) _____

REVIEW ACTIVITIES

CROSSWORD PUZZLE

Check your answers by going back through the frames or checking the solutions in Appendix F.

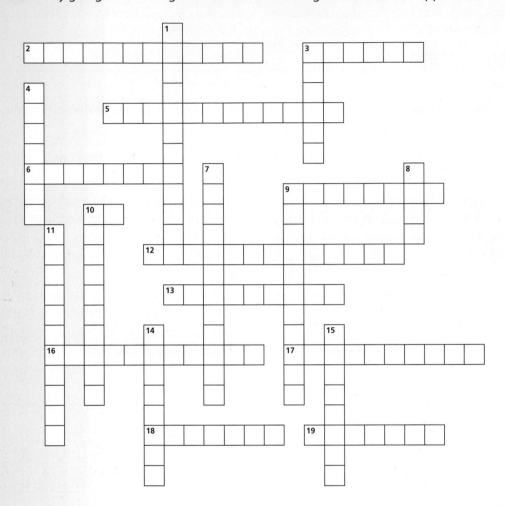

Across

2. subcu. means_____
3. two-headed muscle
5. poor nutritional status
6. a cut made into the body
9. synonym for antenatal
10. after meals (abbr.)
12. partially conscious
13. involving both sides
16. medicines to fight bacteria (plural)
17. born with
18. three-headed muscle
19. to cut apart

Down

1. unable to control urination or defecation
3. sanguinous means___
4. generally poor feeling
7. process of administering medication using drops
8. hemiplegia is paralysis of _____ the body
9. before surgery
10. after delivery (the mother)
11. branched in two (noun)
14. at the site
15. introducing a substance into the body, such as through an IV

REVIEW ACTIVITIES

GLOSSARY

administration	giving a treatment or medication	genitals	reproductive system structures
anorexia	lack of appetite or desire to eat	hemianesthesia	anesthesia involving half the body
antagonistic	oppositional or blocking	hemicardia	half a heart
antefebrile	before a fever	hemigastrectomy	excision of half the stomach
anteflexion	bending forward	hemiplegia	paralysis of one side of the body (right or left) (hemiparalysis)
antemortem	before death		
antenatal	before birth (prenatal)	incise	to cut into
antepartum	before delivery (mother)	incoherent	unable to be understood (speech)
anteposition	in front of	incompatible	not compatible, does not associate well with
antepyretic	before a fever	incompetency	not able to function properly
anteversion	turning toward	incontinence	inability to control urination or defecation
asymptomatic	without symptoms	incubation	original growth of an organism
bicellular	made of two cells	infested	organisms living within or on another organism
biceps	a two-bellied muscle (i.e., b. femoris, b. brachii)	infiltration	penetration of a solution into tissues
bifocal	lens having two focus strengths	inflamed	act of being red, swollen, painful and warm (verb)
bifurcation	branch into two		
binuclear	having two nuclei	inflammation	condition with such symptoms as a red, swollen, and warm area (noun)
bipolar	having two poles	infusion	introducing a substance into a vein through a needle
bisexual	attracted to two sexes		
bulimia	condition of purging after eating	inhale	to breathe in
cachexia	wasting away of the body	injection	procedure of introducing a substance into the body through a needle
congenital	born with		
consanguinity	with blood relationship	insane	not sane
disassociate	to break apart	insemination	process of introducing semen into the uterus or tubes
disinfect	to rid of infectious agents	insomnia	unable to fall asleep
dispense	to give out for use	inspiration	breathing in
dissect	to cut apart	instillation	applying drops
excise	to take out	intercellular	between the cells
exhale	to breathe out	intra-abdominal	within the abdomen
expiration	breathing out	intra-aortic	within the aorta

REVIEW ACTIVITIES

intra-arterial	within the artery	postmortem	after death
intracranial	within the cranium	postnatal	after birth (baby)
intracystic	within the urinary bladder	postoperative	after surgery
intradermal	within the dermal layer	postpartum	after delivery (mother)
intraduodenal	within the duodenum	postprandial	after meals
intrathoracic	within the thorax (thoracic cavity, chest)	preanesthetic	before anesthesia
intravenous	within the vein	precancerous	condition that may lead to cancer
malaise	generally poor feeling, not feeling well	prefrontal	in front of the frontal bone
malaria	infestation of malaria parasite Plasmodium	preoperative	before surgery
malformation	poor formation	prescribe	write an order for before it can be done
malnutrition	poor nutrition, missing essential nutrients	sanguineous	bloody (also, sanguinous)
malodorous	smelling bad	semicircle	half of a circle
mononuclear	having one nucleus	semicomatose	partially in a coma
morbidity	related to illness	semiconscious	partially conscious (half)
mortality	related to death	semiprivate	situation in which a room is shared (patient gets half of the room)
postcibal	after meals	subcutaneous	the layer below the dermis of the skin
postcoital	after intercourse	triceps	a three-headed muscle (i.e., t. femoris, t. brachii)
postesophageal	in back of the esophagus		
postfebrile	after a fever	trifurcation	branch into three
postglucose	after glucose is administered	unicellular	of one cell (also, monocellular)
postmastectomy	after mastectomy surgery	unilateral	one sided
postmenopausal	after menopause is complete	uninuclear	having one nucleus (also, mononuclear)

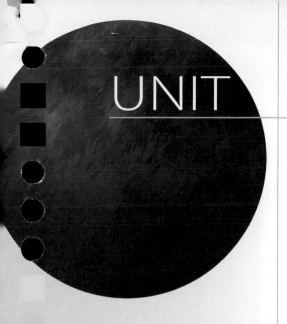

UNIT 13

Respiratory System and Pulmonology

ANSWER COLUMN

13.1

INFORMATION FRAME

The primary function of the re/spir/atory system is the in/spir/ation of life-sustaining oxygen into the lungs and bloodstream and the ex/pir/ation of the gaseous waste carbon dioxide. Air is moistened, warmed, and filtered by the nasal and sinus passages and moves down the pharynx, into the trachea, to the bronchi, and then into the bronchioles and alveoli. Study the illustration of the respiratory system structures on page 491.

13.2

re/spir/atory
res′ pir ə tôr ē
in/spir/ation
ins pir ā′ shun
ex/pir/ation
eks pir ā′ shun

The body system that is responsible for oxygen and carbon dioxide exchange is the _____/_____/_____ system. Inhaling or breathing in is also called _____/_____/_____. Exhaling or breathing out is _____/_____/_____ .

13.3

TAKE A CLOSER LOOK

The alveol/i of the lungs are surrounded by capillaries. Oxygen diffuses through the alveolar wall into the capillaries and is transported via hem/o/glob/in in the red blood cells to the tissues, where it is used to create energy. Carbon dioxide is waste gas produced by metabolism and moves from the tissues into the bloodstream, to the capillaries surrounding the alveoli, then into the alveoli, and finally is exhaled.

STUDYWARE™ CONNECTION

View an animation about *Respiration* on your **StudyWARE™ CD-ROM**.

ANSWER COLUMN

13.4

hem/o/glob/in
hēm' ō glō bin
alveol/i
al vē **ō' lī**

Red blood cells are filled with _____/_____/_____/_____, which carries oxygen through the blood. The _____/_____ are spherical structures surrounded by capillaries through which O_2 and CO_2 exchange occurs.

Use the following table of anatomic terms to build words about the respiratory system:

Combining Form	Meaning	Example
nas/o	nose	nas/o/pharyngeal
rhin/o	nose	rhin/o/rrhea
pharyng/o	pharynx (throat)	pharyng/algia
laryng/o	larynx (voice box)	laryng/itis
trache/o	trachea (windpipe)	trache/o/rrhagia
bronch/o	bronchi (bronchus)	bronch/o/scopy
bronchiol/o	bronchioles	bronchiol/ectasis
alveol/o	alveoli (alveolus)	alveol/o/plasty
phren/o, diaphragmat/o, diaphragm/o	diaphragm	phren/o/plegia diaphragm/atic
pulmon/o	lung	pulmon/ary
pneum/o	air	pneum/o/thorax
pneumon/o	lung	pneumon/ia

13.5

excision of part or all
of a lung
pneumon/o/tomy
nōō' mə **nôt'** ə mē

Pneumon/o is used in medical words concerning lungs.

Pneumon/ectomy means * _____ .

Incision into the lung is a _____/_____/_____ .

13.6

any disease of the lungs

pneumon/o/rrhagia
nōō' mə nō **rā'** jē ə

Pneumon/o/pathy means * _____ .
Form a word meaning hemorrhage of a lung

_____/_____/_____ .

Notice how these word parts about breathing and lungs were built from **pne**.

Word Part	Meaning	Medical Term
pne/o	breathing	**pne/o**/pne/ic
pneum/o	air (lung)	**pneum/o**/thorax
pneumon/o	lung	**pneumon**/ectomy
-pnea (suffix)	breathing	tachy/**pnea**

ANSWER COLUMN

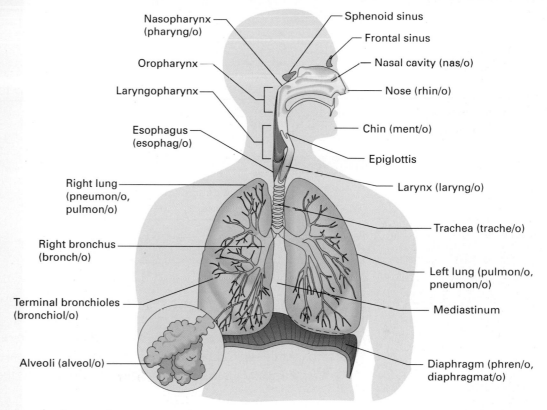

Nasopharynx (pharyng/o)

Sphenoid sinus

Frontal sinus

Oropharynx

Nasal cavity (nas/o)

Laryngopharynx

Nose (rhin/o)

Esophagus (esophag/o)

Chin (ment/o)

Epiglottis

Right lung (pneumon/o, pulmon/o)

Larynx (laryng/o)

Right bronchus (bronch/o)

Trachea (trache/o)

Left lung (pulmon/o, pneumon/o)

Terminal bronchioles (bronchiol/o)

Mediastinum

Alveoli (alveol/o)

Diaphragm (phren/o, diaphragmat/o)

Respiratory system *Delmar/Cengage Learning*

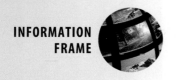

INFORMATION FRAME

13.7

Pneumon/ia is an acute inflammation of the lungs caused by a variety of bacteria, fungi, and viruses. Often antibiotics are used to treat pneumonia. Another word for pneumon/ia is pneumon/itis.

Lung x-ray PA view showing pneumonia
Delmar/Cengage Learning

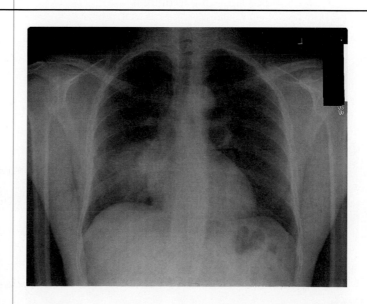

ANSWER COLUMN

13.8

Form words meaning surgical puncture of a lung to remove fluid

pneumon/o/centesis
nōō′ mə nō sen **tē**′ sis

_____/_____/_____.

Surgical puncture of the chest to remove fluid is

thorac/o/centesis
thôr′ ə kō sen **tē**′ sis

_____/_____/_____.

13.9

The two words meaning inflammation of the lungs are

pneumon/ia
nōō **mōn**′ yə

_____/_____ and

pneumon/itis
nōō′ mə **nī**′ tis

_____/_____.

13.10

Pneumocystis carinii pneumonia is an infection caused by a protozoan-like organism. People debilitated by immunodeficiency disease, such as AIDS, are particularly susceptible to this disease, which affects the

lungs

_____.

13.11

SPELL CHECK

Think of the "pn" rule for pronunciation when saying words such as pneumonia. The p is silent when pn begins the word. Also, remember eu makes the "ū" sound. The _e_ is written in front of the _u._

13.12

WORD ORIGINS

In Greek _ateles_ means imperfect and _ektasis_ means expand or dilate. **-ectasia** and **-ectasis** are suffixes used to mean dilation or expansion. Atel/ectasis is the imperfect expansion of the lungs, more commonly known as a collapsed lung. A lung collapse due to trauma

atel/ectasis
at əl **ek**′ ta sis

is _____/_____.

13.13

collapsed

A congenital lung defect may cause atel/ectasis or a _____ lung.

13.14

Prolapsed lung tissue can be surgically attached (fixated) by a procedure called

pneumon/o/pexy
nōō′ mə nō pek′ sē

_____/_____/_____.

ANSWER COLUMN

13.15

Recall that **melan/o** means black. Pneumon/o/melan/osis is a lung disease often found in coal miners in which lung tissue becomes black due to breathing black dust. The word root for black is _____ .

melan

13.16

Pneumon/o/melan/osis literally means a condition of black lungs.
Analyze this word

pneumon/o

melan

osis

_____ / _____ combining form for lung

_____ word root for black

_____ suffix—condition

13.17

The inhalation (breathing) of black dust over time results in

pneumon/o/melanosis
nōō′ mə nō mel′ ə **nō′** sis
pneumon/o/melan/osis

_____ .

The inhalation of soot or black smoke for extended periods can also cause

_____ .

13.18

Pneumon/o/myc/osis is a fungal condition of the lungs. The word root that means fungus is _____ .

myc

13.19

Myces is a Greek word meaning mushroom or fungus. **myc/o** seen any place in a word should make you think of _____ .

fungus (singular) or
fung′ gəs
fungi (plural)
fun′ jī, **fung′** gī

13.20

In high school biology, you read about and/or learned the words mycelium and mycelial. **myc** is the word root for * _____ .

fungi or fungus

13.21

A myc/osis is any condition caused by a fungus. A condition of lung fungus

pneumon/o/myc/osis
nōō **mon′** ō mī kō′ sis

is _____ / _____ / _____ / _____ .

13.22

myc/oid
mī′ koid

myc/o/logy
mī **kol′** ə jē

Build words meaning resembling fungi _____ / _____ ;

science and study of fungi _____ / _____ / _____ .

ANSWER COLUMN

13.23

Build words meaning
fungal disease (condition) of the pharynx (throat)

pharyng/o/myc/osis
fair in' gō mī **kō'** sis

_____/_____/_____/_____ ;

fungal disease (condition) of the nose

rhin/o/myc/osis
rī' nō mī **kō'** sis

_____/_____/_____/_____ ;

fungal disease of the skin

dermat/o/myc/osis
der' mat tō mī **kō'** sis

_____/_____/_____/_____ ;

inflammation of the skin caused by a fungus

myc/o/dermat/itis
mī kō der ma **tī'** tis

_____/_____/_____/_____ .

13.24

INFORMATION FRAME

pneum/o and **pneumon/o** can both refer to the lung. **pneum/o** is derived from the Greek word *pneuma* (for wind or breath). **pneum/o** is also used in words to mean air and breath.

13.25

pneumon/o comes from the Greek word *pneumon* (lung). **pneumon/o** is used

lung or lungs

in words that refer to the * _____ . The lungs are shown on page 491.

13.26

air

pneum/o is used in most words to mean _____ , as in pneumatic drill, but it can also be used to mean lung.

13.27

Thor/ax is a noun and suffix for chest cavity. Your use of **pneum/o** will be in words about air. Pneum/o/derm/a means a collection of air under the skin. A collection of air in the chest cavity (thorax) is a

pneum/o/thorax
no͞o mō **thôr'** aks

_____/_____/_____ .

13.28

Hydro/therapy means treatment with water. Treatment with compressed air is

pneum/o/therapy
no͞o mō **ther'** ə pē

called _____/_____/_____ .

13.29

A spir/o/meter measures lung volume. An instrument that measures air volume is

pneum/o/meter
no͞o **mom'** ə tər

a _____/_____/_____ . The process of measuring lung

spir/o/metry
spir **om'** ə trē

volume is _____/_____/_____ .

ANSWER COLUMN

13.30

A collection of air and serum (**ser/o**) in the chest cavity is pneum/o/ser/o/thorax. A collection of air and pus in the thoracic cavity

pneum/o/py/o/thorax
nōō mō pī ō **thôr′** aks

is a _____/_____/_____/_____/_____,
while a collection of air and blood in this same cavity is a

pneum/o/hem/o/thorax
nōō mō hē′ mō **thôr′** aks

_____/_____/_____/_____/_____.

pneum/o/thorax
nōō mō **thôr′** aks

Air forced into the chest is a _____/_____/_____.

13.31

pulmon/o is another combining form for lung used in only a few words. Pulmonary and pulmonic are both used as adjectives meaning pertaining to the lungs. The heart valve through which blood travels to the lungs is

pulmon/ary
pul′ mon air ē

the _____/_____ valve.

13.32

Blood flows from the heart to the lungs via the

pulmon/ary or pulmon/ic
pul **mon′** ik

_____/_____ artery.
Cardi/o/pulmon/ary refers to the heart

lungs

and the _____ (CPR = cardiopulmonary resuscitation).

Heart with pulmonary arteries and veins *Delmar/ Cengage Learning*

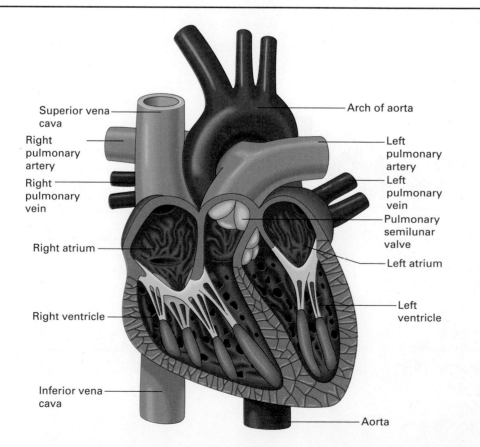

Superior vena cava

Right pulmonary artery

Right pulmonary vein

Right atrium

Right ventricle

Inferior vena cava

Arch of aorta

Left pulmonary artery

Left pulmonary vein

Pulmonary semilunar valve

Left atrium

Left ventricle

Aorta

STUDYWARE™ CONNECTION

View an animation on the *Heart* on your **StudyWARE™ CD-ROM**.

ANSWER COLUMN

13.33

Look up embolus in your dictionary. An embolus (embolism) is a thrombus (clot) that moves. A blood clot moving to the lung is called a

pulmonary embolus
pul' mon air ē **em'** bol us

* _____.

The process or condition of having an embolus is called embolism.

Study the following table of respiratory symptoms:

Term	Symptom
a/pnea	absence of breathing
dys/pnea	difficult breathing
hyper/pnea	increased rate and depth of breathing
tachy/pnea	rapid breathing
brady/pnea	slow breathing
ortho/pnea	able to breathe only when sitting up or standing
hem/o/pty/sis	expectorating (coughing up) blood
hyper/ventil/ation	excessive movement of air in and out of lungs, sighing respirations
hyp/oxia	low oxygen levels in organs and tissues
cyan/osis	bluish color due to hypoxia

13.34

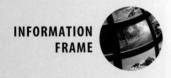

INFORMATION FRAME

pne/o is the combining form for breathing or breath. It is used most often in its suffix form, **-pnea**, to form words about breathing. Normal breathing has a regular rhythm and rate, about 12 to 16 breaths per minute (bpm) for adults. The rates increase with activity and body temperature increases.

13.35

Recall that **orth/o** means straight. Orth/o/pnea is difficulty breathing if laying straight in a horizontal position. For the patient with orthopnea to breath well, it may be necessary to elevate a patient's head and shoulders by propping them up with two or three pillows. This is referred to as two or three pillow

orth/o/pnea
ör **thop'** nē ə

_____/_____/_____.

ANSWER COLUMN

a/pnea
ap' nē ə

brady/pnea
brad ip **nē'** ə

orth/o/pnea
ôr **thop'** nē' ə

13.36

Build breathing words that mean
absence of breathing

_____/_____;

slow breathing

_____/_____;

able to breathe only when sitting up

_____/_____/_____.

CASE STUDY INVESTIGATION (CSI)

COPD

A 62-year-old woman with a two-year history of type 2 diabetes presents with **dyspnea** and a cough. She has a 30-year past history of smoking cigarettes, quitting at age 55. She has a three-year history of chronic obstructive pulmonary disease (COPD) and now has increasing dyspnea with a persistent cough. Her diabetes has been managed with diet and exercise and the last **glycosylated hemoglobin** was 6.8% (normal 4–6%). Physical exam reveals an anxious woman with blood pressure 130/70 mmHg, pulse 120, respiratory rate 24, ht 5"2" weight 165 lb. Lungs are clear to **percussion**, but **bilateral** wheezing is present. No accessory muscles are being used. No cyanosis is present. Lab evaluation: ABG: 7.48; pO_2: 62; pCO_2: 42; O_2 **Sat**: 90%. **CXR**: flat diaphragms hyperinflated, no infiltrates. **Spirometry**: forced vital capacity (**FVC**): 3.2; forced **expiratory** time in 1 second (FeV$_1$): 1.4. Treatment was started with albuterol and a course of prednisone at 40 mg/day for three days, tapering over two weeks.

CSI Vocabulary Challenge

Use a medical dictionary to help you divide the terms into word parts and write the definition of the terms and abbreviations in the space provided.

dyspnea _____

glycosylated _____

hemoglobin _____

percussion _____

bilateral _____

O_2 Sat _____

CXR _____

spirometry _____

FVC _____

expiratory _____

ANSWER COLUMN

INFORMATION FRAME

13.37

Recall that **hem/o** refers to blood. Sputum is a combination of mucus and other fluids and substances that have entered the respiratory tract. **ptyal/o** is used to refer to either saliva or sputum. Hem/o/pty/sis is a condition of bloody sputum. Ptyal/o/rrhea is a flow of saliva.

13.38

hem/o/pty/sis
hēm **op′** tə sis

pty is the word root for sputum. If a patient is coughing up sputum containing

blood, this is called _____/_____/_____/_____.

13.39

ptyal/o/rrhea
tī ə lō rē′ ə

ptyal/o is a combining form for sputum. Someone who drools because of excess

saliva may be said to have _____/_____/_____ or ptyalism.

13.40

SPELL CHECK

pt as a consonant combination is another Greek origin spelling. Watch the pronunciation and spelling. The *p* is silent when at the beginning of the word as when using *pt, ps,* and *pn.*

tī′ əl izm

EXAMPLE: ptyal/ism.
The p is pronounced if it occurs in the middle of the word.

hēm **op′** tə sis

EXAMPLE: hem/o/pty/sis.
Try the following words on your own.
psych/o/logy
pneumon/ia
ptyal/o/rrhea

13.41

nasal cavity

nas/o is used in words about the nasal cavity. Nas/o/antr/itis means inflammation

of the antrum (maxillary sinus) and the * _____.

13.42

chin

Taken from the Latin *mentum,* **ment/o** is the combining form for chin.

Nas/o/ment/al means pertaining to the nasal cavity and _____.

13.43

nas/al
nā′ zəl

Build words meaning
pertaining to the nose (cavity)

_____/_____;

(continued)

ANSWER COLUMN

inflammation of the nose (cavity)

nas/itis
nā **zī′** tis

_____/_____;

instrument to examine the nose (cavity)

nas/o/scope
nā′ zō skōp

_____/_____/_____.

13.44

Build words (you may use your dictionary if necessary) meaning inflammation of nose and pharynx

nas/o/pharyng/itis
nās′ ō far in **jī′** tis

_____/_____/_____/_____;

pertaining to the nasal and frontal bone

nas/o/front/al
nās′ ō **front′** əl

_____/_____/_____/_____;

pertaining to the nose and lacrimal duct

nas/o/lacrim/al
nās′ ō **lak′** rim əl

_____/_____/_____/_____.

WORD ORIGINS

13.45

Epi/staxis is a Greek term built from the prefix **epi-**, which means upon, and staxis meaning dripping or oozing. Although there is no mention of blood in the term, epi/staxis is the medical term for nosebleed or hemorrhage from the nose.

13.46

Hypertension, stress, dryness of membranes, and/or sinusitis may all lead

epi/staxis
e pē **staks′** is

to a nosebleed, also called _____/_____.

13.47

Nas/o/pharyng/eal means pertaining to the

nose and pharynx (throat)

* _____.

Radiologic technologist positioning patient for posteroanterior open-mouth paranasal sinus radiograph *Photo by Timothy J. Dennerll, RT(R), Ph.D., courtesy of Allegiance Health, Jackson, MI*

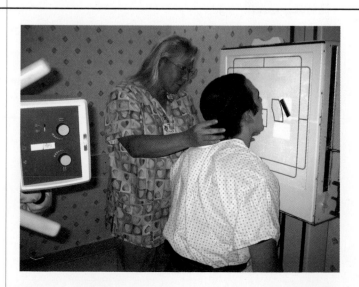

ANSWER COLUMN

13.48

pharynx
far' inks

A pharyng/o/lith (far **ing'** ō lith) is a calculus in the wall of the _____ .

NOTE: Pronounced like *fair* and *inks*. Larynx is pronounced like *lair* and *inks*.

13.49

pharynx (work on the pronunciation)

A pharyng/o/myc/osis (far ing' ō mī **kō'** sis) is a fungal disease of

the _____ .

13.50

Build words meaning
inflammation of the pharynx

pharyng/itis
far' in **jī'** tis

_____/_____ ;

herniation of the pharynx

pharyng/o/cele
fə **ring'** gō sēl

_____/_____/_____ ;

incision of the pharynx

pharyng/o/tomy
far' ing **got'** ə mē

_____/_____/_____ .

13.51

The pharynx is the throat. Build words meaning (you put in slashes):
disease of the pharynx

pharyng/o/pathy

_____ ;

surgical repair of the pharynx

pharyng/o/plasty

_____ ;

instrument to examine the pharynx

pharyng/o/scope
(You pronounce)

_____ .

13.52

laryng/o

laryng/o is used to build words that refer to the larynx. The larynx contains the

vocal cords. When referring to the organ of sound, use _____/_____ .

NOTE: Musical notes make up chords. Ligaments in the body are cords.

Pharyngitis *Courtesy of
the Centers for Disease Control
and Prevention (CDC)*

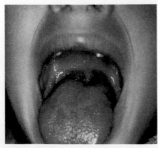

ANSWER COLUMN

13.53

Form a word that means inflammation of the larynx

laryng/itis
lar' in **jī'** tis

_____/_____ .

NOTE: **laryng/o** is also used to indicate throat, as in otorhinolaryngologist (ENT).

13.54

After a bad cold, a patient may have laryngitis with accompanying pain.

laryng/algia
lar' in **gal'** jē ə

Pain in the larynx is called _____/_____ .

13.55

Anything that obstructs the flow of air from the nose to the larynx may call

laryng/o/stomy

for creating a new opening, or a _____/_____/_____ .

13.56

When a temporary opening is wanted into the larynx, the surgical procedure is a laryng/o/tomy. An incision into the larynx is called a

laryng/o/tomy
lar' ing **got'** ə mē

_____/_____/_____ .

Remember the "g" rule for pronunciation in Frames 13.47–13.58.

13.57

herniation of the larynx

A laryng/o/cele is a * _____ .

13.58

Build words meaning
any disease of the larynx

laryng/o/pathy

_____/_____/_____ ;

instrument used to examine the larynx

laryng/o/scope

_____/_____/_____ ;

spasm of the larynx

laryng/o/spasm
(You pronounce)

_____/_____/_____ .

13.59

The trachea (**trache/o**) is the windpipe. Trache/o/py/osis means

a condition of the trachea
with pus formation

* _____

_____ .

13.60

Trache/o/rrhagia means

hemorrhage from the
trachea

* _____

_____ .

ANSWER COLUMN

13.61

Build words meaning
pain in the trachea

trache/algia
trā′ kē **al′** jē ə

_____/_____;

incision into the trachea

trache/o/tomy
trā′ kē **ot′** ə mē

_____/_____/_____;

herniation of the trachea

trache/o/cele
trā′ kē ō sēl

_____/_____/_____.

13.62

Build words meaning
examination of the trachea

trache/o/scopy
trā′ kē **os′** kō pē

_____/_____/_____;

pertaining to the trachea

trache/al
trā′ kē əl

_____/_____;

incision of trachea and larynx

trache/o/laryng/o/tomy
trā′ kē ō lar′ ing **ot′** ō mē

_____/_____/_____/_____/_____;

surgical creation of a new opening in the trachea

trache/ostomy
trā′ kē **os′** tō mē

_____/_____;

within the trachea

endo/trache/al
en′dō **trā′** kē əl

_____/_____/_____.

13.63

inflammation of the
   bronchi

Bronch/itis means * _____
_____.

an instrument to
   examine the bronchi

A bronch/o/scope is * _____
_____.

use of a flexible
   bronchofiberscope
   to examine the
   tracheobronchial tree

Bronch/o/fiber/o/scopy is * _____
_____.

13.64

Build words meaning
calculus in a bronchus

bronch/o/lith
bron′ kō lith

_____/_____/_____;

(continued)

ANSWER COLUMN

bronch/o/scopy
bron **kos′** kə pē

bronch/o/rrhagia
bron′ kô **rā′** jē ə

examination of a bronchus (with instrument)

_____/_____/_____;

bronchial hemorrhage

_____/_____/_____.

13.65

bronch/o/stomy
bron **kos′** tō mē

bronch/o/spasm
bron′ kō spazm

bronch/o/rrhaphy
bron **kôr′** ə fē

Build words meaning
formation of a new opening into a bronchus

_____/_____/_____;

spasm of a bronchus

_____/_____/_____;

suturing of a bronchus

_____/_____/_____.

Several lung conditions are characterized by a distinct type of cough and breathing difficulties. Some are caused by infection and others by deterioration of lung structures due to irritation, allergies, and breathing dirty or smoky air. Study the table below describing four of these conditions.

Disease	Description
croup kroōp	Croup is characterized by a resonant barking cough. Viral infection, allergic reaction, and inhalation of a foreign body are common causes. Croup occurs mostly in children.
asthma **az′** mə	Asthma is brought on by allergies, overexertion through exercise, inhalation of irritants, infection, and emotional distress. Spasms of the bronchi occur causing a wheezing cough and the inability to take a complete breath.
emphysema em fə **sē′** mə	Emphysema is a condition in which the terminal bronchioles and alveoli lose their elasticity and ability to receive and expel air. The person experiences shortness of breath, chronic cough, cyanosis, and wheezing. Long-term prognosis includes congestive heart disease and respiratory failure. The primary cause is smoking cigarettes and breathing dirty, smoky, polluted air.
pertussis per **tu′** sis	Pertussis (whooping cough) is caused by a highly contagious infection. It is characterized by a shrill whooping inspiration and cough. Prevention of pertussis is available through vaccination with DTap for children and Tdap for adults.

13.66

SPELL CHECK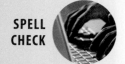

Plural means more than one; **pleural** refers to the membrane around the lungs. The **plural** of **pleura** is **pleurae**.

ANSWER COLUMN

13.67

pertaining to the pleura	Pleur/al means * _____ .
inflammation of the pleura	Pleur/itis means * _____
	_____ .
	Build words meaning
pleur/algia ploo **ral'** jē ə	pain in the pleura _____/_____
	or
pleur/o/dynia ploor' ō **din'** ē ə	_____/_____/_____ ;
	surgical puncturing of the pleura
pleur/o/centesis ploor' ō sen **tē'** sis	_____/_____/_____ .

13.68

	Build words meaning pertaining to the membrane attached to the lung
viscer/o/pleural vis' er ō **ploo'** rəl	_____/_____/_____ ;
	calculus in the pleura
pleur/o/lith **ploor** rō lith	_____/_____/_____ ;
	excision of part of the pleura
pleur/ectomy ploor **ek'** tō mē	_____/_____ .

13.69

TAKE A
CLOSER LOOK

Look up the word pleurisy. Read all your dictionary has to say about this disease. Its synonym is pleuritis. Write the treatment described here:

_____

_____

_____

13.70

pleur/isy **ploor'** ri sē	Inflammation of the pleura is pleuritis or _____/_____ .

13.71

The phrenic nerve controls the diaphragm, which is the muscle that controls breathing. The combining form for diaphragm is **phren/o**. -**plegia** is the suffix for paralysis.

phren/o/plegia fren ō **plē'** jē ə	Paralysis of the diaphragm is _____/_____/_____ .

PROFESSIONAL PROFILE

Respiratory therapists (RRTs or CRTs) perform physiologic (i.e., arterial blood gases) and pulmonary (i.e., breathing) tests to determine respiratory health or impairment. They administer breathing treatment and other respiratory procedures to maintain or improve ventilatory function to patients in hospital and ambulatory care settings. It is also possible for the respiratory therapist to specialize in pulmonary function testing or to be cross-trained to perform cardiopulmonary testing such as stress tests. The National Board for Respiratory Care (NBRC) sets standards for education and credentialing of registered respiratory therapists (minimum two years) and certified respiratory therapists (minimum one year).

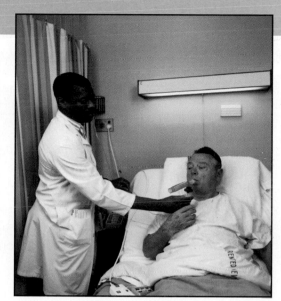

Respiratory therapist (RT) administering nebulizing mist treatment (NMT) *Delmar/Cengage Learning*

ANSWER COLUMN

	13.72
diaphragm/atic di′ ə frag **ma′** tik	**diaphragm/o** is another combining form for the diaphragm. Diaphragm/atic is the adjectival form. Breathing that is automatic as during sleep is controlled by the brain signaling the diaphragm. This is called _____/_____ breathing.
	13.73
diaphragm **di′** ə fram	Singers control their breath during singing by breathing deeply using their _____.
SPELL CHECK	**13.74** Watch your spelling of the word diaphragm. It has a silent *g* in the noun form. In the adjectival form, diaphragmatic, the *g* is pronounced with a hard "g" sound.
phren/ectomy fren **ek′** tō mē phren/ic/ectomy fren i **sek′** tō mē	**13.75** Removal of a portion of the phrenic nerve is a _____/_____ or _____/_____/_____.

ANSWER COLUMN

INFORMATION FRAME

13.76

Many body structures are paired (e.g. right and left arm, right and left leg, right and left kidney, right and left eye, etc). It is important to clarify the location of an injury, disease, or treatment to be given. Errors have been made causing injury to patients because the right and left sides or structures were mixed up.

WORD ORIGINS

13.77

Dexter and *sinister* are Latin words for right and left. From these terms **dextr/o** and **sinistr/o** become the combining forms for right and left. People who were superstitious thought the right side was good and the left side bad. Dextrose is sugar, sweet, or the good. If something is sinister it is bad or evil. Of course there are no scientific facts to justify such a belief. It may help students remember the medical word parts and abbreviations used for right and left, however, if you remember the superstition.

TAKE A CLOSER LOOK

13.78

Study the following Latin abbreviations and phrases:

oculus sinister	os	eye, left
oculus dexter	od	eye, right
auris sinister	as	ear, left
auris dexter	ad	ear, right

13.79

left

In medicine we go back to the original meaning of sinister to find the combining form **sinistr/o**, which means _____ .

13.80

left

ad- as a prefix or **-ad** as a suffix means toward. Sinistr/ad means toward the _____ .

13.81

Using **sinistr/o**, build words meaning
pertaining to the left

sinistr/al
sin' is trəl
_____/_____;

displacement of the heart to the left

sinistr/o/cardi/a
sin' is trō **kär'** dē ə
_____/_____/_____/_____;

pertaining to the left half of the cerebrum

sinistr/o/cerebr/al
sin' is trō **ser'** ə brəl
_____/_____/_____/_____.

13.82

Using manual (hand) and pedal (foot), build words meaning
left-handed

sinistr/o/man/ual
sin' is trō **man'** yōō əl
_____/_____/_____/_____;

(continued)

ANSWER COLUMN	
	left-footed
sinistr/o/ped/al sin' is trō **pē'** dəl	_____/_____/_____/_____ .

13.83

right | The opposite of **sinistr/o** is **dextr/o**. **dextr/o** means _____ .

13.84

right | Dextr/ad means toward the _____ .

13.85

Build words meaning

pertaining to the right

dextr/al
dek' strəl

_____/_____ ;
displacement of the heart to the right

dextr/o/cardi/a
dek' strō **kär'** dē ə

_____/____/_____/_____ ;
displacement of the stomach to the right

dextr/o/gastr/ia
dek' strō **gas'** trē ə

_____/____/_____/_____ .

13.86

Refer to Frame 13.82 if necessary and build words meaning

dextr/o/man/ual

right-handed _____/_____/_____/_____ ;

dextr/o/ped/al
(You pronounce)

right-footed _____/_____/_____/_____ .

13.87

pod/o (Greek) and **ped/i** (Latin) are both combining forms for foot. Two terms for

ped/i/algia
ped ē **al'** jē ə

foot pain are _____/_____/_____
and

pod/algia
pod **al'** jē ə

_____/_____ .

NOTE: Pedialgia is an exception to the rule. The "i" is added to the word root "ped" even though the suffix begins with a vowel.

13.88

ped/i

The two combining forms for foot are _____/_____ and

pod/o

_____/_____ .

13.89

Suffixes **-iatrist** (noun) and **-iatric** (adjective) are used to indicate medical professionals or physicians. A health professional responsible for care of

pod/iatrist
pō **dī'** ə trist

conditions of the feet is a _____/_____ (DPM).
The specialty is called podiatry.

ANSWER COLUMN

**Podiatrist injecting
a toe with cortisone**
*Photo by Timothy J. Dennerll, RT(R), Ph.D.
courtesy of Grant Wiig, DPM*

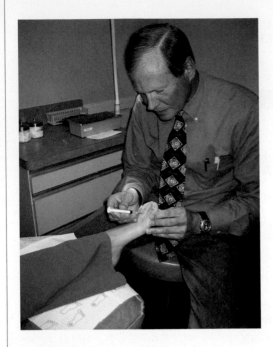

13.90

pod/iatric
pō dē **a'** trik

A hammertoe operation is a type of _____/_____
(adjective) treatment.

13.91

spasm of the hand

chir/o

Cheir is a Greek word for hand. Look up chir/o/spasm; it means

_____.

The combining form for hand is _____/_____.

13.92

hands

Chir/o/practors (doctor of chiropractic [DC]) use their hands to manipulate the
body for therapy. In the adjective chir/o/practic, the word root **chir/o** means

_____.

13.93

chir/o/practic
kī' rō **prak'** tik

Spinal manipulation is a form of _____/_____/_____
(adjective) treatment.

13.94

chir/o/plasty
kī' rō plas tē

Surgical repair of the hand is called _____/_____/_____.

13.95

pedi/a/trician
pē' dē a **tri'** shən

pedi/a is a combining form that comes from the Greek word *pedias*, meaning
child. A physician specialist who treats children is

a _____/_____/_____.

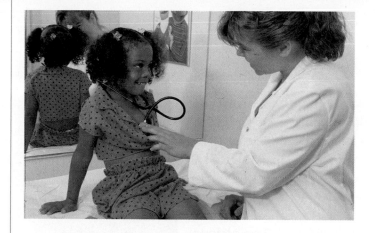

13.96

Recall **-iatric** is a suffix meaning medical or physician. The medical specialty for treatment of diseases of children is _____/_____/_____.

pedi/a/trics
pē′ dē **a**′ triks

13.97

A psych/iatrist is a medical doctor who specializes in the study of diagnosing and treating mental disorders. _____ is the suffix used to indicate a medical professional.

-iatrist

13.98

A psychiatrist provides _____/_____ treatment.

psych/iatric
sī′ kē **a**′ trik

13.99

ger/i means old age. Ger/ont/o/logy is the study of treatment of aging and the elderly. The medical specialty involving treating diseases related to old age is
_____/_____ .
The study of aging is
_____/_____/_____/_____ .

NOTE: Ontology is the study of a developmental process, e.g. embryology or gerontology.

ger/iatrics
jer′ ē **a**′ triks

ger/ont/o/logy
jer′ on **tol**′ ō jē

PROFESSIONAL PROFILE

Registered Health Information Administrators (RHIAs) manage health information departments in hospitals to ensure accurate, complete, orderly, and timely record keeping. They help plan hospital systems for better patient care and provide statistics for research, accreditation, and assistance with financial management.

Registered Health Information Technicians (RHITs) complete, index, code, file, and abstract statistical information and prepare medical records for release. In many institutions they also perform management functions. The American Health Information Management Association (AHIMA) sets standards for education programs (ranging from correspondence courses to bachelor's degrees), registration, and accreditation of medical records professionals.

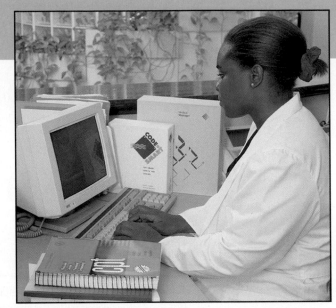

Health information technician *Delmar/Cengage Learning*

ANSWER COLUMN

Abbreviation	Meaning
ABG	arterial blood gases
AD	right ear (auris dexter)
AHIMA	American Health Information Management Association
RHIT	registered health information technician
AS	left ear (auris sinister)
CO_2	carbon dioxide
COLD	chronic obstructive lung disease
COPD	chronic obstructive pulmonary disease
CPR	cardiopulmonary resuscitation
CRT	certified respiratory therapist
DC	doctor of chiropractic medicine
DPM	doctor of podiatric medicine
HIPAA	Health Insurance Portability and Accountability Act of 1996
ICU	intensive care unit
IS	incentive spirometer
NBRC	National Board for Respiratory Care
NMT	nebulizing mist treatment
O_2	oxygen
PD	pulmonary disease

(continued)

ANSWER COLUMN

Abbreviation	Meaning
PE	pulmonary edema, physical exam, pulmonary embolism
Peds	pediatrics
PFT	pulmonary function test
PND	paroxysmal nocturnal dyspnea, postnasal drip
R	respiration (rate)
RHIA	registered health information administrator
RRT	registered respiratory therapist
RT	respiratory therapist
TB	tuberculosis
TC & DB	turn, cough, and deep breath
URI	upper respiratory infection

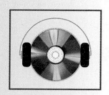

To complete your study of this unit, work the **Review Activities** on the following pages. Also, listen to the Audio CD that accompanies *Medical Terminology: A Programmed Systems Approach*, 10th edition, and practice your pronunciation.

STUDY WARE™ CONNECTION

To help you learn the content in this chapter, take a practice quiz or play an interactive game on your **StudyWARE™ CD-ROM**.

REVIEW ACTIVITIES

CIRCLE AND CORRECT

Circle the correct answer for each question. Then, check your answers in Appendix E.

1. Word root for lung
   a. pnea
   b. pneumonia
   c. pneumon
   d. pulmonary

2. Combining form for fungus
   a. monilo
   b. myo
   c. myco
   d. mycelio

3. Noun for throat
   a. pharynx
   b. trachea
   c. esophagus
   d. phalanx

4. Adjective for kidney
   a. nephriac
   b. nephroc
   c. cystic
   d. renal

5. Which of the following does *not* refer to the lung?
   a. thoraco
   b. pulmonary
   c. pneumono
   d. pneumo

6. Combining form for air:
   a. pneumono
   b. pneumo
   c. pnea
   d. pulmono

7. Combining form for nasal cavity
   a. rhin
   b. mento
   c. naso
   d. antro

8. Singular of pharynges
   a. pharynx
   b. pharyngos
   c. pharyno
   d. pharynge

REVIEW ACTIVITIES

9. Sound made by the g in laryngocele
   - a. s
   - b. k
   - c. j as in job
   - d. g as in goat

10. Combining form for right
    - a. dextro
    - b. dextrose
    - c. dextrous
    - d. dexter

11. Combining form for the windpipe
    - a. esphago
    - b. laryngo
    - c. pharyngo
    - d. tracheo

12. Epistaxis refers to
    - a. upon the stomach
    - b. after dinner
    - c. difficulty breathing
    - d. nose bleed

IMAGE LABELING

Label the structures of the respiratory system by matching them with their correct combining form.

_____ alveol/o

_____ bronch/o

_____ trache/o

_____ laryng/o

_____ rhin/o, nas/o

_____ pharyng/o

_____ phren/o, diaphram/o

_____ pulmon/o

_____ epiglott/o

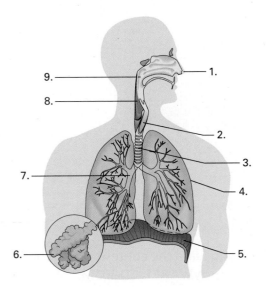

Delmar/Cengage Learning

SELECT AND CONSTRUCT

Select the correct word parts from the following list and construct medical terms that represent the given meaning.

al	algia	ary	atrician	blast	bronch(o)(i)
centesis	chir(o)	constriction	dermat/o	dextr(o)	dilatation
dilation	dynia	ectasis	ectomy	embol	fungi
hist(o)	iatrist	ic	ism	itis	laryn(x)(g)(o)
lith	(o)logy	lysis	manual	melan(o)	mental
myc(o)	nas(o)	oma	osis	pathy	pedal
pedi	pharynx(go)	phren(o)	plegia	pleur(o)(a)	pneumon/o
practor	psych	pulmon/o	rrhagia	scope (y)	sinistr/o
stomy	thorac/o	trache(o)	us		

1. adjective for lung _____

2. black lung disease _____

3. fungal infection of the skin _____

REVIEW ACTIVITIES

4. a moving blood clot _____

5. the study of fungi _____

6. pertaining to the nose and chin _____

7. instrument used to look at the throat _____

8. surgical puncture of the membrane around the lung _____

9. right-footed _____

10. left-handed _____

11. physician specialist for children _____

12. destruction of tissue _____

13. inflammation of the bronchi _____

14. pain in the voice box _____

15. paralysis of the diaphragm _____

16. dilatation of the bronchi _____

17. physician specialist in mental disorders _____

18. making a new opening in the trachea _____

19. doctor using hands to manipulate the spine _____

DEFINE AND DISSECT

Give a brief definition and dissect each term listed into its word parts in the space provided. Check your answers by referring to the frame listed in parentheses and your medical dictionary. Then listen to the Audio CD to practice pronunciation.

1. pneumonocentesis (13.8)   _____/_____/_____
                                                          rt   v   suffix

    meaning
    _____

2. pneumonomelanosis (13.17)   _____/_____/_____/_____
                                                       rt   v   rt   suffix

    _____

3. pharyngomycosis (13.23)   _____/_____/_____/_____
                                                       rt   v   rt   suffix

    _____

REVIEW ACTIVITIES

4. pneumothorax (13.27)

_____/_____/_____
rt   v   rt

_____

5. pulmonary (13.31)

_____/_____
rt   suffix

_____

6. hemoglobin (13.4)

_____/_____/_____/_____
rt   v   rt   suffix

_____

7. pneumohemothorax (13.30)

_____/_____/_____/_____/_____
rt   v   rt   v   rt

_____

8. respiratory (13.2)

_____/_____/_____
pre   rt   suffix

_____

9. embolus (13.33)

_____/_____
rt   suffix

_____

10. pneumonia (13.9)

_____/_____
rt   suffix

_____

11. mycology (13.22)

_____/_____/_____
rt   v   suffix

_____

12. dermatomycosis (13.23)

_____/_____/_____/_____
rt   v   rt   suffix

_____

13. nasitis (13.43)

_____/_____
rt   suffix

_____

14. pharyngomycosis (13.49)

_____/_____/_____/_____
rt   v   rt   suffix

_____

REVIEW ACTIVITIES

15. nasoantritis (13.41)

_____/_____/_____/_____
rt   v   rt   suffix

_____

16. nasopharyngitis (13.44)

_____/_____/_____/_____
rt   v   rt   suffix

_____

17. tracheolaryngotomy (13.62)

_____/_____/_____/_____/_____
rt   v   rt   v   suffix

_____

18. pleurisy (13.70)

_____/_____
rt   suffix

_____

19. bronchorrhaphy (13.65)

_____/_____/_____
rt   v   suffix

_____

20. phrenectomy (13.75)

_____/_____
rt   suffix

_____

21. sinistrocardia (13.81)

_____/_____/_____/_____
rt   v   rt   suffix

_____

22. diaphragmatic (13.72)

_____/_____
rt   suffix

_____

23. podiatric (13.90)

_____/_____
rt   suffix

_____

24. pediatrician (13.95)

_____/_____/_____
rt   v   suffix

_____

25. chiropractor (13.92)

_____/_____/_____
rt   v   rt/suffix

_____

REVIEW ACTIVITIES

26. laryngotomy (13.56)

_____/_____/_____
rt   v   suffix

_____

27. bronchoscopy (13.64)

_____/_____/_____
rt   v   suffix

_____

28. pleurocentesis (13.67)

_____/_____/_____
rt   v   suffix

_____

29. psychiatrist (13.97)

_____/_____
rt   suffix

_____

30. gerontology (13.99)

_____/_____/_____/_____
rt   rt   v   suffix

_____

31. cardiopulmonary (13.32)

_____/_____/_____/_____
rt   v   rt   suffix

_____

32. atelectasis (13.12)

_____/_____
rt   suffix

_____

ABBREVIATION MATCHING

Match the following abbreviations with their definition.

_____ 1. PND   a. intensive care unit

_____ 2. RT   b. partial pressure of oxygen

_____ 3. ICU   c. registered respiratory therapist

_____ 4. AS   d. tuberculosis

(*continued*)

REVIEW ACTIVITIES

_____ 5. URI

_____ 6. ABG

_____ 7. DC

_____ 8. NMT

_____ 9. RRT

_____ 10. CPR

e. current procedures in respiratory therapy

f. postnasal drip

g. urinary tract infection

h. doctor of chiropractic

i. right ear

j. nebulizing mist treatment

k. arterial blood gases

l. left ear

m. upper respiratory infection

n. respiratory therapy (department)

o. arteriobiogram

p. cardiopulmonary resuscitation

q. dentist

ABBREVIATION FILL-IN

Fill in the blanks with the correct abbreviation.

11. pulmonary edema _____

12. pulmonary function test _____

13. carbon dioxide _____

14. respiration (rate) _____

15. chronic obstructive pulmonary disease _____

16. registered health information administrator _____

MATCHING

Match the breathing term on the left with its description on the right.

_____ 1. apnea

_____ 2. hemoptysis

_____ 3. dyspnea

a. difficult (painful) breathing

b. fast breathing

c. slow breathing

(continued)

REVIEW ACTIVITIES

_____ 4. orthopnea   d. bloody sputum

_____ 5. bradypnea   e. absence of breathing

_____ 6. tachypnea   f. breathing best when sitting up

_____ 7. atelectasis   g. collapsed lung

CASE STUDY

Write the term next to its meaning given below. Then draw slashes to analyze the word parts. Note the use of medical abbreviations. Look these up in your dictionary or find them in Appendix B. If you have any questions about the answers, refer to your medical dictionary or check with your instructor for the answers in Appendix E.

CASE STUDY 13-1

Postop Visit

Pt: Male, age 11

Dx: 1. Status **asthmaticus**

2. Probable **viral syndrome**

Peter Puffer is an 11-year-old boy with no known history of asthma, although he does have a history of **bronchitis** during which he has had episodes of wheezing. Peter has had **respiratory symptoms** and fever since Monday morning and now has increasing respiratory distress on the day of admission. He was seen in the office of Dr. Neumo who reported tightness in the chest. **Pulse oximetry** revealed an **O$_2$** saturation of 83**%**. Peter was therefore sent to the hospital, treated overnight with **oxygen, intravenous** aminophylline and Bronkosol, as well as **IV** Zinacef. He appears to be more comfortable at this point with less **tachypnea** and better oxygen saturation.

1. inflammation of the bronchi   _____

2. heart rate   _____

3. fast breathing   _____

4. within a vein   _____

5. measurement of oxygen   _____

6. oxygen symbol   _____

7. percent symbol   _____

8. pertaining to breathing   _____

9. spasms of the bronchi   _____

10. pertaining to a virus   _____

11. O$_2$ _____

12. intravenous   _____

13. feelings and experiences   _____

14. series of symptoms that form a disease   _____

REVIEW ACTIVITIES

CROSSWORD PUZZLE

Check your answers by going back through the frames or checking the solutions in Appendix F.

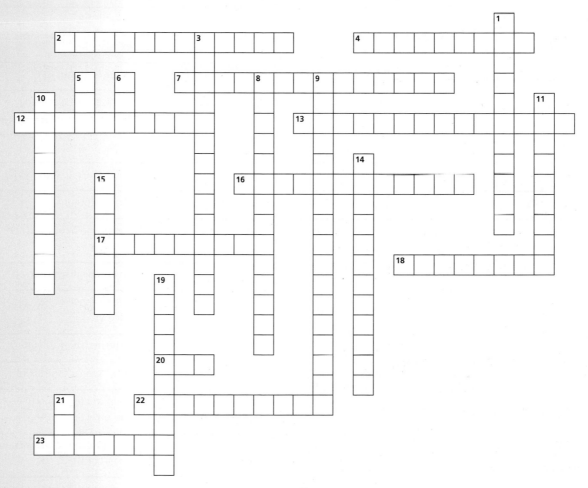

Across

2. instrument to look at the voice box
4. sit up straight to breathe
7. cancer-fighting drugs
12. synonym for gerontology
13. condition known as athlete's foot fungus
16. DC
17. pertaining to lung
18. synonym for pleuritis
20. arterial blood gases (abbr.)
22. inflamed bronchi
23. moving clot

Down

1. right-footed
3. left-handed
5. upper respiratory infection (abbr.)
6. pulmonary function test (abbr.)
8. back of the throat up near the nose (adj.)
9. black lung disease
10. coughing up blood (bloody sputum)
11. study of tissues
14. new permanent opening in the windpipe
15. difficulty breathing
19. foot doctor
21. podiatrist (abbr.)

REVIEW ACTIVITIES

GLOSSARY

apnea	absence of breathing		endotracheal	inside the trachea
asthma	inflammatory lung disease with narrowing of the bronchi		epistaxis	nosebleed
			expiration	exhalation
atelectasis	collapsed lung		fungi	plural of fungus
bradypnea	slow breathing		geriatrics	medical specialty studying aging and related diseases
bronchitis	inflammation of the bronchi			
broncholith	bronchial stone		gerontology	study of aging
bronchorrhagia	hemorrhage of the bronchi		hemoglobin	RBC protein that carries O_2
bronchorrhaphy	suture of the bronchi		hemoptysis	bloody sputum
bronchoscopy	examination of the bronchi with a bronchoscope		hyperpnea	increase in depth and rate of breathing
bronchospasm	uncontrolled contraction of the bronchial muscles		laryngalgia	larynx pain (laryngodynia)
			laryngitis	inflammation of the voice box (larynx)
cardiopulmonary	pertaining to heart and lungs			
chiroplasty	surgical repair of the hand		laryngocele	herniation of the larynx
chiropractic	practice of using hands for therapeutic spinal and skull manipulation, a philosophy of medicine based on musculoskeletal alignment and holistic health practices		laryngopathy	any disease of the larynx
			laryngoscope	an instrument used to examine the larynx
			laryngospasm	uncontrolled contraction of the vocal cords
chiropractor	doctor of chiropractic (DC)		laryngostomy	making a new, permanent opening in the larynx
croup	laryngotracheobronchitis with a hoarse cough			
			laryngotomy	making a temporary incision into the larynx
dermatomycosis	fungal infection of the skin (mycodermatitis)			
			larynx	the voice box
dextral	pertaining to the right		manual	pertaining to the hands
dextrocardia	heart displaced to the right		mycoid	resembling a fungus
dextrogastria	stomach displaced to the right		mycology	the science and study of fungi
diaphragm	breathing muscle below the thoracic cavity		nasoantritis	inflammation of the nose and antrum
dyspnea	difficulty (painful) breathing		nasofrontal	pertaining to the nasal and frontal bones
embolism	process of having an embolus			
embolus	a moving blood clot		nasolacrimal	pertaining to the nose and lacrimal ducts
emphysema	loss of elasticity of terminal bronchioles			
			nasomental	pertaining to the nose and chin

REVIEW ACTIVITIES

nasopharyngeal	pertaining to the nasopharynx (nose and pharynx)		pneumometer	instrument for measuring air volume
nasopharyngitis	inflammation of the nose and pharynx		pneumonectomy	excision of the lung
			pneumonia	inflammation of the lung
nasoscope	instrument used to examine the nose		pneumonocentesis	surgical puncture of the lung to remove fluid (pneumocentesis)
orthopnea	dyspnea when lying down (straight) or any position other than sitting or standing upright		pneumonomelanosis	black lung disease
			pneumonomycosis	fungal infection of the lung
			pneumonopathy	any lung disease
otorhinolaryngologist	physician specialist in diseases of the ear, nose, and throat		pneumonopexy	surgical fixation of a prolapsed lung (pneumonoplasty)
pedal	pertaining to the foot		pneumonorrhagia	hemorrhage of the lung
pedialgia	foot pain (podalgia)		pneumonotomy	incision into the lung
pediatrician	physician specialist in children's diseases and development		pneumotherapy	treatment using air
			pneumothorax	air in the thoracic cavity
pertussis	whooping cough		podiatrist	specialist in care of conditions of the feet; may also perform surgery of the foot
pharyngocele	herniation (weakening of the wall) of the throat			
pharyngomycosis	fungal infection of the throat		psychiatrist	physician specialist in mental disorders
pharyngoplasty	surgical repair of the throat			
pharyngoscope	instrument used to examine the throat		ptyalorrhea	flow of saliva
			pulmonary	pertaining to the lung (pulmonic)
pharynx	throat		respiratory	pertaining to breathing
phrenectomy	excision of part of the phrenic nerve (phrenicectomy)		rhinomycosis	fungal infection in the nose
phrenoplegia	paralysis of the diaphragm		sinistral	pertaining to the left
pleural	pertaining to the pleura		tachypnea	fast breathing
pleuralgia	pleural membrane pain (pleurodynia)		trachea	windpipe
			trachealgia	tracheal pain
pleurectomy	excision of part of the pleura		tracheocele	herniation of the tracheal wall
pleurisy	inflammation of the pleura (pleuritis)		tracheopyosis	condition of pus in the trachea
			tracheorrhagia	hemorrhage of the trachea
pleurocentesis	surgical puncture of the pleura to remove fluid		tracheoscopy	process of inspecting the trachea
pleurolith	stone in the pleural cavity		tracheostomy	surgical creation of an opening in the trachea
pneumohemothorax	air and blood in the thoracic cavity		tracheotomy	incision into the trachea

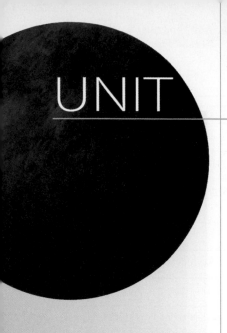

UNIT 14

Word Parts for Night, Sleep, Split, Skeletal System, and Orthopedics

WORD ORIGINS

skeletal
skel′ ə təl

14.1

Bones, joints, and connective tissues support, move, and protect the body. Without the skelet/al system we would be like jellyfish or worms. **skelet/o** comes from the Greek word *skeletos* meaning dried up, which in ancient days may have been how people saw the skeleton after the body had decomposed. It would have seemed hard and dried up. The living skeleton is anything but dried up. It has a blood supply, moist membranes, and is constantly releasing and depositing calcium from its cells.

14.2

muscul/o/skelet/al
mus′ kyoo lo **skel′** ə təl

Movement occurs by muscles pulling on bones to produce movement of the joints. The muscles (muscul/o) attach by tendons to the skeleton at origin and insertion points. The combination of muscle and skeleton is

_____/_____/_____/_____ system.

Study the structures of the skeleton shown in diagram of the skeletal system on the next page to help you build words in the following frames.

ANSWER COLUMN

Skeletal system *Delmar/*
Cengage Learning

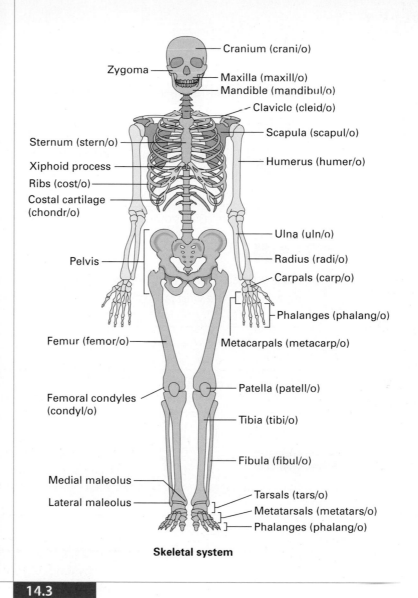

Cranium (crani/o)
Zygoma
Maxilla (maxill/o)
Mandible (mandibul/o)
Clavicle (cleid/o)
Scapula (scapul/o)
Sternum (stern/o)
Humerus (humer/o)
Xiphoid process
Ribs (cost/o)
Costal cartilage (chondr/o)
Ulna (uln/o)
Radius (radi/o)
Pelvis
Carpals (carp/o)
Phalanges (phalang/o)
Femur (femor/o)
Metacarpals (metacarp/o)
Patella (patell/o)
Femoral condyles (condyl/o)
Tibia (tibi/o)
Fibula (fibul/o)
Medial maleolus
Lateral maleolus
Tarsals (tars/o)
Metatarsals (metatars/o)
Phalanges (phalang/o)

Skeletal system

14.3

Recall that an orth/o/pedist treats diseases and performs surgery on the skeletal system. A wrist fracture would be diagnosed and treated by an

orth/o/ped/ist

_____/_____/_____/_____. The specialty

orth/o/ped/ics
(You pronounce)

is _____/_____/_____/_____.

14.4

Carpos is a Greek word meaning wrist. Locate the carpal bones on the diagram of

carpi
kär′ pī

the hand on the next page. The plural of carpus is _____.

14.5

From carpus and carpi, derive a word root that refers to the wrist. It is

carp

_____.

ANSWER COLUMN

14.6

Carpal tunnel syndrome (CTS) is an occupational hazard to those who perform repetitive hand movement, for example, medical transcriptionists. The adjectival

carp/al
kär′ pəl

form for carpus is _____/_____.

14.7

Look at the words (in your medical dictionary) that begin with **carp**. The

carp/o

combining form that is used in words about the wrist is _____/_____.

14.8

Close your dictionary. Build words meaning
pertaining to the wrist (adjective)

carp/al
kär′ pəl

_____/_____;

pertaining to the wrist and metacarpals

carp/o/meta/carp/al
kär′ pō **met′** ə kär pəl

_____/_____/_____/_____/_____;

excision of all or part of the wrist

carp/ectomy
kär **pek′** tə mē

_____/_____.

14.9

Recall that **meta-** means beyond. The bones in the hand "beyond" the carpals are

meta/carp/als
met′ ə **kär′** palz

called the _____/_____/_____.

Bones of the left hand *Delmar /Cengage Learning*

Bones of the left hand

ANSWER COLUMN

14.10

Refer to the illustration of the bones of the foot. **tars/o** is the combining form for the tarsal bones in the ankle. From what you already know about the prefix meta-, name the bones that are located beyond the tarsals:

meta/tars/als
met' ə **tar'** salz

_____/_____/_____.

14.11

Locate the following bones

wrist

carpal _____;

ankle

tarsal _____.

14.12

TAKE A CLOSER LOOK

A mallet is a large hammer. The malle/us bone in the middle ear is shaped like a hammer. The names for the inner and outer ankle bone landmarks come from this same word root. The medial malleolus is a bony process on the inner distal end of the tibia. The lateral malleolus is a bony process on the outer distal end of the fibula. Both of these resembled a mallet to those ancient anatomists that named them. Study the diagrams of the foot (on the next page) and skeleton (on page 523) to locate these structures.

14.13

bones of the fingers
and/or toes

Locate the phalang/es. They are the * _____

_____.

14.14

phalanges
fə **lan'** jēs

Phalang/o is the combining form for _____ or (plural).

phalanx
fā' lanks

The singular form of phalanges is _____ .

PROFESSIONAL PROFILE

Registered occupational therapists (OTR)—The American Occupational Therapy Association (AOTA) information brochure defines occupational therapy as "the use of purposeful activity with individuals who are limited by physical injury or illness, psychosocial dysfunction, developmental or learning disabilities, poverty and cultural differences, or the aging process to maximize independence, prevent disability, and maintain health. The practice encompasses evaluation, treatment, and consultation." Preparation for this profession requires completion of a masters or doctorate degree from an approved college including an internship experience. An occupational therapist may specialize in a particular area of expertise such as hand therapy or substance abuse rehabilitation.

ANSWER COLUMN

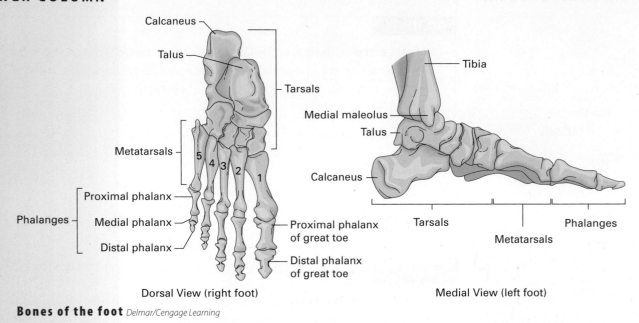

Bones of the foot *Delmar/Cengage Learning*

14.15

Build words meaning
inflammation of phalanges

phalang/itis
fal' an **ji'** tis   _____/_____;
                                           excision of a phalanx (singular)
phalang/ectomy
fal' an **jek'** tə mē   _____/_____.

14.16

scapula   Locate the acromi/on process. It is a projection of the _____
                                           (check a dictionary if necessary). **acromi/o** is the combining form.

14.17

acromi/o   The combining form for the acromion is _____/_____ .

14.18

Find words in your dictionary meaning
pertaining to the acromion

acromi/al
ə **krō'** mē əl   _____/_____;
                                           pertaining to the acromion and humerus

acromi/o/humer/al
ə krō' mē ō **hyōō'** mər əl   _____/_____/humer/al;
                                           pertaining to the acromion and the clavicle

acromi/o/clavicul/ar
ə krō' mē ō kla **vik'** yōō lar   _____/_____/_____/_____.

ANSWER COLUMN

14.19

humer/o

Look at Frame 14.18. Can it start you looking for another combining form? Try.

It is _____/_____.

14.20

humerus

humer/o is used in words to refer to the bone of the upper arm, which is named

the _____.

14.21

DICTIONARY EXERCISE

Find four words in your dictionary that begin with humer or **humer/o**.

_____

_____

_____

_____

14.22

radi/o/uln/ar
rā′ dē ō **ul**′ nar

The radius (**radi/o**) and ulna (**uln/o**) are located in the forearm.
If both are fractured, it would be described as a

_____/_____/_____/_____ fracture.
(Abbreviation: FxBB, fracture of both bones.)

14.23

TAKE A CLOSER LOOK

A fracture is a break or crack. There are at least ten different types of bone fractures. Fracture wounds may be open or closed and are described by the type and location of break that has occurred. Study the table of fracture facts below. Then, take a "break"!

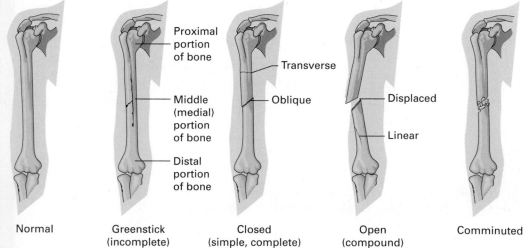

Proximal portion of bone
Middle (medial) portion of bone
Distal portion of bone
Transverse
Oblique
Displaced
Linear

Normal   Greenstick (incomplete)   Closed (simple, complete)   Open (compound)   Comminuted

Types of bone fractures *Delmar/Cengage Learning*

Pediatric left-leg femur fracture *Image prepared by Timothy J. Dennerll, RT(R), Ph.D., courtesy of Allegiance Health, Jackson, MI*

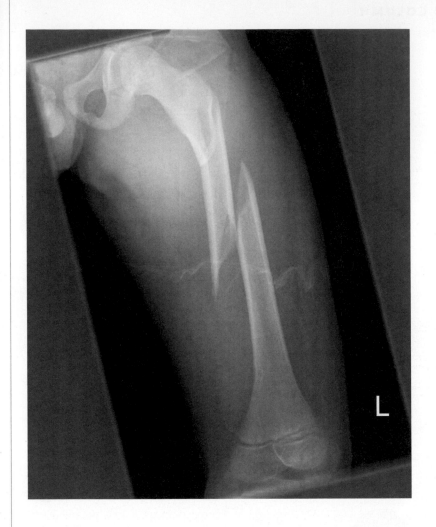

Fracture Facts	
complete	break through the width of the bone
incomplete	break not through the width of the bone
closed	[simple fracture] skin is not broken
open	[compound fracture] bone ends protrude through the skin
pathologic fracture	diseased area that weakens the bone

Fracture Reduction and Fixation

closed manipulation	movement of body part to cause bone ends to align without surgery
internal fixation	screws or nails in bone under the skin (ORIF)
external fixation	screws attached to an external bar (OREF)

14.24

condyl

Refer back to the drawing of the skeleton on page 523. Locate a condyle. A condyle is a rounded process that occurs on many bones. The word root for condyle is _____.

ANSWER COLUMN

14.25

Two rounded processes at the medial and lateral distal ends of the femur are the

condyles
kon' dīlz

femoral _____.

14.26

In Latin *femur* means thigh. **femor/o** is the combining form for the longest bone

in the body, the femur (thigh bone—notice the spelling). Look at the illustration

femur
fē' mer

of the skeleton. The proximal end of the _____ is part of the hip joint.

The artery that supplies blood to the leg is called the

femor/al
fem' er əl

_____/_____ artery.

14.27

SPELL
CHECK

Watch the spelling of fem*ur* as it changes to **femor/o** to make the combining

form.

14.28

The tibia is the shin bone. Use **tibi/o** as the combining form. The fibula is a thin,

long bone lateral to the tibia. Use **fibul/o** for the fibula. If both bones are broken in

tibi/o/fibul/ar
ti' bē ō **fib'** yōō lär

the same injury, it would be a _____/_____/_____/_____

fracture.

14.29

One way to remember the location of the tibia and fibula is to think of the tibia

aligned with the big toe (both start with t). The fibula is aligned with the little toe,

and a little lie is a fib. In any case, the thicker shin bone on the big toe side is the

tibia
ti' bē ə
fibula
fib' yōō la

_____ and the thinner, lower leg bone on the little toe side

is the _____.

14.30

A rounded bony process on any bone is a condyle.
Build words meaning
excision of a condyle

condyl/ectomy
kon' di **lek'** tō mē

_____/_____;

resembling a condyle

condyl/oid
kon' di loid

_____/_____;

upon a condyle

epi/condyle
ep i **kon'** dīl

_____/_____.

ANSWER COLUMN

14.31

condyle

condyle

Condyl/ar is an adjective meaning pertaining to a _____. The femoral _____ is a rounded end of the bone.

14.32

calcanea
kal **kā'** nē ə

Locate the calcaneus bone (also calcaneum). The plural of calcaneus is _____.

14.33

calcane

From calcaneus and calcanea, derive the word root for the heel _____.

14.34

calcane/o

In your medical dictionary, look at the words beginning with calcane. Derive the combining form that is used in words that refer to the heel:

_____/_____ .

14.35

Close your dictionary. Now build words meaning
pertaining to the heel

calcane/al
kal **kā'** nē əl

_____/_____ ;

pain in the heel

calcane/o/dynia
kal kā' nē ō **din'** ē ə

_____/_____/_____

or

calcane/algia
kal kā nē **al'** jē ə

_____/_____ .

14.36

The bones of the pelvis include the ischium, ilium, and pubis. Locate them and their combining forms in the illustration below.
Write the combining forms below.

ischi/o

ischium _____/_____

ili/o

ilium _____/_____

pub/o

pubis _____/_____

14.37

SPELL
CHECK

It is easy to confuse ilium with ileum because they are pronounced the same and differ in spelling by only one letter. Remember i-l-**e**-um is part of the small intestine of the digestive system and the *e* reminds us of eat. The combining forms are also spelled differently, **ile/o** for ileum (small intestine) and **ili/o** for ilium (one of the pelvic bones).

ANSWER COLUMN

Anterior view of bones of the pelvis *Delmar/Cengage Learning*

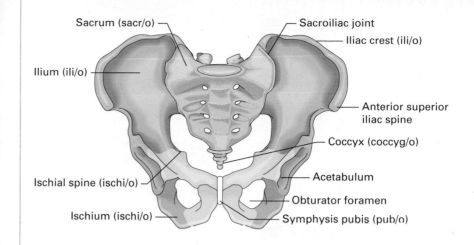

Sacrum (sacr/o)
Sacroiliac joint
Iliac crest (ili/o)
Ilium (ili/o)
Anterior superior iliac spine
Coccyx (coccyg/o)
Acetabulum
Ischial spine (ischi/o)
Obturator foramen
Ischium (ischi/o)
Symphysis pubis (pub/o)

14.38

From what you have just learned, try this question. In which body system would you find the ile/o/cecal valve?

digestive system

_____

In which body system would you find the iliac crest?

skeletal system

_____

Good!

14.39

CONGRATULATIONS!

You are now finding your own combining forms. Feels good, doesn't it? Let's do some more.

14.40

ischia
is′ ke ə

Locate the ischium. The plural of ischium is _____. Refer to the illustration of the pelvis.

14.41

ischi
ischi/o

From ischium and ischia, derive a word root that refers to the part of the hip bone on which the body rests when sitting. The word root is _____; the combining form is _____/_____ .

STUDYWARE™ CONNECTION

Remember, after completing this unit, you can complete a crossword puzzle or other interactive game on your **StudyWARE™ CD-ROM** that will help you learn the content in this chapter.

ANSWER COLUMN

14.42

In your dictionary, find words meaning
pertaining to ischium and rectum

ischi/o/rect/al
is′ kē ō **rek′** təl

_____/_____/_____/_____ ;

neuralgic pain in the hip (synonym is sciatica)

ischi/o/neur/algia
is′ kē ō nōō **ral′** jē ə

_____/_____/_____/_____ ;

pertaining to the ischium and pubis

ischi/o/pub/ic
is′ kē ō **pyōō′** bik

_____/_____/_____/_____ .

14.43

Close your dictionary. Build words meaning
pertaining to the ischium

ischi/al
is′ kē əl

_____/_____ ;

herniation through the ischium

ischi/o/cele
is′ kē ō sēl

_____/_____/_____ .

14.44

ischi/o in a word refers to the part of the hip bone known as the

ischium
is′ kē əm

_____ .

14.45

Locate the pubis in the illustration of the pelvis. The plural of pubis

pubes
pyōō′ bēz

is _____ .

pub/o

The combining form is _____/_____ .

supra/pub/ic
sōō pra **pyoo′** bik

A _____/_____/_____ incision is made above
the pubis.

14.46

Close your dictionary. Recall that **femor/o** is the combining form for femur. Using
pub/o and **femor/o**, build a word meaning pertaining to the pubis and femur:

pub/o/femor/al
pyōō bō **fem′** ər əl

_____/_____/_____/_____ .

14.47

Using the illustration of the skeletal system on page 523, locate the sternum.

stern/o

The combining form for sternum is _____/_____ .

ANSWER COLUMN

Types of abdominal incisions *Delmar/Cengage Learning*

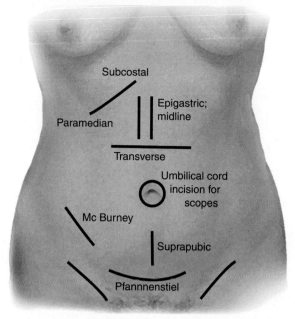

14.48

With your dictionary open, find words meaning pertaining to the sternum and pericardium

stern/o/peri/cardi/al
stûr′ nō per i **kärd′** ē əl

_____/_____/_____/_____/_____;

pertaining to the sternum and ribs

stern/o/cost/al
stûr′ nō **kos′** təl

_____/_____/_____/_____.

14.49

Close your dictionary. Build words meaning pertaining to the sternum

stern/al

_____/_____;

pain in the sternum

stern/algia

_____/_____ or

stern/o/dynia
(You pronounce)

_____/_____/_____.

14.50

sternum

breastbone

stern/o in a word makes you think of the _____, which is the _____.

14.51

Recall **cost/o** refers to ribs. The xiphoid (from the Greek *xiphos,* meaning sword) process is the projection at the inferior end of the sternum. **xiph/o** is the combining form. A word meaning pertaining to the xiphoid process and the ribs

xiph/o/cost/al
zi′ fō **kos′** təl

is _____/_____/_____/_____.

ANSWER COLUMN

14.52

The plural of gangli/on is gangli/a. A gangli/on is a collection of nerve cell bodies. Now that you have a system, form the word root/combining form for

gangli/o

ganglion: _____/_____.

14.53

ganglia

The main cerebral nerve centers are called the cerebral _____.

14.54

gangli/on

gangli/a

Any one of three neural masses found in the cervical region is called a

cervical _____/_____, whereas all three are referred to as

the cervical _____/_____.

14.55

You are now ready to find word roots and their combining forms by another method. Look up spine in your dictionary. A synonym for spine is

backbone

_____.

14.56

Look in your dictionary for words beginning with rach. rach is the word root

spine

for _____.

14.57

There are two word roots that mean spine. One is rach (**rachi/o**), the other is spondyl (**spondyl/o**). Build a word that means inflammation of the spine:

rach/itis *or*

rā **kī'** tis

spondyl/itis

spon di **lī'** tis

_____/_____.

14.58

Words beginning with the combining forms **rachi/o** or **spondyl/o** refer to the

spine

_____.

14.59

Using **rachi/o**, build words meaning

spine pain

rachi/algia

rā' kē **al'** jē ə

_____/_____;

incision into the spine

rachi/o/tomy

rā' kē **ot'** ō mē

_____/_____/_____.

ANSWER COLUMN

14.60

Using **rachi/o**, build words meaning
a synonym for rachialgia

rachi/o/dynia
rā' kē ō **din'** ē ə

_____/_____/_____;

instrument to measure spinal curvature

rachi/o/meter
rā' kē **om'** ə tər

_____/_____/_____;

spinal paralysis

rachi/o/plegia
rā' kē ō **plē'** jē ə

_____/_____/_____.

14.61

-schisis is a suffix meaning split. Using **rach/i**, build words meaning
fissure of the spine (split spine)

rachi/schisis
rā **kis'** kis is

_____/_____;

inflammation of the spine

rach/itis
rā **kī'** tis

_____/_____.

Spinal column *Delmar/ Cengage Learning*

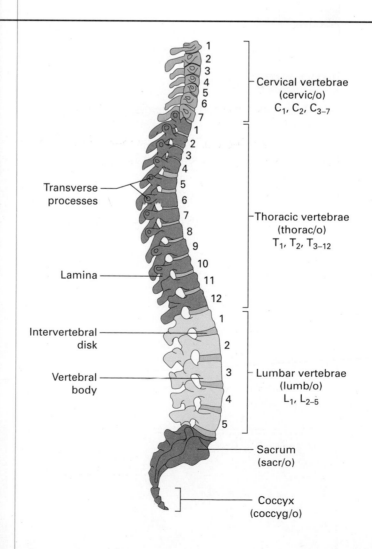

Transverse processes

Lamina

Intervertebral disk

Vertebral body

Cervical vertebrae
(cervic/o)
C_1, C_2, C_{3-7}

Thoracic vertebrae
(thorac/o)
T_1, T_2, T_{3-12}

Lumbar vertebrae
(lumb/o)
L_1, L_{2-5}

Sacrum
(sacr/o)

Coccyx
(coccyg/o)

ANSWER COLUMN

TAKE A CLOSER LOOK
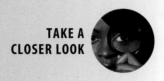

14.62

The three basic types of spinal curvature are kyphosis (posterior curvature), lordosis (anterior curvature), and scoliosis (lateral curvature). Refer back to the illustration in Unit 12, on page 471.
The following word parts refer to regions of the spine.

Combining Form	Adjective
cervic/o	cervical
thorac/o	thoracic
lumb/o	lumbar
sacr/o	sacral
coccyg/o	coccygeal

14.63

cervical

A device used to immobilize the neck is a _____ collar.

14.64

neck

Cervic/al traction is applied as a treatment for an injured _____.

14.65

Recall that the cervix is the neck of the uterus. The plural of cervix is

cervices

_____.

14.66

Build a combining form for cervix. The combining form takes **o**.

cervic/o
sûr′ vi kō

The combining form is _____/_____.

14.67

Build words meaning
excision of the cervix

cervic/ectomy
sûr′ vi **sek**′ tō mē

_____/_____;

inflammation of the cervix

cervic/itis
sûr′ vi **sī**′ tis

_____/_____;

pertaining to the cervix

cervic/al
sûr′ vi kəl

_____/_____.

CASE STUDY INVESTIGATION (CSI)

Cervical Radiology Report

Radiographs provided: **AP**, APOM, neutral **lateral** C spine. Slightly reduced **cervical lordosis** is present. The right angle of the **mandible** projects inferior to the left with mild **scoliosis** at the apex of **C5**. Normal bone density is noted. A minor **retrolisthesis** of C3 is present. The **intervertebral** disc spaces, facet and joints are normal. All pre-vertebral soft tissue spaces are within normal limits. The visualized **apical** lung is normal. No other abnormalities are detected.

CSI Vocabulary Challenge

Use a medical dictionary to help you divide the terms into word parts and write the definition of the terms and abbreviations in the space provided.

AP _____

lateral _____

cervical _____

lordosis _____

mandible _____

scoliosis _____

C5 _____

retrolisthesis _____

intervertebral _____

apical _____

ANSWER COLUMN

14.68

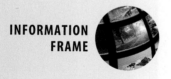

INFORMATION FRAME

cervic/o can mean the neck, the neck of the uterus as well as several other types of anatomic necks. In usage you are not likely to confuse them. The next frames will make the point. Refer to the previous illustration of the spinal column.

14.69

neck

neck

neck

Cervic/o/faci/al means pertaining to the face and _____.

Cervic/o/brachi/al means pertaining to the arm and _____.

Cervic/o/thoracic means pertaining to the chest and _____.

14.70

Study these phrases that refer to a necklike structure.

cervix of the axon—constriction between the cell body and the axon

cervix dentis—neck of the tooth

cervix uteri—neck of the uterus

cervix vesicae urinariae—neck of the urinary bladder

ANSWER COLUMN

14.71

cervix
ser' viks

In the previous phrases, the term that means neck is _____.

14.72

arm

arm

brachi/o is the combining form for arm. It is used to describe bones and blood vessels in the arm. The biceps brachii is a muscle in the _____.

The brachial artery is an artery in the _____.

14.73

brachi/o/radi/alis
brā' kē ō rā dē **al'** is

The muscle that extends from the upper arm to the radial bone is

the _____/_____/_____/_____ muscle.

14.74

brachi/al
brā' kē əl

brachi/o/radi/alis
brā' kē ō rā dē **al'** is

brachi/o/cephal/ic
brā' kē ō se **fal'** ik

Build words that mean pertaining to the
artery of the arm

_____/_____;

arm and radius muscle

_____/_____/_____/_____;

arm and head

_____/_____/_____/_____.

14.75

sacr/o/ili/ac
sak rō **il'** ē ak

The joint between the sacrum and the ilium is the

_____/_____/_____/_____ joint.

14.76

thorac/o/lumbar
thôr' ə kō **lum'** bär

sacr/o/sciat/ic
sak' rō sī **a'** tik

coccyg/ectomy
kok' si **jek'** tō mē

Build terms meaning
pertaining to the thorax and lumbar spines

_____/_____/_____;
pertaining to the sacrum and the sciatic nerve

_____/_____/_____/_____;
removal of the coccyx

_____/_____.

14.77

cervic/al

Provide the adjectival forms for

cervix _____/_____;

(continued)

ANSWER COLUMN

thorac/ic

sacr/al

coccyg/eal

thorax _____/_____ ;

sacrum _____/_____ ;

coccyx _____/_____ .

14.78

A lamina (**lamin/o**) is a thin, flat sheet, plate, or membrane. A lamin/ectomy is the removal of the lamina of the vertebral posterior arch that has been ruptured (ruptured disk). One treatment to repair an intervertebral disk herniation may be

lamin/ectomy
lam' in **ek**' tō mē

_____/_____ .

14.79

Disk is the word root for intervertebral disk. A myel/o/gram (spinal x-ray) is used to diagnose disk herniation. Removal of a herniated disk is called a

disk/ectomy
dis **kek**' tō mē

myel/o/gram
mī' el ō gram

_____/_____ after which a spinal fusion may be performed. The x-ray that can be used to view the spine is a

_____/_____/_____ .

14.80

There are two combining forms that mean night. One is Latin, **noct/i,** the other is Greek, **nyct/o**. Noct/i/luca are microscopic marine animals that make the ocean glow during the _____ .

night

14.81

Those of you who have studied music know that a noct/urne is dreamy music, sometimes called _____ _____ music.

night

14.82

WORD ORIGINS

In Greek mythology sleep and death were related to night. Somnus (Sleep) and Thanatos (Death) were the sons of Nox (Night).

Herniated disk with nerve root and spinal cord displaced by bulging disk (transverse section) Delmar/Cengage Learning

Spine of vertebra

Spinal cord

Spinal nerve root

Nucleus

Intervertebral disk

Bulging nucleus creates pressure on spinal nerves

ANSWER COLUMN

14.83

ambul, from the Latin *ambulare,* is a word root meaning walk. Look up the meaning of these terms about walking.

able to walk

ambul/atory * _____ ;

a vehicle for transporting
the sick (who
cannot walk)

ambul/ance * _____ .

14.84

ambul is the word root for walk. Noct/ambul/ism literally means walking at night. Sleepwalking is what you mean when you use the word

noct/ambul/ism
nokt **am'** byo͞o lizm

_____/_____/_____ .

14.85

somn is the word root for sleep. A common term for sleepwalking is

somn/ambul/ism
som **nam'** byo͞o lizm

_____/_____/_____ .

14.86

Sleepwalking can occur at any age but childhood is the most common age for

somnambulism

_____ .

14.87

Sleep studies have revealed that somnambulism is a condition in which a series of complex motor activity occurs during a lighter cycle of sleep, not during rapid eye motion (REM) sleep. Getting out of bed, walking around, or doing other activities

somnambulism

with no recall during sleep is _____ .

14.88

nyct/o is another combining form for night. It comes from the Greek word *nyx.*

night

Nyct/algia means pain during the _____ .

14.89

Nyct/albumin/uria means the presence of albumin in the urine only during the

night

_____ .

14.90

Nyct/al/opia means night blindness or difficulty in seeing at night.
Vitamin A is associated with night vision. Lack of vitamin A in the diet is one

nyct/al/opia
nik' tə **lō'** pē ə

cause of _____/_____/_____ .

ANSWER COLUMN

14.91

WORD ORIGINS

al comes from the Greek *alaos,* meaning blind. Nyctalopia literally means night blind vision.

14.92

nyctalopia

Nyct/al/opia has several causes. Retinal fatigue from exposure to very bright light is a cause of _____.

14.93

nyctalopia

Retinitis pigmentosa is another cause of _____.

14.94

nyct/o/phobia
nik′ tō **fō′** bē ə

noct/i/phobia
nok′ ti **fō′** bē ə

nyct/o/philia
nik′ tō **fil′** ē ə

noct/i/philia
nok′ ti **fil′** ē ə

Using **nyct/o** and **noct/i** build two words that mean abnormal fear of night

_____/_____/_____

_____/_____/_____;
unusual attraction to the night

_____/_____/_____

_____/_____/_____.

14.95

nycturia
nikt **yōōr′** ē ə

Noct/uria means excessive urination during the night. Another word that means the same as nocturia is _____/_____.

14.96

nyct/uria

noct/uria

Two words that mean excessive urination during the night are

_____/_____ and

_____/_____.

14.97

immovable eyelids

ankyl/o means immovable or fixed. Ankylosed means stiffened. Ankyl/o/blephar/on means adhesions resulting in

*_____.

14.98

immobility

Ankyl/osis, such as in ankylosing spondylitis, is a condition of

_____ of the spine.

ANSWER COLUMN

Use the following table to build words for Frames 14.99–14.101.

Combining Form	Noun or Suffix
aden/o (gland)	aden/ia
cardi/o (heart)	cardi/a
cheil/o (lips)	cheil/ia
dactyl/o (digits)	dactyl/ia
dent/o (teeth)	dent/ia
derm/o (skin)	derm/a
	-derm/ia
gastr/o (stomach)	gastr/ia
gloss/o (tongue)	gloss/ia
onych/o (nails)ᵃ	onych/ia
ophthalm/o (eyes)ᵃ	ophthalm/ia
ot/o (ears)	ot/ia
phag/o (eat)	**-phag/ia**
pneumon/o (lung)	pneumon/ia
proct/o (anus + rectum)	proct/ia
urethr/o (urethra)	urethr/a
ᵃnew in Unit 15	

NOTE: The **-ia** suffix means conditon.

14.99

Ankyl/o/stoma means lockjaw (stiff mouth). Build words meaning (remember, you may look back) adhesions of lips (immovable lips)

_____/_____/_____/_____;

ankyl/o/cheil/ia
ang′ ki lō **kī′** lē ə

closure (immobility) of the anus and rectum

_____/_____/_____/_____;

ankyl/o/proct/ia
ang′ ki lō **prok′** shē ə

abnormal fear of ankylosis

_____/_____/_____/_____.

ankyl/o/phob/ia
ang′ ki lō **fō′** bē ə

14.100

Build words meaning
tongue tied (stiff tongue)

_____/_____/_____/_____;

ankyl/o/gloss/ia
ang′ ki lō **glos′** ē ə

adhesions of fingers (immovable fingers) or toes

_____/_____/_____/_____.

ankyl/o/dactyl/ia
ang′ ki lō dak **til′** ē ə

14.101

noun

condition

-ia is a(n) (choose one) _____ (noun/adjective/verb) suffix meaning

_____.

STUDY WARE™ CONNECTION

After completing this unit, you can play a Spelling Bee game to help you learn the pronunciation of terms presented in the chapter or play other interactive games on your **StudyWARE™ CD-ROM** that will help you learn the content in this chapter.

ANSWER COLUMN

14.102

-stasis is used as a suffix and means stopping or controlling. To say that you control an organ or what that organ produces, use the combining form for organ

-stasis

viscer/o/stasis

vi′ ser **os**′ tə sis

(**viscer/o**) plus the suffix _____ to form

_____/_____/_____ .

14.103

stopped or controlled

Fung/i/stasis is a condition in which the growth of fungi is

* _____ .

14.104

control or stopping
bile flow

Chol/e/stasis means

* _____ .

14.105

Read Frame 14.102 again. Build words meaning
controlling the small intestine

enter/o/stasis

en′ tə **ros**′ tə sis

py/o/stasis

pī **os**′ tə sis

_____/_____/_____ ;

stopping the formation of pus

_____/_____/_____ .

14.106

**TAKE A
CLOSER LOOK**

Acceptable alternative pronunciations of terms with **-stasis** as a suffix include
arteri/o/stasis　　ar tĕr ē ō **stā**′ sis;
enter/o/stasis　　en ter ō **stā**′ sis;
hem/o/stasis　　hēm ō **stā**′ sis.

14.107

hem/o/stasis

hē **mos**′ tə sis

Build words meaning
controlling the flow of blood

_____/_____/_____ ;

(continued)

ANSWER COLUMN

phleb/o/stasis *or*
fleb **os'** tə sis
ven/o/stasis
vēn **os'** tə sis

arteri/o/stasis
är tir' ē **os'** tə sis

checking flow in the veins

_____/_____/_____;

checking flow in the arteries

_____/_____/_____.

14.108

schizo- (prefix), schisto- (prefix), and **-schisis** (suffix) have a complicated evolution from the Greek language. They mean split, cleft, or fissure. Build words meaning split speech (incomprehensible speech)

_____/_____/_____;

split nails (**onych/o**)—condition

_____/_____/_____.

NOTE: schizo- and schisto- are combining forms used as prefixes.

schizo/phas/ia
skit' zō **fā'** zē ə

schiz/onych/ia
skit' zō **nik'** ē ə

14.109

Schiz/o/phren/ia literally means split mind. It is actually a group of severe mental disorders in which thinking, emotions, and behavior are disturbed. A person with delusions of persecution, jealousy, and hallucinations may suffer from paranoid

_____/_____/_____.

schizo/phren/ia
skit' zō **fre'** nē ə

14.110

Anti/psych/otic medications and psych/o/therapy are treatments used for those

with _____.

schizophrenia

14.111

A fissure is a troughlike cleft in a structure.
Build words using **schisto**-:
split tongue condition

_____/_____/_____;

schisto/gloss/ia
shis' tō **glos'** ē ə

(continued)

Cleft palate *Courtesy of Dr. Joseph Konzelman, School of Dentistry, Medical College of Georgia*

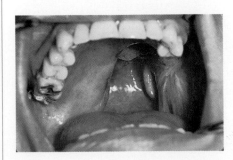

ANSWER COLUMN

split cell (cell with a fissure)

schist/o/cyte
shis′ tō sīt   _____ / _____ / _____ ;

schist/o/thorax   split chest (fissure)

shis′ tō **thôr′** aks   _____ / _____ / _____ .

14.112

Build words using **-schisis** as a suffix:
cleft palate (**palat/o**)

palat/o/schisis
pal ə **tos′** ki sis   _____ / _____ / _____ ;

uran/o/schisis   cleft palate (**uran/o**)

yōōr ə **nos′** ki sis   _____ / _____ / _____ ;

rach/i/schisis   split spine (**rach/i**)

rā **kis′** ki sis   _____ / _____ / _____ .

14.113

**TAKE A
CLOSER LOOK**

Look up spina bifida in your dictionary. This condition is synonymous with rachischisis. Read about the two types and write notes here.

_____

_____

14.114

In your dictionary, read about the disease schistosomiasis and *Schistosoma japonicum*. Schistosomiasis is an important disease in terms of world health. Because of increased worldwide travel, all people should be concerned with the

schisto/som/iasis   disease _____ / _____ / _____ .
shis′ tō sō **mī′** ə sis

14.115

As a review, test what you have learned by building terms that mean
a physician specialist in bone and joint disorders

orthopedist   _____ ;

the bones of the hand beyond the wrist

metacarpals   _____ ;

excision of a toe bone

phalangectomy   _____ ;

pertaining to the radius and ulna

radioulnar   _____ ;

location upon a condyle

epicondyle   _____ ;

a fissure or split in the spine

rachischisis   _____ .

Good work.

ANSWER COLUMN

Abbreviation	Meaning
AMB	ambulate, ambulatory
AOTA	American Occupational Therapy Association
C_1, C_2, C_{3-7}	cervical vertebrae 1–7
DPM	podiatrist (doctor of podiatric medicine)
Fx	fracture
FxBB	fracture of both bones
L_1, L_2, L_{3-5}	lumbar vertebrae 1–5
LP	lumbar puncture
lt, L	left
OREF	open reduction external fixation
ORIF	open reduction internal fixation
ORTH	orthopedist, orthopedics
OTR	registered occupational therapist
rt, R	right
T_1, T_2, T_{3-12}	thoracic vertebrae 1–12
y/o, yr	year(s) old, year(s)

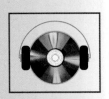

To complete your study of this unit, work the **Review Activities** on the following pages. Also, listen to the Audio CD that accompanies *Medical Terminology: A Programmed Systems Approach,* 10th edition, and practice your pronunciation.

STUDYWARE™ CONNECTION

To help you learn the content in this chapter, take a practice quiz or play an interactive game on your **StudyWARE™ CD-ROM**.

REVIEW ACTIVITIES

CIRCLE AND CORRECT

Circle the correct answer for each question. Then, check your answers in Appendix E.

1. Combining form for night
   a. narco
   b. necro
   c. nycto
   d. noct

2. Suffix meaning in the urine
   a. -uro
   b. -uremia
   c. -urine
   d. -uria

3. Word root for immovable or fixed
   a. syn
   b. ankyl
   c. stasis
   d. spondyl

4. Noun ending
   a. -ia
   b. -ic
   c. -ous
   d. -ed

5. Prefix for inward
   a. exo-
   b. meso-
   c. inner-
   d. eso-

6. Suffix for split
   a. -stasis
   b. -schiz
   c. -schisis
   d. -schist

REVIEW ACTIVITIES

7. Adjectival form for wrist bones
   - a. carpi
   - b. carpal
   - c. carpus
   - d. metacarpal

8. Combining form for one of the pelvic bones
   - a. ischium
   - b. ileo
   - c. ilio
   - d. ishci

9. Word root for walk
   - a. somn
   - b. duct
   - c. kines
   - d. ambul

10. Suffix for control or stopping
    - a. -rrhexis
    - b. -stasis
    - c. -schisis
    - d. -ectasis

11. Bony process at the end of the sternum
    - a. amnion
    - b. acromion
    - c. xiphoid
    - d. phalanx

12. Combining form for spine
    - a. rachi/o
    - b. spondyl
    - c. myel/o
    - d. ischi/o

SELECT AND CONSTRUCT

Select the correct word parts from the following list and construct medical terms that represent the given meaning.

ac	acromi/o(on)	al	algia	ambul/o/ism	ankylo
ar	arteri/o	ate	brachi/o(al)	calcane/o	carp(o)(al)
cephalic	cervic/o(al)	chondr/o	clavicul/o(ar)	condyl/o(ar)	cost/o(al)
dactyl/ia/o	dynia	ectomy	femor/o	fibul/o	fungi
humer/o(al)	ili/o	ischi/o	ism	itis	meta
myco	noct/i	nyct/o	opia	palat/o	patell/o
phas/o/ia	pub(o)(is)(ic)	rachi/o	scapul/o(ar)	schisis	schizo
somno/ia	stasis	stern/o(al)	tars/o	tomy	urano
uria	xiph/o(oid)				

1. breast bone pain _____

2. pertaining to the arm and head _____

3. control of fungal growth _____

4. including the ischium and pubis _____

5. excision of a rounded bony process _____

6. split spine (spina bifida) _____

7. cleft palate _____

8. pertaining to the cartilage end of the sternum and the ribs _____

9. the bones of the hand beyond the wrist _____

10. split speech (incomprehensible) _____

11. sleepwalking _____

12. night blindness _____

13. excessive urination at night _____

14. stiffened fingers _____

15. pertaining to the ilium _____

REVIEW ACTIVITIES

16. pertaining to the pubis _____

17. pertaining to the thighbone _____

18. pertaining to the kneecap _____

19. pertaining to the fibula _____

20. the bones of the ankle _____

21. the bones of the foot (not toes) _____

22. the heel bone _____

23. the ribs _____

24. pertaining to cartilage _____

FIND THE FORM

Give the correct combining form and adjectival form for each of the following bones.

		Combining Form	Adjectival Form
skull	1.	_____	_____
first seven vertebrae	2.	_____	_____
clavicle	3.	_____	_____
scapula	4.	_____	_____
acromion process	5.	_____	_____
humerus	6.	_____	_____
sternum	7.	_____	_____
xiphoid process	8.	_____	_____
ulna	9.	_____	_____
radius	10.	_____	_____
carpus	11.	_____	_____
metacarpus	12.	_____	_____
phalanx	13.	_____	_____
ischium	14.	_____	_____
ilium	15.	_____	_____
pubis	16.	_____	_____
femur	17.	_____	_____
patella	18.	_____	_____

REVIEW ACTIVITIES

		Combining Form	Adjectival Form
tibia	19.	_____	_____
fibula	20.	_____	_____
tarsus	21.	_____	_____
metatarsus	22.	_____	_____
calcaneus	23.	_____	_____
ribs	24.	_____	_____
cartilage	25.	_____	_____

DEFINE AND DISSECT

Give a brief definition, and dissect each term listed into its word parts in the space provided. Check your answers by referring to the frame listed in parentheses and your medical dictionary. Then listen to the Audio CD to practice pronunciation.

1. noctambulism (14.84)

_____/_____/_____
      rt   rt   suffix

meaning _____

2. nyctalopia (14.90)

_____/_____/_____
      rt   rt   suffix

_____

3. somnambulism (14.85)

_____/_____/_____
      rt   rt   suffix

_____

4. ankylodactylia (14.100)

_____/_____/_____/_____
      rt   v   rt   suffix

_____

5. nycturia (14.95)

_____/_____
      rt   suffix

_____

6. enterostasis (14.105)

_____/_____/_____
      rt   v   suffix

_____

REVIEW ACTIVITIES

7. schizophrenia (14.109)

_____/_____/_____
pre   rt   suffix

_____

8. schistosomiasis (14.114)

_____/_____/_____
pre   rt   suffix

_____

9. palatoschisis (14.112)

_____/_____/_____
rt   v   suffix

_____

10. calcaneodynia (14.35)

_____/_____/_____
rt   v   suffix

_____

11. carpometacarpal (14.8)

_____/_____/ _____/_____/_____
rt   v   pre   rt   suffix

_____

12. ischioneuralgia (14.42)

_____/_____/_____/_____
rt   v   rt   suffix

_____

13. sternopericardial (14.48)

_____/_____/ _____/_____/_____
rt   v   pre   rt   suffix

_____

14. acromiohumeral (14.18)

_____/_____/_____/_____
rt   v   rt   suffix

_____

15. epicondyle (14.30)

_____/_____
pre   rt/suffix

_____

16. ganglion (14.52)

_____/_____
rt   suffix

_____

17. xiphocostal (14.51)

_____/_____/_____/_____
rt   v   rt   suffix

_____

REVIEW ACTIVITIES

18. laminectomy (14.78)

_____/_____
            rt   suffix

19. diskectomy (14.79)

_____/_____
            rt   suffix

20. fungistasis (14.103)

_____/_____/_____
            rt   v   suffix

21. rachischisis (14.61)

_____/_____
            rt   suffix

22. antipsychotic (14.110)

_____/_____/_____
           pre   rt   suffix

23. metatarsal (14.10)

_____/_____/_____
           pre   rt   suffix

24. radioulnar (14.22)

_____/_____/_____/_____
            rt   v   rt   suffix

25. pubofemoral (14.46)

_____/_____/_____/_____
            rt   v   rt   suffix

26. cervicobrachial (14.69)

_____/_____/_____/_____
            rt   v   rt   suffix

27. tibiofibular (14.28)

_____/_____/_____/_____
         rt   v   rt   suffix

28. musculoskeletal (14.2)

_____/_____/_____/_____
         rt   v   rt   suffix

REVIEW ACTIVITIES

IMAGE LABELING

Label the structures of the skeleton by writing the number in front of the correct word part and write the body part indicated.

_____ xiph/o   _____

_____ condyl/o   _____

_____ femor/o   _____

_____ cleid/o   _____

_____ phalang/o   _____

_____ carp/o   _____

_____ radi/o   _____

_____ humer/o   _____

_____ cost/o   _____

_____ scapul/o   _____

_____ uln/o   _____

_____ metatars/o   _____

_____ tibi/o   _____

_____ fibul/o   _____

_____ vertebr/o   _____

_____ stern/o   _____

_____ crani/o   _____

_____ ili/o   _____

_____ ischi/o   _____

_____ patell/o   _____

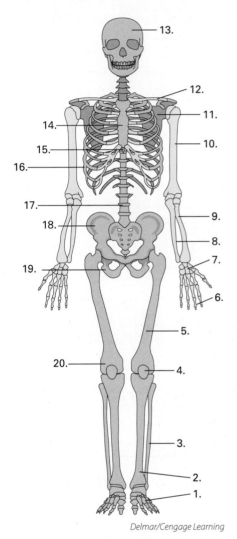

Delmar/Cengage Learning

REVIEW ACTIVITIES

ABBREVIATION MATCHING

Match the following abbreviations with their definition.

_____	1. ORTH	a.	noctambulism
_____	2. FxBB	b.	first thoracic vertebra
_____	3. yr	c.	fracture
_____	4. AMB	d.	orthodontist
_____	5. LP	e.	year
_____	6. L_1	f.	fracture of both bones
_____	7. Fx	g.	ambulate
_____	8. T_3	h.	first lumbar vertebra
		i.	twice a night
		j.	long-playing record
		k.	lumbar puncture
		l.	orthopedist
		m.	third thoracic vertebra

ABBREVIATION FILL-IN

Fill in the blanks with the correct abbreviation.

9. third cervical vertebra _____

10. fracture of both bones _____

11. registered occupational therapist _____

12. American Occupational Therapy Association _____

13. right _____

14. years old _____

15. open reduction internal fixation _____

CASE STUDY

Write the term next to its meaning. Then draw slashes to analyze the word parts. Note the use of medical abbreviations. Look these up in your dictionary or find them in Appendix B. If you have any questions about the answers, refer to your medical dictionary or check with your instructor for the answers in Appendix E.

REVIEW ACTIVITIES

CASE STUDY 14-1

Operative Report

Pt: **M,** 15 y/o

Dx: **Fracture lateral** condyle, **right** elbow

Procedure: Open **reduction, internal fixation** of fracture. Carl Cracken was **anesthetized**; the skin was prepped with Betadine, **sterile** drapes were applied, and the **pneumatic** tourniquet inflated around the right arm. An **incision** was made around the area of the lateral **epicondyle** through a Steri-drape, and this was carried through **subcutaneous** tissue, and the fracture site was easily exposed. **Inspection** revealed the fragment to be rotated in two planes about 90 degrees. It was possible to **manually** reduce this quite easily, judicious manipulation resulted in an almost **anatomic** reduction. This was fixed with two pins driven across the **humerus**. These pins were cut off below skin level. The wound was closed with some plain catgut subcutaneously and 5-0 nylon in the skin. Dressings were applied to Mr. Cracken and the tourniquet released. A long arm cast was applied. The patient was transfered to **PAR** in good condition.

1. looking   _____

2. using the hands   _____

3. toward the side   _____

4. cut into   _____

5. free of microorganisms   _____

6. below the skin   _____

7. pertaining to body structures   _____

8. inside   _____

9. Fx   _____

10. uses air (adjective)   _____

11. made to have no sensation   _____

12. surgery to restore position   _____

13. hold in place   _____

14. upon the condyle   _____

15. upper arm bone   _____

16. male   _____

17. years old   _____

18. Rt   _____

19. Post Anesthesia Recovery   _____

REVIEW ACTIVITIES

CROSSWORD PUZZLE

Check your answers by going back through the frames or checking the solutions in Appendix F.

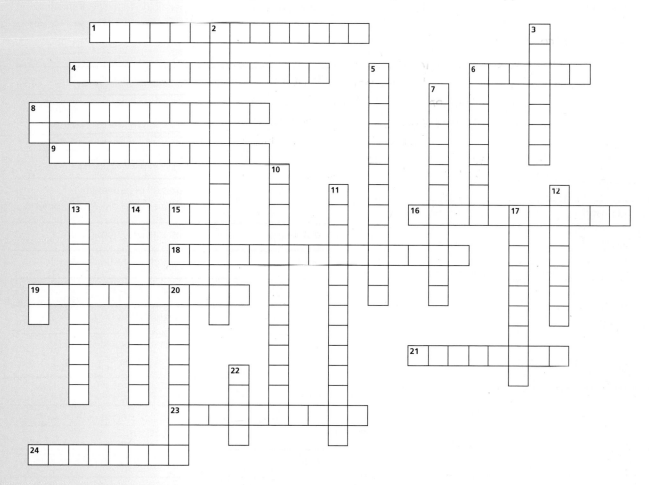

Across

1. including the upper arm bone and the shoulder blades
4. severe mental disorder with hallucinations
6. __ tunnel syndrome
8. synonym for spina bifida cystica
9. excision of herniated lamina of a disk
15. podiatrist (abbr.)
16. foot bones beyond the tarsals
18. muscle from upper arm to radius bone
19. synonym for mycostasis
21. group of nerve cell bodies
23. night blindness
24. walk (verb)

Down

2. sleeping sickness caused by a liver fluke
3. process at the end of the sternum
5. sleepwalking
6. plural for heel bone
7. physician specialist in skeletal disorders
8. right (abbr.)
10. pertaining to neck and face
11. cleft palate
12. bone you sit on
13. pain in the breast bone
14. stop blood flow
17. condition of stiffening
19. fracture (abbr.)
20. vehicle for emergency transport
22. orthopedist (abbr.)

REVIEW ACTIVITIES

GLOSSARY

acromioclavicular	joint between the collar bone and the acromion process
acromiohumeral	joint between the acromion process and the humerus
acromion	the bony projection on the scapula at the humeroscapular joint
ambulance	vehicle used to transport patients
ambulatory	able to walk, walking (ambulate)
ankyloblepharon	stiffened, adhered eyelids
ankylocheilia	adhesion of the upper and lower lips, making them stiff
ankylodactylia	adhesion of two or more digits, making them stiff
ankyloglossia	limited movement (stiffness) of the tongue
ankylophobia	abnormal fear of ankylosis
ankyloproctia	closure (immobility) of the anus and rectum
ankylosis	condition of stiffening, loss of mobility
arteriostasis	control of arterial flow
brachial	pertaining to the arm
brachiocephalic	pertaining to the arm and head
brachioradialis	muscle that extends from the upper arm to the radial bone
calcaneodynia	heel pain (calcanealgia)
calcaneum, calcaneus, calcanea	heel bone
carpi, carpus, carpal	wrist bones
cervical	pertaining to the neck, neck of the uterus, other necklike structure
cervicectomy	excision of the cervix of the uterus
cervicitis	inflammation of the cervix of the uterus

cervicobrachial	pertaining to the neck and arm
cervicofacial	pertaining to the neck and the face
cholestasis	control of bile flow
condyle, condylar	a rounded process on a bone end
condylectomy	excision of a condyle
condyloid	resembling a condyle
diskectomy	excision of herniated intervertebral disk (discectomy)
distal	distant, away from the origin
enterostasis	control of intestinal flow
epicondyle	upon a condyle
femur, femoral	the thigh bone
fibula	small, long bone in lower leg lateral to tibia
fracture	break or crack
fungistasis	control or stop growth of a fungus (mycostasis)
ganglion	a collection of nerve cell bodies
hemostasis	control of blood flow (hematostasis)
humeroradial	pertaining to the humerus and the radius
humeroscapular	pertaining to the humerus and the scapula
humeroulnar	pertaining to the humerus and the ulna
ileum	third part of the small intestine
ilium	upper pelvic bone
intervertebral	between the vertebrae
ischiocele	herniation through the ischial bone
ischioneuralgia	pain in the nerves near the ischium (sciatica)

REVIEW ACTIVITIES

ischiopubic	pertaining to the ischium and the pubis		rachischisis	split spine (spina bifida cystica)
ischiorectal	pertaining to the ischium and the rectum		rachitis	inflammation of the spine (spondylitis)
kyphosis	posterior curvature of the thoracic spine		radioulnar	pertaining to the radius and the ulna
laminectomy	excision of the lamina of the vertebral posterior arch		retrolisthesis	posterior displacement of a vertebra
lordosis	anterior curvature of the lumbar spine		sacral	pertaining to the sacrum
medial	toward the middle		scapula	shoulder blade
metacarpi, metacarpals	hand bones distal to the carpi		schistoglossia	split tongue (fissure)
metatarsals, metatarsi	foot bones distal to the tarsals		schistosomiasis	infestation with *Schistosoma* (*mansoni, japonicum, haematobium*) flukes
noctambulism	sleepwalking (somnambulism)		schizonychia	split finger nails or toenails
noctalbuminuria	excretion of albumin in urine at night		schizophasia	split speech (incomprehensible)
nyctalgia	pain during the night		schizophrenia	severe mental disorder in which thinking, emotions, and behavior are disturbed (includes paranoia, hallucination, delusion, persecution, and jealousy)
nyctalopia	night blindness			
nyctophobia	abnormal fear of the night (noctiphobia)			
nycturia	excessive urination during the night (nocturia)		scoliosis	lateral curvature of the spine
orthopedist	bone and joint specialist		skeletal	pertaining to bones
palatoschisis	cleft palate (uranoschisis)		sternalgia	sternal pain (sternodynia)
phalagitis	inflammation of the phalanges		sternopericardial	pertaining to the sternum and the pericardium
phlebostasis	control of venous flow		tarsi, tarsus, tarsal	bones of the ankle (not including the tibia)
pubofemoral	pertaining to the pubic bone and the femur		tibia	shin bone, medial to fibula
pyostasis	control of pus formation		tibiofibular	pertaining to the tibia and fibula
rachialgia	spinal pain (rachiodynia)		viscerostasis	control of an organ
rachiometer	instrument to measure spinal curvature		xiphocostal	pertaining to the xiphoid process and the ribs
rachioplegia	spinal paralysis		xiphoid (process)	cartilage bony projection on the distal end of the sternum

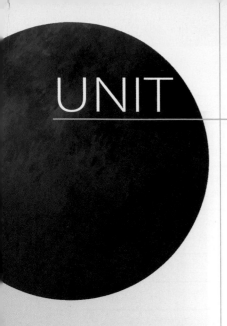

UNIT 15

Ophthalmology, Endocrinology, and Medical Specialties

ANSWER COLUMN

15.1

ophthalm/o is used in words to mean eye. Ophthalm/itis means

inflammation of the eye

* _____ .

pertaining to the eye

Ophthalm/ic means * _____ .

ocul/ar
ok' yoo lər

Ocular also means pertaining to the eye. _____ pain is eye pain.

15.2

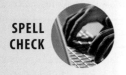

SPELL
CHECK

Watch your spelling on this one. Before building words with this root, be sure you have the "phth" order of **ophthalm/o** straight. Pronounce it: off **thal'** mō.

15.3

Ophthalm/algia and ophthalm/o/dynia both mean

pain in the eye

* _____ .

15.4

Build words meaning
herniation of an eye (abnormal herniation or protrusion—three possible)

ophthalm/o/ptosis *or*
off thal' mop **tō'** sis

_____/_____/_____;

ophthalm/o/cele *or*
off **thal'** mo sel

exophthalmos
eks of **thal'** mōs

(continued)

ANSWER COLUMN

ophthalm/o/meter
off′ thal **mom′** ə ter

ophthalm/algia *or*
off′ thal **mal′** gē ə
ophthalm/o/dynia
off thal mō **din′** ē ə

instrument for measuring the eye

_____/_____/_____ ;

ocular pain

_____/_____ .

15.5

Build words meaning
any ocular disease

ophthalm/o/pathy
off thal **mop′** ə thē

ophthalm/o/plasty
off **thal′** mō plas tē

ophthalm/o/plegia
off thal mō **plē′** jē ə

_____/_____/_____ ;

plastic surgery of the eye

_____/_____/_____ ;

paralysis of the eye (muscles)

_____/_____/_____ .

15.6

Ophthalm/o/logy is the medical specialty studying eye disease and surgery of the eye. We call the physician who practices this specialty an

ophthalm/o/logist
off thal **mol′** ō jist

_____/_____/_____ .

**External structures
of the right eye**
Delmar/Cengage Learning

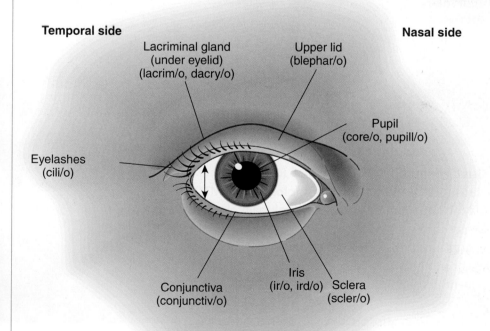

Temporal side   Nasal side

Lacriminal gland
(under eyelid)
(lacrim/o, dacry/o)

Upper lid
(blephar/o)

Pupil
(core/o, pupill/o)

Eyelashes
(cili/o)

Conjunctiva
(conjunctiv/o)

Iris
(ir/o, ird/o)

Sclera
(scler/o)

RIGHT EYE

ANSWER COLUMN

15.7

Ophthalm/o/scopy is the examination of the interior of the eye.
The instrument used for this examination is an

ophthalm/o/scope
off **thal'** mō skōp

_____ / _____ / _____ .

The process of performing an examination of the eye with a scope is

ophthalm/o/scopy
off thal **mos'** kō pē

_____ / _____ / _____ .

The following table analyzes word parts pertaining to the eye and vision.

Word Part	Use
-op/ia	suffix for vision
opt/ic	adjective—pertaining to vision
opt/o	combining form for vision
ophthalm/o	combining form for eye
ophthalm/ic	adjective—pertaining to eye

15.8

opt/o refers to vision. Use **opt/o** to build words meaning
one who measures visual acuity

opt/o/metrist
op' **tom'** ə trist

_____ / _____ / _____ ;

the cranial nerve for vision (adjective)

opt/ic
op' tik

_____ / _____ ;

the measurement of vision (practice of assessing vision disorders)

opt/o/metry
op **tom'** e trē

_____ / _____ / _____ .

NOTE: Optometrists are licensed to prescribe corrective lenses and treat some
eye diseases.

PROFESSIONAL PROFILE

Certified ophthalmic assistants (COAs), technicians (COTs), and **medical technologists (COMTs)** play an important role in assisting ophthalmologists by assessing visual acuity, performing diagnostic tests (e.g., glaucoma screening), assisting with minor and major ophthalmic surgical procedures, and providing patient education. The Joint Commission on Allied Health Personnel in Ophthalmology (JCAHPO) is the certifying agency for ophthalmic medical personnel.

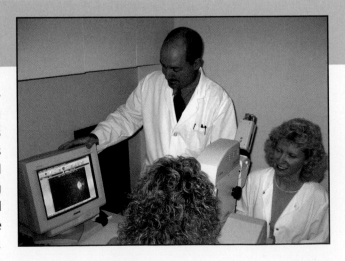

Optometrist and ophthalmic technician performing a retina photo *Delmar/Cengage Learning*

ANSWER COLUMN

TAKE A CLOSER LOOK

15.9

Notice the difference between the following
ophthalmologist—physician (MD or DO) specialist in treating diseases of the eye and performing surgery; and
optometrist—licensed practitioner (OD) limited to eye examinations and prescribing corrective lenses.
Both are called doctor, having received doctorate degrees from schools of medicine or optometry.

15.10

ophthalm/ic
off **thal'** mik

A special technician who assists ophthalmologists with eye exams and helps fit corrective lenses is called a certified _____/_____ technician (COT).

15.11

Recall word roots indicating colors. **-opia** is a suffix denoting a vision condition. Cyan/opia is a defect in vision that causes objects to appear blue.
Form words meaning
yellow vision

xanth/opia
zan **thō'** pē ə

_____/_____;

green vision

chlor/opia
klor **ō'** pē ə

_____/_____;

red vision

erythr/opia
er i **thrō'** pē ə

_____/_____.

15.12

nearsightedness

farsightedness

loss of accommodation

double vision

Look up the following terms and note the type of vision they describe.

my/opia _____;

hyper/opia _____;

presby/opia * _____;

dipl/opia * _____.

**(A) Myopia
(nearsightedness)**
Light rays focus in front of the retina
**(B) Hyperopia
(farsightedness)**
Light rays focus beyond the retina
Delmar/Cengage Learning

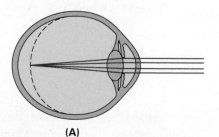

(A)

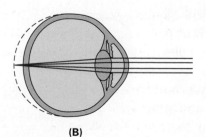

(B)

ANSWER COLUMN

15.13

heart

double

double

diplo- means double. Diplo/cardia means having a double _____.

Diplo/genesis means production of _____ parts

or _____ substances.

15.14

dipl/opia

dip lō′ pē ə

-opia is an involved form that we can use as a suffix. -opia means vision.

Build a word meaning double vision: _____/_____.

15.15

diplopia

There are many kinds of diplopia. Crossed eyes causes one kind of

_____.

15.16

diplopia

When both eyes fail to record the same image on the brain,

_____ occurs.

15.17

-opia

If you can see close objects but not distant ones, you may have my/opia or close vision. Presby/opia is experienced by older people as a loss of accommodation by the lens. The word literally means old vision. In each of these terms the suffix for

vision is _____.

15.18

both

ambi- means both or both sides. Ambi/later/al means pertaining to

_____ sides.

15.19

both

An ambi/dextr/ous person can work well with _____ hands.

15.20

ambi/opia

am bē ō′ pē ə

A word that means both eyes (OU—both eyes) forming separate images (vision)

is _____/_____.

NOTE: Ambiopia is a term not commonly used in optometry.

15.21

dipl/opia

(You pronounce)

dipl- and diplo- are prefixes meaning double. The result of separate vision from both eyes is a double image or double vision. Medically, double vision can be

expressed as _____/_____.

NOTE: diplo- and ambi- are combining forms used as prefixes.

ANSWER COLUMN

	15.22
	Hyper/opia means farsightedness (able to focus on objects at a distance)
my/opia mī ō′ pē ə	The opposite of hyperopia is nearsightedness, or _____/_____.
	15.23
	Look up ambivalence in any dictionary. Read its meaning. Analyze this word and the word ambivalent.
ambi/valence am **biv′** ə ləns ambi/valent am **biv′** ə lənt	_____/_____ _____/_____
	15.24
	Recall that a diplo/bacillus is a bacillus that occurs in pairs. A coccus that grows in
diplo/coccus dip lō **kok′** əs	pairs is a _____/_____.
	15.25
TAKE A CLOSER LOOK	Light travels through the lens of the eye, it is refracted, and an image is focused on the retina. **-opter** is a suffix meaning visible. A di/opter (Greek: *dia*, meaning through, and *optos*, meaning that which sees) is a unit of measurement of refraction in the eye.
	15.26
	Glasses or contact lenses are used to correct myopia, hyperopia, or presbyopia. A prescription written for corrective lenses that reads OS + 1 D means left eye
di/opter **dī′** op ter	one _____/_____.
	15.27
	A micr/o/scope is an instrument for examining something small. An instrument
dia/scope **dī′** ə skōp	used for examining (looking) through is a _____/_____.
	15.28
	A diascope is a glass plate held against the skin. The skin is examined through the diascope to see superficial lesions (erythematous and others). The prefix for
dia-	through is _____.
	15.29
WORD ORIGINS	**-tropia** is from the Greek *tropē* meaning turning. In ophthalmology, when the eyes appear to be turned in an abnormal position while open, it is referred to as a strabismus or squint. The medical terms used indicating the malposition of the eye include exo/tropia, eso/tropia, hyper/tropia, hypo/tropia, and cyclo/tropia.

ANSWER COLUMN

15.30

exo- means outward. eso- means toward. hypo- means downward.
hyper- means upward. From what you have just learned, build words that mean
eyes pointing outward

exo/tropia
eks ō **trō'** pē ə

_____/_____;

eyes pointing inward

eso/tropia
es ō **trō'** pē ə

_____/_____;

eyes pointing upward

hyper/tropia
hī per **trō'** pē ə

_____/_____;

eyes pointing downward

hypo/tropia
hī pō **trō'** pē ə

_____/_____.

Good!

15.31

Write the abnormal direction of the eye positions indicated below

upward

hypertropia _____

downward

hypotropia _____

inward

esotropia _____

outward

exotropia _____

15.32

Hyper/tropia results when an eye muscle moves one eye upward. When one eye

hypo/tropia
hī pō **trō'** pē ə

turns downward, we call it _____/_____.

15.33

Another term for exotropia, esotropia, hypertropia, and hypotropia is

strabismus
stra **bis'** mus
or squint

_____.

15.34

phor(ia) means to carry or bear. Dys/phoria means a feeling of depression—you
carry with you an ill (bad) feeling. The word that means feeling of well-being

eu/phoria
yōō **fôr'** ē ə

is _____/_____.

15.35

When your diet is good, you have enough rest, and the world is a wonderful

euphoria

place in which to be, you are enjoying a state of _____.

ANSWER COLUMN

(A) Esotropia
(B) Exotropia
Delmar/Cengage Learning

OD right eye

OS left eye

(A)   (B)

15.36

A phor/opt/er is an instrument used to determine the prescription strength needed for corrective lenses. An optometrist may use a

_____/_____/_____.

The unit measure for vision is the _____/_____.

phor/opt/er
for **op′** ter
dī **op′** ter
di/opter

15.37

Blephar/o/ptosis means prolapse of an eyelid. The combining form for eyelid is

_____/_____.

blephar/o

15.38

Edema is swelling due to fluid retention. Blephar/edema means swelling

of the _____. blephar/o seen anywhere makes you think of

the _____.

Edema makes you think of _____.

eyelid

eyelid

swelling

15.39

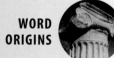

WORD ORIGINS

The word edema is related to the name of the Greek tragic hero Oedipus the king, whose father bound and pierced his feet as a child and left him to die. Oedipus comes from the Greek verb *oidein* (to become swollen) and literally translated means swollen foot. After a bizarre series of events, Oedipus kills his father and marries his own mother. Freud named his Oedipus complex theory after this story. The oe in Oedipus was later changed to e, and the modern English medical term became edema: Edema/tous is the adjectival form for swollen.

15.40

Blephar/edema means swelling of the eyelid. Build words that mean inflammation of an eyelid

_____/_____;

incision of an eyelid

_____/_____/_____.

blephar/itis
blef′ ə **rī′** tis

blephar/o/tomy
blef′ ə **rot′** ə mē

Lateral view of eyeball interior *Delmar/Cengage Learning*

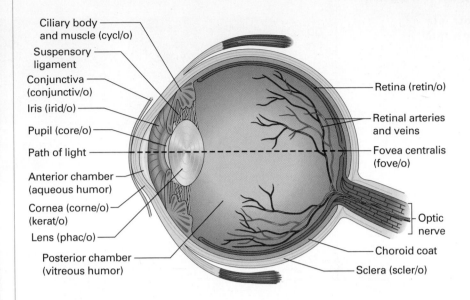

Ciliary body and muscle (cycl/o)
Suspensory ligament
Conjunctiva (conjunctiv/o)
Iris (irid/o)
Pupil (core/o)
Path of light
Anterior chamber (aqueous humor)
Cornea (corne/o) (kerat/o)
Lens (phac/o)
Posterior chamber (vitreous humor)
Retina (retin/o)
Retinal arteries and veins
Fovea centralis (fove/o)
Optic nerve
Choroid coat
Sclera (scler/o)

15.41

Build words that mean
excision of lesions on the eyelid

blephar/ectomy
blef' ər **ek'** tō mē

_____/_____;

surgical repair of an eyelid

blephar/o/plasty
blef' ə rō plas tē

_____/_____/_____;

twitching of an eyelid

blephar/o/spasm
blef' ə rō spaz əm

_____/_____/_____;

prolapse of an eyelid (droopy eyelid)

blephar/o/ptosis
blef' ər op **tō'** sis

_____/_____/_____;

suture of the eyelid

blephar/o/rrhaphy
blef' ər **or'** ə fē

_____/_____/_____.

15.42

The conjunctiva is the membrane that lines the eyelids (palpebral conjunctiva) and the sclera (bulbar conjunctiva). Look up conjunctivitis in your dictionary. There are over thirty types of inflammation of the conjunctiva or

conjunctiv/itis
kon junk' ti **vī'** tis

_____/_____.

STUDY**WARE**™ CONNECTION

View an animation on *Vision* on your **StudyWARE™ CD-ROM.**

ANSWER COLUMN

15.43

DICTIONARY EXERCISE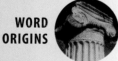

corne/o

Look up cornea in your dictionary. Look at the words that begin with corne.

A combining form for cornea is _____/_____.

Write the meaning and analyze by inserting the slashes for the following terms:

corneal

_____/_____, _____;

                                  meaning

corneoiritis

_____/_____/_____/_____, _____;

                                  meaning

corneoscleral

_____/_____/_____/_____, _____;

                                  meaning

15.44

ir, scler

From the preceding frame identify two word roots that mean iris and sclera.

They are _____ and _____.

15.45

phac/o/cele
fā′ kō sēl

Locate the lens on the illustration on page 566. **phac/o** is the combining form for the crystalline lens of the eye. Recall that **-cele** is used for herniation or dislocation. Build a word that means protrusion of the lens:

_____/_____/_____.

15.46

WORD ORIGINS

The lens is shaped like a lentil. In Greek, *phacos* means lentil. Lentils have a biconvex shape just like the crystalline lens of the eye.

15.47

phac/o
fā′ kō
cataracts
kat′ ə raktz

Cataracts are opacities that develop on the lens of the eye. Cataracts can be treated with an ultrasonic device to emulsify the lens for removal. This procedure

is called _____/_____ emulsification. Lens implants are used

to surgically treat _____.

NOTE: Phacoemulsification is part of a lens implant surgical procedure.

15.48

TAKE A CLOSER LOOK

sclera
sklair′ ə

Look up the first word in your dictionary beginning with scler.

It is _____. Read about the sclera.

Does the word root plus the Greek word *scleras*, meaning hard, from which it is derived, suggest an already familiar combining form to you?

(continued)

ANSWER COLUMN

scler/o/sis
condition of hardness

It is _____/_____/_____ , which means

* _____ .

(Remember sclerosis.)

15.49

The sclera of the eye is the white, "hard" outer coat of the eye.
Build words meaning
pertaining to the sclera (adjective)

scler/al
sklair′ əl

_____/_____ ;

excision of the sclera (or part)

scler/ectomy
sklair ek′ tō mē

_____/_____ ;

formation of an opening into the sclera

scler/o/stomy
sklair os′ tə mē

_____/_____/_____ ;

inflammation of the sclera

scler/itis
sklair ī′ tis

_____/_____ .

15.50

iris
ī′ ris

Look at the diagram of the eye on page 566. The colored part of the eye is

the _____ .

15.51

TAKE A CLOSER LOOK

Look up iris in your dictionary. ir and irid are word roots for the iris. **ir/o** and **irid/o** are both combining forms for iris. ir has limited use, usually with **-itis**, indicating inflammation of the iris. Also, look up the plural form of iris.

15.52

With the information in Frame 15.51 and the word root you found,
build words meaning
inflammation of the iris

ir/itis

_____/_____ ;

inflammation of the cornea and iris

corne/o/ir/itis

_____/_____/_____/_____ ;

inflammation of the sclera and iris

scler/o/ir/itis
(You pronounce)

_____/_____/_____/_____ .

15.53

You may have found in your dictionary the plural of iris.

ir/ides
ir′ i dēz, ī′ ri dēz

It is _____/_____ .

irid/o

The combining form for iris is _____/_____ .

ANSWER COLUMN

15.54

Using **irid/o**, build words meaning
protrusion of the iris (dislocation)

irid/o/cele
i **rid′** ō sēl (ī **rid′** ō sel)

_____/_____/_____;

pain in the iris

irid/algia
ir′ i **dal′** jē ə (ī ri **dal′** jē ə)

_____/_____;

excision of part or all of the iris

irid/ectomy
ir′ i **dek′** tə mē
(ī′ ri **dek′** tə mē)

_____/_____.

15.55

Build words meaning (you insert the slashes)
prolapse of the iris

irid/o/ptosis
ī′ rid op **tō′** sis

_____;

softening of the iris

irid/o/malacia
ī′ rid ō mal **ā′** shə

_____;

rupture of the iris

irid/o/rrhexis
ī′ rid ō **rek′** sis

_____.

15.56

The two words to express paralysis of the iris are

irid/o/plegia
ī rid ō **plē′** jē ə
irid/o/paralysis
ī rid ō pə **ral′** ə sis

_____/_____/_____ and

_____/_____/_____.

15.57

The following forms make you think of

iris

ir _____

iris

irid/o _____

sclera (hard)

scler/o _____

cornea

corne/o _____

15.58

Look up retina in your dictionary. Read about the retina and look at the words
beginning with retin in your dictionary. The combining form for words about the

retin/o

retina is _____/_____.

ANSWER COLUMN

15.59

Build words meaning
pertaining to the retina

retin/al
ret′ i nəl

_____/_____ ;
inflammation of the retina

retin/itis
ret i **nī′** tis

_____/_____ ;
fixation of a detached retina (repair)

retin/o/pexy _or_
ret′ i nō pek sē
retin/o/plasty
ret′ i nō **plas′** tē

_____/_____/_____ .

15.60

The instrument used to examine the refractive error of the eye (retina) is the

retin/o/scope
ret′ i nō skōp

_____/_____/_____ .
The process of using a

retin/o/scopy
ret i **nos′** kə pē

retinoscope is _____/_____/_____ .

NOTE: The proper term for retinoscopy is skiascopy. Look it up!

15.61

INFORMATION FRAME

Macul/ar de/gen/eration is a common cause of blindness in the elderly. In ophthalmology the macula lutea is an area of the retina near the optic nerve that has many blood vessels. Deterioration of the macula leads to central vision loss.

15.62

A photo of the retina may be taken to detect aging changes that may lead to

de/gen/eration
dē jen er **ā′** shun

macular _____/_____/_____ .

15.63

One treatment for macular degeneration is to perform an intra/ocular injection.

eye

Medication is injected into the _____ to slow down the progression

of disease.

15.64

INFORMATION FRAME

Glaucoma is a disease of the eye in which the intraocular pressure is increased. If glaucoma is not treated, the person will become blind. The three basic types of glaucoma are open angle, angle closure, and congenital.

15.65

One part of a complete eye exam includes checking the intraocular pressure.

glaucoma
glou **cō′** ma

This is done to look for signs of _____ .

ANSWER COLUMN

INFORMATION FRAME

15.66

The pupil in the eye is the opening in the iris through which light passes. Identify the pupil in the illustration of the eye on page 559. The word root for pupil is cor.

15.67

cor/ect/opia
kôr′ ek **tō′** pe ə

cor/e/lysis
kôr′ **el′** ə sis

cor/ectasia (is)
kôr′ ek **tā′** zhə

anis/o/cor/ia
an ī′ sō **kôr′** ē ə

One combining form for pupil is **cor/e**.
Build words meaning
pupil out of place

_____/_____/_____;

destruction of the pupil

_____/_____/_____;

dilatation (stretching) of the pupil

_____/_____;

unequal pupil size

_____/_____/_____/_____.

15.68

core/o/meter or
kôr ē **om′** ə ter

pupill/o/meter
pyōō pil **om′** ə ter

core/o/metry or
kôr ē **om′** ə trē

pupill/o/metry
pyōō pil **om′** ə trē

core/o/plasty
kôr ē ō **plas′** tē

core/o is used also as a combining form for pupil. Using **core/o**, build words meaning
instrument for measuring the pupil

_____/_____/_____;

measurement of the pupil

_____/_____/_____;

plastic surgery of the pupil

_____/____/_____

NOTE: Pupill/o is also used to build terms about the pupil.

15.69

cor

Whether **cor/e** or **core/o** is used, the word root for pupil of the eye is

_____.

15.70

corne

You have already learned one word root for cornea. It is _____.
Another word root for cornea is kerat, and it is the more commonly used form. (Think of kerats [carrots] and corn.)

15.71

kerat

kerat/o

The word root most commonly used for cornea is _____.

The combining form is _____/_____.

ANSWER COLUMN

15.72

Using **kerat/o**, build words meaning

forward bulging (dilatation) of the cornea

kerat/ectasia (is)
ker ə tek **tā′** zhə

_____/_____;

kerat/o/cele
ker′ ə tō sēl

herniation of the cornea (protrusion of the cornea)

_____/_____/_____;

kerat/o/plasty
ker′ ə tō plas tē

plastic operation of the cornea (corneal transplant)

_____/_____/_____.

15.73

Again using **kerat/o**, build words meaning

incision of the cornea

kerat/o/tomy
ker ə **to′** tō mē

_____/_____/_____;

kerat/o/rrhexis
ker′ ə tō **rek′** sis

corneal rupture

_____/_____/_____;

kerat/o/scler/itis
ker′ ə tō skler **ĭ′** tis

inflammation of cornea and sclera

_____/_____/_____/_____.

15.74

kerat/o/tomy

Making small incisions into the cornea to improve vision for those with myopia is
called radial _____/_____/_____.

15.75

**TAKE A
CLOSER LOOK**

The combining form for ciliary body is **cycl/o**. Cilia are hairlike structures. Turn to
cycl/o words in your dictionary. *Cyclos* is Greek for circle. The ciliary body encircles
the inside of the iris with muscle fibers that look like hairs.

15.76

Find words meaning

paralysis of the ciliary body (noun)

cycl/o/plegia
sī klō **plē′** jē ə

_____/_____/_____;

paralysis of the ciliary body (adjective)

cycl/o/pleg/ic
sī klō **plē′** jik

_____/_____/_____/_____;

ciliary body and cornea inflammation

cycl/o/keratitis
sī klō ker ə **tī′** tis

_____/_____/_____/_____.

15.77

The following combining forms make you think of

iris

irid/o _____

retina

retin/o _____

(continued)

ANSWER COLUMN

pupil	**cor/e** _____
pupil	**core/o** _____
cornea	**kerat/o** _____
cornea	**corne/o** _____
ciliary body	**cycl/o** _____

15.78

tears

Look up lacrim/al in your dictionary. Lacrimal means pertaining

to _____.

tearing

Lacrim/ation is _____.

15.79

lacrim/al
lak' ri məl

The gland that secretes tears is the _____/_____ gland.

15.80

lacrimal

The sac that collects lacrimal fluid is the _____ sac.

15.81

nas/o/lacrim/al
nā zō **lak'** ri məl

Lacrimal fluid is drained into the nasal cavity by means of the

_____/_____/_____/_____ duct.

15.82

Lacrimal fluid keeps the surface of the eye moistened. It is continually forming and being drained. When there is more formed than can be drained through a duct, you say the person is

crying or tearing

* _____.

15.83

dacry
-rrhea

Lacrimation means crying. Excessive lacrimation is called dacry/o/rrhea. This word gives you another word root for tear. It is _____, and the suffix for flow is _____.

15.84

lacrimation
lak ri **ma'** shun

dacry/o/rrhea
da'krē ō **rē'** ə

Flow of tears is either _____ or

_____/_____/_____.

ANSWER COLUMN

15.85

Analyze (you insert the slashes and define)
dacryocystitis

dacry/o/cyst/itis
dak′ rē ō sis **tī′** tis
tear sac inflammation

_____,

* _____;

dacryoadenalgia

dacry/o/aden/algia
dak′ rē ō ad′ ə **nal′** jē ə
pain in a tear gland

_____,

* _____;

dacryoma

dacry/oma
dak′ rē **ō′** mə
tumor of the tear duct
   or gland

_____,

* _____.

15.86

Insert the slashes and define
dacryopyorrhea

dacry/o/py/o/rrhea
discharge of pus from
   tear gland

_____,

* _____;

dacryocystocele

dacry/o/cyst/o/cele

hernia of the tear sac

_____,

* _____;

dacryolith

dacry/o/lith

stone in the tear sac
(You pronounce)

_____,

* _____.

15.87

If necessary you may use your dictionary to complete the following
dacryorrhea means

excessive flow of tears

* _____.

dacryocystoptosis means

prolapse of the tear sac

* _____.

a dacryocystotome is

an instrument for cutting
   (incising) the tear sac

* _____.

15.88

Look in your dictionary for words beginning with **onych**. These words refer to

nails

the _____.

ANSWER COLUMN

15.89

onych/o

By studying words beginning with onych, you can find its combining form.
The combining form that refers to nail is _____/_____.

15.90

SPELL
CHECK

Watch your spelling and pronunciation. The y is pronounced with a short "i" sound and the ch like a "k": o-n-y-c-h.

15.91

onych/oid
on' i koid

onych/oma
on i **kō'** mə

onych/osis
on i **kō'** sis

Build words meaning
resembling a fingernail or toenail

_____/_____ ;

tumor of the nail (or nail bed)

_____/_____ ;

any nail condition

_____/_____ .

15.92

onych/o/malac/ia
on' i kō ma **lā'** shə

onych/o/myc/osis
on' i kō mī **kō'** sis

onych/o/phagia
on' i kō **fā'** jē ə

Build words meaning
softening of the nails

_____/_____/_____/_____ ;

fungus infection (condition) of the nails

_____/_____/_____/_____ ;

nail biting (eating)

_____/_____/____ _____ .

15.93

hidden nail or condition
of nail being hidden

Recall that crypt means hidden. Onych/o/crypt/osis means literally

* _____ .

15.94

ingrown nail (usually
a toenail)

Look up onychocryptosis (on' i kō krip **tō'** sis) in your dictionary. It refers to an

* _____ .

15.95

par/onych/ia
par' ō **nik'** ē ə

Par/onych/ia is a condition of infection in the tissues around the nail. If the cuticle around the nail is infected, this is called _____/_____/_____ , also known as a "run around." To see this condition look at the pictures on the next page.

ANSWER COLUMN

(A) Paronychia,
infection of tissues
around the nail
Delmar/Cengage Learning

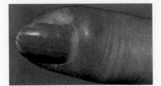

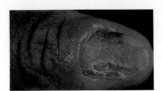

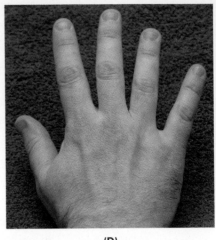

(B) Onychomycosis,
caused by parasitic
fungus *Delmar/Cengage Learning*

(C) Onychocryptosis,
ingrown nail *Delmar/Cengage Learning*

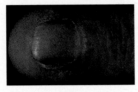

(A)

(B)

(C)

(D)

(D) Onychophagy, onychophagia,
bitten nails *Delmar/Cengage Learning*

15.96

hair

trich/o is used in words to mean hair. A trich/o/genous (trik **o'** jen us) substance promotes the growth of _____.

15.97

hair

Lith/iasis is the formation of calculi. Trich/iasis is the formation of _____ (in the wrong places).

15.98

Using **trich/o**, build words meaning
hairy tongue (noun)

trich/o/glossia
trik' ō **glos'** ē ə

_____/_____/_____;
resembling hair

trich/oid
trik' oid

_____/_____;
abnormal fear of hair

trich/o/phobia
trik' ō **fō'** bē ə

_____/_____/_____;
any hair disease

trich/o/pathy
trik **op'** ə thē

_____/_____/_____.

15.99

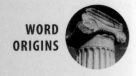

**WORD
ORIGINS**

Alopex is a Greek word meaning "like a fox with mange," referring to the hair loss due to a skin infection. Alopec/ia (al ō **pē'** shə) is the medical term for a condition of baldness.

ANSWER COLUMN

Alopecia *Courtesy of Robert A. Silverman, MD, Pediatric Dermatology, Georgetown University*

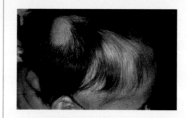

DICTIONARY EXERCISE

15.100

Look up alopecia in your dictionary. Read about some of the types of baldness listed below and describe each.

alopecia areata

_____

alopecia congenitalis

_____

alopecia medicamentosa

_____

Good work.

15.101

eat or swallow

eating or swallowing

Recall that **phag/o** means * _____ , and

phagia is a condition of * _____ .

15.102

eats (or ingests)

eating (or ingesting)

A phag/o/cyte is a cell that _____ microorganisms.

Phag/o/cyt/osis is the process of the cells _____
microorganisms.

15.103

phag/o/cyte

phag/o/cyt/osis
(You pronounce)

A cell that eats cells is a _____/_____/_____ .

The process is _____/_____/_____/_____ .

15.104

the ingestion of cells
   by phagocytes or
   phagocytosis

Cyt/o/phagy is another way of saying * _____

_____ .

15.105

cyt/o/meter
sī **tom'** ə tər

cyt'/ō/metry
sī **tom'** ə trē

Recall that an instrument for measuring (counting) cells is a

_____/_____/_____ , and the process of measuring

(counting) cells is _____/_____/_____ .

ANSWER COLUMN

15.106

Stopping or controlling cells is called

cyt/o/stasis
sī **tos'** tə sis

_____/_____/_____.

Examination of cells is

cyt/o/scopy
sī **tos'** kə pē

_____/_____/_____.

15.107

A large phagocyte is called a macr/o/phage. A small phagocyte is called a

micr/o/phage
mī' krō fāj

_____/_____/_____.

15.108

Onychophagia (on i kō **fā'** jē ə) is nail biting. A word that means

trich/o/phagy (ia)
tri **kof'** ə jē

hair swallowing is _____/_____/_____.
Air swallowing is

aer/o/phagy (ia)
air **of'** ə jē

_____/_____/_____.

Nail biting or eating is

onychophagy (ia)
on i **ko'** fa jē

_____/_____/_____.

15.109

Recall the prefix **endo-** means inside. Endo/crine literally means to secrete inside.

endo/crine
en' dō krin

Hormones are secreted from the _____/_____ glands.

15.110

The medical specialty studying the endocrine system is called

endo/crin/o/logy
en' dō krin **o'** lō jē

_____/_____/_____/_____.

The specialist (physician) in the study of the endocrine system is called an

endo/crin/o/logist
en' dō krin **ol'** ō jist

_____/_____/_____/_____.

The following table analyzes word parts related to the endocrine system. Refer to the illustration on page 579.

Combining Form	Meaning	Example
thyroid/o, thyr/o	thyroid gland	thyroidectomy
thym/o	thymus gland	thymosin
adren/o	adrenal gland	adrenalin
pancreat/o	pancreas	pancreatitis
oophor/o	ovary	oophoroma
testic/, orchid/o, orchi/o	testis	testicular

Review the male and female reproductive systems, in Unit 6.

ANSWER COLUMN

Endocrine system structures *Delmar/Cengage Learning*

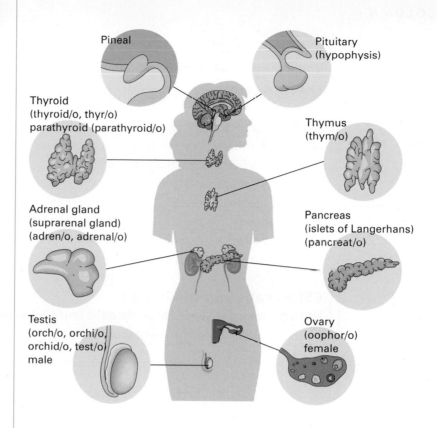

Pineal

Pituitary (hypophysis)

Thyroid (thyroid/o, thyr/o) parathyroid (parathyroid/o)

Thymus (thym/o)

Adrenal gland (suprarenal gland) (adren/o, adrenal/o)

Pancreas (islets of Langerhans) (pancreat/o)

Testis (orch/o, orchi/o, orchid/o, test/o) male

Ovary (oophor/o) female

15.111

Analyzing the following hormones, name the gland by which they are produced
adren/o/corticoid (cortisone)

adrenal gland (adrenal cortex)

_____ ;

thyr/o/xine, or thyr/o/xin

thyroid gland

_____ ;

test/o/sterone

testes

_____ .

See how much you have learned about word building!

15.112

Hyper/thyroid/ism is an overactive thyroid. An underactive (slow-acting) thyroid

hypo/thyroid/ism
hī pō **thī'** roid izm

condition is called _____/_____/_____ .

STUDY **WARE**™ CONNECTION

View an animation on the *Endocrine System* on your **StudyWARE™ CD-ROM.**

CASE STUDY INVESTIGATION (CSI)

Thyroidectomy

A 57-year-old woman presented with a 6.5 cm right sided painless neck mass and right recurrent **laryngeal palsy**. Magnetic resonance imaging (**MRI**) scan of the neck showed a mass with high signal intensity arising from the right lobe of the thyroid, displacing the **trachea** and encasing the right **internal** jugular vein (IJV). Right cervical lymph nodes were enlarged from levels 2–4. A highly **vascular** tumor was revealed during surgery extending down into the superior **mediastinum**, compressing and displacing the **IJV**. Total **thyroidectomy** and neck **dissection** were performed. Pathology revealed a wide **infiltrating** follicular **carcinoma** of the thyroid.

CSI Vocabulary Challenge

Use a dictionary if needed to analyze the terms listed below from the case study. Write the definition in the space provided.

laryngeal   _____

palsy   _____

MRI   _____

trachea   _____

internal   _____

vascular   _____

mediastinum   _____

IJV   _____

thyroidectomy   _____

dissection   _____

infiltrating   _____

carcinoma   _____

15.113

Build terms meaning
any disease condition of the adrenal glands

adren/o/pathy
ad′ rēn **op**′ ath ē

_____/_____/_____;

enlargement of the adrenal glands

adren/o/megaly
ad rēn′ ō **meg**′ əl ē

_____/_____/_____;

destruction of adrenal tissue

adren/o/lysis
ad′ rēn **ol**′ ə sis

_____/_____/_____.

ANSWER COLUMN

15.114

The adrenal glands are also called the supra/renal glands because they are above the kidneys. Epi/nephr/ine is a hormone produced by the supra/renal glands. Define these two terms

supra/renal

above the kidneys
(adrenal)

* _____ .

a hormone produced
upon the kidney

epi/nephr/ine

* _____ .

15.115

**TAKE A
CLOSER LOOK**

Nor/epinephr/ine is a neur/o/transmitter hormone that stimulates autonomic nervous system response. Adren/erg/ic receptors are activated by norepinephrine, epinephrine, and adrenergic drugs. Adrenergic literally means pertaining to adrenal work. The adrenal glands stimulate the autonomic nervous system.

15.116

A bronchodilator medication may be given to treat an asthma attack. Epinephrine dilates the bronchi by working on the nerves and is used as an

adren/erg/ic
ə dren **er′** jik

_____ / _____ / _____ drug.

15.117

Epinephrine and norepinephrine are naturally produced in the medulla of the

adrenal
ə **drē′** nəl

_____ glands.

15.118

There are many hormones produced by the pituitary gland. Look up pituitary in your dictionary and read about its function. The pituitary gland (hypophysis) has

anterior

front and back lobes. These are called the _____ lobe and the

posterior

_____ lobe.

15.119

**INFORMATION
FRAME**

Our bodies synthesize natural steroid hormones from cholesterol in the ovaries, testes, and adrenal glands. Steroids are lipid hormones and work by entering through the cell membrane and into the nucleus to affect the function of the cell. Once in the nucleus, their main function is to code RNA for the production of proteins. Because of this ability to stimulate protein synthesis, steroid hormone injections are used by some body builders and athletes to enhance muscle structure.

ANSWER COLUMN

	15.120
ster/oid **stair'** oid	Estrogen, progesterone, and testosterone are _____/_____ hormones.
testosterone tes **tos'** ter ōn	Sexual dysfunction or lack of libido in a male may be due to a low _____ level.
estrogen **es'** trō jen	Infertility in a female may be due to a low _____ level.

	15.121
insulin **in'** sə lin	Nonsteroidal hormones are protein-based hormones that link up to receptors on the surface of the cell membrane. Insulin is a protein hormone manufactured in the pancreas. Insulin causes the cell membrane to become permeable to glucose so that glucose can enter the cell and be used to create energy. The nonsteroidal hormone that allows glucose to enter the cell is _____.

	15.122
hyper/glyc/emia hi' per glī **se'** mē ə dia/betes dī ə **bē'** təs	Lack of or low insulin production causes glucose to build up in the blood and not enter the cells. Recall that high blood sugar is called _____/_____/_____ and may be a sign of _____.

	15.123
insulin	Type I diabetes mellitus is a condition in which the person does not produce enough _____.

	15.124
condition of the blood or in the blood	For another review recall that **-emia** is a suffix that means * _____.

	15.125
leuk/emia lōō **kē'** mē ə	Isch/emia (is **kē'** mē ə) is a condition in which blood flow is interrupted. Blood cancer (a sign being abnormally increased leukocyte count) is called _____/_____.

	15.126
blood	A transient isch/emic attack (TIA) is a temporary interruption of _____ flow, usually occurring in the brain.

ANSWER COLUMN

15.127

Build words meaning
reduction in red blood cells

an/emia
e **nē'** mē ə

_____/_____;

hyper/emia
hī pər **ē'** mē ə

too much blood (in one part)

_____/_____;

ur/emia
yōō **rē'** mē ə

urine constituents in the blood

_____/_____.

15.128

-emia is used as a suffix meaning in the blood. **hemat/o** is a combining form used as a prefix meaning blood. Build words meaning
blood in the urine

hemat/ur/ia
hēm at **yōō'** rē ə

_____/____/_____;

ur/emia
yōō **rē'** mē ə

urine constituents in the blood

_____/_____.

15.129

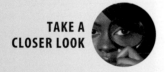

TAKE A CLOSER LOOK

You now know many prefixes, suffixes, and combining forms. You even know how to find combining forms and form singular and plural forms of a word. You also know several ways to find combining forms in your dictionary.

PROFESSIONAL PROFILE

Emergency medical technicians (EMTs) provide basic emergency medical care including first aid, CPR, immobilizing injuries, extricating accident victims from unsafe environments, and providing transportation. They may work directly in the field or in emergency departments. **Paramedics (EMT-Ps)** provide advanced life support such as using monitors and defibrillators, administering intravenous medications, as well as basic emergency care. Licensure requirements vary greatly throughout North America, and education ranges from private short course instruction to college-based programs offering associate degrees.

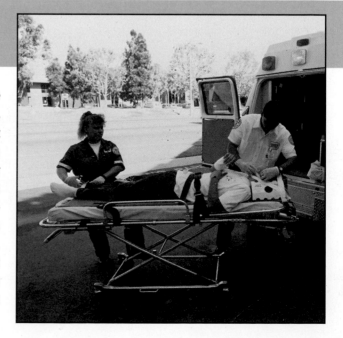

Emergency medical personnel aiding a patient *Delmar/Cengage Learning*

ANSWER COLUMN

15.130

To prove it again, look up trauma in your dictionary. It means a

wound or injury

* _____ .

15.131

Traumat/o/logy is the study of wound care. The combining form for trauma is

traumat/o

_____ / _____ .

15.132

The study of caring for wounds is called

traumat/o/logy
trô mə **tol'** ə jē

_____ / _____ / _____ .
Pertaining to wounds or woundedness is

traumat/ic
trô **ma'** tik

_____ / _____ .

15.133

A trauma center may provide 24-hour care for treatment of

wounds or injuries
trauma

* _____ . Physicians can specialize

in treatment of emergency cases including _____ .

15.134

TAKE A CLOSER LOOK

A trauma can produce many injuries. Look up the following in the dictionary and
write their definitions

abrasion * _____ ;

contusion * _____ ;

evulsion * _____ ;

puncture * _____ ;

fracture * _____ ;

laceration * _____ .

These are all types of wounds. Getting wounded is traumat/ic.

As a final review, notice that each of these medical specialties uses medical
terminology. Use your knowledge of word-building systems to fill in the blanks
in the following table. Check your answers in the second part of the table.

Specialty	Specialist	Limits of Field
pathology (15.136) _____	(15.135) _____ dermatologist	diseases—nature and causes (15.137) _____
neurology (15.139) _____	(15.138) _____ gynecologist	nervous system diseases female diseases
urology (15.141) _____	(15.140) _____ endocrinologist	male diseases and all urinary diseases glands of internal secretion
oncology (15.143) _____	(15.142) _____ (15.144) _____	neoplasms (new growths) heart
ophthalmology (15.146) _____	(15.145) _____ otorhinolaryngologist	eye (15.147) _____
obstetrics (15.149) _____	(15.148) _____ geriatrician	pregnancy, childbirth, and puerperium old age
pediatrics (15.151) _____	(15.150) _____ orthopedist	children bones and muscles
psychiatry (15.153) _____	(15.152) _____ audiologist	mental disorders hearing function
radiology (15.155) _____	(15.154) _____ chiropractor	diagnostic imaging therapeutic x-ray (15.156) _____
(15.157) _____	podiatrist	diseases of the foot

	pathologist (15.135)	
dermatology (15.136)		skin (15.137)
	neurologist (15.138)	
gynecology (15.139)		
	urologist (15.140)	
endocrinology (15.141)		
	oncologist (15.142)	
cardiology (15.143)	cardiologist (15.144)	
	ophthalmologist (15.145)	
otorhinolaryngology (15.146)		ear-nose-throat (15.147)
	obstetrician (15.148)	
geriatrics (15.149)		
	pediatrician (15.150)	
orthopedics (15.151)		
	psychiatrist (15.152)	
audiology (15.153)		
	radiologist (15.154)	
chiropractic (15.155)		manipulation therapy (15.156)
podiatry (15.157)		

15.158

Great!
See, you really are competent in the study of systematic medical terminology.

ANSWER COLUMN

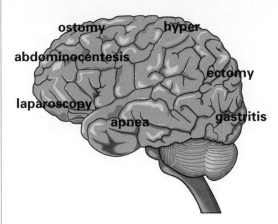

Delmar/Cengage Learning

Abbreviation	Meaning
ACTH	adrenocorticotropic hormone
AOA	American Optometric Association
COA	certified ophthalmic assistant
COMT	certified ophthalmic medical technologist
COT	certified ophthalmic technician
d, D	diopter
EMT	emergency medical technician
EMT-P	EMT—paramedic
ENT	ear, nose, throat
EOMI	extraocular movement intact (muscles)
FSH	follicle-stimulating hormone
Fx	fracture
HCG	human chorionic gonadotropin
IJV	internal jugular view
L&A, L and A	light and accommodation
laser	light amplification by stimulated emission of radiation
mg	milligram(s) (0.001 gram)
mm	millimeter(s) (0.001 meter)
MRI	maganetic resonance imaging
OAG	open-angle glaucoma
OB	obstetrician, obstetrics
OD*	right eye (oculus dexter)
OD	doctor of optometry
OS*	left eye (oculus sinister)
OU*	both eyes (oculus uterque)
PERRLA	pupils equal, round, reactive to light and accommodation
T_3, T_4	triiodothyronine, tetraiodothyronine (thyroid function tests)
TIA	transient ischemic attack
TSH	thyroid-stimulating hormone

*Abbreviations use warning. These abbreviations have been judged dangerous and should not be used.

ANSWER COLUMN

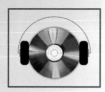

Now work the last **Review Activities** on the following pages. Also, listen to the Audio CD that accompanies *Medical Terminology: A Programmed Systems Approach,* 10th Edition, and practice your pronunciation.

Congratulations on your completion of this programmed study of medical terminology! May what you have learned in this course of study sustain you throughout your experiences in the health care field. Do not forget to celebrate your success!

STUDY**WARE**™ C O N N E C T I O N

To help you learn the content in this chapter, take a practice quiz or play an interactive game on your **StudyWARE™ CD-ROM.**

REVIEW ACTIVITIES

CIRCLE AND CORRECT

Circle the correct answer for each question. Then check your answers in Appendix E.

1. Prefix meaning inward
   a. inter-   b. exo-
   c. infra-   d. eso-

2. Suffix for vision
   a. -ophthalmic   b. -metry
   c. -opia   d. -ophthic

3. Combining form for yellow
   a. jaundice   b. xantho
   c. chloro   d. yello

4. Which of the following means nearsightedness?
   a. myopia   b. hyperopia
   c. presbyopia   d. exophoria

5. Combining form for eye
   a. optalmo   b. opthalmo
   c. optic   d. ophthalmo

6. Word root for lens
   a. lens   b. phac
   c. kerat   d. corne

7. Combining form for nail
   a. onycho   b. omphalo
   c. optic   d. onchyo

8. Word root for suprarenal glands
   a. aden   b. glandul
   c. genit   d. adren

9. Prefix meaning overactive
   a. hyper-   b. ultra-
   c. supra-   d. meta-

10. Combining form for eyelid
    a. maculo   b. cyclo
    c. lacrimo   d. blepharo

11. Which of the following does not have to do with tearing?
    a. lacrimation   b. cycloplegia
    c. dacryorrhea   d. dacryocystitis

12. Word root for hair
    a. omphal   b. trich
    c. cyclo   d. onycho

13. Combining form for double
    a. onycho   b. bi
    c. diplo   d. di

14. One combining form for cornea
    a. kerato   b. irido
    c. cyclo   d. coreo

REVIEW ACTIVITIES

SELECT AND CONSTRUCT

Select the correct word parts from the list below and construct medical terms that represent the given meaning.

adren	al	aniso	blephar	cardia
cele	cor(ne)(ia)	crypt	cyclo	dacry/o
diplo	disk	ectas(ia)(is)	ectomy	emia
emulsification	epi	eso	hyper	hypo
in(e)	ir	irid/o	itis	kerat (corne)
lacrim	lamin/o	(o)logy	lysis	malacia
megaly	metry	my	myco	naso
nephrine	onych/o	oophoro	ophthalmo	opia
opt(ic)(o)	orchid	osis	otomy	pathy
phac/o	phobia	phoria	plasty	plegia
presby/o	ptosis	retin(o)	rrhea	rrhexia
scope	thym/o	thyro(oid)	tomy	traumat/o
trich/o	trop/ia			

1. specialty measuring vision _____

2. paralysis of the ciliary body _____

3. softening of the nails _____

4. inflammation of the iris _____

5. excessive flow of tears _____

6. removal of the lens through a destruction procedure _____

7. hormone produced by the glands above the kidneys _____

8. farsightedness _____

9. instrument to examine the retina _____

10. study of wounds _____

11. surgical repair of the eye _____

12. dilatation of the pupil _____

13. prolapse of the eyelid _____

14. incision into the cornea _____

15. enlargement of the thyroid _____

16. unequal pupil size _____

17. inward crossed eyes _____

18. old eye (vision) _____

19. ingrown (hidden) nail _____

20. surgical repair of the retina _____

REVIEW ACTIVITIES

DEFINE AND DISSECT

Give a brief definition and dissect each term listed into its word parts in the space provided. Check your answers by referring to the frame listed in parentheses and your medical dictionary. Then listen to the Audio CD to practice pronunciation.

1. exotropia (15.30)

    _____/_____
                   pre   rt/suffix

    meaning _____

2. phoropter (15.36)

    _____/_____/_____
           rt   rt   suffix

    _____

3. paronychia (15.95)

    _____/_____/_____
          pre   rt   suffix

    _____

4. ophthalmologist (15.6)

    _____/_____/_____
          rt   v   suffix

    _____

5. myopia (15.12)

    _____/_____
              rt   suffix

    _____

6. optometrist (15.8)

    _____/_____/_____
          rt   v   rt/suffix

    _____

7. blepharoplasty (15.41)

    _____/_____/_____
          rt   v   suffix

    _____

8. corneoiritis (15.43)

    _____/_____/_____/_____
       rt   v   rt   suffix

    _____

9. phacocele (15.45)

    _____/_____/_____
          rt   v   suffix

    _____

10. retinoscopy (15.60)

    _____/_____/_____
          rt   v   suffix

    _____

REVIEW ACTIVITIES

11. corelysis (15.67)

_____/_____/_____
rt　　　　　　v　　　　　　suffix

_____

12. keratoscleritis (15.73)

_____/_____/_____/_____
rt　　　　　　v　　　　　　rt　　　　　　suffix

_____

13. nasolacrimal (15.81)

_____/_____/_____/_____
rt　　　　　　v　　　　　　rt　　　　　　suffix

_____

14. dacryocystocele (15.86)

_____/_____/_____/_____/_____
rt　　　　　　v　　　　　　rt　　　　　　v　　　　　　suffix

_____

15. onychophagia (15.92)

_____/_____/_____
rt　　　　　　v　　　　　　suffix

_____

16. trichopathy (15.98)

_____/_____/_____
rt　　　　　　v　　　　　　suffix

_____

17. phagocytosis (15.102)

_____/_____/_____/_____
rt　　　　　　v　　　　　　rt　　　　　　suffix

_____

18. endocrinologist (15.110)

_____/_____/_____/_____
pre　　　　　　rt　　　　　　v　　　　　　suffix

_____

19. adrenocorticoid (15.111)

_____/_____/_____
rt　　　　　　v　　　　　　rt/suffix

_____

20. hypothyroidism (15.112)

_____/_____/_____
pre　　　　　　rt　　　　　　suffix

_____

21. adrenomegaly (15.113)

_____/_____/_____
rt　　　　　　v　　　　　　suffix

_____

REVIEW ACTIVITIES

22. uremia (15.127)

_____/_____
           rt   rt/suffix

_____

23. pathologist (15.135)

_____/_____/_____
        rt   v   suffix

_____

24. oncology (15.142)

_____/_____/_____
        rt   v   suffix

_____

25. otorhinolaryngologist (15.146)

_____/_____/_____/_____/_____/_____/_____
      rt   v   rt   v   rt   v   suffix

_____

26. orthopedist (15.152)

_____/_____/_____/_____
        rt   v   rt   suffix

_____

27. radiology (15.154)

_____/_____/_____
        rt   v   suffix

_____

28. chiropractor (15.155)

_____/_____/_____
        rt   v   rt/suffix

_____

29. podiatry (15.157)

_____/_____
          rt   suffix

_____

30. audiology (15.153)

_____/_____/_____
        rt   v   suffix

_____

31. thyroidectomy (case study)

_____/_____
          rt   suffix

_____

32. degeneration (15.62)

_____/_____/_____
        pre   rt   suffix

_____

REVIEW ACTIVITIES

33. alopecia (15.99)

_____/_____
rt   suffix

_____

34. neurotransmitter (15.115)

_____/_____/_____/_____
rt   v   rt   suffix

_____

IMAGE LABELING

Label the structures of the eye by matching the number with the combining form. Then write the structure name in the blank.

_____ corne/o, kerat/o   _____

_____ retin/o   _____

_____ scler/o   _____

_____ cycl/o   _____

_____ core/o   _____

_____ phac/o   _____

_____ irid/o   _____

_____ blephar/o   _____

_____ conjunctiv/o   _____

_____ lacrim/o, dacry/o   _____

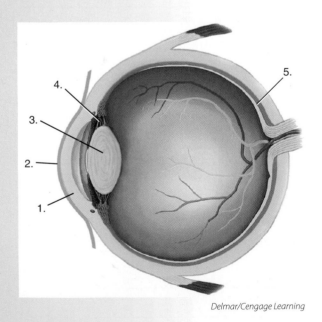

Delmar/Cengage Learning

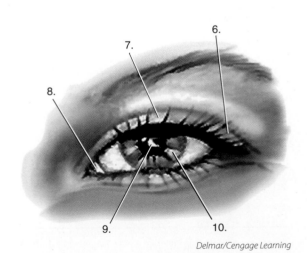

Delmar/Cengage Learning

REVIEW ACTIVITIES

ABBREVIATION MATCHING

Match the following abbreviations with their definition.

_____ 1. COT	a.	otorhinolaryngologist
_____ 2. TIA	b.	both eyes
_____ 3. OU	c.	living and well
_____ 4. TSH	d.	extraocular (muscles) movement intact
_____ 5. PERRLA	e.	light and accommodation
_____ 6. ENT	f.	thyroid-stimulating hormone
_____ 7. OB	g.	right eye
_____ 8. OD	h.	certified occupational therapy assistant
_____ 9. EOMI	i.	doctor of optometry
_____ 10. OAG	j.	fasting sugar
	k.	left ear
	l.	open-angle glaucoma
	m.	obstetrician
	n.	certified ophthalmic technician
	o.	follicle-stimulating hormone
	p.	pupils equal, round, reactive to light and accommodation
	q.	acute glaucoma
	r.	transient ischemic attack

ABBREVIATION FILL-IN

Fill in the blanks with the correct abbreviation.

11. American Optometric Association _____

12. emergency medical technician _____

13. follicle-stimulating hormone _____

14. thyroid function tests _____

15. right eye _____

16. light and accommodation _____

REVIEW ACTIVITIES

CASE STUDY

Write the term next to its meaning. Then draw slashes to analyze the word parts. Note the use of medical abbreviations. Look these up in your dictionary or find them in Appendix B. If you have any questions about the answers, refer to your medical dictionary or check with your instructor for the answers in Appendix E.

CASE STUDY 15-1

Phacoemulsification

Surgeon: P.H. Ernest, M.D.

Preoperative and postoperative diagnoses

1. **cataract OD**, with low **corneal** endothelial cell count.

2. **myopia OD**

Operation performed: **Phacoemulsification** of right eye with insertion of foldable **intraocular** lens of 22 power.

Summary: 2% Xylocaine and Wydase administered by peribulbar injection. A Honan balloon was placed on the eye for 20 minutes at 5-minute intervals. Betadine drops were instilled into the cul-de-sac and cornea. A temporal approach was made. A **paracentesis** incision was made and Viscoelastic was used to replace the aqueous. At the limbus, a temporally approached 3.2-mm incision and then dissection into the cornea was made with crescent blade. A 2.3-mm **keratome** was used to make an internal corneal cut through Descemet's membrane creating a square wound. Under Viscoelastic, multiple sphincterotomies were performed. A 360-degree **capsulorrhexis** was performed. Hydrocortical cleavage and hydrodelineation was performed. Using phacoemulsification, the nucleus was sculpted into perpendicular grooves. Using an Ernest nuclear cracker, the nucleus was cracked into four quadrants. The **epinucleus** and any residual cortex was removed using pulsed phaco, irrigation, and aspiration. Under Viscoelastic, a foldable intraocular lens was inserted and positioned within the capsular bag. All Viscoelastic was removed both anterior and posterior from the intraocular lens using irrigation and aspiration. 500-cc balanced salt, 20-mg Vancomycin and 10-mg Tobramicin was instilled. The wound was tested to ensure no wound leaks. Maxitrol ointment and a shield was applied over the eye to ensure no inadvertent corneal **abrasion**. The patient was sent to the recovery room in good condition.

1. breakup of the lens _____

2. scrape wound _____

3. rupture of the capsule _____

4. within the eye _____

5. instrument used to cut thin slices of the cornea _____

6. nearsightedness _____

7. cloudy lesion on the lens _____

8. upon the nucleus _____

9. pertaining to the cornea _____

10. puncture for the removal of fluid _____

11. abbreviation, right eye _____

REVIEW ACTIVITIES

CROSSWORD PUZZLE

Check your answers by going back through the frames or checking the solutions in Appendix F.

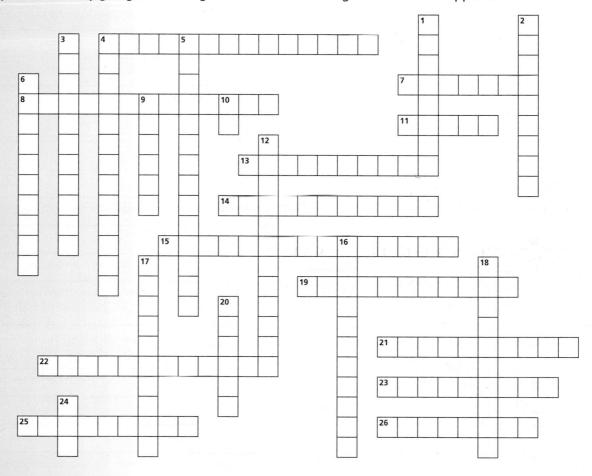

Across

4. instrument to look into the eye
7. unit of measurement for lens prescription
8. study of hormones and glands
11. pertaining to vision
13. seeing red
14. synonym for dacryorrhea
15. hormone from the adrenal cortex
19. adrenal medulla hormone
21. tear duct stone
22. swollen eyelid
23. cross-eyed
25. bruise
26. a tearing wound

Down

1. synonym for diplopia
2. thyroid hormone
3. prolapsed iris
4. soft nails
5. slow thyroid
6. fix the retina
9. inflamed iris
10. optometrist (abbr.)
12. hair eating
16. hair disease
17. pertaining to the eye
18. unequal pupils
20. white of the eye
24. otorhinolaryngologist (abbr.)

REVIEW ACTIVITIES

GLOSSARY

abrasion	scrape
adrenergic	activated by epinephrine
adrenocorticoid	hormone manufactured in the adrenal cortex
adrenolysis	destruction of the adrenal glands
adrenomegaly	enlarged adrenal glands
ambiopia	separate images from each eye
alopecia	baldness
ambivalence	unable to decide, wavering on both sides
anisocoria	pupils of unequal size
blepharedema	swelling of the eyelid
blepharoplasty	plastic surgery of the eyelid
blepharoptosis	prolapse of the upper eyelid (drooping)
blepharorrhaphy	suturing of the eyelid
blepharospasm	twitching eyelid
cataract	opacity on the lens
chloropia	seeing green
contusion	bruise
corectasia	dilation of the pupil
corectopia	displaced pupil
corelysis	destruction of the pupil
coreometer	instrument used to measure pupil size
coreoplasty	plastic surgery of the pupil
corneitis	inflammation of the cornea (keratitis)
corneoiritis	inflammation of the cornea and the iris
corneoscleral	pertaining to the cornea and the sclera
cyclokeratitis	inflammation of the ciliary body and the cornea
cycloplegia	paralysis of the ciliary body

cytophagy	destruction of other cells by phagocytes (cytophagia, phagocytosis)
dacryoadenalgia	pain in the tear gland
dacryocystitis	inflammation of the tear sac
dacryocystocele	herniation of a tear sac
dacryocystoptosis	prolapse of the tear sac
dacryocystotome	instrument for incision of a tear sac
dacryolith	calculus in the tear duct or sac
dacryoma	tumor of the lacrimal tissue
dacryopyorrhea	discharge of pus from the tear gland
degeneration	breakdown due to aging
diabetes	disease characterized by hyper-glycemia and lack of insulin
diascope	a glass plate used to look through to examine the skin
diopter	measurement unit of refraction
diplopia	double vision (ambiopia)
edema	swelling
endocrine	glands that secrete hormones
endocrinologist	specialist in the study and treatment of disorders of the endocrine system
endocrinology	the science studying the endocrine system
epinephrine	hormone produced by the adrenal medulla
erythropia	seeing red
esotropia	condition in which the eyes point inward (cross-eyed)
estrogen	female hormone (steroid)
euphoria	feeling good
evulsion	a tearing away
exotropia	condition in which the eyes point outward
fracture	break

REVIEW ACTIVITIES

glaucoma	condition in which the intraocular aqueous humor pressure is high
hormones	substances secreted by endocrine glands that affect body processes
hyperglycemia	high blood sugar
hyperopia	farsightedness
hypertropia	condition in which the eyes point upward
hyperthyroidism	overactive thyroid condition
hypotropia	condition in which the eyes point downward
hypothyroidism	underactive thyroid condition
insulin	pancreatic protein hormone
iridalgia	iris pain
iridectomy	excision of the iris
iridocele	herniation of the iris
iridomalacia	softening of the iris
iridoplegia	paralysis of the iris (iridoparalysis)
iridoptosis	prolapse of the iris
iridorrhexis	rupture of the iris
keratectasia	protrusion of a thin scarred cornea
keratorrhexis	rupture of the cornea
keratoscleritis	inflammation of the cornea and sclera
keratotomy	incision into the cornea
laceration	a cut (verb form lacerate)
lacrimal	pertaining to tearing
lacrimation	tearing (dacryorrhea)
macrophage	large phagocyte
macular	pertaining to the macula of the eye
microphage	small phagocyte
myopia	nearsightedness
nasolacrimal	pertaining to the nasal passages and the tear ducts

onychocryptosis	ingrown nail
onychoid	resembling a nail
onychoma	nail tumor
onychomalacia	softening of the nails
onychomycosis	fungus infection of the nail
onychophagia	nail biting
ophthalmalgia	eye pain (ophthalmodynia)
ophthalmic	pertaining to the eye
ophthalmocele	herniation of the eye
ophthalmologist	physician specialist in treatment of eye disease
ophthalmometer	instrument used to measure the eye
ophthalmopathy	any eye disease
ophthalmoplasty	surgical repair of the eye
ophthalmoplegia	ocular muscle paralysis
ophthalmoscope	instrument used to examine the interior of the eye
ophthalmoscopy	process of using an ophthalmoscope
optic	pertaining to vision
optometrist	specialist in assessing and treating visual acuity problems and other eye diseases (limited license)
optometry	the measurement of vision and the practice performed by the optometrist
paronychia	condition of infection around a nail
phacocele	protrusion of the lens of the eye
phacoemulsification	procedure to disintegrate the lens for insertion of lens implant
phagocyte	cell that eats cells (macrophage, leukocyte)
phorometer	instrument used to measure ocular muscle movement
phoropter	instrument used to measure prescription strength for lenses
presbyopia	old eye, loss of accommodation

REVIEW ACTIVITIES

puncture	to make a hole	thyroidectomy	excision of the thyroid
retinal	pertaining to the retina	thyroxine	thyroid hormone
retinitis	inflammation of the retina	traumatology	the study of wound treatment
retinopexy	fixation of a detached retina (retinoplasty)	trichoglossia	condition of hair growth on the tongue
retinoscope	instrument used to look at the retina	trichoid	resembling hair
sclerectomy	excision of the sclera	trichopathy	any hair disease
sclerostomy	make an opening in the sclera	trichophagia	condition in which the person bites on or eats hair
steroid	lipid bioregulator hormone	trichophobia	fear of hair growth (i.e., facial hair on women) or touching hair
strabismus	malposition of the eye		
suprarenal	upon the kidney, refers to the adrenal glands	uremia	urine products in the blood
testosterone	hormone produced in the testes (androgen)	xanthopia	see yellow

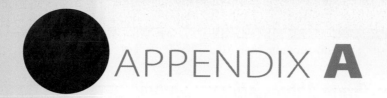

APPENDIX A

ISMP'S LIST OF ERROR-PRONE ABBREVIATIONS, SYMBOLS, AND DOSE DESIGNATIONS

The appendix that follows is reprinted with permission of the Institute for Safe Medication Practices (www.ismp.org).

ISMP's List of *Error-Prone Abbreviations, Symbols,* and *Dose Designations*

The abbreviations, symbols, and dose designations found in this table have been reported to ISMP through the ISMP Medication Errors Reporting Program (MERP) as being frequently misinterpreted and involved in harmful medication errors. They should NEVER be used when communicating medical information. This includes internal communications, telephone/verbal prescriptions, computer-generated labels, labels for drug storage bins, medication administration records, as well as pharmacy and prescriber computer order entry screens.

The Joint Commission (TJC) has established a National Patient Safety Goal that specifies that certain abbreviations must appear on an accredited organization's do-not-use list; we have highlighted these items with a double asterisk (**). However, we hope that you will consider others beyond the minimum TJC requirements. By using and promoting safe practices and by educating one another about hazards, we can better protect our patients.

Abbreviations	Intended Meaning	Misinterpretation	Correction
μg	Microgram	Mistaken as "mg"	Use "mcg"
AD, AS, AU	Right ear, left ear, each ear	Mistaken as OD, OS, OU (right eye, left eye, each eye)	Use "right ear," "left ear," or "each ear"
OD, OS, OU	Right eye, left eye, each eye	Mistaken as AD, AS, AU (right ear, left ear, each ear)	Use "right eye," "left eye," or "each eye"
BT	Bedtime	Mistaken as "BID" (twice daily)	Use "bedtime"
cc	Cubic centimeters	Mistaken as "u" (units)	Use "mL"
D/C	Discharge or discontinue	Premature discontinuation of medications if D/C (intended to mean "discharge") has been misinterpreted as "discontinued" when followed by a list of discharge medications	Use "discharge" and "discontinue"
IJ	Injection	Mistaken as "IV" or "intrajugular"	Use "injection"
IN	Intranasal	Mistaken as "IM" or "IV"	Use "intranasal" or "NAS"
HS	Half-strength	Mistaken as bedtime	Use "half-strength" or "bedtime"
hs	At bedtime, hours of sleep	Mistaken as half-strength	
IU**	International unit	Mistaken as IV (intravenous) or 10 (ten)	Use "units"
o.d. or OD	Once daily	Mistaken as "right eye" (OD-oculus dexter), leading to oral liquid medications administered in the eye	Use "daily"
OJ	Orange juice	Mistaken as OD or OS (right or left eye); drugs meant to be diluted in orange juice may be given in the eye	Use "orange juice"
Per os	By mouth, orally	The "os" can be mistaken as "left eye" (OS-oculus sinister)	Use "PO," "by mouth," or "orally"
q.d. or QD**	Every day	Mistaken as q.i.d., especially if the period after the "q" or the tail of the "q" is misunderstood as an "i"	Use "daily"
qhs	Nightly at bedtime	Mistaken as "qhr" or every hour	Use "nightly"
qn	Nightly or at bedtime	Mistaken as "qh" (every hour)	Use "nightly" or "at bedtime"
q.o.d. or QOD**	Every other day	Mistaken as "q.d." (daily) or "q.i.d. (four times daily) if the "o" is poorly written	Use "every other day"
q1d	Daily	Mistaken as q.i.d. (four times daily)	Use "daily"
q6PM, etc.	Every evening at 6 PM	Mistaken as every 6 hours	Use "6 PM nightly" or "6 PM daily"
SC, SQ, sub q	Subcutaneous	SC mistaken as SL (sublingual); SQ mistaken as "5 every;" the "q" in "sub q" has been mistaken as "every" (e.g., a heparin dose ordered "sub q 2 hours before surgery" misunderstood as every 2 hours before surgery)	Use "subcut" or "subcutaneously"
ss	Sliding scale (insulin) or ½ (apothecary)	Mistaken as "55"	Spell out "sliding scale;" use "one-half" or "½"
SSRI	Sliding scale regular insulin	Mistaken as selective-serotonin reuptake inhibitor	Spell out "sliding scale (insulin)"
SSI	Sliding scale insulin	Mistaken as Strong Solution of Iodine (Lugol's)	
i/d	One daily	Mistaken as "tid"	Use "1 daily"
TIW or tiw	3 times a week	Mistaken as "3 times a day" or "twice in a week"	Use "3 times weekly"
U or u**	Unit	Mistaken as the number 0 or 4, causing a 10-fold overdose or greater (e.g., 4U seen as "40" or 4u seen as "44"); mistaken as "cc" so dose given in volume instead of units (e.g., 4u seen as 4cc)	Use "unit"

Dose Designations and Other Information	Intended Meaning	Misinterpretation	Correction
Trailing zero after decimal point (e.g., 1.0 mg)**	1 mg	Mistaken as 10 mg if the decimal point is not seen	Do not use trailing zeros for doses expressed in whole numbers"
"Naked" decimal point (e.g., .5 mg)**	0.5 mg	Mistaken as 5 mg if the decimal point is not seen	Use zero before a decimal point when the dose is less than a whole unit

ISMP's List of *Error-Prone Abbreviations, Symbols,* and *Dose Designations* (continued)

Dose Designations and Other Information	Intended Meaning	Misinterpretation	Correction
Drug name and dose run together (especially problematic for drug names that end in "l" such as Inderal40 mg; Tegretol300 mg)	Inderal 40 mg Tegretol 300 mg	Mistaken as Inderal 140 mg Mistaken as Tegretol 1300 mg	Place adequate space between the drug name, dose, and unit of measure
Numerical dose and unit of measure run together (e.g., 10mg, 100mL)	10 mg 100 mL	The "m" is sometimes mistaken as a zero or two zeros, risking a 10- to 100-fold overdose	Place adequate space between the dose and unit of measure
Abbreviations such as mg. or mL. with a period following the abbreviation	mg mL	The period is unnecessary and could be mistaken as the number 1 if written poorly	Use mg, mL, etc. without a terminal period
Large doses without properly placed commas (e.g., 100000 units; 1000000 units)	100,000 units 1,000,000 units	100000 has been mistaken as 10,000 or 1,000,000; 1000000 has been mistaken as 100,000	Use commas for dosing units at or above 1,000, or use words such as 100 "thousand" or 1 "million" to improve readability

Drug Name Abbreviations	Intended Meaning	Misinterpretation	Correction
ARA A	vidarabine	Mistaken as cytarabine (ARA C)	Use complete drug name
AZT	zidovudine (Retrovir)	Mistaken as azathioprine or aztreonam	Use complete drug name
CPZ	Compazine (prochlorperazine)	Mistaken as chlorpromazine	Use complete drug name
DPT	Demerol-Phenergan-Thorazine	Mistaken as diphtheria-pertussis-tetanus (vaccine)	Use complete drug name
DTO	Diluted tincture of opium, or deodorized tincture of opium (Paregoric)	Mistaken as tincture of opium	Use complete drug name
HCl	hydrochloric acid or hydrochloride	Mistaken as potassium chloride (The "H" is misinterpreted as "K")	Use complete drug name unless expressed as a salt of a drug
HCT	hydrocortisone	Mistaken as hydrochlorothiazide	Use complete drug name
HCTZ	hydrochlorothiazide	Mistaken as hydrocortisone (seen as HCT250 mg)	Use complete drug name
MgSO4**	magnesium sulfate	Mistaken as morphine sulfate	Use complete drug name
MS, MSO4**	morphine sulfate	Mistaken as magnesium sulfate	Use complete drug name
MTX	methotrexate	Mistaken as mitoxantrone	Use complete drug name
PCA	procainamide	Mistaken as patient controlled analgesia	Use complete drug name
PTU	propylthiouracil	Mistaken as mercaptopurine	Use complete drug name
T3	Tylenol with codeine No. 3	Mistaken as liothyronine	Use complete drug name
TAC	triamcinolone	Mistaken as tetracaine, Adrenalin, cocaine	Use complete drug name
TNK	TNKase	Mistaken as "TPA"	Use complete drug name
ZnSO4	zinc sulfate	Mistaken as morphine sulfate	Use complete drug name

Stemmed Drug Names	Intended Meaning	Misinterpretation	Correction
"Nitro" drip	nitroglycerin infusion	Mistaken as sodium nitroprusside infusion	Use complete drug name
"Norflox"	norfloxacin	Mistaken as Norflex	Use complete drug name
"IV Vanc"	intravenous vancomycin	Mistaken as Invanz	Use complete drug name

Symbols	Intended Meaning	Misinterpretation	Correction
ʒ ♏	Dram Minim	Symbol for dram mistaken as "3" Symbol for minim mistaken as "mL"	Use the metric system
x3d	For three days	Mistaken as "3 doses"	Use "for three days"
> and <	Greater than and less than	Mistaken as opposite of intended; mistakenly use incorrect symbol; "< 10" mistaken as "40"	Use "greater than" or "less than"
/ (slash mark)	Separates two doses or indicates "per"	Mistaken as the number 1 (e.g., "25 units/10 units" misread as "25 units and 110" units)	Use "per" rather than a slash mark to separate doses
@	At	Mistaken as "2"	Use "at"
&	And	Mistaken as "2"	Use "and"
+	Plus or and	Mistaken as "4"	Use "and"
°	Hour	Mistaken as a zero (e.g., q2° seen as q 20)	Use "hr," "h," or "hour"

**These abbreviations are included on TJC's "minimum list" of dangerous abbreviations, acronyms and symbols that must be included on an organization's "Do Not Use" list, effective January 1, 2004. Visit www.jointcommission.org for more information about this TJC requirement.

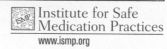

Institute for Safe Medication Practices

www.ismp.org

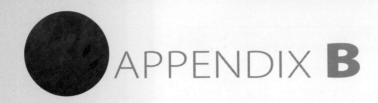

APPENDIX B

ABBREVIATIONS

The following lists of abbreviations are grouped by topic. To assist you in learning, they are arranged in columns. Column 1 lists the abbreviation, column 2 the meaning, and column 3 is left blank as a work space. Study the abbreviation and its meaning. Then cover the abbreviation and read the meaning. Write the abbreviation correctly in the blank. You may use the same method to learn the meanings by covering the meaning and reading the abbreviation. Write the meaning correctly on a separate piece of paper. Abbreviations that correspond to word parts presented in the frames are also listed at the end of each unit.

WEIGHTS AND MEASURES

Metric:

kg	kilogram(s) (1000 g)
hg	hectogram (100 g)
dag	decagram (10 g)
gm or g	gram
dg	decigram (0.1 g)
cg	centigram (0.01 g)
mg	milligram (0.001 g)
mcg, μg	microgram (0.001 mg)

Standard:

lb, #	pound
oz, ℥	ounce
dr, ℨ	dram
gr	grain

Volume:

cu mm	cubic millimeter (mm³)
cc	cubic centimeter (cm³)
cu m	cubic meter (m³)
cu in	cubic inch (in³)
cu ft	cubic foot (ft³)
cu yd	cubic yard (yd³)

Apothecary:

ī, īī, īīī	one, two, three
īV, V̄, etc.	four, five, etc.
īss	one and one half

Lengths:

in, ″	inch (2.54 cm)
ft, ′	foot (12 in)
yd	yard (36 in)
μm	micrometer (0.000001 m)
mm	millimeter (0.001 m)
cm	centimeter (0.01 m)
m	meter
km	kilometer (1000 m)

ABBREVIATIONS

Liquid Volume:

t, tsp	teaspoon
T, Tbsp	tablespoon
c	cup
m, min	minim
ml	milliliter (0.001 L)
cc	cubic centimeter (1 ml)
cl	centiliter (0.01 L)
dl	deciliter (0.1 L)
L	liter (1000 ml)
dal	decaliter (10 L)
hl	hectoliter (100 L)
fl dr, fl 3	fluid dram (60 min)
fl oz, fl 3	fluid ounce (8 fl dr)
pt	pint (16 oz)
qt	quart (32 oz)
gal, °	gallon (4 qt)
gt	drop (1 min)
gtt	drops

Miscellaneous:

at wt	atomic weight
C, kcal	calorie
c, Ci	curie
ht	height
mA	milliampere
mEq	milliequivalent
MHz	megahertz
mg%	milligram percent
mm Hg	millimeters of mercury
mw	molecular weight
ms	millisecond
IU	international units
U	units
°C	degrees Celsius
°F	degrees Fahrenheit

Chemical Symbols

Ag	silver (argentum—Latin)
$AgNO_3$	silver nitrate
Al	aluminum
Ar	argon
As	arsenic
Au	gold
B	boron
Ba	barium
Br	bromine
C	carbon
$C_6H_{12}O_6$	glucose
Ca	calcium (Ca^{++} ion)
Cd	cadmium
Cl	chlorine (Cl^- ion)
Co	cobalt
CO_2	carbon dioxide
Cr	chromium

ABBREVIATIONS

Cu	copper (Cu^{++} ion)	
F	fluorine	
Fe	iron (ferrum—Latin)	
H	hydrogen	
H_2O	water	
HCl	hydrochloric acid	
He	helium	
Hg	mercury (hydrargyrum—Latin)	
I	iodine (I^{131} radioactive)	
K	potassium (kalium—Latin, K^+ ion)	
Kr	krypton	
Li	lithium	
Mg	magnesium	
Mn	manganese	
N	nitrogen	
Na	sodium (natrium—Latin Na^+ ion)	
NaCl	sodium chloride (table salt)	
Ne	neon	
O	oxygen (O_2 molecule)	
P	phosphorus	
Pb	lead (plumbum—Latin)	
pCO_2	partial pressure carbon dioxide	
pO_2	partial pressure oxygen	
Ra	radium	
S	sulfur	
Se	selenium	
Si	silicon	
U	uranium	
Zn	zinc	

Diagnoses

AB 1, 2, 3 . . .	abortion one, two, three . . .	
ABE	acute bacterial endocarditis	
ACVD	acute cardiovascular disease	
AF (Afib)	atrial fibrillation	
AI	aortic insufficiency	
AID	acute infectious disease	
	artificial insemination donor	
AIDS	acquired immunodeficiency syndrome	
AIH	artificial insemination husband	
ALL	acute lymphocytic leukemia	
ALS	amyotrophic lateral sclerosis	
AMI	acute myocardial infarction	
AML	acute myelocytic leukemia	
AOD	arterial occlusive disease	
ARC	AIDS-related complex (conditions)	
ARD	acute respiratory disease	
ARF	acute respiratory failure	
	acute renal failure	
	acute rheumatic fever	
ARV	AIDS-related virus	
AS	aortic stenosis	
	arteriosclerosis	
	left ear (*auris sinistra*)	
ASCVD	arteriosclerotic cardiovascular disease	

ABBREVIATIONS

ASHD	arteriosclerotic heart disease	
AV, A-V	arteriovenous, atrioventricular	
BCC	basal cell carcinoma	
BO	body odor	
BPH	benign prostatic hyperplasia (hypertrophy)	
CA	cancer	
CAD	coronary artery disease	
CD	childhood disease	
CE	cardiac enlargement	
CF	cystic fibrosis	
CHD	congestive heart disease	
	congenital hip dislocation	
	congenital or coronary heart disease	
CHF	congestive heart failure	
CIS	carcinoma in situ	
CLD	chronic liver disease	
	chronic lung disease	
COLD	chronic obstructive lung disease	
COPD	chronic obstructive pulmonary disease	
CP	cerebral palsy	
	cor pulmonale	
CPD	cephalopelvic disproportion	
CRF	chronic renal failure	
CT	carpal tunnel (syndrome)	
	coronary thrombosis	
CVA	cerebrovascular accident (stroke)	
CVD	cardiovascular disease	
DNR	do not resuscitate	
DOA	dead on arrival	
DRG	diagnostic-related group	
DTs	delirium tremens	
Dx	diagnosis	
EOMI	extraocular movement intact (muscles)	
ESRD	end stage renal disease (failure)	
FAS	fetal alcohol syndrome	
FB	foreign body	
FOD	free of disease	
FTND	full-term normal delivery	
FTT	failure to thrive	
FUO	fever of unknown origin	
Fx	fracture	
FxBB	fracture both bones	
GERD	gastroesophageal reflux disease	
GNID	gram-negative intracellular diplococci	
G, Grav 1 2, 3 . . . , G1, G2	pregnancy one, two, three . . .	
HA	headache	
	hearing aid	
	hemolytic anemia	
	hepatitis A	
HAA	hepatitis-associated antigen	
HAV	hepatitis A virus	
HBV	hepatitis B virus	
HC	Huntington's chorea	
HCV	hepatitis C virus	
HCVD	hypertensive cardiovascular disease	

ABBREVIATIONS

HD	Hodgkin's disease	
HDN	hemolytic disease of newborn	
HF	heart failure	
HH	hiatal hernia	
	hard of hearing	
HIV	human immunodeficiency virus	
HLV	herpes-like virus	
HPV	human papilloma virus	
HSV	herpes simplex virus	
HTLV/III	human T-cell lymphotropic virus/three	
HTN	hypertension	
HUS	hemorrhagic uremic syndrome	
Hx	history	
IDDM	insulin-dependent diabetes mellitus	
IHD	ischemic heart disease	
IM	infectious mononucleosis	
LAV	lymphadenopathy-associated virus	
LE	lupus erythematosus	
LGB	Landry-Guillain-Barré syndrome	
LOA	left occiput anterior	
MBD	minimal brain dysfunction	
MD	manic depression	
	muscular dystrophy	
	myocardial disease	
met., metas., mets.	metastasis, metastases	
MI	myocardial infarction	
mono	mononucleosis	
MP	metacarpophalangeal (joint)	
MRSA	methicillin-resistant *Staphylococcus aureus*	
MS	mitral stenosis	
	multiple sclerosis	
MVP	mitral valve prolapse	
NMT	nebulizing mist treatment	
OA	osteoarthritis	
OAG	open-angle glaucoma	
OCD	obsessive-compulsive disorder	
OM	otitis media	
P (1, 2, 3 . . .)	preterm parity 1, 2, 3	
PAC	premature atrial contraction	
PAR	perennial allergic rhinitis	
	postanesthesia recovery	
para	paraplegic	
para 1, 2, 3 . . .	live births (one, two, three . . .)	
PAT	paroxysmal atrial tachycardia	
PCD	polycystic disease	
PD	Parkinson's disease	
	pulmonary disease	
PE	pulmonary edema	
	pulmonary embolism	
PERRLA	pupils equal, round, reactive to light and accommodation	
PID	pelvic inflammatory disease	
PKU	phenylketonuria	
PMS	premenstrual syndrome	

ABBREVIATIONS

PND	paroxysmal nocturnal dyspnea
	postnasal drip
PPS	post-polio syndrome
preg	pregnant
PVC	premature ventricular contraction
Px	prognosis
RA	rheumatoid arthritis
ROP	right occiput posterior
S-C disease	sickle cell hemoglobin-c disease
SCZ, SZ	schizophrenia
SIDS	sudden infant death syndrome
staph	staphylococcus
STD	sexually transmitted disease
STI	sexually transmitted infection
strep	streptococcus
T (1, 2, 3)	Term parity 1, 2, 3
Tb	tubercle bacillus
Top	termination of pregnancy
type 1	diabetes (insulin dependent)
type 2	diabetes (noninsulin, noninsulin dependent)
TB	tuberculosis
TCS	transcavital sonography
thal	thalassemia
TEE	transesophageal echocardiography
TIA	transient ischemic attack
TSD	Tay-Sachs disease
TVS	transvaginal sonography
URI	upper respiratory infection
UTI	urinary tract infection
VD	venereal disease (old, use. STD or STI)
VZV	varicella zoster virus

Procedures

A, B, O, AB	blood typing groups
AB	abortion
ABG	arterial blood gas
ACT	activated clotting time—Lee-White
ACTH	adrenocorticotropic hormone (test)
AFB	acid-fast bacillus
AID	artificial insemination donor
AIH	artificial insemination husband
ALT	alanine aminotransferase (liver enzyme)
ANA	antinuclear antibodies (RIA)
AST	aspartate aminotransferase (liver enzyme)
A&P	auscultation and percussion
BaEn, BE	barium enema
BP	blood pressure
BUN	blood urea nitrogen
Bx	biopsy
C-section	cesarean section
CABG	coronary artery bypass graft
CAD	computer-aided design
CAPD	continuous ambulatory peritoneal dialysis
CAT, CAT scan	computerized axial tomography (scan)

ABBREVIATIONS

cath	catheter	
CBC	complete blood count	
CH, chol	cholesterol	
CPAP	continuous positive airway pressure	
CPK	creatine phosphokinase	
CPR	cardiopulmonary resuscitation	
CSF	cerebrospinal fluid	
cTn I	Troponin I	
cTn T	Troponin T	
CT	computerized tomography (scan)	
CXR	chest x-ray	
cysto	cystoscopy	
C&S	culture and sensitivity	
DAW	dispense as written	
del	delivery	
DHT	dihydrotestosterone	
DNA	deoxyribonucleic acid	
DPT DTP, DTaP	diphtheria-pertussis-tetanus (vaccine)	
D&C	dilation and curettage	
ECG, EKG	electrocardiogram	
ECHO	echocardiogram	
ECT	electroconvulsive therapy	
EEG	electroencephalogram, electroencepholography	
EGD	esophagogastroduodenoscopy	
EMG	electromyogram	
ENG	electronystagmography	
EP	evoked potential	
ERCP	endoscopic retrograde cholangiopancreatography	
ERG	electroretinogram	
ESR	erythrocyte sedimentation rate (sed. rate)	
ESWL	extracorporeal shockwave lithotripsy	
exam	examination	
exc	excision	
FBS	fasting blood sugar	
FDG	fluorodeoxyglucose	
FME	full mouth extraction	
FOB	fecal occult blood (test)	
FSH	follicle-stimulating hormone	
GA	gastric analysis	
GHB	glycosolated hemoglobin	
GTT	glucose tolerance test	
GxT	graded exercise test	
HA	hearing aid, headache	
HAA	hepatitis-associated antigen (test)	
HAI	hemagglutination inhibition—rubella test	
HAV	hepatitis A virus	
Hb, Hgb	hemoglobin	
Hb Alc, Hgb Alc	hemoglobin Alc (test)	
HBV	hepatitis B virus	
HCG (hcg)	human chorionic gonadotropin	
Hct	hematocrit	
HCV	hepatitis C virus	
HDL	high-density lipoprotein	
HepB	hepatitis B vaccine	

ABBREVIATIONS

HGH	human growth hormone
Hib	*Hemophilus influenzae* vaccine
HPV	human papilloma virus
HSG	hysterosalpingogram
Hx	history
H&P	history and physical
IABP	intra-aortic balloon pump
ICAT	indirect Coomb's test
ICSH	interstitial cell-stimulating hormone
ID	intradermal (injection), identification
Ig	immunoglobulin, gamma (A, E, D, G, or M)
IM	intramuscular (injection)
inf	infusion
instill	instillation (drops)
IPPB	intermittent positive pressure breathing
IPV	inactivated polio virus vaccine (injectable)
IUD	intrauterine device
IV	intravenous (injection)
IVC	intravenous catheter
	intravenous cholangiogram
IVP	intravenous pyelogram
I&D	incision and drainage
I&O	intake and output
KUB	kidney-ureter-bladder (x-ray)
lab	laboratory
LASER	light amplification by stimulated emission of radiation
LAVH	laparoscopically assisted vaginal hysterectomy
LDH	lactose dehydrogenase (cardiac enzyme)
LDL	low-density lipoprotein
LH	luteinizing hormone
LP	lumbar puncture
MASER	microwave amplification by stimulated emission of radiation
MFT	muscle function test
MMRV	measles, mumps, rubella vaccine
MRI	magnetic resonance imaging
NCS	nerve conduction studies
OC	office call
OMT	osteopathic manipulative therapy
OPG	oculoplethysmography
OPV	oral polio vaccine
OREF	open reduction external fixation
ORIF	open reduction internal fixation
O&P	ova and parasites test
P+V	pyloroplasty and vagotomy
Pap	Papanicolaou test (smear)
Pap	pulmonary artery pressure
PBI	protein bound iodine
PCTA	percutaneous transluminal angioplasty
PCV	packed cell volume, pneumococcal vaccine
PE	physical examination
PET	positron emission tomography
PFT	pulmonary function test

ABBREVIATIONS

pH	hydrogen ion concentration, acid/base	_____
PO	by mouth (per os)	_____
postop	postoperative	_____
pro time, pt	prothrombin time	_____
PSA	prostate specific antigen	_____
PSG	polysomnogram	_____
PTCA	percutaneous transluminal coronary angioplasty	_____
PTT	partial thromboplastin time	_____
2hr pc	two-hour postcibal blood glucose	_____
2hr pg	two-hour postglucose blood glucose	_____
2hr pp	two-hour postprandial blood glucose	_____
P&A	percussion and auscultation	_____
RATx	radiation therapy	_____
RBC	red blood cell (count)	_____
RIA	radioimmunoassay	_____
RPG	retrograde pyelogram	_____
RPR	syphilis test (also: DRT, VDRL, STS)	_____
Rx	take, prescribe	_____
S/A, S&A	sugar and acetone	_____
SALT (old SGPT)	serum alanine aminotransferase	_____
SAST (old SGOT)	serum aspartate aminotransferase	_____
Sc, subcu, subq, sq	subcutaneous (injection)	_____
SOP	standard operating procedure	_____
SPECT	single photon emission computed tomography	_____
sp gr, SpG	specific gravity (urine)	_____
T, temp	temperature	_____
T3	thyroid test (triiodothyronine)	_____
T4	thyroid test (tetraiodothyronine)	_____
tab	tablet(s)	_____
TAH	total abdominal hysterectomy	_____
Td	tetanus	_____
TENS	transcutaneous electrical nerve stimulation	_____
TSE	testicular self-exam	_____
TSH	thyroid-stimulating hormone	_____
TUR (TURP)	transurethral resection (of the prostate)	_____
Tx	treatment, traction, transplant	_____
UA	urinalysis	_____
UV	ultraviolet (light)	_____
V, Y, W, Z, -plasty	various types of plastic surgery	_____
Var, VAR	chickenpox vaccine (_Varicella zoster_)	_____
VCG	vectorcardiogram	_____
VDRL	Venereal Disease Research Laboratory (syphilis test)	_____
WBC	white blood cell (count)	_____
XM	crossmatch for blood (type and crossmatch)	_____
XR	x-ray	_____
YAG	yttrium-aluminum-garnet (laser)	_____

Health Professions and Groups

AA	Alcoholics Anonymous	_____
AAD	American Academy of Dermatology	_____
AAFP	American Academy of Family Physicians	_____
AAMA	American Association of Medical Assistants	_____
AAMT	American Association of Medical Transcriptionists	_____
AANA	American Association of Nurse Anesthetists	_____

ABBREVIATIONS

AAP	American Academy of Pediatrics
AAPA	American Academy of Physician Assistants
AART	American Association of Rehabilitation Therapy
ACOA	Adult Children of Alcoholics
ACPMR	American Congress of Physical Medicine and Rehabilitation
ACS	American Cancer Society
	American College of Surgeons
ADA	American Dental Association
	American Diabetes Association
	American Dietetic Association
AHA	American Heart Association
AHIMA	American Health Information Management Association
AL-Anon, Alateen	Families of Alcoholics Groups
AMA	American Medical Association
ANA	American Nurses Association
	American Neurologic Association
AOA	American Optometric Association
	American Osteopathic Association
APA	American Psychiatric Association
APTA	American Physical Therapy Association
ARDMS	American Registry of Diagnostic Medical Sonographers (Sonography)
ARRT	American Registry of Radiologic Technologists
ART	Accredited Records Technician
ASCP	American Society of Clinical Pathologists
ASRT	American Society of Radiologic Technologists
BSN	Bachelors of Science in Nursing
CDC	Centers for Disease Control
CENA, CNA	Certified Nursing Assistant, Competency
CHUC	Certified Health Unit Coordinator (Clerk)
CLA	Certified Laboratory Assistant
CMA	Certified Medical Assistant
CMT	Certified Medical Transcriptionist
COMA	Certified Ophthalmic Medical Assistant
COMT	Certified Ophthalmic Medical Technician
COTA	Certified Occupational Therapy Assistant
CRNA	Certified Registered Nurse Anesthetist
CRTT	Certified Respiratory Therapy Technician
CST	Certified Surgical Technologist
CT (ASCP)	Cyto technologist (American Society of Clinical Pathology)
DC	Doctor of Chiropractic
DDS	Doctor of Dental Surgery
DO	Doctor of Osteopathy
DPM	Doctor of Podiatric Medicine
EENT	Eye, Ear, Nose, and Throat specialist
EMT	Emergency Medical Technician
EMT-P	Emergency Medical Technician Paramedic
ENT	Ear, Nose, and Throat specialist
FACP	Fellow of the American College of Physicians
FACS	Fellow of the American College of Surgeons
GYN	Gynecologist

ABBREVIATIONS

HMO	health maintenance organization	_____
ICU	intensive care unit	_____
LPN	Licensed Practical Nurse	_____
LVN	Licensed Vocational Nurse	_____
MD	Doctor of Medicine	_____
MLT	Medical Laboratory Technician	_____
MSN	Masters of Science in Nursing	_____
MT (ASCP)	Medical Technologist (American Society of Clinical Pathologists)	_____
NAHUC	National Association of Health Unit Coordinators (Clerks)	_____
NANDA	North American Nursing Diagnosis Association	_____
NLN	National League for Nursing	_____
NP	Nurse Practitioner	_____
OA	Overeaters Anonymous	_____
OB	Obstetrician	_____
ORTH	Orthopedist	_____
OSHA	Occupational Safety and Health Administration	_____
OT	Occupational Therapy	_____
OTR	Occupational Therapist Registered	_____
PA	Physician's Assistant	_____
Pharm D	Doctor of Pharmacy	_____
PT	Physical Therapy (Therapist)	_____
RD	Registered Dietician	_____
RDCS	Registered Diagnostic Cardiac Sonographer	_____
RDMS	Registered Diagnostic Medical Sonographer	_____
RN	Registered Nurse	_____
R.Ph	Registered Pharmacist	_____
RRA	Registered Records Administrator	_____
RRT	Registered Respiratory Therapist	_____
RT (MR)	Registered Technologist (Magnetic Resonance Imaging)	_____
RT (R)	Registered Technologist (Radiography)	_____
RT (N)	Registered Technologist (Nuclear)	_____
RT (T)	Registered Technologist (Radiation Therapy)	_____
RVT	Registered Vascular Technologist	_____
USP	United States Pharmacopeia	_____

Charting Abbreviations

aa	of each	_____
ac	before meals (ante cibum)	_____
AD	right ear (auris dextra)	_____
adj	adjective	_____
ADLs	activities of daily living	_____
ad lib	as desired (at liberty)	_____
adm	admission	_____
AE	above the elbow	_____
AJ	ankle jerk	_____
AK	above the knee	_____
am	before noon (ante meridiem)	_____
AMA	against medical advice	_____
AMB	ambulate	_____
ant	anterior	_____
ANS	autonomic nervous system	_____

ABBREVIATIONS

AP	anteroposterior
approx	approximately
ASAP	as soon as possible
AS or LE	left ear (*auris sinistra*), arteriosclerosis
AU	both ears (*auris uterque*)
AV	atrioventricular
AX	axillary
BE	below the elbow
bid	twice a day (*bis in die*)
bin	twice a night (*bis in nocte*)
BK	below the knee
BM	bowel movement
BMR	basal metabolic rate
BP	blood pressure
BRP	bathroom privileges
$\bar{c}$	with (Latin: *cum*)
$C_1, C_2, C_3 \ldots C_7$	cervical vertebrae first, second, third . . . seventh
$C_1, C_2 \ldots C_8$	cervical spinal nerve pairs
C	centigrade, celsius, or large calorie (kilocalorie)
cap(s)	capsules
CBR	complete bed rest
CC	chief complaint
CCU	cardiac care unit (coronary care unit)
c/o	complains of
cont	continue
D	diopter (ocular measurement)
dc	discontinue
DC	discharge from hospital
DNA	does not apply
DNR	do not resuscitate
DNS	did not show
Dr	doctor
D/W	dextrose in water
Dx	diagnosis
EOM	extraocular movement
ER	emergency room
Ex	examination
F	Fahrenheit
FHS	fetal heart sounds
FHT	fetal heart tones
GR	Greek
GB	gallbladder
GI	gastrointestinal
GU	genitourinary
h, hr, °	hour
Hb, Hgb	hemoglobin
hpf	high power field
hs	hour of sleep, bedtime (*hora somni*)
hypo	hypodermic injection
ICU	intensive care unit
IJV	Internal jugular vein
IM	intramuscular
I&O	intake and output

ABBREVIATIONS

$\overline{\text{iss}}$	one and one half
IU	international units
IV	intravenous
L	Latin
L, lt	left
L_1, L_2, L_3 ... L_5	lumbar vertebrae first, second, third ... fifth (spinal nerve pairs)
L&A	light and accommodation
LAT	lateral
L&W	living and well
LLQ	left lower quadrant
LMP	last menstrual period
LOA	left occipitoanterior
LPF	low power field (10x)
LUQ	left upper quadrant of abdomen
MTD	right ear drum (*membrana tympani dexter*)
MTS	left ear drum (*membrana tympani sinister*)
n	noun
neg	negative
NG	nasogastric
NPO	nothing by mouth
NS	norm saline
OD	right eye (*oculus dexter*)
OP	outpatient
OR	operating room
OS or OL	left eye (*oculus sinister, oculus laevus*)
OU	each eye (*oculus uterque*)
	both eyes (*oculi unitas*)
P	pulse
PA	posteroanterior
pc	after meals (*post cibum*)
PDR	Physicians' Desk Reference
PI	present illness
pl	plural
pm	afternoon or evening (*post meridiem*)
PNS	peripheral nervous system
po	by mouth (*per os*)
PO	postoperative
prn	as needed or desired (*pro re nata*)
q	every (*quaque*)
qd	every day (*quaque die*)
qh	every hour (*quaque hora*)
q2h, q4h	every two hours, every four hours
qid	four times a day (*quater in die*)
qm	every morning (*quaque mane*)
qn	every night (*quaque nocte*)
R, rt	right, respiration
RBC	red blood cell, erythrocyte count
Rh	blood factor, Rh+ or Rh−
RLQ	right lower quadrant (abdomen)
R/O	rule out
ROM	range of motion
RPO	right occiput oblique
RUQ	right upper quadrant (abdomen)

ABBREVIATIONS

S	singular
$S_1, S_2 \ldots S_5$	sacral spinal nerve pairs
s̄	without (sine)
sc, subcu, sq, subq	subcutaneously (into fat layer)
sed rate	sedimentation rate (erythrocyte)
SOB	short of breath
SOS	if necessary (*si opus sit*)
s̄s, ½, .5	half (Latin: *semis*)
staph	staphylococcus
stat	immediately (statim)
strep	streptococcus
Sx	symptoms
$T_1, T_2, T_3 \ldots T_{12}$	thoracic vertebrae: first, second, third … twelfth (thoracic spinal nerve pairs)
T, temp	temperature
tab(s)	tablets
TC&DB	turn, cough, and deep breathe
tid	three times a day (*ter in die*)
tinct	tincture
TPN	total parenteral nutrition
trans	transverse
ULQ	upper left quadrant (abdomen)
ung	ointment (unguentum)
URQ	upper right quadrant (abdomen)
v	verb
VS	vital signs
WBC	white blood cell, leukocyte count
wm, bm	white male, black male
wf, bf	white female, black female
x	times, power
y/o, yr	year(s) old, year(s)
−	negative
F, ♀	female
M, ♂	male
+/−	positive or negative
*	birth
†	death
p̄	after (post—Latin)
ā	before (ante—Latin)
#	pound, number
↑	increase
↓	decrease
>	greater than
<	less than

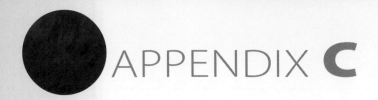

ADDITIONAL WORD PARTS

Following are word parts in addition to those presented in your study of the frames. Use these lists, your knowledge of word building, and your medical dictionary to enrich your medical vocabulary.

1. Pick a word part from the alphabetic list that interests you.
2. Look for it in your medical dictionary.
3. Find words that begin or end with this part and make a list.
4. Write the meanings of the new words you discovered.
5. Use the key in your dictionary to decipher the correct pronunciation, and practice saying the new words.

Word Part	Meaning	Example
acid/o	acid	acid/osis
acne	point	acne vulgaris
actin/o	ray (radiation)	actin/o/dermat/itis
acu	needle	acu/puncture
adnex/al	adjacent, accessory	adnex/ectomy
albin/o	white	albin/ism
alkal/o	base	alkal/osis
all/o	other, different	all/o/pathy, all/ergy
ambly/o	dim, dull	ambly/opia
amyl/o	starch	amyl/ase
andr/o	man	andr/o/gen
aneurysm	abnormal dilation	aneurysm/o/rrhaphy
aort/o	aorta	aort/o/graphy
atel/o	imperfect, collapsed	atel/ectasis
bil/i	bile	bil/i/rubin
cat/a	down, downward	cat/a/tonic
celi/o	abdominal region	celi/ac artery
cerumin	wax	cerumin/o/lysis
chalas/ia	relaxation	a/chalas/ia
chron/o	time	chronological, chronic
chym/o	juice	ec/chym/o/sis
cirrhos	orange-yellow	cirrh/o/sis
clasia	breaking down	arthr/o/clasia
cleisis	closure, occlusion	colp/o/cleis/is
coll/o	glutinous, jellylike	coll/agen
cry/o	freezing	cry/o/surgery
decub/o	lying down	decubit/us ulcer
eczem/o	boil out	eczem/a
glomerul/o	glomerulus	glomerul/o/nephr/itis
gonad/o	ovaries, testes	gonad/o/tropin
halit/o	breath	halit/o/sis
kal/i	potassium	hyper/kal/emia
kary/o	nucleus	kary/o/type

Word Part	Meaning	Example
ket/o	ketones	ket/o/sis
klept/o	stealing	klept/o/mania
mediastin/o	mediastinum	mediastin/al
muscul/o	muscle	muscul/o/skelet/al
natr/i	sodium	hyper/natr/emia
pach/y	thick	pach/y/dermat/ous
-poiesis	produce, form	hemat/o/poies/is
poikil/o	irregular shape	poikil/o/cyt/o/sis
prax/ia	action	a/prax/ia
prur/i	itch	prur/itis
pteryg/o	wing	pteryg/o/mandibul/ar
ptyal/o	saliva	ptyal/in
radicul/o	root	radicul/o/neur/itis
roentgen/o	x-ray	roentgen/o/graphy
scot/o	darkness	scot/oma
seb/o	fatty, sebum	seb/o/rrhea
sial/o	saliva	sial/aden/itis
somat/o	body	psych/o/somat/ic
sphygm/o	pulse	sphygm/o/man/o/meter
sphyxis	pulse (related to O_2)	a/sphyxia
stere/o	solid, three-dimensional	stere/o/metry
steth/o	chest	steth/o/scope
sthenia	strength	my/e/sthen/ia
stigma	point	a/stigmat/ism
stigmat/o	mark, point	a/stigmat/ism
taxia	muscle coordination	a/tax/ia
tel/e	distant, far	tel/e/metry
terat/o	monster, wonder	terat/o/genic
thel/o	nipple	thel/o/rrhagia
varic/o	twisted vein	varic/o/sity
vulv/o	vulva	vulv/o/vagin/itis
xen/o	strange, foreign	xen/o/phob/ia
xer/o	dry	xer/o/derma

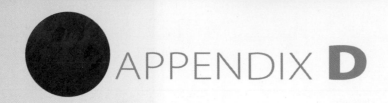

APPENDIX D

GLOSSARY OF PROPER NAMES OF DISEASES AND PROCEDURES

Addison's disease	deficiency in adrenocortical hormones caused by a progressive destruction of the adrenal glands	Cushing's syndrome	hypersecretion of the adrenal cortex causing excessive production of glucocorticoids; may be caused by a tumor
Bartholin cyst	cyst of the gland located in the cleft between the labia minora and the hymenal ring that secretes mucous lubricant	Down syndrome	extra chromosome (trisomy) of 21 or 22, variety of signs and symptoms including retardation, sloping forehead, flat nose or absent bridge, and generally dwarfed physique
Bell's palsy	idiopathic facial palsy of CN VII resulting in asymmetry of the palpebral fissures, nasolabial folds, mouth, and facial expression on the affected side	Electra complex	girls' sexual attraction toward their fathers and rivalry with their mothers
Biot's respirations	irregular respiratory pattern caused by damage to the medulla	Fallopian tubes	uterine tubes
Bouchard's node	bony enlargement of the proximal interphalangeal joint of the finger	Giardia	genus of protozoan flagellate causing dysentery
Braxton Hicks contractions	uterine contractions that are irregular and painless; also known as false labor	Glasgow Coma Scale	international scale used in grading neurologic response
Brushfield's spots	small, white flecks located around the perimeter of the iris and associated with Down syndrome	Graafian follicle	mature vesicular follicle of the ovary, matures ovum and secretes estrogen and progesterone
Cesarean section	delivery of the fetus by abdominal surgery (hysterotomy)	Graves' disease	disease characterized by hyperthyroidism, exophthalmic goiter, and thyromegaly, and dermopathy
Chadwick's sign	blue soft cervix occurring normally during pregnancy	Guillain-Barre syndrome	autoimmune inflammation causing destruction to the myelin sheath
Chandelier's sign	cervix motion tenderness on palpation	Harlequin color change	one half of the newborn's body is red or ruddy and the other half appears pale
Cheyne-Stokes respirations	crescendo/decrescendo respiratory pattern interspersed between periods of apnea	Heberden's node	enlargement of the distal interphalangeal joint of the finger
Cooley's anemia	thalasemia major	HELLP syndrome	pregnancy-induced hypertension, hemolysis, elevated liver enzymes, and low platelets
Coombs' test	postnatal blood test of cord blood for antibodies against fetal blood type (Rh neg mother, Rh pos fetus)	Hirsutism	excessive body hair
		Hodgkin's disease	cancerous lymphoreticular tumor
Cullen's sign	bluish color encircling the umbilicus and indicative of blood in the peritoneal cavity	Homans' sign	pain in the calf when the foot is dorsiflexed

Horner's syndrome	paralysis of the cervical sympathetic nerve causing contracted pupil and blepharoptosis
Korotkoff's sounds	sounds generated when the flow of blood through an artery is altered by the inflation of a blood pressure cuff around the extremity
Korsakoff's syndrome	polyneuritic psychosis caused by chronic alcoholism
Kussmaul's respirations	respirations characterized by extreme increased rate and depth, as in diabetic ketoacidosis
Lou Gehrig's disease	amyotrophic lateral sclerosis
Mantoux test	test for tuberculosis
McBurney's point	anatomic location that is approximately at the normal location of the appendix in the RLQ; point of increased tenderness in appendicitis
Mongolian spots	various irregularly sized areas of deep bluish pigmentation on the upper back, shoulders, buttocks, and lumbosacral area of newborns of African, Latino, and Asian descent
Mongolism	obsolete term for Down syndrome
Montgomery's tubercles	sebaceous and milk glands present on the areola that produce secretions during breastfeeding
Murphy's sign	abnormal finding elicited during abdominal palpation in the RUQ and revealing gallbladder inflammation, patient will abruptly stop inspiration and complain of a sharp pain
Nabothian cysts	small, round, yellow lesions on the cervical surface
Non-Hodgkin's lymphoma	lymphoma that arises directly from the thymus gland
Oedipus complex	boys' sexual attraction to their mothers and feelings of rivalry toward their fathers

Paget's disease	1. malignant neoplasm of the mammary ducts 2. osteitis deformans
Papanicolaou test	Pap smear, tissue slide examination to detect cervical cancer
Parkinson's disease	chronic degenerative nerve disease characterized by palsy, muscle stiffness and weakness, tremor, and fatigue and malaise
Persian Gulf syndrome	variety of symptoms experienced by veterans of the Persian Gulf War including respiratory, gastrointestinal, joint, and muscle discomforts, fatigue, and memory loss
Rosving's sign	technique to elicit referred pain indicative of peritoneal inflammation
Skene's glands	paraurethral glands
Snellen chart	chart used for testing distance vision using standardized numbers and letters of various sizes
Stensen's ducts	openings from the parotids glands
Tay-Sachs disease	autosomal recessive trait inherited causing lack of hexosaminase A; disease is characterized by mental and physical retardation, blindness, convulsions, cephalomegaly, and death by age 4
Tourette's syndrome	symptoms include lack of muscle coordination, spasms, tics, grunts, barks, involuntary swearing, and coprolalia
Weber's test	tuning fork used to measure hearing loss and determine if it is conductive or sensoneural
Wharton's ducts	openings to the submaxillary glands

Reference: Estes, *Health Assessment & Physical Examination*. Delmar 1997, and *Tabor's Cyclopedic Medical Dictionary*, 18th Ed. F. A. Davis 1993.

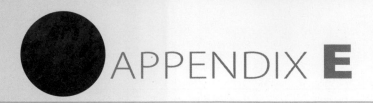

APPENDIX E

ANSWERS TO UNIT REVIEW ACTIVITIES AND CASE STUDIES

UNIT 1

Circle and Correct

1. d   2. a   3. d   4. c   5. a   6. d   7. a   8. c   9. c   10. a   11. c   12. d   13. a   14. c   15. c   16. b

Select and Construct

1. acromegaly
2. microscope
3. anemic
4. radiographer
5. acrodermatitis
6. hydrophobia
7. thermometer
8. microsurgery
9. gastroduodenoscopy
10. cytometer

Plural/Singular Forms

1. bursae
2. cocci
3. carcinomata
4. protozoa
5. crises
6. appendices
7. ova
8. phalanges

Adjective Forms

1. cyanotic
2. anemic
3. duodenal
4. mucous
5. arthritic
6. injectable
7. emetic
8. condylar

Matching

1. d   2. a   3. f   4. b   5. e   6. c   7. g

UNIT 2

Circle and Correct

1. b   2. d   3. b   4. c   5. c   6. d   7. b   8. a   9. b   10. c   11. a   12. d   13. d   14. c   15. b

Select and Construct

1. gastrectomy
2. gastroduodenostomy
3. cyanoderma
4. dermopathy (dermatopathy)
5. erythrocyte
6. melanoblast
7. thrombocytopenia
8. gastromegaly (megalogastria)
9. megalomania
10. electrocardiograph
11. duodenotomy
12. cardiac
13. echography (sonography)
14. echocardiogram
15. radiographer
16. leukocytosis
17. acromegaly
18. tomogram
19. xanthosis, xanthoderma
20. cytology

Abbreviation Matching

1. l   2. k   3. d   4. b   5. h   6. g   7. m   8. n   9. i   10. c

Abbreviation Fill-in

11. CBC   12. RBC   13. MRI   14. RT(R), radiologic   15. EKG   16. CCU, ER, ED   17. ECHO   18. ALL

Case Study

1. acute
2. cardiac
3. echocardiogram
4. telemetry
5. CBC
6. cardiologist
7. CCU
8. angiography
9. Troponins
10. hypertension

ANSWERS

UNIT 3

Circle and Correct

1. a   2. c   3. b   4. a   5. c   6. c   7. b   8. b   9. d   10. b   11. c   12. a   13. c   14. b   15. d   16. d

Select and Construct

1. encephalocele
2. electroencephalograph
3. cranioplasty
4. cerebrospinal
5. adenocarcinoma
6. mucoid
7. lipoma
8. craniomalacia
9. cerebrotomy
10. meningitis
11. oncologist
12. sarcoma
13. lymphadenoma, lymphoma
14. hypertrophy
15. hypotension
16. histologist
17. neoplasms
18. antineoplastic
19. histoblast
20. neonatal

Tumor Terminology Matching

1. j   2. g   3. h   4. c   5. d   6. b   7. e   8. i   9. a   10. f

Image Labeling

6—myel/o
4—crani/o
5—mening/o

2,3—cerebr/o
2,3—encepha/o
1 cephal/o

Abbreviation Matching

1. d   2. l   3. g   4. c   5. n   6. k   7. h   8. i   9. m   10. b

Abbreviation Fill-in

11. MLT   12. BP, mmHg, HCVD   13. TIA, CVA   14. BCC

UNIT 4

Circle and Correct

1. c   2. d   3. a   4. b   5. c   6. a   7. d   8. b   9. c   10. d   11. d   12. b   13. c   14. a   15. d

Select and Construct

1. osteomalacia
2. abduction
3. hydrocyst
4. hydrocephalic
5. suprapubic
6. intercostal
7. abdominocentesis
8. arthroscopy
9. aberrant
10. orthodontist
11. tendinitis (tendonitis)
12. pelvimeter
13. cephalopelvic
14. orthopedist
15. osteosarcoma
16. hypertrophy
17. dysplasia
18. chondrodysplasia
19. amniocentesis
20. thoracic, supralumbar

Image Labeling 1

4	pelv/i/o	pelvis
1	crani/o	cranium, skull
2	thorac/o	chest, thoracic cavity, thorax
3	abdomin/o	abdomen, abdominal cavity
5	lumb/o	lumbar spine
6	oste/o	bone
7	arthr/o	joint

ANSWERS

Image Labeling 2

1	tendin/o	tendon
4	chondr/o	cartilage
2	my/o	muscle
5	arthr/o	joint
7	oste/o	bone
3		fascia
6		ligament

Image Labeling 3

1. right and left hypochondriac regions
2. epigastric region
3. right and left lumbar regions
4. umbilical region
5. right and left iliac (inguinal) region
6. hypogastric (pubic) region

Abbreviation Matching

1. d   2. n   3. h   4. p   5. r   6. b   7. m   8. k   9. o   10. c

Abbreviation Fill-in

11. DTs   12. RUQ   13. OMT   14. DDS   15. ORTHO (ORTH)

Case Study

1. inflammation
2. arthroscope
3. mediolateral
4. meniscectomy
5. chondromalacia
6. arthritis
7. arthroscopic
8. patella
9. orthopedic
10. medial
11. pyorrhea
12. incision
13. arthrotomy
14. arthroplasty

UNIT 5

Circle and Correct

1. b   2. a   3. d   4. b   5. b   6. a   7. d   8. c   9. d   10. a   11. b   12. d   13. b   14. a   15. c   16. c   17. c   18. a   19. d   20. b   21. b   22. a

Select and Construct

1. bradycardia
2. tachyphagia
3. staphylitis (uvulitis)
4. cholelithiasis
5. otodynia (otalgia)
6. audiometry
7. dyspepsia
8. pyogenic
9. rhinorrhea
10. tympanogram
11. tympanites
12. cholecystogram
13. apnea
14. diathermy
15. polydipsia
16. synergy (synergistic)
17. microcephalus
18. macrocyte
19. prodromal
20. hypothermia

Mix and Match

1. f   2. d   3. a   4. c   5. b   6. e   7. g   8. h

Abbreviation Matching

1. r   2. l   3. f   4. a   5. q   6. p   7. d   8. s   9. n   10. o   11. i   12. m

Case Study

1. ductal
2. edematous
3. gallbladder
4. cholelith
5. cholangiogram
6. cm
7. epigastric
8. RUQ
9. cholecystectomy
10. ultrasound
11. T 99.6°F

UNIT 6

Circle and Correct

1. b   2. c   3. d   4. b   5. a   6. d   7. b   8. b   9. c   10. a   11. c   12. a   13. b   14. c   15. c   16. d   17. b   18. d

ANSWERS

Select and Construct

1. pyelonephritis
2. ureterorrhaphy
3. cystoscopy
4. nephroptosis
5. renogram, renograph
6. cystopexy
7. urethrorrhagia
8. nephrolysis
9. cystostomy
10. endometritis
11. hysteroptosis (metroptosis)
12. cryptorchidism
13. prostatectomy
14. gynecologist
15. oogenesis
16. balanorrhea
17. colpalgia (colpodynia)
18. hysteroscope
19. urologist
20. hysterosalpingogram
21. orchidopexy (orchiopexy)
22. colposcopy
23. endocervical

Image Labeling

Male Reproductive System

6—rect/o, rectum
3—cyst/o, urinary bladder
10—urethr/o, urethra
1—balan/o, glans penis
7—prostat/o, prostate gland
4—vas/o, vas deferens (ductus deferens)
8—orchid/o, testis
2—pen/o, penis
5—ureter/o, ureter
9—scrot/o, scrotum

Female Reproductive System

11—colp/o, vagina
5—hyster/o, uterus
7—oophor/o, ovary
13—metr/o, uterine tissue
6—salping/o, uterine tubes, fallopian tubes
10—cervic/o, cervix
9—rect/o, rectum
3—clitor/o, clitoris
1—labi/o, labium
2—urethr/o, urethra
14—an/o, anus
8—ureter/o, ureter
12—cystovagin/o, cystovaginal wall
4—cyst/o, urinary bladder

Abbreviation Matching

1. q   2. s   3. g   4. h   5. i   6. m   7. o   8. p   9. n   10. b   11. e   12. l   13. a   14. d

Abbreviation Fill-in

15. MD   16. PSA   17. KUB   18. AIH   19. ESRD   20. Pap (smear)

Case Study

1. mg qid
2. benign
3. pathology
4. hyperplasia
5. prostatitis
6. chronic
7. H&P
8. hydronephrosis
9. TUR
10. hematuria
11. afebrile
12. cystoclysis
13. catheter
14. postoperative
15. transurethral

UNIT 7

Circle and Correct

1. d   2. c   3. b   4. b   5. c   6. d   7. a   8. b   9. c   10. d   11. d   12. c

Select and Construct

1. stomatomycosis
2. sublingual (hypoglossal, subglossal)
3. cheiloplasty
4. gingivitis
5. enterorrhagia
6. esophagogastroduodenoscopy
7. enteroptosis
8. rectoclysis
9. proctoplegia
10. pancreatolith
11. splenomegaly
12. gastrectasia
13. sigmoidoscope
14. hepatitis
15. rectocele
16. esophagogastric (gastroesophageal)
17. cholangiopancreatography
18. colorectal

Image Labeling

12—hepat/o, liver
4—gastr/o, stomach
6—col/o, colon
3—esophag/o, esophagus
1—stomat/o, mouth
5—pancreat/o, pancreas
7—sigmoid/o, sigmoid colon
2—pharyng/o, pharynx
11—cholecyst/o, gallbladder
8—rect/o, rectum
10—duoden/o, duodenum
9—appendic/o, appendix

ANSWERS

Abbreviation Matching

1. f 2. k 3. i 4. j 5. g 6. h 7. o 8. q 9. r 10. e 11. a

Suffix Matching

1. j 2. e 3. a 4. f 5. h 6. c

Case Study

1. anterior
2. vomiting
3. hemorrhage
4. nasogastric
5. endoscope
6. mucosal
7. aspirate
8. isotonic
9. ulcer
10. gastrointestinal
11. melenic
12. hypotensive
13. duodenal
14. thrombi
15. EGD

UNIT 8

Circle and Correct

1. c 2. a 3. d 4. a 5. c 6. a 7. b 8. c 9. d 10. d 11. c 12. c 13. a 14. a

Select and Construct

1. arteriosclerosis
2. phlebectasia
3. enterorrhexis
4. angiogram (angiograph)
5. esthesiometer
6. anesthesiologist
7. analgesic
8. parahepatitis
9. neurosis, psychoneurosis
10. myograph, myometer
11. dyskinesia, kinesialgia
12. pharmacist
13. psychotropic
14. paraplegia
15. fibromyoma
16. atherosclerosis
17. angioplasty
18. thrombosis
19. myospasm
20. fibroneuroma
21. thrombophlebitis
22. neurologist
23. cardiomyopathy
24. myocardial

Abbreviation Matching

1. k 2. t 3. l 4. j 5. g 6. c 7. p 8. n 9. d 10. r

Abbreviation Fill-in

11. HDL 12. MI 13. PT 14. CABG 15. IV 16. hct 17. MD 18. TENS 19. PND 20. OCD

Case Study

1. hypothyroidism
2. incontinence
3. psychiatric
4. obsessive compulsive disorder
5. UTI
6. EST
7. diarrhea
8. BP, T, R
9. Ua with C+S
10. paranoia

UNIT 9

Circle and Correct

1. b 2. d 3. b 4. c 5. d 6. c 7. a 8. c 9. a 10. c 11. b 12. c 13. a 14. d 15. c 16. b

Select and Construct

1. gastroscopy
2. retroperitoneal
3. dialysis, hemodialysis
4. endoderm
5. ectopic
6. posteroanterior
7. procephalic
8. diagnosis
9. omphalitis
10. lateroanterior, anterolateral, ventrolateral, lateroventral
11. cephalocaudal
12. apepsia
13. pseudocyesis, pseudopregnancy
14. euphoria
15. euthanasia
16. dysmenorrhea
17. visceropleura, visceral pleura
18. hemostasis
19. aerobic
20. chromophilic
21. peritoneum, visceroperitoneum
22. omphalorrhea
23. syphilophobia
24. mediolateral
25. ectogenous

Diagram Labeling

1. cephalic (cephalad)
2. superior (hyper, super, supra)
3. inferior (hypo, sub, infra)
4. anterior, ventral (pre, pro, ante)
5. circum
6. posterior, dorsal (retro, post)
7. abduct (lateral)
8. adduct (medial)
9. distal
10. proximal
11. sagittal

ANSWERS

Abbreviation Matching

1. h   2. l   3. k   4. m   5. e   6. n   7. p   8. f   9. c   10. d

Abbreviation Fill-in

11. LOA   12. STD   13. RPR (VDRL)   14. LAT   15. LMP   16. PA   17. OT   18. TB

Case Study

1. catheterization
2. apnea
3. IDDM DM Type 1
4. URI
5. narcolepsy
6. CPAP
7. hypoventilation
8. syndrome
9. symptoms
10. U
11. hypoglycemic
12. analgesic
13. cephalalgia
14. dyspnea
15. ventilatory

UNIT 10

Prefix and Word

1. ab, abduct
2. de, descending
3. ex, excise
4. iso, isotonic
5. aniso, anisocytosis
6. dia, diathermy
7. per, percussion
8. peri, pericardium
9. circum, circumduction
10. sub, sublingual, subglossal (hypo, hypoglossal)

Circle and Correct

1. b   2. d   3. a   4. b   5. d   6. c   7. b   8. b   9. c   10. d

Count with Prefixes

1. nulli, nulligravida
2. primi, primipara
3. mono, monocyte
4. bi, bifurcate, birfurcation
5. tri, trilateral
6. quad, quadriplegia
7. quint, quintuplets
8. sexti, sextigravida
9. septi, septipara
10. octo, octogenarian
11. noni, nonigravida
12. deca, decaliter
13. centi, centimeter
14. kilo, kilocalorie
15. multi, multiglandular

Select and Construct Part I

1. laparoscope
2. pyrosis
3. hyperhidrosis (hidrosis, hidrorrhea)
4. glycolysis
5. pericystitis
6. hypoglycemia
7. glucolipid (glycolipid)
8. decagram
9. millimeter
10. retromammary

Select and Construct Part II

1. excretion
2. abort
3. narcolepsy
4. mastocarcinoma
5. abrade
6. perihepatitis
7. narcotic
8. decalcification
9. isotonic
10. circumcision
11. ablation
12. percussion
13. anisocytosis
14. ablactation
15. dehydration
16. perfusion
17. circumduction
18. exhale, expiration
19. abrasion, abrade
20. pericardium

Matching

1. c   2. h   3. g   4. d   5. a   6. b   7. f   8. e

Abbreviation Matching Part I

1. d   2. g   3. f   4. b   5. a   6. h   7. o   8. t   9. q   10. r   11. p   12. s   13. j

Abbreviations—Weights and Measures

1. kg
2. mg
3. cc
4. dL
5. mm
6. mcg, μg

Abbreviation Matching Part II

1. g   2. h   3. m   4. i   5. f   6. j   7. c   8. b

ANSWERS

Abbreviation Fill-in

9. q4h   10. D/W   11. NS   12. qid   13. †

Case Study

1. subcuticular
2. anesthesia
3. multifocal
4. carcinoma in situ
5. dissected
6. axillary
7. hemostasis
8. mastectomy
9. mammogram
10. sterile
11. retraction
12. microcalcifications
13. biopsy

UNIT 11

Circle and Correct

1. c   2. d   3. a   4. d   5. a   6. b   7. c   8. a   9. d   10. b

Select and Construct

1. antibiotic (antiseptic)
2. contraceptive
3. homosexual
4. anisocytosis
5. sympodia
6. substernal (infrasternal)
7. mammography
8. ultrasonographer (sonographer)
9. epidural
10. extracystic
11. trilateral
12. metastasis

Prefix and Word

1. homo, homosexual
2. hetero, heterogeneous (heterogenous)
3. sym, sympodia
4. super, superficial
5. supra, suprarenal
6. a/an, amenorrhea
7. a/an, anesthesia
8. epi, epigastric
9. extra, extracellular
10. infra, infrasternal (substernal)
11. meta, metacarpals
12. ultra, ultrasound (ultrasonic)
13. bi, bilateral
14. anti, antiarthritic
15. contra, contraindicated
16. trans, transurethral

Abbreviation Matching

1. g   2. f   3. i   4. h   5. a   6. j   7. l   8. c

Abbreviation Fill-in

9. AAMA   10. s̄   11. inf   12. XM   13. subcu, subq, s.c.   14. ftm   15. TURP

Case Study

1. subdural
2. anesthesiologist
3. incision
4. hemostasis
5. subcutaneous
6. pericranium
7. retracted
8. perforator
9. dura mater
10. transferred
11. hemiparesis
12. temporoparietal

UNIT 12

Circle and Correct

1. c   2. d   3. b   4. d   5. c   6. d   7. c   8. a

Prefix and Word

1. ex, exhale
2. in, incise
3. in, incompetent
4. mal, malnutrition
5. tri, trigeminal
6. bi, bifocal
7. uni, unilateral
8. semi, semiconscious
9. hemi, hemiplegia
10. con, congenital
11. dis, disinfectant
12. post, postmastectomy
13. pre, presurgical
14. pre, prefrontal
15. retro, retroesophageal post, postesophageal
16. ante, antefebrile
17. intra, intradermal
18. inter, intercellular
19. sub, subcutaneous

Select and Construct

1. antenatal (prenatal)
2. postpartum
3. hemicardia
4. semicomatose
5. unicellular
6. uninuclear
7. precancerous
8. inject
9. incontinent
10. insane
11. malformation
12. malaria
13. postcoital
14. antefebrile, prefebrile
15. postcibal

ANSWERS

Abbreviation Matching

1. g   2. f   3. i   4. c   5. h   6. k   7. l   8. b

Abbreviation Fill-in

9. exc   10. AIH   11. ID   12. iii   13. am   14. inf   15. prn

Case Study

1. bilateral
2. endometriomata
3. incised
4. transversely
5. visceroperitoneum
6. preoperative
7. dissected
8. posterior
9. intracystic
10. appendectomy
11. salpingo-oophorectomy
12. adhesions
13. postoperative
14. dissection

UNIT 13

Circle and Correct

1. c   2. c   3. a   4. d   5. a   6. b   7. c   8. a   9. d   10. a   11. d   12. d

Image Labeling

1. rhin/o
2. laryng/o
3. trache/o
4. pulmon/o
5. phren/o, diaphragm/o
6. alveol/o
7. bronch/o
8. epiglott/o
9. pharyng/o

Select and Construct

1. pulmonary (pulmonic)
2. pneumonomelanosis
3. dermatomycosis (mycodermatitis)
4. embolus
5. mycology
6. nasomental
7. pharyngoscope
8. pleurocentesis
9. dextropedal
10. sinistromanual
11. pediatrician
12. histolysis
13. bronchitis
14. laryngalgia (laryngodynia)
15. phrenoplegia
16. bronchiectasis (bronchodilation)
17. psychiatrist
18. tracheostomy
19. chiropractor

Abbreviation Matching

1. f   2. n   3. a   4. l   5. m   6. k   7. h   8. j   9. c   10. p

Abbreviation Fill-in

11. PE   12. PFT   13. CO_2 14. R   15. COPD   16. RHIA

Matching

1. e   2. d   3. a   4. f   5. c   6. b   7. g

Case Study

1. bronchitis
2. pulse
3. tachypnea
4. intravenous
5. oximetry
6. O_2
7. %
8. respiratory
9. asthmaticus
10. viral
11. oxygen
12. IV
13. symptoms
14. syndrome

UNIT 14

Circle and Correct

1. c   2. d   3. b   4. a   5. d   6. c   7. b   8. c   9. d   10. b   11. c   12. a

Select and Construct

1. sternalgia (sternodynia)
2. brachiocephalic
3. mycostasis (fungistasis)
4. ischiopubic
5. condylectomy
6. rachischisis
7. palatoschisis (uranoschisis)
8. xiphocostal
9. metacarpals
10. schizophasia
11. somnabulism (noctambulism)
12. nyctalopia
13. nycturia (nocturia)
14. ankylodactylia
15. iliac
16. pubic
17. femoral
18. patellar

ANSWERS

19. fibular
20. tarsals
21. metatarsals
22. calcaneus, calcaneum
23. cost/o, costal
24. chondral

Find the Form

1. cranio, cranial
2. cervico, cervical
3. cleido, clavicular
4. scapulo, scapular
5. acromio, acromial
6. humero, humeral
7. sterno, sternal
8. xipho, xiphoid
9. ulno, ulnar
10. radio, radial
11. carpo, carpal
12. metacarpo, metacarpal
13. phalango, phalangeal
14. ischio, ischial
15. ilio, iliac
16. pubo, pubic
17. femoro, femoral
18. patello, patellar
19. tibio, tibial
20. fibulo, fibular
21. tarso, tarsal
22. metatarso, metatarsal
23. calcaneo, calcaneal
24. costo, costal
25. chondro, chondral

Image Labeling

15—xiph/o, xiphoid
20—condyl/o, condyle
5—femor/o, femur
12—cleid/o, clavicle
6—phalang/o, phalanx
7—carp/o, carpus
9—radi/o, radius
10—humer/o, humerus
16—cost/o, rib
11—scapul/o, scapula
8—uln/o, ulna
1—metatars/o, metatarsal
2—tibi/o, tibia
3—fibul/o, fibula
17—vertebr/o, vertebra
14—stern/o, sternum
13—crani/o, cranium
18—ili/o, ilium
19—ischi/o, ischium
4—patell/o, patella

Abbreviation Matching

1. l   2. f   3. e   4. g   5. k   6. h   7. c   8. m

Abbreviation Fill-in

9. C_3 10. FxBB   11. OT(R), OTR   12. AOTA   13. R, rt   14. y/o (yr)   15. ORIF

Case Study

1. inspection
2. manually
3. lateral
4. incision
5. sterile
6. subcutaneous
7. anatomic
8. internal
9. fracture
10. pneumatic
11. anesthetized
12. reduction
13. fixation
14. epicondyle
15. humerus
16. M
17. y/o
18. right
19. par

UNIT 15

Circle and Correct

1. d   2. c   3. b   4. a   5. d   6. b   7. a   8. d   9. a   10. d   11. b   12. b   13. c   14. a

Select and Construct

1. optometry
2. cycloplegia
3. onychomalacia
4. iritis
5. dacryorrhea
6. phacoemulsification
7. adrenalin (epinephrine)
8. hyperopia
9. retinoscope
10. traumatology
11. ophthalmoplasty
12. corectasis (corectasia)
13. blepharoptosis
14. keratotomy
15. thyromegaly
16. anisocoria
17. esotropia
18. presbyopia
19. onychocryptosis
20. retinoplasty

Image Labeling

1—corne/o, kerat/o cornea
5—retin/o, retina
8—lacrim/o, lacrimal
4—cycl/o, ciliary body
9—core/o, pupil
3—phac/o, lens
10—irid/o, iris
7—blephar/o, eyelid
2—conjunctiv/o, conjunction
6—scler/o, sclera

ANSWERS

Abbreviation Matching

1. n   2. r   3. b   4. f   5. p   6. a   7. m   8. i, g   9. d   10. l

Abbreviation Fill-in

11. AOA   12. EMT   13. FSH   14. T3, T4   15. OD   16. L&A

Case Study

1. phacoemulsification
2. abrasion
3. capsulorrhexis
4. intraocular
5. keratome
6. myopia
7. cataract
8. epinucleus
9. corneal
10. paracentesis
11. OD

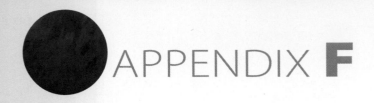

PUZZLE SOLUTIONS

UNIT 1

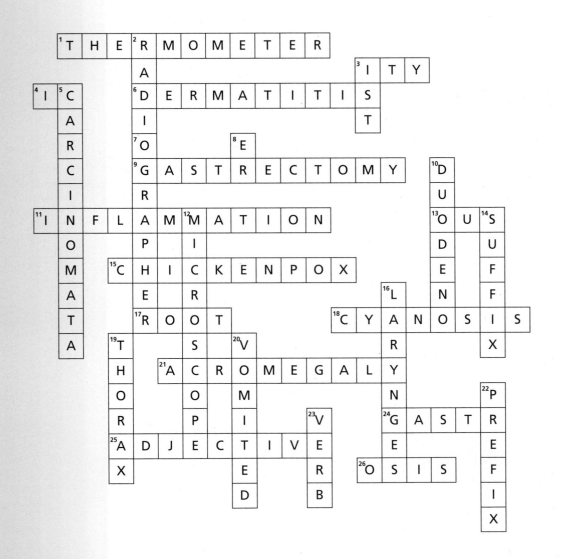

PUZZLE SOLUTIONS

UNIT 2

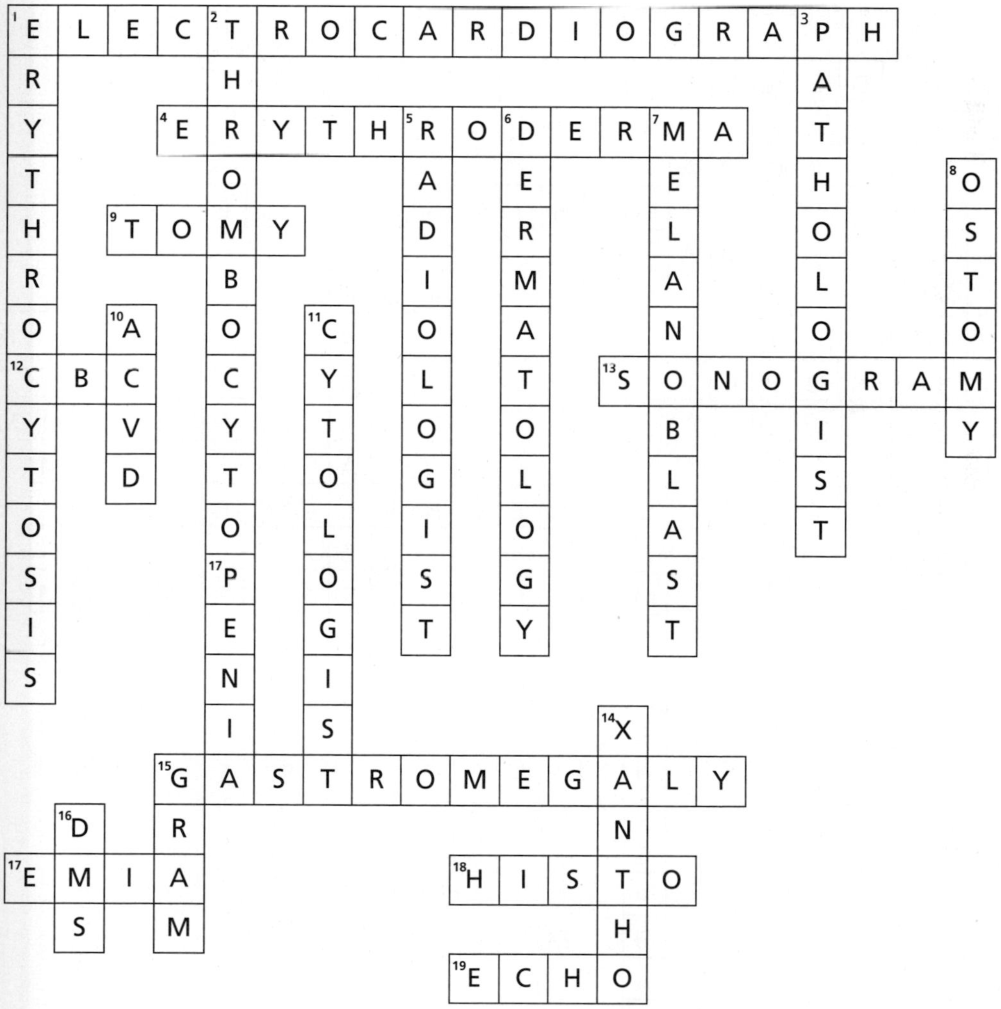
1 ELECTROCARDIOGRAPH
1 ERYTHROCYTOSIS
2 THROMBOCYTOPENIA
3 PATHOLOGIST
4 ERYTHRODERMA
5 RADIOLOGIST
6 DERMATOLOGY
7 MELANOBLAST
8 OSTOMY
9 TOMY
10 ACVD
11 CYTOLOGIST
12 CBC
13 SONOGRAM
14 XANTHO
15 GASTROMEGALY
15 GRAM
16 DMS
17 EMIA
18 HISTO
19 ECHO

PUZZLE SOLUTIONS

UNIT 3

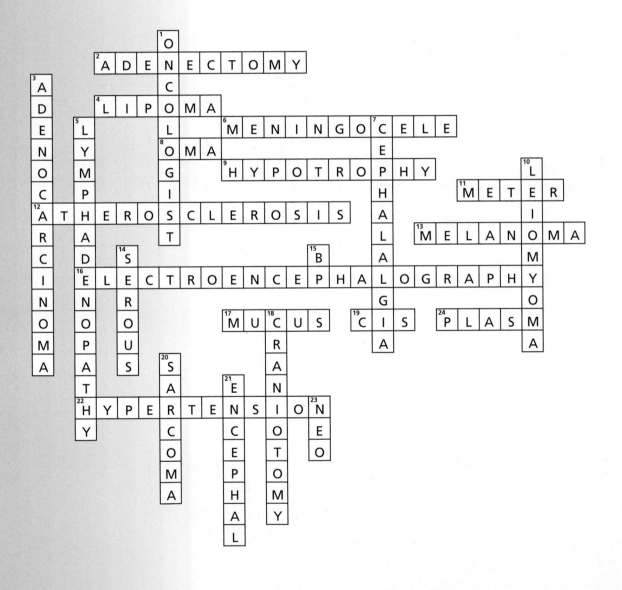

PUZZLE SOLUTIONS

UNIT 4

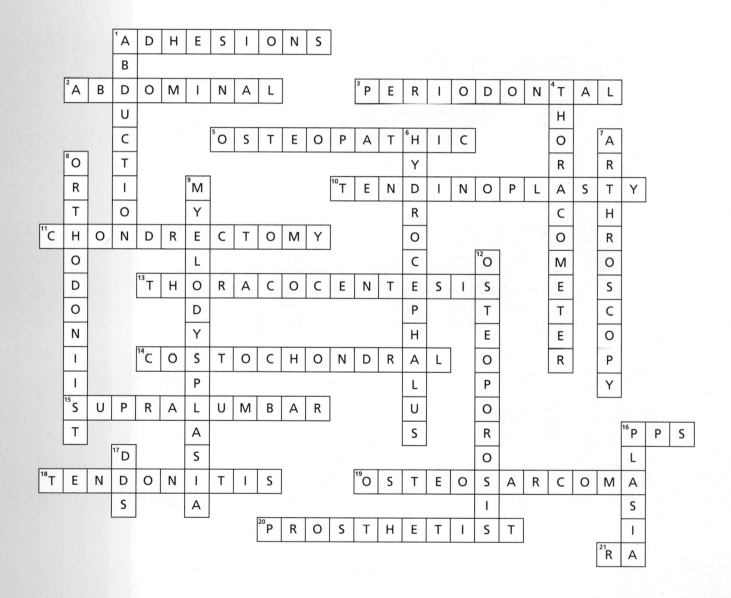

PUZZLE SOLUTIONS

UNIT 5

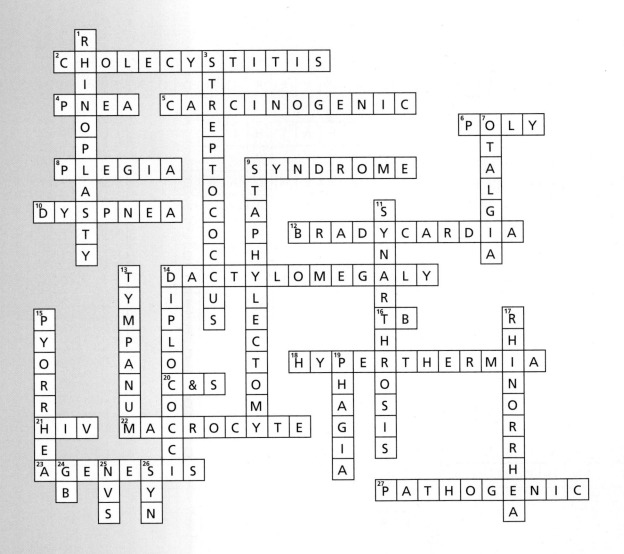

PUZZLE SOLUTIONS

UNIT 6

Across:
1. CYSTORRHAPHY
3. PENILE
5. NEPHROPYELITIS
8. ENDOMETRIOSIS
12. BALANORRHEA
13. OLIGURIA
21. ORCHIOPEXY
23. URETEROLITH
25. TESTICULAR

Down:
2. PROSTATECTOMY
4. TUP
6. HYSTPHAGA
7. NEPHROPTOSIS
9. ORCHIDOPLASTY
10. URETINE
11. RENAL
14. METROPA
15. MENORR
16. HYSTEY
17. OOPRILTISA
18. POLYOTIA
19. COLPALGIA
20. HMATURIA
22. CRYP
24. P

PUZZLE SOLUTIONS

UNIT 7

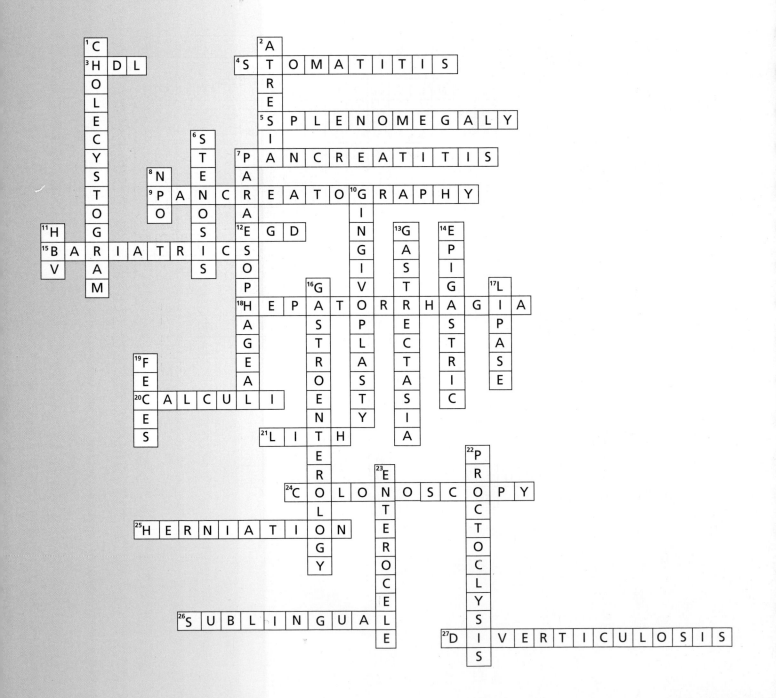

PUZZLE SOLUTIONS

UNIT 8

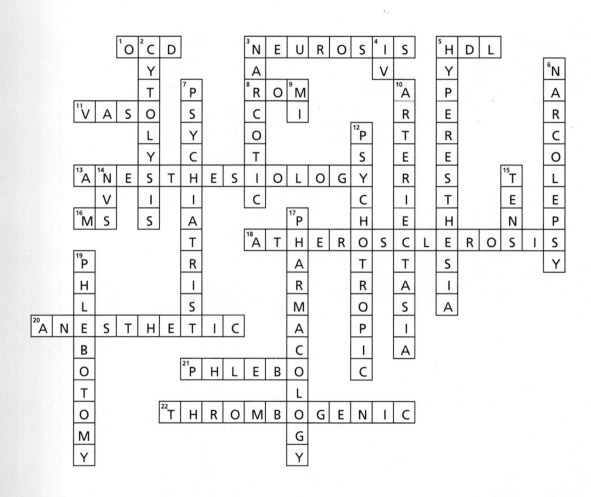

PUZZLE SOLUTIONS

UNIT 9

Across and down answers shown in grid:

- 1 Down: MENORRHAGIA
- 2 Across: ACHROMOPHILIC
- 2 Down: ANTEROLATERA
- 3 Down: CHINDRYDYSPL
- 4 Across: PARAPLEGIA
- 5 Down: PRERIST... (PRERI...)
- 6 Down: EUTHANASIA
- 7 Across: RETROPERITONITIS
- 8 Across: RETROVERSION
- 9 Across: DORSOCEPHALAD
- 10 Down: AMENORRHEA
- 11 Across: ANTEFLEXION
- 12 Down: LI...
- 13 Down: BIOELEC (BIOE...)
- 14 Across: ECTOGENOUS
- 15 Down: MEDIAL
- 16 Across: ANAEROBIC
- 17 Across: DORSAL
- 18 Across: PARACYSTITIS
- 19 Down: CELI... / CEPHAL
- 20 Down: INFERIOR
- 21 Down: ECT...
- 22 Down: LATERAL
- 23 Down: DY...
- 24 Across: HYPOPLASIA
- 25 Down: DISTAL
- 26 Across: DIALYSIS
- 27 Across: ENDOSCOPY
- 28 Down: DIARRRH (DIARRH...)
- 29 Down: DIAGNOSIS
- 30 Across: ECTOPIC
- 31 Across: DYSPNEA
- 32 Down: VENTRAL
- 33 Across: EUGENICS
- 34 Down: COROAL (CO...ROAL)
- 35 Across: MENOPAUSE
- 36 Across: MENSES

PUZZLE SOLUTIONS

UNIT 10a

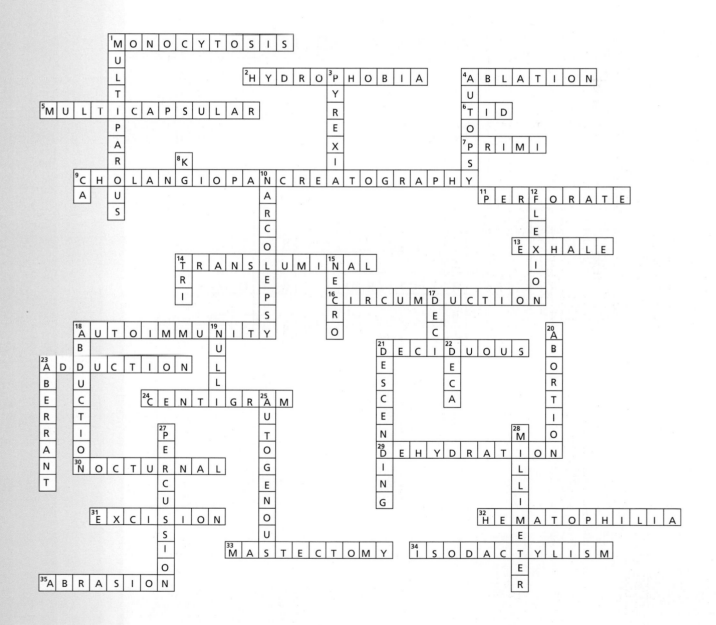

PUZZLE SOLUTIONS

UNIT 10b

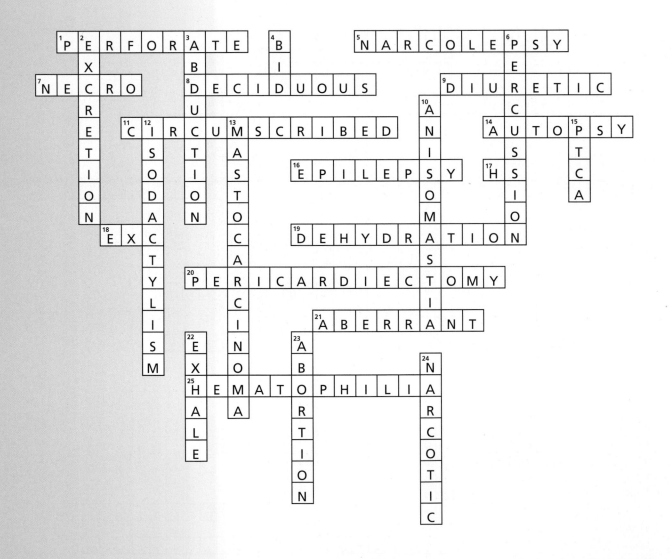

PUZZLE SOLUTIONS

UNIT 11

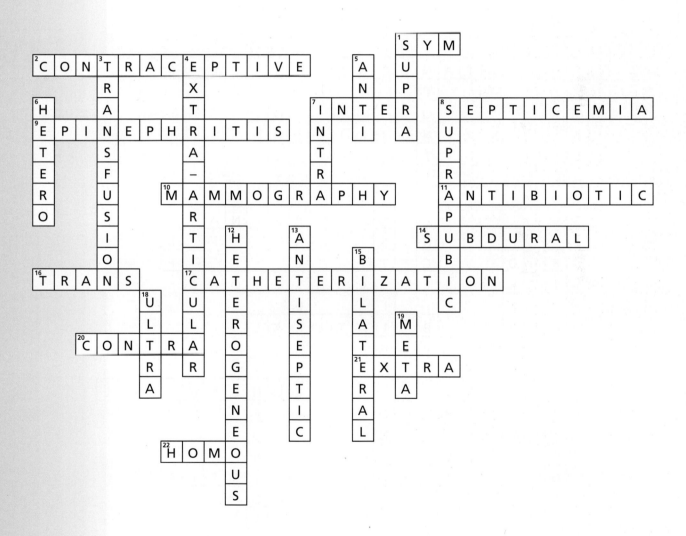

UNIT 12

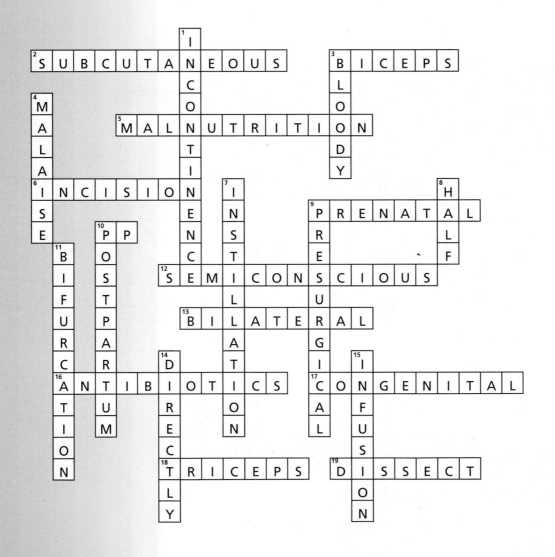

PUZZLE SOLUTIONS

UNIT 13

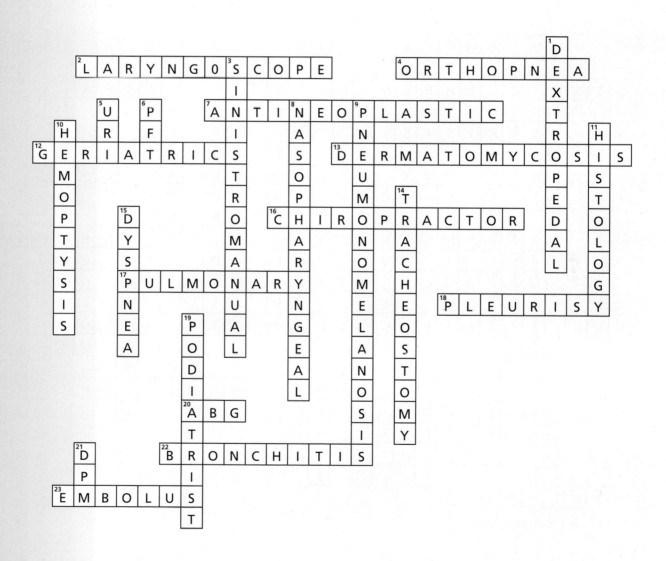

PUZZLE SOLUTIONS

UNIT 14

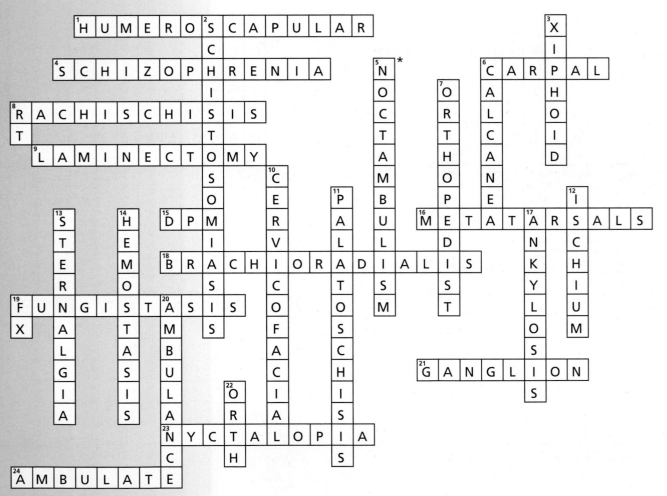

* 5. Down also somnambulism

PUZZLE SOLUTIONS

UNIT 15

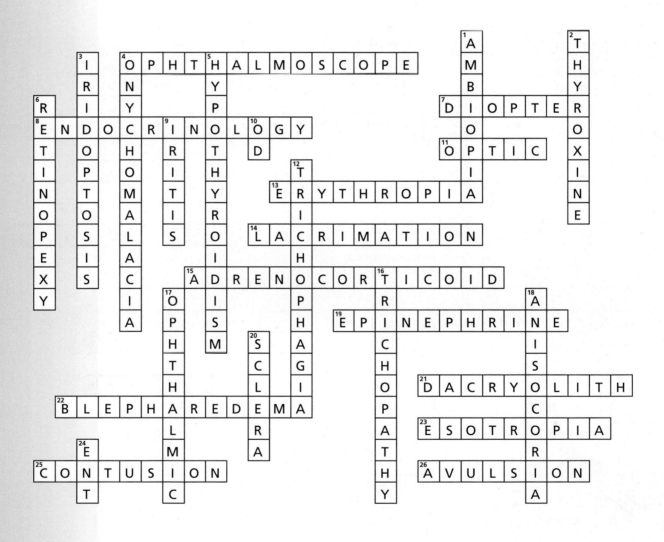

INDEX OF WORD PARTS LEARNED

UNIT 1
suffix
er
ist
ism
ity

UNIT 1
cyano
cyanosis
cyanotic

UNIT 1
acro
acrodermatitis
acromegaly

UNIT 1
verb
ed
ing

UNIT 1
dermatitis
dermatology

UNIT 1
adjective
anemic
mucous
duodenal

UNIT 1
cytometer
micrometer
thermometer

UNIT 1
microbe
microscope
microsurgery

UNIT 1
Singular nouns:
appendix
bacillus
bacterium
larynx
vertebra

UNIT 1
practitioner
radiographer

UNIT 1
adeno
lympho
lymphadenopathy

UNIT 1
compound word
chickenpox
microfilm
brainstem

UNIT 1
inflammation
contraction

UNIT 1
injection
injected
injectable

combining form for blue
condition of blueness (caused
    by low oxygen to tissues)
adjective for cyanosis

follows a word root to change
    its meaning or part of speech
suffix for one who
suffix for specialist
suffix for condition or theory
suffix for quality

inflammation of the skin
study of the skin—specialty

part of speech that shows
    action
verb suffix indicating past tense
verb suffix indicating present
    tense

combining form for extremities
inflammation of the skin on the
    extremities
enlargement of the extremities

small organism
instrument used to look at very
    small objects
delicate surgery performed
    using magnification

instrument that measures
    (counts) cells
instrument that measures small
    objects
instrument that measures
    temperature

part of speech that describes or
    modifies nouns
adjective form for anemia
adjective form for mucus
adjective form for duodenum

combining form for gland
combining form for lymph
    (fluid, ducts, system)
general term for disease of the
    lymphatic glands

one who practices (usually a
    professional)
one who makes images using
    x-rays

Plural nouns:
appendices
bacilli
bacteria
larynges
vertebrae

noun for inject, put in using a
    needle
past tense verb for inject
able to be injected (adjective
    form)

condition of redness, swelling,
    and heat
condition of shortening or
    tensing a body part such as a
    muscle

word made of two or more
    word roots
varicella virus infection
film process used that reduces
    size of documents for storage
posterior base of the brain
    (midbrain, medulla
    oblongata, pons)

UNIT 1
gastric
gastroduodenoscopy
gastroduodenostomy

UNIT 2
electro
electrocardiography
electrocardiograph

UNIT 2
jaundice
xanthemia

UNIT 1
-itis
-ectomy
-ostomy
-pathy

UNIT 2
erythema
erythremia
erythroderma

UNIT 2
inflammation
inflamed
inflammatory

UNIT 2
blastocyte
cytology
cytometry

UNIT 2
etiology
diagnosis

UNIT 2
mania
megalomania

UNIT 2
cardio
cardiologist
cardiomegaly

UNIT 2
gastralgia
gastromegaly
gastroduodenostomy

UNIT 2
melanocyte
melanoblast
melanoderma

UNIT 2
dermo, dermato
dermatome
dermatology

UNIT 2
histoblast
histology
histologist

UNIT 2
patho
pathology
pathologist

yellow color of the skin caused
    by high blood bilirubin
yellow color of the blood and
    skin due to high carotene
    levels (carotenemia)

combining form for electricity
process of making an image
    of heart function using
    electricity
instrument used to produce an
    electrocardiogram

pertaining to the stomach
    (adjective)
looking into the stomach with
    a scope
making a new surgical opening
    in the stomach

condition of redness, swelling,
    heat
past tense verb pertaining to
    inflammation
something that causes
    inflammation

condition of redness (skin)
condition of too many red
    blood cells (erythrocytosis)
condition of redness of the skin
    (erythema)

Suffixes for:
inflammation
excision (to cut out)
make a surgical opening that
    will remain open
general suffix for any disease

condition of madness
abnormally enlarged self-image
    to the point of madness

study of the origin of a disease
identification of a disease
    through signs and symptoms

immature cell
study of cells
measurement (counting) of
    cells

pigmented cell
immature melanocyte
dark pigmentation to the skin
    (patches)

stomach pain
enlargement of the stomach
making a surgical opening in
    the stomach

combining form for heart
physician heart specialist
enlargement of the heart

combining form for disease
study of disease (specialty)
physician specialist in disease

immature tissues
study of tissues
specialist in tissue studies

combining form for skin
instrument used to cut thin
    slices of skin
study of skin

UNIT 2
radio
radiogram
radiography

UNIT 3
athero
atheroma
atherosclerosis

UNIT 3
encephalo
encephalomalacia
encephalitis

UNIT 2
sono
sonographer
sonography

UNIT 3
carcino
carcinoma
carcinogenic

UNIT 3
hyper
hypertension
hypertrophy

UNIT 2
thrombo
thrombocytopenia
thrombocytosis

UNIT 3
cephalo
cephalalgia
cephalic

UNIT 3
hypo
hypotension
hypotrophy

UNIT 3
adeno
adenitis
adenoma
adenopathy

UNIT 3
cerebro
cerebral
cerebrospinal
cerebrovascular

UNIT 3
lipo
lipoid
lipoma

UNIT 3
neo
neoplasm
antineoplastic

UNIT 3
cranio
craniectomy
craniomalacia
craniotomy

UNIT 3
mal
malignant

combining form for brain (inside
    the head)
softening of the brain
inflammation of the brain

combining form for fatty or
    porridge-like fat
tumor composed of fat in the
    blood vessels
hardening for a blood vessel
    caused by fat

combining form for x-ray
image made using x-rays
process of producing a radiogram

prefix for above, abnormally
    high, increased
abnormally high blood pressure
overdevelopment, enlarged

combining form for cancer
    (epithelial origin)
cancerous tumor (epithelial
    origin)
pertaining to cancer development

sound waves
one who uses sound waves to
    create an image
process of producing a
    sonogram

prefix for below, abnormally low,
    decreased
abnormally low blood pressure
underdevelopment, loss of size
    (atrophy)

combining form for head
pain the head, headache
pertaining to the head

combining form for blood clot
condition of low number of
    thrombocytes
condition of high number of
    thrombocytes

combining form for fat (superficial fat)
resembling fat
tumor composed of fat
    tissue

combining form for cerebrum
    (brain)
adjective for cerebrum
pertaining to cerebrum (brain)
    and spine
pertaining to cerebrum (brain)
    and blood vessels

combining form for gland
inflammation of a gland
glandular tumor
any disease of a gland

prefix meaning bad
bad, worsening, leading to
    death

combining form for skull
excision (cut out) of the skull
softening of the skull
incision (cut) into the skull

combining form for new
abnormal new growth (tumor)
agent that fights tumor growth

UNIT 3
melanocyte
melanocarcinoma
melanoma

UNIT 4
ab
abduction
aberrant
abnormal

UNIT 4
costo
costochondral
intercostal

UNIT 3
meningo
meningitis
meningocele

UNIT 4
ad
addiction
adduction
adhesions

UNIT 4
cysto
cystocele
cystotomy
cystitis

UNIT 3
meta
metastasis
metastasize
metastatic

UNIT 4
arthro
arthritis
arthroplasty
arthroscope

UNIT 4
dento
dentalgia
dentist
dentoid

UNIT 3
onco
oncologist
oncology

UNIT 4
bursa
bursectomy
bursitis

UNIT 4
dys
dysplasia
chondrodysplasia

UNIT 4
abdomino
abdominocentesis
-centesis

UNIT 4
chondro
chondrodynia
chondrectomy

UNIT 4
hydro
hydrocele
hydrocephalus
(hydrencephalus)
hydrophobia

combining form for rib
pertaining to rib and rib
    cartilage
between the ribs

prefix for away from
movement away from the
    midline or body
wandering from the normal
    path
deviating from the expected

pigmented cell (containing
    melanin)
cancer originating from
    melanocytes
malignant melanocyte tumor

combining form for urinary
    bladder or a fluid-filled sac
herniation of the urinary
    bladder
incision into the urinary bladder
inflammation of the urinary
    bladder

prefix for toward
compulsive attraction to a
    substance or habit
movement toward the midline
    or body
tissues that stick together,
    normally apart

combining form for meninges
    (membrane)
inflammation of the meninges
herniation of the meninges

combining form for tooth or
    teeth
tooth pain
specialist in care of teeth
resembling a toothlike structure

combining form for joint
inflammation of a joint
surgical repair of a joint
instrument used to look into a
    joint

prefix for beyond
tumor or condition that
    spreads beyond its origin
action of becoming a
    metastasis (verb)
pertaining to metastases
    (adjective)

prefix for defective or painful
defective development
    (abnormal tissues)
defective development of
    cartilage

serous sac in a joint
excision of a bursa
inflammation of a bursa

combining form for tumors
    and cancer
physician specialist in
    treatment of cancer and
    tumors
study of cancer and tumors

combining form for water
herniation containing fluid or
    water
abnormal amount of fluid inside
    the head
fear of water (symptom of
    rabies)

combining form for cartilage
cartilage pain (chondralgia)
excision of cartilage

combining form for abdomen
surgical puncture for removal
    of fluid from the abdomen
suffix: surgical puncture of a
    cavity for fluid/cell removal

UNIT 4
tendino
tendinitis
tendinoplasty

UNIT 5
a- an-
amenorrhea
apepsia
aphasia
aphonia

UNIT 5
bacillus
bacilli
streptobacillus
diplobacillus

UNIT 4
myelo
myelocyte
myelodysplasia

UNIT 5
audio
audiogram
audiology
audiometry

UNIT 5
dactylo
dactylospasm
dactylomegaly

UNIT 4
ortho
orthodontist
orthopedist
orthotic

UNIT 5
brady
bradycardia
bradyphasia
bradypnea

UNIT 5
dyslexia
dysrhythmia
dysphagia

UNIT 4
osteo
osteoma
osteopenia
osteopathy

UNIT 5
chole
cholecystitis
cholecystogram
cholelithiasis

UNIT 5
hyperthermia
thermoesthesia
thermoplegia

UNIT 4
peri
pericardium
periosteum
periodontal

UNIT 5
coccus
diplococcus
staphylococcus
streptococcus

UNIT 5
macro
macroblast
macrocephalus

rod-shaped bacterium (singular)
rod-shaped bacteria (plural)
bacillus growing in twisted
    chains
bacillus growing in pairs

prefix for not, absence or lack of
absence of menstruation
unable to digest food
unable to speak
no voice

combining form for tendon
inflammation of a tendon
surgical repair of a tendon

---

combining form for digit
    (fingers, toes)
contracture or spasm of a digit
enlarged fingers or toes

combining form for hearing
image of hearing function
study of hearing (specialty)
measurement of hearing function

combining form for spinal cord
    or bone marrow
bone marrow cell that produces
    blood cells
defective development of the
    spinal cord

---

condition causing difficulty with
    reading
irregular rhythm (heart)
difficulty swallowing (eating)

prefix for abnormally slow
slow heart rate
slow speech
slow breathing

combining form for straighten
dental specialist that straightens
    teeth
physician bone and joint
    specialist and surgeon
device used to straighten and
    support joints

---

abnormally high body
    temperature (fever)
oversensitivity to feeling heat
paralysis caused by high
    temperature

word root for bile (gall)
inflammation of the gallbladder
x-ray image of the gallbladder
infestation with gallstones

combining form for bone
bone tumor
bone loss (degeneration)
practice of an osteopathic
    physician

---

combining form for large (used
    as a prefix)
large cell
abnormally large head

round spherical-shaped bacteria
coccus found growing in pairs
coccus found growing in
    bunches (like grapes)
coccus found growing in twisted
    chains

prefix for around or surrounding
membrane around the heart
membrane around the bone
tissues around the teeth (gums)

UNIT 5
micro
microrhinia
microcardia
microgram

UNIT 6
hematuria
oliguria
glycosuria
dysuria

UNIT 6
hystero
hysterectomy
hysteropexy
hysterosalpingogram

UNIT 5
oto
otic
otorrhea
otoscope

UNIT 6
cervico
cervicitis
endocervical

UNIT 6
nephro
nephritis
nephrorrhaphy
nephroptosis

UNIT 5
poly
polydactylism
polydipsia

UNIT 6
colpo
colpoptosis
colposcopy
colpalgia

UNIT 6
oophoro
oophoroma
oophoroptosis
oophoritis

UNIT 5
pyo
pyogenic
pyothorax
pyorrhea

UNIT 6
metro
endometriosis
metrocele
metrorrhea

UNIT 6
orchido
orchidocele
orchidalgia
orchidoplasty

UNIT 5
tympano
tympanitis
tympanotomy
tympanites

UNIT 6
gyneco
gynecologist
gynephobia

UNIT 6
penile
penitis
penoscrotal

combining form for uterus
excision of the uterus
fixation of a prolapsed uterus
x-ray image of the uterus and
    fallopian tubes

blood in the urine
scant or slight amount of urine
glucose (sugar) in the urine
difficult or painful urination

combining form for small (used as
    a prefix)
small nose
small heart
one-millionth of a gram (mcg)

combining form for kidney
inflammation of the kidney
suturing of the kidney
prolapse or displaced kidney

combining form for the neck of
    the uterus (cervix)
inflammation of the cervix
inner core of the cervix

combining form for ear
pertaining to the ear (adjective)
discharge or flow from the ear
instrument used to examine
    the ear

combining form for ovary
ovarian tumor
prolapse of the ovary
inflammation of the ovary

combining form for vagina
prolapse or displaced vagina
process of using a scope to look
    through the vagina
vaginal pain

prefix for many or too many
condition of having too many
    fingers or toes
condition of excessive thirst

combining form for testis
herniation of a testis
testicular pain
surgical repair of a testis

combining form for tissues of
    the uterus
endometrial tissues found
    growing outside the uterus
herniation of the uterine tissues
discharge from the uterine
    tissues

combining form for pus
formation of pus (adjective)
pus in the chest cavity
flow or discharge of pus

pertaining to the penis
inflammation of the penis
pertaining to the penis and
    scrotum

combining form for pertaining
    to women
physician specialist in treatment
    of women
fear of women

combining form for eardrum
inflammation of the eardrum
incision into the eardrum
abdomen distended with gas
    (tight as a drum)

UNIT 6
polycystic
polyneuralgia
polyotia
polyphagia

UNIT 6
uretero
ureterolith
ureterorrhagia

UNIT 7
esophageal
esophagogastric
esophagostenosis

UNIT 6
prostato
prostatectomy
prostatitis
prostatorrhea

UNIT 7
mastication
ingestion
digestion
absorption
elimination

UNIT 7
gingival
gingivitis
gingivoglossitis

UNIT 6
pyelo
pyelogram
pyelonephritis
pyeloplasty

UNIT 7
cheilo
cheilosis
cheilostomatoplasty
cheilorrhaphy

UNIT 7
hepato
hepatodynia
hepatolith
hepatitis

UNIT 6
salpingo
salpingo-oophoritis
salpingo-oophorocele
salpingostomy

UNIT 7
colo
coloclysis
colopexy
colostomy

UNIT 7
hypoglossal
sublingual
subglossal

UNIT 6
semen
spermatolysis
spermicide

UNIT 7
entero
dysentery
enterectasia
enterorrhagia

UNIT 7
lipase
lactase
amylase

pertaining to the esophagus
pertaining to the esophagus
  and stomach
narrowing of the esophagus

combining form for ureter
stone in a ureter
hemorrhage of the ureter

having many cysts
pain in many nerves
having more that two ears
excessive eating or frequent
  eating

pertaining to the gums
inflammation of the gums
inflammation of the gums and
  tongue

chewing
take in orally by swallowing,
  eating
breaking down food physically
  and chemically
movement of substances
  such as nutrients into the
  bloodstream
removal of waste (urine or feces)

combining form for prostate
  gland
excision of the prostate gland
inflammation of the prostate
flow or discharge from the
  prostate

combining form for liver
liver pain (hepatalgia)
stone in the liver
inflammation of the liver

combining form for lips
condition of the lips
surgical repair of the lips and
  mouth
suturing of the lips

combining form for renal pelvis
x-ray image of the renal pelvis
inflammation of the renal pelvis
  and kidney
surgical repair of the renal pelvis

below the tongue

combining form for colon
irrigation or washing of the
  colon
fixation of a prolapsed colon
make a new opening in the
  colon (abdominal)

combining form for fallopian
  tube
inflammation of the fallopian
  tube and ovary
herniation of the fallopian tube
  and ovary
making a surgical opening in
  the fallopian tube

enzyme that breaks down fat
  (lipids)
enzyme that breaks down
  lactose
enzyme that breaks down
  starch

combining form for small
  intestine
painful intestinal condition
  (diarrhea, pain, inflammation)
stretching or dilation of the small
  intestine
hemorrhage of the small
  intestine

fluid containing sperm,
  ejaculate
destruction of sperm
agent that kills sperm

UNIT 7
pancreato
pancreatolysis
pancreatopathy
pancreatolith

UNIT 7
stomato
stomatoplasty
stomatoscope

UNIT 8
arterio
arteriofibrosis
arteriomalacia
arteriosclerosis

UNIT 7
procto
proctologist
proctoplegia
proctoscopy

UNIT 7
recto
rectoclysis
rectoplasty
rectourethral

UNIT 8
afferent
affect
accept

UNIT 7
anorexia
obesity
bariatrics

UNIT 8
algesia
algesimeter
analgesia

UNIT 8
efferent
effect
except

UNIT 7
spleno
splenomegaly
splenopexy
splenorrhagia

UNIT 8
esthesio
anesthesia
anesthesiologist
anesthetist

UNIT 8
autonomic
sympathetic
parasympathetic

UNIT 7
ulcer
occult blood
nausea

UNIT 8
angio
angiography
hemangioma
angiorrhexis

UNIT 8
cystorrhexis
angiorrhexis
phleborrhexis
arteriorrhexis

combining form for artery
condition of fibrous tissue and
    arteries
softening of arteries
hardening of arteries

combining form for mouth
surgical repair of the mouth
instrument used to look into the
    mouth

combining form for pancreas
destruction of the pancreas
any disease of the pancreas
stone in the pancreas

inflowing
influence, cause change
include

combining form for rectum
washing or irrigation of the
    rectum
surgical repair of the rectum
pertaining to the rectum and
    urethra

combining form for anus and
    rectum
paralysis of the anus and rectum
examination of the anus and
    rectum with a scope

out-flowing
result, end product
exclude, reject

painful condition
instrument that measures pain
    intensity
without pain

loss of appetite
quality of being overweight for
    body type
specialty that studies treatment
    of obesity

self-controlling stress response
    that is part of
    the nervous system
nerves that respond during
    stress (autonomic)
nerves that return the body to
    pre-stress state
    (autonomic)

combining form for feeling or
    sensation
without feeling or sensation,
    numb
physician specialist in
    administration of anesthesia
person who administers
    anesthesia

combining form for spleen
enlargement of the spleen
prolapse of the spleen
hemorrhage of the spleen

rupture of the urinary
    bladder
rupture of a vessel
rupture of a vein
rupture of an artery

combining form for vessel (duct)
process of making an image of a
    vessel
tumor composed of a number of
    blood vessels
rupture of a vessel

crater-like sore
hidden blood or bleeding
feeling like one is going to
    vomit

UNIT 8
hematocrit
hematologist
hematolysis
hematophobia

UNIT 8
neuro
neurologist
neurosurgeon
neurotripsy

UNIT 9
antero
anterolateral
anteromedial
anteroposterior

UNIT 8
ischemia
infarction
occlusion

UNIT 8
phlebo
phlebectasia
phlebotomy
phleboplasty

UNIT 9
axillary
midaxillary
midsagittal

UNIT 8
myo
myoblast
myocardial
myocarditis

UNIT 8
psycho
psychomotor
psychotherapy
psychotropic
psychiatrist

UNIT 9
cephalad
cephalocaudal
coronal

UNIT 8
myography
myosclerosis
myopathy

UNIT 9
aero
aerophobia
aerotherapy
anaerobic

UNIT 9
dia
dialysis
diarrhea
diagnosis

UNIT 8
narco
narcolepsy
narcosis
narcotic

UNIT 9
chromo
chromophilic
achromophilic
chromolysis

UNIT 9
dorsal
dorsocephalad
dorsoventral

combining form for front
    (ventral)
pertaining to front and side
pertaining to front and middle
direction from front to back

combining form for nerve
physician specialist in nervous
    system disorders
physician who performs surgical
    treatment on the nervous
    system
surgical crushing of a nerve

measurement of % formed
    elements of blood
physician specialist in treatment
    of blood disorders
destruction of blood
fear of blood

pertaining to the armpit area
pertaining to the middle of the
    armpit
vertical plane that divides the
    body into right and left
    halves

combining form for vein
stretching or dilation of a vein
incision into a vein
    (venipuncture)
surgical repair of a vein

condition of stopping or
    slowing down blood flow
tissue death (necrosis) due to
    ischemia
blockage, closing

toward the head
pertaining to a head to tail
    (distal spine)
crown, lateral suture line of the
    skull

combining form for mind,
    mental processes
mental process that controls
    movement
treatment for mental disorders
medication that affects mental
    processes
physician specialist in treatment
    of mental disorders

combining form for muscle
immature muscle cell
pertaining to heart muscle
inflammation of the
    myocardium

prefix for through
destruction through (filtration
    using an artificial kidney)
flow through, watery stool
    (feces)
identification of a disease
    through its symptoms and
    signs

combining form for air
    (containing oxygen)
fear of air
therapy using air (respiratory
    therapy)
able to live without air (oxygen)

making an image of muscle
    function
hardening of muscle tissue
any muscle disease

pertaining to the back
    (posterior)
toward the back of the head
direction from back to front

combining form for color
attraction of color (stain)
not absorbing color (stain)
destruction of color

combining form for sleep
seizures of uncontrolled sleep
condition of being affected by
    narcotics
controlled substance drug
    that produces analgesia
    and sleep

UNIT 9
ecto
ectocytic
ectogenous
ectopic

UNIT 9
omphalo
omphalectomy
omphalitis
omphalocele

UNIT 10
centi
centigram
centimeter

UNIT 9
endo
endoderm
endogenous
endoscopy

UNIT 9
para
pseudo
retro
pro

UNIT 10
circum
circumduction
circumscribed
circumocular

UNIT 9
eu
eugenics
eupnea
euthanasia

UNIT 9
syphilo
syphilophobia
syphilopsychosis
syphilotherapy

UNIT 10
de
dehydration
descending

UNIT 9
inferior
superior
lateral
medial

UNIT 10
ablactation
ablation
aboral
abortion

UNIT 10
ex
excision
excretion
exhale
extraction

UNIT 9
meno
menopause
menorrhagia
dysmenorrhea

UNIT 10
auto
autograft
autogenous
autoimmunity

UNIT 10
iso
isometric
isodactylism
isotonic

prefix for one hundredth
one hundredth of a gram
one hundredth of a meter

combining form for umbilicus
   (navel)
excision of the umbilicus
inflammation of the navel
herniation of the navel

combining form (prefix) for
   outer, outside
outside the cell
produced or generated outside,
   not from one's own body
located outside the normal area,
   such as a tubal pregnancy

prefix for encircling
moving as to describe a circle
encircling or in a circular shape
encircling the eye

prefixes:
around, near
false
behind, in back of
before, in front of

combining form (prefix) for
   inner, inside
inner embryonic (stem cells)
made inside one's own body
looking into the body (cavity or
   tube) with a scope

prefix for down from, resulting
   in less than
resulting in less that normal
   amount of water
in a downward direction or
   moving downward

combining form for syphilis
fear of contracting syphilis
severe mental condition caused
   by untreated syphilis
treatment for syphilis

prefix for easy or good
choosing the good genes for
   reproduction
easy breathing
good death, easy death

prefix for out from
removal, cutting out
removal of waste
breath out
pull out, remove

weaning a nursing baby, away
   from the breast milk
taking away tissue by cutting or
   cautery
away from the mouth
termination of pregnancy

below, under
above, over
side
middle

prefix meaning same or equal
measuring equal or the same
   on both sides
fingers or toes all an even
   length
osmotic pressure the same as
   a cell

combining form for self
tissue grafting with one's own
   tissues
one's own generated substance
   or tissue
immune response (sensitivity) to
   one's own tissues

combining form for menses
   (menstruation)
permanent cessation of
   menstruation
hemorrhaging during
   menstruation
difficult and painful menses

UNIT 10

masto
mastectomy
mastocarcinoma

UNIT 10

mono
monomyoplegia
mononuclear
mononucleosis

UNIT 10

glycogenesis
glycohemoglobin
hyperglycemia
hypoglycemia

UNIT 10

multi
multiglandular
multinuclear
multipara

UNIT 10

necro
necrotic
necrotomy
necropsy

UNIT 10

peri
periarticular
pericardiectomy
peritonsillar

UNIT 10

primi
primigravida
primipara

UNIT 10

per
percussion
percutaneous
perfusion
perforation

UNIT 10

pyro
pyrexia
pyrolysis
pyrotoxin

UNIT 11

anti
antiarthritics
antibiotic
antidepressant
antirheumatic

UNIT 11

antiseptic
disinfectant
sanitization
sterilization

UNIT 11

epi
epidural
epigastrorrhaphy
epinephrectomy

UNIT 11

hetero
heterogeneous
heteropsia
heterosexual

UNIT 11

infra
infracostal
inframammary
infrapatellar

UNIT 11

meta
metatarsals
metacarpals

agent that cleans to protect
    from infections (used
    externally)
chemical agent used to kill
    organisms on surfaces
cleaning, washing with soaps
    and friction
complete destruction of organisms

prefix for around, surrounding
around a joint
excision of the pericardial
    membrane
around the tonsil

combining form for breast
excision of the breast
cancer of breast tissue

prefix for upon
upon the dura mater
    (meninges)
suturing of an area above the
    stomach
excision of tissues upon the
    kidney (adrenal)

prefix for first
first pregnancy
first birth

prefix (combining form) for one
paralysis of one muscle
having one nucleus
condition of increase in
    monocytes (viral infection)

combining form (prefix) for
    different
made of different tissues or
    substances
visual acuity different in each
    eye
sexually attracted to the
    opposite sex

prefix for through
striking through (tapping)
through the skin
supplying blood through tissues
puncturing, making a hole
    through

formation of sugar or glycogen
glucose attached to
    hemoglobin
high blood glucose level
low blood glucose level

prefix for below
below the ribs
below the breast
below the patella (kneecap)

combining form for fever (fire)
condition of high temperature,
    fever
destruction of tissue caused by
    fever
poisons created by metabolism
    during fever

prefix (combining form) for
    many
pertaining to many glands
having many nuclei in one cell
having many (more that one)
    births

prefix for beyond
bones of the foot beyond the
    tarsal bones
bones of the hand beyond the
    carpal bones

prefix for against
agent that works against arthritis
agent that works against bacteria
agent that elevates mood to treat
    depression
agent that works against
    rheumatic disease

combining form for dead (dead
    tissue)
pertaining to dead tissue
incision into dead tissue
inspection of dead tissue
    (autopsy)

UNIT 11
subaural
subcutaneous
subdural

UNIT 11
bilateral
symmetry
sympathetic

UNIT 12
a-, an-
anorexia
asymptomatic
antagonistic

UNIT 11
supralumbar
suprarenal
suprapubic

UNIT 11
super
superciliary
superinfection
superficial

UNIT 12
ante
antefebrile
anteflexion
antemortem
antepartum

UNIT 11
trans
transdermal
transcatheter
transposition
transvaginal

UNIT 11
contra
contraceptive
contravolitional

UNIT 12
bi
bicellular
bipolar
bisexual

UNIT 11
ultra
ultrasonography
ultraviolet

UNIT 11
septicemia
septopyemia
asepsis

UNIT 12
cachexia
bulimia

UNIT 11
homo
homosexual
homoglandula
homogeneous

UNIT 11
mammo
mammogram
mammography
mammoplasty

UNIT 12
con
congenital
consanguinity

prefix for not or lack of
condition of loss of appetite
without symptoms
works against or in opposition

pertaining to both sides
measures or looks the same on
    both sides, balanced
sharing the same feelings

below the ear
below the skin
below the dura mater
    (meninges)

prefix for in front or before
before a fever
bending forward
before death
before birth (referring to the
    mom)

prefix for above or over
above the ciliary body (of the
    eye)
infection on top of another
    infection
pertaining to on the surface

above the lumbar spine
above the kidney
above the pubic bone area

prefix for two or both
consisting of two cells
two poles, mental disorder
    manic/depressive
sexually attracted to both males
    and females

prefix for against
agent that prevents conception
    (pregnancy)
against one's will

prefix for across or through
across (through) the dermis
across (through) a flexible tube
    (catheter)
placed across to the opposite
    side
across (through) the vagina

wasting away of the body
eating disorder of purging after
    eating

infection in the blood
infection and pus in the blood
without poisons or infection

prefix for above or over
making images using reflected
    high frequency sound
light frequency above violet

prefix for with
pertaining to born with
quality of blood relationship

combining form for breast
x-ray image of the breast
process of making a
    mammogram
surgical repair of the breast

prefix (combining form) for
    same
sexual attraction to the same
    sex
pertaining to the same glandular
    tissue
make of the same tissue or
    items

UNIT 12
dis
disinfect
dissect
disassociate

UNIT 12
intra-abdominal
intra-aortic
intra-arterial
intrathoracic
intravenous

UNIT 12
semi
semicomatose
semiconscious
semiprivate

UNIT 12
ex
exhale
excise
expiration

UNIT 12
mal
malaise
malformation
malnutrition

UNIT 12
triceps
trifurcation
unicellular
unilateral
uninuclear

UNIT 12
hemi
hemianesthesia
hemicardia
hemiplegia

UNIT 12
morbidity
mortality

UNIT 13
-pnea
apnea
dyspnea
orthopnea
bradypnea

UNIT 12
incompetency
incontinence
incubation
infested
infiltration

UNIT 12
postcibal
postcoital
postfebrile
postmortem
postnatal

UNIT 13
bronchitis
bronchorrhaphy
bronchoscopy
bronchospasm

UNIT 12
infusion
injection
insomnia
instillation

UNIT 12
pre
prefrontal
preoperative
prescribe

UNIT 13
pulmonic
pneumonal
pulmonary
cardiopulmonary

prefix for half or partially
partially in a coma
partially conscious
half private (two to a room)

within the abdomen
within the aorta
within an artery
within the chest (thorax)
within a vein

prefix for undo or take apart
to rid of infectious agents
to cut apart (for examination)
to split up, may be personality
    splits

prefix for three
three-bellied muscle (posterior
    upper arm)
having three branches
made of one cell
one sided
having one nucleus

prefix for bad
feeling bad, general poor
    feeling
poorly formed, deformed
poor nutrition, missing nutrients

prefix for out
breathe out
cut out
breathing out

suffix for breathing
not breathing
difficult or painful breathing
breathing well only when sitting
    upright
abnormally slow breathing

quality of illness or disease
quality of death

prefix for half
anesthesia blocking sensation in
    half the body
half of a heart
paralysis on one side of the
    body

inflammation of the bronchi
suturing of the bronchi
examining the bronchi using a
    scope
uncontrolled twitching or
    contractions of the bronchi

following a meal (breakfast)
after intercourse (coitus)
after a fever
after death
after birth (referring to the baby)

not competent
unable to control urination or
    defecation
original growth time (grow
    within)
organism living within another
    organism
penetration of a solution into
    tissues

pertaining to lungs
pertaining to lungs
pertaining to lungs
pertaining to the heart and
    lungs

prefix for before or in front
in front of the frontal bone or
    lobe of the brain
before surgery
write an order before treatment

introduction of a substance into a
    vein (IV)
introduction of a substance
    through a needle
unable to sleep
put in by drops

UNIT 13

chiro
chiroplasty
chiropractor
chiropractic

UNIT 13

laryngitis
laryngalgia
laryngoscope
laryngotomy

UNIT 13

pneumonia
pneumonomelanosis
pneumonopathy
pneumonorrhagia

UNIT 13

dextral
dextrocardia
dextrogastria
dextromanual

UNIT 13

nasofrontal
paranasal
nasopharyngeal
nasolacrimal

UNIT 13

sinistral
sinistrocardia
sinistromanual

UNIT 13

phreno
phrenoplegia
phrenic
diaphragm

UNIT 13

otorhinolaryngologist
pediatrician
podiatrist

UNIT 13

trachealgia
tracheopyosis
tracheostomy
endotracheal

UNIT 13

epistaxis
hemoptysis
ptyalorrhea

UNIT 13

pharyngomycosis
pharyngoplasty
pharynx

UNIT 14

acromion process
acromioclavicular
acromiohumeral

UNIT 13

myco
mycology
pneumonomycosis
mycoderma

UNIT 13

pleural
pleurectomy
pleurisy
pleurocentesis

UNIT 14

ambulance
ambulate
noctambulism

inflammation of the lungs
    (pneumonitis)
black lung disease
any disease of the lung
hemorrhage of the lung

inflammation of the larynx
pain in the larynx
instrument used to examine the
    larynx
incision into the larynx

combining form for hand
surgical repair of the hand
practitioner that uses
    manipulative therapy
    (Doctor of Chiropractic)
the practice of the chiropractor

pertaining to the left
heart displaced to the left
left handed

pertaining to the nose and
    frontal bones
area around the nasal bones
    (sinuses)
pertaining to the nose and
    throat
pertaining to the nose and tear
    ducts

pertaining to the right
heart displaced to the right
stomach displaced to the right
right handedness

pain in the trachea (windpipe)
pus condition in the trachea
make a new surgical opening in
    the trachea
inside the trachea

physician specialist in ear, nose,
    and throat disorders
physician specialist in treating
    children
specialist caring for feet (Doctor of
    Podiatric Medicine)

combining form for the diaphragm
    (muscle)
paralysis of the diaphragm
nerve that enervates the
    diaphragm for breathing
large breathing muscle inferior to
    the lungs

bony bump where the clavicle
    meets the scapula
pertaining to the acromion and
    collar bone
pertaining to the acromion and
    humerus

fungus condition of the throat
surgical repair of the throat
singular of pharynges

nosebleed
bloody sputum or saliva
excessive flow of saliva

vehicle used to transport
    people in emergencies
walk
sleep walking (somnambulism)

pertaining to the membrane
    around the lungs (pleura)
excision of the pleura
inflammation of the pleura
    (pleuritis)
surgical puncture of the pleura to
    remove fluid

combining form for fungus
the study of fungi
fungus condition in the lungs
fungus condition of the skin

UNIT 14
brachial
brachiocephalic
brachioradialis
humeroradial
humeroscapular

UNIT 14
fibula
tibia
tibiofibular

UNIT 14
phalanges
phalagitis
interphalangeal

UNIT 14
calcaneus
calcaneodynia
calcaneal

UNIT 14
ileum
ilium
ilial
iliosacral

UNIT 14
rachialgia
rachiometer
rachischisis
rachitis

UNIT 14
cervical
cervicobrachial
cervicofacial

UNIT 14
ischial
ischioneuralgia
ischiopubic
ischiorectal

UNIT 14
schistosomiasis
schistoglossia
schizonychia
schizophrenia

UNIT 14
condyle
condylectomy
condyloid
epicondyle

UNIT 14
laminectomy
diskectomy
intervertebral

UNIT 14
scoliosis
kyphosis
lordosis

UNIT 14
femur
femoral
pubofemoral

UNIT 14
carpi
carpometacarpal
carpal
metacarpals
metatarsals

UNIT 15
abrasion
contusion
laceration
avulsion (evulsion)
fracture

plural of phalanx (finger or toe bone)
inflammation of the phalanges
between two phalanges (joint)

small bone lateral to the tibia in the lower leg
large bone medial to the tibia in the lower leg
pertaining to both the tibia and the fibula

pertaining to the arm
pertaining to the arm and head
muscle that extends from upper arm to radius bone
pertaining to the humerus and radius
pertaining to the humerus and scapula

pain in the spine
instrument used to measure the spine
split in the spine (spina bifida)
inflammation of the spine

the third part of the small intestine
the upper outer pelvic bone
pertaining to the ilium
pertaining to the ilium and sacrum

heel bone
heel bone pain
pertaining to the heel bone

infestation with a parasite with a split in its body, *Schistosoma*
split tongue
split nails (toe or finger nails)
sever mental disorder causing a break with reality

pertaining to the bottom bones of the pelvis (sit bones)
nerve pain near the ischium
pertaining to the ischium and pubis
pertaining to the ischium and rectum

pertaining to the area of the spine called the neck (7 vertebrae)
pertaining to the cervical spine and the arm
pertaining to the cervical spine and the face

lateral curvature of the spine
posterior curvature of the thoracic spine (hunchback)
anterior curvature of the lumbar spine (swayback)

excision of the lamina of an intervertebral disk
excision of an intervertebral disk between vertebrae

rounded bony process (normal structure bump)
excision of a condyle
resembling a condyle
structure upon a condyle

scrape
bruise
cut
gauge (flap of tissue)
break

wrist bones (plural)
joint between the carpal bones and the metacarpals
pertaining to the wrist bones
bones of the hand beyond (distal to) the carpals (wrist)
bones of the foot beyond (distal to) the tarsals (ankle)

thigh bone
pertaining to the femur
pertaining to the pubis and femur

UNIT 15

adrenal
adrenocorticoid
adrenolysis
adrenomegaly

UNIT 15

corneitis
corneoiritis
corneoscleral
corneotomy

UNIT 15

onychocryptosis
onychoma
onychomalacia
paronychia

UNIT 15

ambi
ambivalence
ambiopia
hyperopia
myopia

UNIT 15

dacryoadenalgia
dacryocystocele
dacryocystoptosis
dacryoma

UNIT 15

ophthalmic
ophthalmologist
ophthalmometer
ophthalmoscope

UNIT 15

blepharedema
blepharoplasty
blepharoptosis
blepharorrhaphy

UNIT 15

endocrine
endocrinology
exocrine

UNIT 15

optic
optometrist
optometry

UNIT 15

cataract
glaucoma
strabismus

UNIT 15

hypertropia
hypotropia
hyperthyroidism
hypothyroidism

UNIT 15

phacocele
phacoemulsification
macular

UNIT 15

corectopia
corelysis
coreometer
coreoplasty

UNIT 15

iridocele
iridomalacia
iridoplegia
iridoptosis

UNIT 15

trichoid
trichopathy
trichiasis
trichophagia

ingrown toe or finger nail
nail tumor
softening of the nails
condition of the tissue
    around the nails

inflammation of the cornea
    (keratitis)
inflammation of the cornea and
    iris (keratoiritis)
pertaining to the cornea and
    sclera (keratoscleral)
incision into the cornea
    (keratotomy)

pertaining to the adrenal glands
cortisone hormone produced
    by the adrenal glands
destruction of the adrenal gland
enlarged adrenal gland

pertaining to the eye (
    ophthalmal)
physician specialist in eye
    diseases and surgery
instrument used to measure
    the eye
instrument used to look into
    the eye

condition of the tear gland
    (lacrimal gland)
herniation of the tear gland
    (lacrimal gland)
prolapse of the tear gland
    (lacrimal gland)
tear gland tissue tumor (lacrimal tumor)

prefix for both
undecided, seeing both sides
different vision in each eye
    (diplopia)
farsightedness
nearsightedness

pertaining to vision
specialist that measures vision
measurement of vision

glands that secrete hormones
    into the bloodstream
study of the endocrine glands
    and hormones
glands that secrete substances
    into ducts directly for use

swelling of the eyelid
surgical repair of the eyelid
droopy or prolapsed eyelid
suturing of the eyelid

herniation of the lens
destruction of the lens for lens
    implant
pertaining to the macula of the
    retina

malposition of the eye pointed
    upward
malposition of the eye pointed
    downward
overactive thyroid function
underactive thyroid function

cloudy spots or opacities on the
    lens of the eye
high vitreous humor pressure in
    the front of the eye
malposition of the eye (squint)

resembling hair
any disease of the hair
infestation or growth of hair not
    in normal locations
eating hair, biting or chewing
    on hair

herniation of the iris
softening of the iris
paralysis of the iris
prolapse of the iris

dilation of the pupil
destruction of the pupil
instrument used to measure
    pupil size
surgical repair of the pupil